NASM Essentials of
Personal Fitness Training

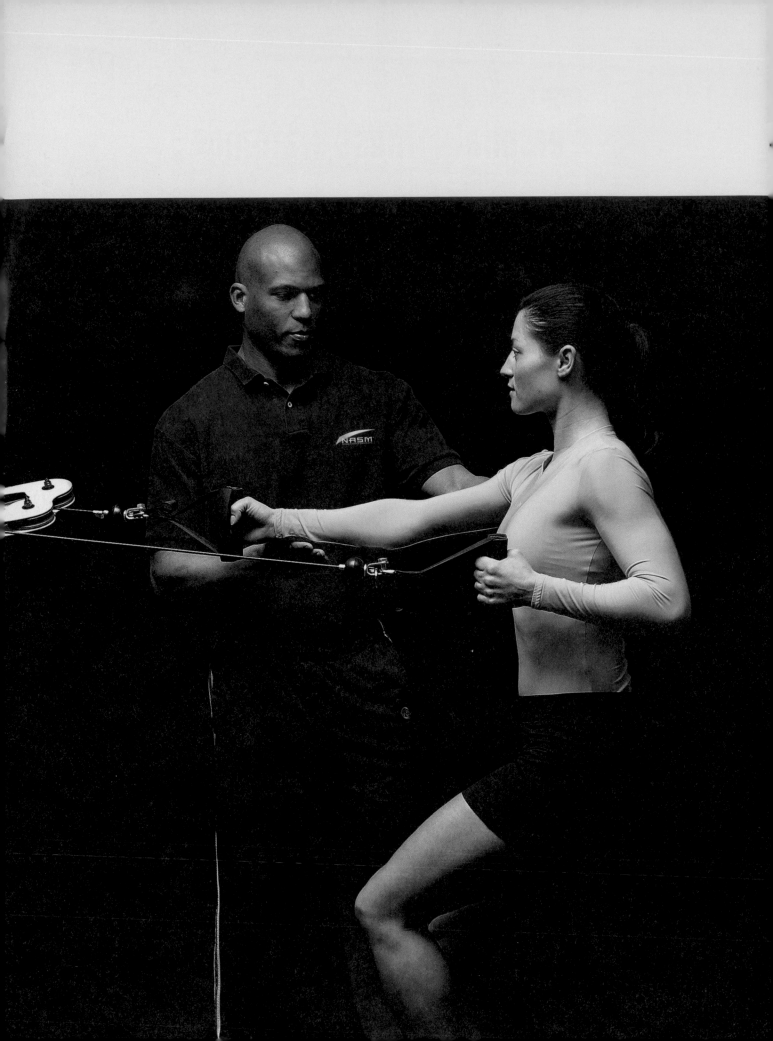

NASM Essentials of
Personal Fitness Training

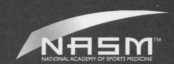

THIRD EDITION

Micheal A. Clark, DPT, MS, PES, CES
President and CEO
National Academy of Sports Medicine
Calabasas, CA

Scott Lucett, MS, PES, CES, NASM-CPT
Director of Education
National Academy of Sports Medicine
Calabasas, CA

Rodney J. Corn, MA, PES, CES, CPT
Training and Development Manager
National Academy of Sports Medicine
Calabasas, CA

Wolters Kluwer | Lippincott Williams & Wilkins
Health

Philadelphia · Baltimore · New York · London
Buenos Aires · Hong Kong · Sydney · Tokyo

Acquisitions Editor: Emily Lupash
Managing Editor: Matthew J. Hauber
Marketing Manager: Christen D. Murphy
Production Editor: Jennifer P. Ajello
Designer: Risa Clow
Art & Illustration: Dragonfly Media Group
Compositor: Aptara, Inc.
Printer: R. R. Donnelley & Sons—Willard

351 West Camden Street
Baltimore, MD 21201

530 Walnut Street
Philadelphia, PA 19106

Printed in the United States of America

Library of Congress Cataloging-in-Publication Data

NASM Essentials of Personal Fitness Training : course manual. —3rd ed.
    p.   cm.
ISBN   978-0-7817-8291-3
1. Personal trainers—Training of—United States—Handbooks, manuals, etc.   2. Personal trainers—Vocational guidance—United States—Handbooks, manuals, etc.   3. Personal trainers—Certification—United States—Study guides.   4. Physical education and training—United States—Handbooks, manuals, etc.   I. National Academy of Sports Medicine.
GV428.7.N37   2008
613.7′11023—dc22

2006102963

To purchase additional copies of this book, call our customer service department at **(800) 638-3030** or fax orders to **(301) 223-2320**. International customers should call **(301) 223-2300**.

Visit Lippincott Williams & Wilkins on the Internet: http://www.LWW.com. Lippincott Williams & Wilkins customer service representatives are available from 8:30 am to 6:00 pm, EST.

08 09 10 11
4 5 6 7 8 9 10

The NASM Mission

NASM's mission is to empower individuals to live a healthy life.

Code of Ethics

The following code of ethics is designed to assist certified and noncertified members of the National Academy of Sports Medicine (NASM) to uphold (both as individuals and as an industry) the highest levels of professional and ethical conduct. This Code of Ethics reflects the level of commitment and integrity necessary to ensure that all NASM members provide the highest level of service and respect for all colleagues, allied professionals, and the general public.

PROFESSIONALISM

Each certified or noncertified member must provide optimal professional service and demonstrate excellent client care in his or her practice. Each member shall:

1. Abide fully by the NASM Code of Ethics.

2. Conduct themselves in a manner that merits the respect of the public, other colleagues, and NASM.

3. Treat each colleague and client with the utmost respect and dignity.

4. Not make false or derogatory assumptions concerning the practices of colleagues and clients.

5. Use appropriate professional communication in all verbal, nonverbal, and written transactions.

6. Provide and maintain an environment that ensures client safety that, at a minimum, requires that the certified or noncertified member:

   a. Shall not diagnose or treat illness or injury (except for basic first aid) unless the certified or noncertified member is legally licensed to do so and is working in that capacity at that time.

   b. Shall not train clients with a diagnosed health condition unless the certified or noncertified member has been specifically trained to do so, is following procedures prescribed and supervised by a valid licensed medical professional, or is legally licensed to do so and is working in that capacity at that time.

   c. Shall not begin to train a client before receiving and reviewing a current health-history questionnaire signed by the client.

   d. Shall hold a CPR and AED certification at all times.

7. Refer the client to the appropriate medical practitioner when, at a minimum, the certified or noncertified member:

   a. Becomes aware of any change in the client's health status or medication.

   b. Becomes aware of an undiagnosed illness, injury, or risk factor.

   c. Becomes aware of any unusual client pain or discomfort during the course of the training session that warrants professional care after the session has been discontinued and assessed.

8. Refer the client to other healthcare professionals when nutritional and supplemental advice is requested unless the certified or noncertified member has been specifically trained to do so or holds a credential to do so and is acting in that capacity at the time.

9. Maintain a level of personal hygiene appropriate for a health and fitness setting.

10. Wear clothing that is clean, modest, and professional.

11. Remain in good standing and maintain current certification status by acquiring all necessary continuing-education requirements (see NASM Board of Certification Candidate Handbook).

CONFIDENTIALITY

Each certified and noncertified member shall respect the confidentiality of all client information. In his or her professional role, the certified or noncertified member should:

1. Protect the client's confidentiality in conversations, advertisements, and any other arena, unless otherwise agreed to by the client in writing, or as a result of medical or legal necessity.
2. Protect the interest of clients who are minors by law, or who are unable to give voluntary consent by securing the legal permission of the appropriate third party or guardian.
3. Store and dispose of client records in secure manner.

LEGAL AND ETHICAL

Each certified or noncertified member must comply with all legal requirements within the applicable jurisdiction. In his or her professional role, the certified or noncertified member must:

1. Obey all local, state, provincial, or federal laws.
2. Accept complete responsibility for his or her actions.
3. Maintain accurate and truthful records.
4. Respect and uphold all existing publishing and copyright laws.

BUSINESS PRACTICE

Each certified or noncertified member must practice with honesty, integrity, and lawfulness. In his or her professional role, the certified or noncertified member shall:

1. Maintain adequate liability insurance.
2. Maintain adequate and truthful progress notes for each client.
3. Accurately and truthfully inform the public of services rendered.
4. Honestly and truthfully represent all professional qualifications and affiliations.
5. Advertise in a manner that is honest, dignified, and representative of services that can be delivered without the use of provocative or sexual language or pictures.
6. Maintain accurate financial, contract, appointment, and tax records including original receipts for a minimum of 4 years.
7. Comply with all local, state, federal, or providence laws regarding sexual harassment.

NASM expects each member to uphold the Code of Ethics in its entirety. Failure to comply with the NASM Code of Ethics may result in disciplinary actions including but not limited to, suspension or termination of membership and certification. All members are obligated to report any unethical behavior or violation of the Code of Ethics by other NASM members.

Preface: Letter from the President

I applaud you on your dedication and commitment to helping others live healthier lives, and thank you for entrusting the National Academy of Sports Medicine (NASM) with your education.

By following the techniques in this book, *NASM Essentials of Personal Fitness Training*, you will gain the information, insight, and inspiration you need to change the world as a health and fitness professional.

Since 1987, NASM has been the leading authority in certification, continuing education, solutions, and tools for health and fitness, sports performance, and sports medicine professionals. Our systematic and scientific approach to fitness continues to raise the bar as the "gold standard" in the industry. Today, we serve as the global authority in more than 80 countries, serving more than 100,000 members! Tomorrow, our possibilities are endless . . . .

Our industry is on the verge of massive changes, such as an aging and diverse population, globalization, healthcare-industry convergence, oversight and regulation, consumer-driven choice, and as always, the rapidly developing world of technology. These industry shifts will continue to provide unlimited opportunities for you as an elite NASM-certified professional.

Today's health and fitness consumer has an increasingly high level of expectations. They want the best and the brightest who can provide unparalleled results. To meet these expectations and better deliver quality, innovation, and evidence-based health and fitness solutions to the world, NASM has developed new and exciting solutions with best-in-class partners from the education, healthcare, sports and entertainment, and technology industries. NASM was recently named the number-one organization to shape the future of fitness.[1] With the help of our best-in-class partnerships—and top professionals like you—we will continue to live up to the expectations placed on us and strive to raise the bar in our pursuit of excellence!

Flexibility is important in fitness, and the new NASM reflects our ability to remain flexible in an ever-changing world. Amidst all of the change, we will always stay true to our mission and values: delivering evidence-based solutions driven by excellence, innovation, and results. This is essential to our long-term success as a company, and to your individual career success as a health and fitness professional.

Scientific research and techniques also continue to advance, and, as a result, you must remain on the cutting edge to remain competitive. The NASM education continuum—certification, specialization, and continuing and higher education—is based on a foundation of comprehensive, scientific research supported by leading institutes and universities. As a result, NASM offers scientifically validated education, evidence-based solutions, and user-friendly tools that can be applied immediately.

The tools and solutions in the OPT™ methodology help put science into practice to create amazing results for clients. OPT™ is an innovative, systemic approach, used by thousands of fitness professionals and athletes worldwide. NASM's techniques work, creating a dramatic difference in training programs and their results.

One of the most influential people of the 20th century told us that "a life is not important except for the impact it has on other lives."[2] For us as health and fitness professionals in the 21st century, the truth behind this wisdom has never been greater.

There is no quick fix to a healthy lifestyle. However, NASM's education, solutions, and tools can positively impact behavior by allowing the masses to participate in practical, customized, evidence-based exercise.

[1]Men's Health Magazine, October 2005

[2]Jackie Robinson, Hall of Fame baseball player and civil rights leader (1919–1972)

The future of fitness is upon us all, and there is much work to be done. With that, I welcome you to the NASM community of health and fitness professionals. If you ever need assistance from one of our subject matter experts, or simply want to learn more about our new partnerships and evidence-based health and fitness solutions, please call us at 800-460-NASM or visit us online at www.nasm.org.

We look forward to working with you to help shape the future of fitness.

Now let's go out together and empower individuals to live healthy lives!

Micheal A. Clark, DPT, MS, PT, PES, CES
President and CEO

NEW CONTENT

Although the overall structure of the textbook has not changed, there are several key updates to highlight. They are as follows:

1. **Streamlined OPT™ Model**—The OPT™ model has been simplified to include five of the most commonly used phases of training for fitness goals, versus the previous seven-phase model. The two phases of training that are not highlighted in this text, Corrective Exercise Training and Maximal Power Training, are specialized forms of training that would be used in very specific situations. Corrective Exercise Training would be used for individuals who have come off an injury and *prepares* one to enter into the OPT™ model. Maximal Power Training would be used for a very select population of extremely high-level athletes (a training population the typical health and fitness professional would not be working with).

2. **Revised Model Nomenclature**—We have also renamed the phases so it is easier to understand the exact function and desired adaptation for that phase of training.

3. **Movement Compensation Table**—In Chapter 5, we have simplified the movement compensation table to focus on the major compensations that are very commonly seen when performing movement assessments.

4. **Corrective Solutions Tables**—We have also updated the corrective solutions tables in Chapter 6 to include the exact strategies in dealing with these movement deficiencies in an easy to understand manner.

5. **Research Updates**—In Chapters 6, 8, 9, 10, and 13 we have included some of the most current and relevant research that further validates the rationale for flexibility, core, balance, reactive training, and periodized program design and their incorporation into an integrated training program.

6. **Glossary of Terms**—We have updated our glossary of terms to include a larger number of terms and definitions. We have also updated our index for easy navigation when searching for topics, concepts, or programming strategies.

NEW PEDAGOLOGICAL FEATURES

The new textbook comes with a variety of new educational features. These features include the following:

- New illustrations that visually emphasize muscle imbalances
- Updated tables
- New anatomical images
- Stretch your knowledge sections containing relevant research
- End of chapter review questions
- Updated photos
- Exercise technique and safety tips

Many of the changes above reflect the feedback received from health and fitness professionals regarding our 2nd edition textbook. We hope these additions will assist in the learning process and experience, thus making you a more confident and successful professional!

Acknowledgments

Writers:
Micheal A. Clark, DPT, MS, PES, CES
Scott C. Lucett, MS, PES, CES, NASM-CPT
Rodney J. Corn, MA, PES, CES, NASM-CPT
Reed Humphrey, PhD, PT, FACSM
Stephen J. Kraus, PhD
Alan Titchenal, PhD
Paul Robbins, MS
Robert Cappuccio

Contributors:
The Apex Fitness Group
www.apexfitness.com

Primal Anatomy Ltd.
www.primalpictures.com

Nautilus, Inc.
www.nautilus.com

Photographer:
Gene Smith
Gene Smith Studio Advertising Photography
www.genesmithstudio.com

Art and Illustration:
Dragonfly Media Group

Models:
Monica Carlson
Mike Chapin
Naim Hasan
Marge Gale
Ric Miller
Sonata Polanco
Alexcia Tsu
Seth Tyler

User's Guide

This User's Guide introduces you to the many features of **NASM Essentials of Personal Fitness Training, Third Edition.** Taking full advantage of these features, you will be able to have a better understanding of the material and more effectively design exercise programs to train clients safely and effectively.

Each chapter is loaded with features that help you focus on the key points, deepen your knowledge, and apply your new skills.

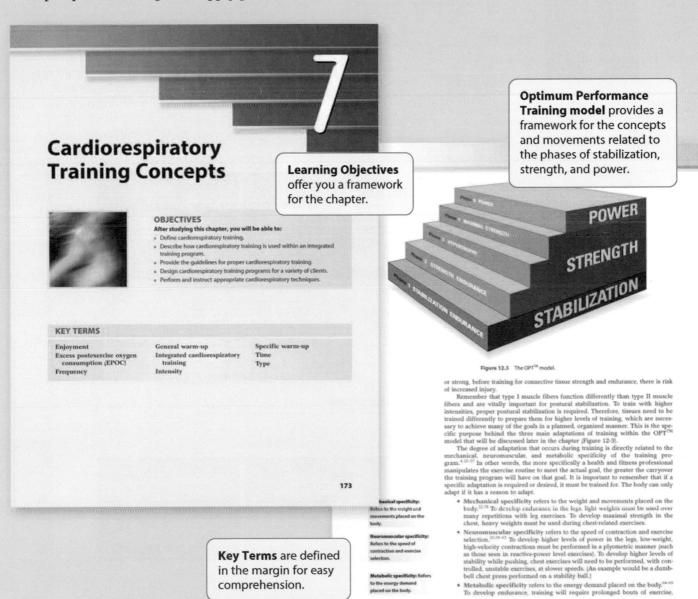

7

Cardiorespiratory Training Concepts

> **Learning Objectives** offer you a framework for the chapter.

OBJECTIVES

After studying this chapter, you will be able to:

- Define cardiorespiratory training.
- Describe how cardiorespiratory training is used within an integrated training program.
- Provide the guidelines for proper cardiorespiratory training.
- Design cardiorespiratory training programs for a variety of clients.
- Perform and instruct appropriate cardiorespiratory techniques.

KEY TERMS

Enjoyment	General warm-up	Specific warm-up
Excess postexercise oxygen consumption (EPOC)	Integrated cardiorespiratory training	Time
Frequency	Intensity	Type

173

> **Optimum Performance Training model** provides a framework for the concepts and movements related to the phases of stabilization, strength, and power.

POWER

STRENGTH

STABILIZATION

Figure 12.3 The OPT™ model.

or strong, before training for connective tissue strength and endurance, there is risk of increased injury.

Remember that type I muscle fibers function differently than type II muscle fibers and are vitally important for postural stabilization. To train with higher intensities, proper postural stabilization is required. Therefore, tissues need to be trained differently to prepare them for higher levels of training, which are necessary to achieve many of the goals in a planned, organized manner. This is the specific purpose behind the three main adaptations of training within the OPT™ model that will be discussed later in the chapter (Figure 12-3).

The degree of adaptation that occurs during training is directly related to the mechanical, neuromuscular, and metabolic specificity of the training program.[4,12-17] In other words, the more specifically a health and fitness professional manipulates the exercise routine to meet the actual goal, the greater the carryover the training program will have on that goal. It is important to remember that if a specific adaptation is required or desired, it must be trained for. The body can only adapt if it has a reason to adapt.

Mechanical specificity: Refers to the weight and movements placed on the body.

Neuromuscular specificity: Refers to the speed of contraction and exercise selection.

Metabolic specificity: Refers to the energy demand placed on the body.

- Mechanical specificity refers to the weight and movements placed on the body.[52-79] To develop endurance in the legs, light weights must be used over many repetitions with leg exercises. To develop maximal strength in the chest, heavy weights must be used during chest-related exercises.
- Neuromuscular specificity refers to the speed of contraction and exercise selection.[80,98-43] To develop higher levels of power in the legs, low-weight, high-velocity contractions must be performed in a plyometric manner (such as those seen in reactive-power level exercises). To develop higher levels of stability while pushing, chest exercises will need to be performed, with controlled, unstable exercises, at slower speeds. (An example would be a dumbbell chest press performed on a stability ball.)
- Metabolic specificity refers to the energy demand placed on the body.[64-65] To develop endurance, training will require prolonged bouts of exercise,

> **Key Terms** are defined in the margin for easy comprehension.

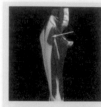

TENSOR FASCIA LATAE (TFL)

ORIGIN
- Outer surface of the iliac crest just posterior to the anterior-superior iliac spine of the pelvis

INSERTION
- Proximal one third of the iliotibial band

ISOLATED FUNCTION
- Concentrically accelerates hip flexion, abduction, and internal rotation

INTEGRATED FUNCTION
- Eccentrically decelerates hip extension, adduction, and external rotation
- Isometrically stabilizes the lumbo-pelvic-hip complex

GLUTEUS MAXIMUS

ORIGIN
- Outer ilium of the pelvis, posterior side of sacrum and coccyx, and part of the sacrotuberous and posterior sacroiliac ligament

INSERTION
- Gluteal tuberosity of the femur and iliotibial tract

ISOLATED FUNCTION
- Concentrically accelerates hip extension and external rotation

INTEGRATED FUNCTION
- Eccentrically decelerates hip flexion and internal rotation
- Decelerates tibial internal rotation via the iliotibial band
- Isometrically stabilizes the lumbo-pelvic-hip complex

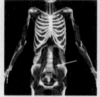

PSOAS

ORIGIN
- Transverse processes and lateral bodies of the last thoracic and all lumbar vertebrae including intervetebral disks

INSERTION
- Lesser trochanter of the femur

ISOLATED FUNCTION
- Concentrically accelerates hip flexion and external rotation
- Concentrically extends and rotates lumbar spine

INTEGRATED FUNCTION
- Eccentrically decelerates hip internal rotation
- Eccentrically decelerates hip extension
- Isometrically stabilizes the lumbo-pelvic-hip complex

> **Muscle tables** show detailed illustrations of isolated muscles and present Origin, Insertion, and Function.

> **Exercise boxes** demonstrate core exercises to use with clients. A starting position and finishing position are often included to illustrate good technique.

Ball Crunch

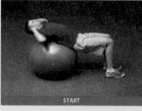

START   FINISH

PREPARATION

1. Lie supine on a stability ball (ball under low back) with knees bent at a 90-degree angle. Place feet flat on floor with toes shoulder-width apart and pointing straight ahead. Allow back to extend over curve of ball. Cross arms across chest.

MOVEMENT

2. Draw navel in and activate gluteals.
3. Slowly crunch upper body forward, raising shoulder blades off the ball and tucking chin to chest.
4. Slowly lower upper body over the ball, maintaining a drawn-in position.
5. Repeat as instructed.
6. To progress, perform as a long-lever exercise.

Safety   Make sure to keep the chin tucked while performing the exercise. This will take stress off of the muscles of the cervical spine.

Back Extension

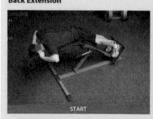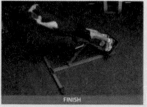

START   FINISH

> **Safety Tips** and **Technique Tips** present important safety considerations, warnings, or cautions and notes on proper exercise technique.

Full-color illustrations and photographs demonstrate concepts and help you learn proper technique.

64 CHAPTER 4

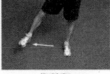

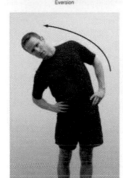

Eversion

Hip abduction

Lateral flexion

Shoulder abduction

Figure 4.7

lengthen.⁴·⁵ In actuality, the lengthening of the muscle usually refers to its return to a resting length and not actually increasing in its length as if it were being stretched.⁵

Eccentric muscle action is also known as 'a negative' in the health and fitness industry. The term "negative" was derived from the fact that in eccentric movement,

FLEXIBILITY TRAINING CONCEPTS 145

joint motion causes altered length-tension relationships. This affects the joint and causes poor
...ple, externally rotating the feet when squatting
...o externally rotate. This alters length-tension rela-
...knee and hips, putting the gluteus maximus (ago-
...decreasing its ability to generate force. This caus-
...rmis (synergists) to become synergistically domi-
...relationships (recruitment patterns), altering
...and increasing stress to the knees and low back.¹⁷
...o pain, which can further alter muscle recruitment

...cy

...scular efficiency is the ability of the neuromuscu-
...muscles to produce force (concentrically), reduce
...nically stabilize (isometrically) the entire kinetic
...on. Because the nervous system is the controlling
...s important to mention that *mechanoreceptors* (or
...e muscles and tendons help to determine muscle
...echanoreceptors include the muscle spindles and

...scle spindles are the major sensory organ of the
...roscopic fibers that lie parallel to the muscle fiber.
...are sensitive to change in length and rate of length
...one side of a joint is lengthened (owing to a short-
...le), the spindles of the lengthened muscle are
...nsmitted to the brain and spinal cord, exciting the
...cle fibers to contract. This often results in muscle
...¹,³,⁶

...xample of this response when the pelvis is rotat-
...6-5). This means that the anterior superior iliac
...e downward (inferiorly) and the ischium (bottom
...here the hamstrings originate) moves upward
...of the hamstrings is moved superiorly, it increas-
...o attachment sites and lengthens the muscle. In
... need to be statically stretched because they are
...n. When a lengthened muscle is stretched, it

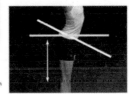

Figure 6.5 Effect of the hamstring with an anteriorly rotated pelvis.

146 CHAPTER 6

later in the chapter.)

Another example includes an individual wh...
rotate during an overhead squat. The underactiv...
(hip abductor and external rotator). Thus, one...
gluteus medius, but instead stretch the adductor...
overactive, pulling the femur into excessive a...
Individuals with protracted (rounded) shoulders...
and the middle and lower trapezius (underactive...
tive muscles, pulling them into this position (pe...
and latissimus dorsi).

GOLGI TENDON ORGANS

As also mentioned in Chapter 2, Golgi tendon organs are located within the *musculotendinous junction* (or the point where the muscle and the tendon meet) and
are sensitive to changes in muscular tension and rate of the tension change.⁵,¹⁸⁻²⁵
When excited, the Golgi tendon organ causes the muscle to relax. This prevents
the muscle from being placed under excessive stress, which could result in
injury.

Prolonged Golgi tendon organ stimulation provides an inhibitory action to
muscle spindles (located within the same muscle). This neuromuscular phenomenon is called autogenic inhibition and occurs when the neural impulses sensing
tension are greater than the impulses causing muscle contraction.¹⁴ The phenomenon is termed "autogenic" because the contracting muscle is being inhibited by its
own receptors.

MEMORY JOGGER

Autogenic inhibition is one of the main principles used in flexibility training, particularly with static stretching when one holds a stretch for a prolonged period of time
(20–30 seconds). Holding a stretch creates tension in the muscle. This tension stimulates the Golgi tendon organ, which overrides muscle spindle activity in the muscle
being stretched, causing relaxation in the overactive muscle and allowing for optimal lengthening
of the tissue.

Memory Joggers call out core concepts and program design instructions.

SUMMARY

Flexibility training may decrease the chance of muscle imbalances, joint dysfunctions, and overuse injuries. It is important to have proper range of motion in all
three planes. This can be achieved by implementing an integrated approach toward
flexibility training.

All segments of the kinetic chain must be properly aligned to avoid postural
distortion patterns, decreased neuromuscular efficiency, and tissue overload. The
adaptive potential of the kinetic chain is decreased by limited flexibility. This
forces the body to move in an altered fashion, leading to relative flexibility.

Muscle imbalances result from altered length-tension relationships, force-
couple relationships, and arthrokinematics. These imbalances can be caused by
poor posture, poor training technique, or previous injury. These muscle imbalances
result in altered reciprocal inhibition, synergistic dominance, and arthrokinetic
dysfunction, which in turn lead to decreased neuromuscular control.

Summaries wrap up each section and remind you of crucial material.

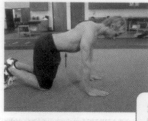

202   CHAPTER 8

REQUIREMENTS FOR CORE TRAINING

The core-stabilization system (transverse abd...
floor musculature, diaphragm, transversospina...
marily of slow-twitch, type I muscle fibers, w...
tension.⁶⁸ This means that these muscles need...

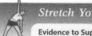

Stretch Your Knowledge

Evidence to Support the Use of Core-Stabilization Training

- Cosio-Lima et al. (2003) in a randomized controlled trial with 30 subjects demonstrated increased abdominal and back extensor strength and single leg balance improvements with a 5-week stability ball training program compared with conventional floor exercises.[1]
- Mills and Taunton (2003) in a randomized controlled trial with 36 subjects demonstrated that agility and balance were improved after a 10-week specific spinal stabilization training program compared with the control group performing an equivalent volume of traditional, nonspecific abdominal exercises.[2]
- Vera-Garcia et al. (2000) in a single-subject design with 8 subjects found that performing abdominal exercises on a labile surface increased activation levels, suggesting increased demand on the motor control system to help stabilize the spine.[3]
- Hahn et al. (1998) in a randomized controlled trial with 35 female subjects demonstrated that traditional floor exercises and stability ball exercises significantly increased core strength during a 10-week training period.[4]
- O'Sullivan et al. (1997) in a randomized clinical trial demonstrated that pain and function improve initially and at 1- and 3-year follow-up in patients with low back pain undergoing specific stabilizing exercises.[5]

1. Cosio-Lima LM, Reynolds KL, Winter C, et al. Effects of physioball and conventional floor exercises on early phase adaptations in back and abdominal core stability and balance in women. J Strength Cond Res 2003;17(4):721–725.
2. Mills JD, Taunton JE. The effect of spinal stabilization training on spinal mobility, vertical jump, agility and balance. Med Sci Sports Exerc 2003;35(5 Suppl).
3. Vera-Garcia FJ, Grenier SG, McGill SM. Abdominal muscle response during curl-ups on both stable and labile surfaces. Phys Ther 2003;80(6):564–594.
4. Hahn S, Stanforth D, Stanforth PR, Philips A. A 10 week training study comparing resistaball and traditional trunk training. Med Sci Sports Exerc 1998;30(5):199.
5. O'Sullivan PB, Twomey L, Allison GT. Evaluation of specific stabilizing exercises in the treatment of chronic low back pain with radiological diagnosis of spondylosis and spondylolisthesis. Spine 1997;22(24):2959–2967.

Stretch Your Knowledge boxes present findings from contemporary research to help you expand your knowledge of the material.

---

216   CHAPTER 8

Review Questions

1 *The movement system should be trained before the s...*

   a. True

   b. False

2 *In core stabilization training, exercises involve little ...*
   spine and pelvis.

   a. True

   b. False

3 *Indicate whether the following exercises are stabiliza...*
   power exercises.

   i. Stabilization

   ii. Strength

   iii. Power

   ...
   ...row

   ...exercises would you choose for a client...

   ...

   c. Core power

5 *Research shows that individuals who have chronic lo...*
   an increased activation of the transversus abdominis,
   pelvic floor muscles, multifidus, diaphragm, and deep...

   a. True

   b. False

REFERENCES

1. Aaron G. The use of stabilization training in the rehabilitation of th...
   Therapy Home Study Course. 1996.
2. Dominguez RH. Total Body Training. East Dundee, IL: Moving Force S...
3. Gracovetsky S, Farfan H. The optimum spine. Spine 1986;11:543–573.
4. Gracovetsky S, Farfan H, Heuller C. The abdominal mechanism. Spine...
5. Panjabi MM. The stabilizing system of the spine. Part I: function, dy...
   enhancement. J Spinal Disord 1992;5:383–389.
6. Panjabi MM, Tech D, White AA. Basic biomechanics of the spine. Neurosurgery 1980;7:76–93.
7. Sahrmann S. Posture and muscle imbalance: faulty lumbo-pelvic alignment and associated musculoskeletal pain syndromes. Orthop Div Rev Can Phys Ther 1992;12:13–20.
8. Sahrmann S. Diagnosis and Treatment of Muscle Imbalances and Musculoskeletal Pain Syndrome. Continuing Education Course. St. Louis: 1997.

Review Questions test your knowledge of the chapter. An answer key is provided at the end of the book.

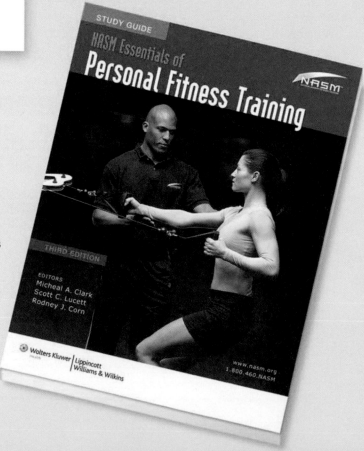

Corresponding Study Guide helps you test your knowledge and reinforce what you have learned. This separate resource includes matching, vocabulary, short answer, and multiple choice exercises.

Figure Credits List

2.5, 2.6
Modified from Premkumar K. The Massage Connection, Anatomy and Physiology, 2nd Ed. Baltimore: Lippincott Williams & Wilkins, 2004.

2-8 to 2-15, 2-26, 2-27, 8-1, and 3D anatomical series in Chapter 4 Reprinted with permission. Copyright© 2007 Primal Pictures Ltd.

2.28, 2.32
From Premkumar K. The Massage Connection, Anatomy and Physiology, 2nd Ed. Baltimore: Lippincott Williams and Wilkins, 2004.

2.18
Modified from Oatis Carol A. Kinesiology – The Mechanics and Pathomechanics of Human Movement. Baltimore: Lippincott Williams & Wilkins, 2004.

2.19-2.25
Modified from LifeART collection. Copyright© 2007 Lippincott Williams & Wilkins. All rights reserved.

2.30
From Bear MF, Connors BW, and Parasido, MA. Neuroscience – Exploring the Brain, 2nd Ed. Philadelphia: Lippincott Williams & Wilkins, 2001.

3.2
Asset provided by Anatomical Chart Co.

3.3
From Smeltzer SCO, Bare BG. Brunner and Suddarth's Textbook of Medical-Surgical Nursing. 9th Ed. Philadelphia: Lippincott Williams & Wilkins, 2002.

3.5
From McArdle WD, Katch FI, Katch VL. Essentials of Exercise Physiology, 2nd Ed. Baltimore: Lippincott Williams & Wilkins, 2000.

3.7
Modified from Stedman's Medical Dictionary, 27th Ed. Baltimore: Lippincott Williams & Wilkins, 2000.

Contents

PART 1 FUNDAMENTALS OF HUMAN MOVEMENT SCIENCE   1

PART **2** ASSESSMENTS, TRAINING CONCEPTS, AND PROGRAM DESIGN **97**

13 Program Design Concepts   325

PART 3   NUTRITION AND SUPPLEMENTATION   417

PART 4 CLIENT INTERACTION AND PROFESSIONAL DEVELOPMENT   463

FUNDAMENTALS OF HUMAN MOVEMENT SCIENCE

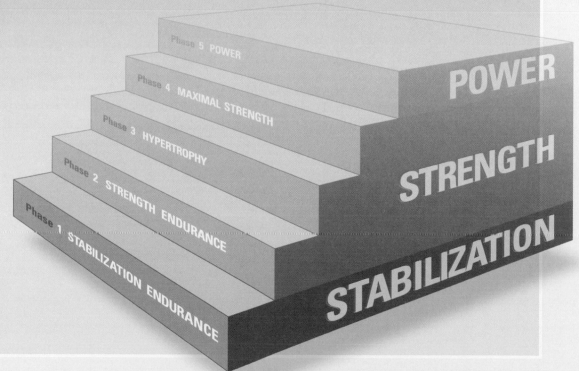

The Scientific Rationale for Integrated Training

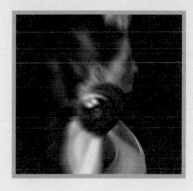

OBJECTIVES

After studying this chapter, you will be able to:

- Explain the history of personal training.
- Understand today's typical client.
- Rationalize the need for integrated program design.
- Describe the Optimum Performance Training (OPT™) model.

KEY TERMS

Deconditioned
Muscular endurance
Neuromuscular efficiency
Phase of training

Prime mover
Proprioception
Proprioceptively enriched
  environment

Rate of force production
Superset

The Personal Training Industry

OVERVIEW OF THE PERSONAL TRAINING INDUSTRY

Personal training is one of the fastest growing occupations in the United States. A recent survey from IDEA Health and Fitness Association has noted a significant growth rate in the personal training industry.[1] However, the origin of personal training is undocumented and anecdotal, at best. It is necessary to investigate the known beginnings of this occupation to better understand the rationale for current training concepts and their effect on clientele.

The Past

During the 1950s and 1960s, gym members were predominantly men who were training for specific goals, such as increased size (bodybuilders), strength (power lifters), explosive strength (Olympic lifters), or a combination of all of these goals (athletes). However, by the end of the 1960s, society's view of exercise began to change.

By the 1970s, going to the gym (and training to become fit) had become much more socially acceptable. It provided a structured way to achieve social interaction and health simultaneously. Fitness training did not require high levels of skill (as did sport forms of exercise) and was used to augment existing activity levels. Simply, it was an active outlet for anyone, regardless of physical ability, that could be utilized year-round, day or night and without concern for weather conditions. It was also perceived as a way to directly alter physical characteristics, in a society that had become very appearance-conscious.

Thus, the number of new gym members increased to include a large number of people who were uneducated about training and the gym environment. This brought about the desire to seek out help and guidance from an "expert."

Essentially, the expert of the 1970s was the person in the gym who had been training the longest, looked the most fit, or was the strongest. However, these qualities are primarily genetic in nature and are not necessarily based on training knowledge. Often, a new member would approach one of the perceived experts and offer that person money in exchange for his or her training knowledge and guidance. Hence, the fitness professional was born.

Although, for the most part, these individuals were probably able to provide good information on the acute variables of training such as loads, sets, reps, and so forth, the understanding and application of human movement science (functional anatomy, functional biomechanics, and motor behavior) is something very different. It was not usual practice to assess a new client for past medical conditions, training risk factors, muscle imbalances, goals, and such. This resulted in training programs that simply mimicked those of the current fitness professional or instructor. Programs were rarely designed to meet an individual client's goals, needs, and abilities.

At the time, the typical health-club member was probably better prepared for activity. The work and home environments were not as inundated with automation, personal computers, cell phones, and other technology that are more prevalent today. Housekeepers, gardeners, remote controls, and video games did not run a household. Furthermore, mandated activity, such as physical education in school, was not yet compromised. The activity level of daily life was still somewhat brisk.

The Present

From the mid-1980s to the present, the wealth of technology and automation in the United States has begun to take a toll on public health. In 1985, the International

Obesity Task Force deemed the prevalence of obesity an epidemic. Today, approximately 33% of adults are estimated to be obese. This carries over to the adolescent population, with 16% of teenagers considered overweight.[2]

The American population is also living longer. The U.S. Census Bureau reported that the proportion of the population older than 65 is projected to increase from 12.4% in 2000 to 19.6% in 2030. The number of individuals older than 80 is expected to increase from 9.3 million in 2000 to 19.5 million in 2030. This leads to the number of individuals developing chronic diseases and disability. In the United States, approximately 80% of all persons older than 65 have at least one chronic condition, and 50% have at least two. One in five adults report having doctor-diagnosed arthritis, and this is a leading cause of disability.[3]

Meanwhile, daily activity levels continue to decline.[4] People are less active and are no longer spending as much of their free time engaged in physical activity. Physical education and after-school sports programs are being cut from school budgets, further decreasing the amount of physical activity in children's lives. This new environment is producing more inactive and nonfunctional people.[5]

EVIDENCE OF MUSCULAR DYSFUNCTION AND INCREASED INJURY

Research suggests that musculoskeletal pain is more common now than it was 40 years ago.[6] This lends support to the concept that decreased activity may lead to muscular dysfunction and, ultimately, injury. Some of the major topics studied include low back pain, knee injuries, chronic diseases in the adult population, and musculoskeletal injuries.

Low Back Pain. Low back pain is one the major forms of musculoskeletal degeneration seen in the adult population, affecting nearly 80% of all adults.[7,8] Research has shown low back pain to be predominant among workers in enclosed workspaces (such as offices),[9,10] as well as in people engaged in manual labor (farming).[11] Low back pain is also seen in people who sit for periods of time greater than 3 hours[10] and in individuals who have altered lumbar lordosis (curve in the lumbar spine).[12]

Knee Injuries. The incidence of knee injuries is also a concern. An estimated 80,000 to 100,000 anterior cruciate ligament (ACL) injuries occur annually in the general U.S. population. Approximately 70% of these are noncontact injuries.[13] In addition, ACL injuries have a strong correlation to acquiring arthritis in the affected knee.[14]

Most ACL injuries occur between 15 and 25 years of age.[13] This comes as no surprise when considering the lack of activity and increased obesity occurring in this age group. U.S. teenagers have an abundance of automation and technology, combined with a lack of mandatory physical education in schools.[5]

Fortunately, research suggests that enhancing neuromuscular stabilization (or body control) may alleviate the high incidence of noncontact injuries.[15]

Chronic Diseases in the Adult Population. The U.S. Centers for Disease Control and Prevention reported that chronic diseases were responsible for five of the leading six causes of disease in the United States in 2002. One of these chronic diseases, obesity, is now a worldwide epidemic leading to many other chronic diseases including cancer, cardiovascular disease, arthritis, and diabetes.[16]

Physical activity has been proven to reduce the risk of chronic diseases and disorders that are related to lifestyle, such as increased triglycerides and cholesterol levels, obesity, glucose tolerance, high blood pressure, coronary heart disease, and strokes.[17] More importantly, some research indicates that discontinuing (or significantly decreasing) physical activity can actually lead to a higher risk of chronic diseases that are related to lifestyle.[18]

Musculoskeletal Injuries. In 2003, musculoskeletal symptoms were the number two reason for physician visits. Approximately 31 million visits were made to physicians' offices because of back problems in 2003, including more than 10 million visits for low back problems. Approximately 19 million visits in 2003 were made because of knee problems, 14 million for shoulder problems, and 11 million for foot and ankle problems.[19]

Unnatural posture, caused by improper sitting, results in increased neck, mid- and lower back, shoulder, and leg pain. Of work-related injuries, more than 40% are sprains and strains. More than one third of all work-related injuries involve the trunk, and of these, more than 60% involve the low back. These work-related injuries cost workers approximately 9 days per back episode or, combined, more than 39 million days of restricted activity. The monetary value of lost work time as a result of these musculoskeletal injuries was estimated to be approximately $120 billion.[20]

It has become much more important in today's society to focus on health and well-being. Many individuals realize that they need to exercise, and although statistics show an increase of prevalence of physical activity in 41 of the United States and U.S. territories in the last few years, only nine states showed a significant increase. On the other hand, 12 states (or territories) showed a decrease, and it is estimated that approximately 54% of U.S. adults did not engage in the minimum recommended level of physical activity (at least 30 minutes of moderate-intensity physical activity on most days).[21] Moreover, Americans older than 55 and younger than 18 are the fastest-growing age groups among health-club members. This translates to a relatively large number of inactive persons entering the fitness population.

With this growing population of untrained or undertrained individuals it is important to ensure that all components of their bodies are properly prepared for the stress that will be placed on them. Unfortunately, many training programs and apparatus used to condition the musculoskeletal system often neglect proper training guidelines. These include training essential areas of the body, such as the stabilizing muscles of the hips, upper and lower back, and neck, and using a proper progression of acute variables. This neglect can result in a weakened structure and lead to injury.

Simply put, the extent to which we condition our musculoskeletal system directly influences our risk of injury. The less conditioned our musculoskeletal systems are, the higher the risk of injury.[22] Therefore, as our daily lives include less physical activity, the less prepared we are to partake in recreational and leisure activities such as resistance training, weekend sports, or simply playing on the playground.

CURRENT TRAINING PROGRAMS

Research has been conducted on the effectiveness of training programs on sedentary adults. It has been shown that the intensity of activity required by a sedentary person trying to improve cardiorespiratory fitness might put that person into a state of excessive overload.[23] In the initial 6 weeks of a study that physically trained sedentary adults, there was a 50 to 90% injury rate.[24] This occurred even though programs were specifically designed to minimize risk of injury. Researchers concluded that the musculoskeletal system is very easily overtrained when it is **deconditioned**.

It is important to note that deconditioned does not simply mean a person is out of breath on climbing a flight of stairs or that they are overweight. It is a state in which a person may have muscle imbalances, decreased flexibility, or a lack of core and joint stability. All of these conditions can greatly affect the ability of the human body to produce proper movement and can eventually lead to injury.

Most training programs do not emphasize multiplanar movements (or movement in different degrees of the various planes of the body) through the full muscle action spectrum (concentric, eccentric, and isometric muscle contractions) in an environment that enriches **proprioception**. A **proprioceptively enriched** environment is one that challenges the internal balance and stabilization mechanisms of the body. (Examples of this include performing a dumbbell chest press while on a stability ball or performing a single-leg squat.)

Deconditioned: A state of lost physical fitness, which may include muscle imbalances, decreased flexibility, and a lack of core and joint stability.

Proprioception: The cumulative sensory input to the central nervous system from all mechanoreceptors that sense body position and limb movement.

Proprioceptively enriched environment: An unstable (yet controllable) physical situation in which exercises are performed that causes the body to use its internal balance and stabilization mechanisms.

The Future

There is a general inability to meet the needs of today's client. The fitness industry has only recently recognized the trend toward nonfunctional living. Fitness professionals are now noticing a decrease in the physical functionality of their clients and are beginning to address it.

This is a new state of training, in which the client has been physically molded by furniture, gravity, and inactivity. The continual decrease in everyday activity has contributed to many of the postural deficiencies seen in people.[25] Today's client is not ready to begin physical activity at the same level that a typical client could 20 years ago. Therefore, today's training programs cannot stay the same as programs of the past.

The new mindset in fitness should cater to creating programs that address functional capacity, as part of a safe program designed especially for each individual person. In other words, training programs must consider each person, their environment, and the tasks that will be performed. This is best achieved by introducing an integrated approach to program design. It is on this premise that the National Academy of Sports Medicine (NASM) presents the rationale for integrated training and the Optimum Performance Training (OPT™) model.

SUMMARY

The typical gym members of the 1950s were mainly athletes, and, in the 1970s, those involved in recreational sports. The first fitness professionals were physically fit individuals who did not necessarily have education in human movement science. They did not design programs to meet the specific goals, needs, and abilities of their clients.

Today, more people work in offices, have longer work hours, use better technology and automation, and are required to move less on a daily basis. This new environment produces more inactive and nonfunctional people and leads to dysfunction and increased incidents of injury including low back pain, knee injuries, chronic diseases in the adult population, and musculoskeletal injuries.

In working with today's typical client, who is likely to be deconditioned, the fitness professional must take special consideration when designing programs. An integrated approach should be used to create safe programs that consider functional capacity for each individual person. They must address factors such as appropriate forms of flexibility, increasing strength and endurance, and training in different types of environments. These are the bases for NASM's OPT™ model.

Integrated Training and the OPT™ Model

Integrated training is a concept that incorporates all forms of training in an integrated fashion as part of a progressive system. These forms of training include flexibility training, cardiorespiratory training, core training, balance training, reactive training, speed, agility, and quickness training, and resistance training. This system was developed by NASM and is termed Optimum Performance Training (OPT™).

WHAT IS THE OPT™ MODEL?

The OPT™ model was conceptualized as a training program for a society that has more physical structural imbalances and susceptibility to injury than ever before. It is a process of programming that systematically progresses any client to any goal. The OPT™ model (Figure 1-1) is built on a foundation of principles that progressively

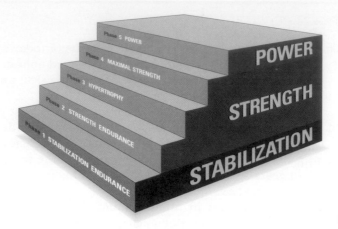

Figure 1.1   OPT™ Model.

and systematically allow any client to achieve optimum levels of physiologic, physical, and performance adaptations, including:

Physiologic Benefits
- Improves cardiorespiratory efficiency
- Enhances beneficial endocrine and serum lipid adaptations
- Increases metabolic efficiency
- Increases tissue tensile strength
- Increases bone density

Physical Benefits
- Decreases body fat
- Increases lean body mass (muscle)

Performance Benefits
- Strength
- Power
- Endurance
- Flexibility
- Speed
- Agility
- Balance

The OPT™ model is based on the scientific rationale of human movement science. Each stage has a designated purpose that provides the client with a systematic approach for progressing toward his or her individual goals, as well as addressing his or her specific needs. Now, more than ever, it is imperative that fitness professionals fully understand all components of programming as well as the right order in which those components must be addressed to help their clients achieve success.

THE OPT™ MODEL

Phases of training: Smaller divisions of training progressions that fall within the three building blocks of training.

The OPT™ model is divided into three different building blocks of training—stabilization, strength, and power (Figure 1-1). Each building block contains specific **phases of training**. It is imperative that the fitness professional understands the scientific rationale behind each building block to properly use the OPT™ model.

Stabilization Level

Muscular endurance: A muscle's ability to contract for an extended period of time.

Stabilization level consists of one phase of training—Phase 1: Stabilization Endurance Training. The main focus of this form of training is to increase **muscular endurance**

Neuromuscular efficiency:
The ability of the neuromuscular system to enable all muscles to efficiently work together in all planes of motion.

and stability while developing optimal communication between one's nervous system and muscular system (**neuromuscular efficiency**).

The progression for this block of training is proprioceptively based. This means that difficulty is increased by introducing more challenge to the balance and stabilization systems of the body (versus simply increasing the load).

Stabilization and neuromuscular efficiency can only be obtained by having the appropriate combination of proper alignment of the kinetic chain and the stability strength necessary to maintain that alignment.[26-28] Training provides the needed stimuli to acquire stabilization and neuromuscular efficiency through the use of proprioceptively enriched exercises and progressions. The goal is to increase the client's ability to stabilize their joints and posture.

It must be noted that stabilization training must be done before strength and power training. Research has shown that inefficient stabilization can negatively affect the way force is produced by the muscles, increase stress at the joints, overload the soft tissues, and, eventually, cause injury.[22,29-31]

Stabilization endurance training not only addresses the existing structural deficiencies, it also provides a superior way to alter body composition. By performing exercises in a proprioceptively enriched environment (controlled, unstable), the body is forced to recruit more muscles to stabilize itself. In doing so, more calories are potentially expended.[32,33]

GOALS AND STRATEGIES OF STABILIZATION LEVEL TRAINING

Phase 1: Stabilization Endurance Training
- Goals
  - Improve muscular endurance
  - Enhance joint stability
  - Increase flexibility
  - Enhance control of posture
  - Improve neuromuscular efficiency (balance, stabilization)
- Training Strategies
  - Corrective flexibility
  - Training in unstable, yet controllable environments (proprioceptively enriched)
  - Low loads, high repetitions

Strength Level

The strength level of training follows the successful completion of stabilization training. The emphasis is to maintain stabilization endurance while increasing **prime mover** strength. This is also the block of training an individual will progress to if his or her goals are *hypertrophy* (increasing muscle size) or *maximal strength* (lifting heavy loads). The Strength Level in the OPT™ model consists of three phases.

Prime mover: The muscle that acts as the initial and main source of motive power.

Superset: Set of two exercises that are performed back-to-back, without any rest time between them.

In Phase 2: Strength Endurance training, the goal is to enhance stabilization endurance while increasing prime mover strength. These two adaptations are accomplished by performing two exercises in a **superset** sequence (or back-to-back without rest) with similar joint dynamics (Table 1-1). One exercise is a more traditional strength exercise performed in a more stable environment, whereas the other is an integrated exercise performed in a less stable (yet controllable) environment. The principle behind this method is to work the prime movers predominantly in the first exercise to elicit prime mover strength. Then, immediately follow with an exercise that challenges the stabilization muscles. This produces an increased ability to maintain postural stabilization and dynamic joint stabilization.

Phase 3: Hypertrophy training is designed for individuals who have the goal of maximal muscle growth. Phase 4: Maximal Strength Training works toward the goal of maximal prime mover strength by lifting heavy loads. These two components of

Table 1.1

Phase 2 Example Supersets

Body Part	Strength Exercise	Stabilization Exercise
Chest	1. Barbell bench press	2. Stability ball push-up
Back	1. Seated cable row	2. Stability ball dumbbell row
Shoulders	1. Shoulder press machine	2. Single-leg dumbbell press
Legs	1. Leg press	2. Single-leg squat

training can be used as more special forms of training and as progressions within strength level training.

GOALS AND STRATEGIES OF STRENGTH LEVEL TRAINING

Phase 2: Strength Endurance Training

- Goals
  - Improve stabilization endurance and increase prime mover strength
  - Improve overall work capacity
  - Enhance joint stabilization
  - Increase lean body mass
- Training Strategies
  - Active flexibility
  - Moderate loads and repetitions (8–12)
  - Superset: one traditional strength exercise and one stabilization exercise per body part in the resistance training portion of the program

Phase 3: Hypertrophy Training *(optional phase, depending on client goals)*

- Goal
  - Achieve optimum levels of muscular hypertrophy
- Training Strategies
  - Active flexibility
  - High volume, high loads, moderate or low repetitions (6–10)

Phase 4: Maximum Strength Training *(optional phase, depending on client goals)*

- Goals
  - Increase motor unit recruitment
  - Increase frequency of motor unit recruitment
  - Improve peak force
- Training Strategies
  - Active flexibility
  - High loads, low repetitions (1–5), longer rest periods

Power Level

Power level training should only be entered after successful completion of the two previous training blocks. This block of training emphasizes the development of speed and power. This is achieved through one phase of training simply named Phase 5: Power Training.

Table 1.2		
Phase 5 Example Supersets		
Body Part	**Strength Exercise**	**Power Exercise**
Chest	1. Incline dumbbell press	2. Medicine ball chest pass
Back	1. Pull-up	2. Soccer throw
Shoulders	1. Overhead dumbbell press	2. Scoop toss
Legs	1. Barbell squat	2. Squat jump

Rate of force production:
How quickly a muscle can generate force.

The premise behind this phase of training is the execution of a more traditional strength exercise superset with a power exercise of similar joint dynamics. This is to enhance prime mover strength while also improving the **rate of force production** (Table 1-2).

GOALS AND STRATEGIES OF POWER LEVEL TRAINING

Phase 5: Power Training
- Goals
  - Enhance neuromuscular efficiency
  - Enhance prime mover strength
  - Increase rate of force production (power)
  - Enhance speed strength
- Training Strategies
  - Dynamic flexibility
  - Superset: one strength and one power exercise per body part in the resistance training portion of the program
  - Perform all power exercises as fast as can be controlled

THE PROGRAM TEMPLATE

The uniqueness of the OPT™ model is that it packages scientific principles into an applicable form of programming. This is a direct result of testing within NASM's clinical setting, used on actual clients. NASM has developed a template that provides health and fitness professionals with specific guidelines for creating an individualized program (Figure 1-2).

HOW TO USE THE OPT™ MODEL

Chapters later in this text will be specifically dedicated to explaining how to use the OPT™ model in the fitness environment and detail the necessary components of an integrated training program. They include:
- Client assessments
- Flexibility training
- Cardiorespiratory training
- Core training
- Balance training
- Reactive training
- Speed, agility, and quickness training
- Resistance training
- Program design

NASM™
NATIONAL ACADEMY OF SPORTS MEDICINE

OPT For Fitness

Name:	Month:
Date:	Week:
Professional:	Day:

Program Goal:

STEP 1

A. Foam Roll

Foam Roll	Sets	Duration

B. Stretch

Exercise	Sets	Duration

C. Cardiovascular

STEP 2

A. Core

Exercise	Sets	Reps	Tempo	Rest

B. Balance

Exercise	Sets	Reps	Tempo	Rest

C. Reactive

Exercise	Sets	Reps	Tempo	Rest

STEP 3

Resistance Training Program

Body Part	Exercise	Sets	Reps	Intensity	Tempo	Rest
Total Body						
Chest						
Back						
Shoulder						
Legs						

STEP 4

Cool-Down

Repeat Steps 1A and 1B

Figure 1.2 NASM Program Template.

Each of these chapters explains how each component specifically fits into the OPT™ model and how to realistically apply the information given. Other chapters in this textbook review:

- Applied exercise science
- Nutrition
- Supplementation
- Special populations
- Behavior modification
- Professional development

All of this combined information should provide any individual with all of the tools necessary to become a skilled and well-rounded fitness professional.

SUMMARY

The Optimum Performance Training (OPT™) model provides a system for properly and safely progressing any client to his or her goals, by using integrated training methods. It consists of three building blocks—stabilization, strength, and power.

The stabilization level addresses muscular imbalances and attempts to improve the stabilization of joints and overall posture. This is a component that most training programs leave out even though it is the most important in ensuring proper neuromuscular functioning. This training block has one phase of training—Phase 1: Stabilization Endurance Training.

The strength level focuses on enhancing stabilization while increasing muscle size or maximal strength. Most traditional programs begin at this point and, as a result, often lead to injury. This training block has three phases—Phase 2: Strength Endurance Training, Phase 3: Hypertrophy Training, and Phase 4: Maximum Strength Training.

The power level is designed to target specific forms of training that are necessary for maximal force production. This stage has one phase of training—Phase 5: Power Training.

All of these phases of training have been specifically designed to follow biomechanical, physiologic, and functional principles of the kinetic chain. They should provide an easy-to-follow systematic progression that minimizes injury and maximizes results. To help ensure proper organization and structure, NASM has developed a program template that guides fitness professionals through the process.

Review Questions

1 *Today, approximately what percentage of adults are estimated to be obese:*

  a. 15%

  b. 22%

  c. 30%

2 *A proprioceptively enriched environment is one that challenges the internal balance and stabilization mechanisms of the body.*

  a. True

  b. False

3 *Name the three building blocks of training.*

4 *In which building block does the phase of Hypertrophy Training belong?*

5 *Which phase of training enhances prime mover strength and improves the rate of force production concurrently?*

REFERENCES

1. [Anonymous]. Fitness trends outlined. 2003 IDEA Fitness Programs & Equipment Survey; Oct. 30, 2003.
2. Katz DL, O'Connell M, Yeh M, et al. Public health strategies for preventing and controlling overweight and obesity in school and worksite settings. MMWR Morb Mortal Wkly Rep 2005;54(RR-10):1–11.
3. Centers for Disease Control and Prevention. Summary health statistics for US adults: National Health Interview Survey, 2002. Vital Health Stat 10 2004;10(222). <http://www.cdc.gov/nchs/data/series/sr_10/sr10_222acc.pdf>.

4. Centers for Disease Control and Prevention. Prevalence of physical activity, including lifestyle activities among adults—United States, 2000–2001. MMWR Morb Mortal Wkly Rep 2003;52(32): 764–769.

5. The burden of obesity in the United States: a problem of massive proportions. Chronic Dis Notes Rep 2005;17(2):4–9.

6. Harkness EF, Macfarlane GJ, Silman AJ, McBeth J. Is musculoskeletal pain more common now than 40 years ago? Two population-based cross-sectional studies. Rheumatology (Oxf) 2005; 44(7):831–833.

7. Walker BF, Muller R, Grant WD. Low back pain in Australian adults: prevalence and associated disability. J Manipulative Physiol Ther 2004;27(4):238–244.

8. Cassidy JD, Carroll LJ, Cote P. The Saskatchewan Health and Back Pain Survey. The prevalence of low back pain and related disability in Saskatchewan adults. Spine 1998;23(17):1860–1866.

9. Volinn E. The epidemiology of low back pain in the rest of the world. A review of surveys in low- and middle-income countries. Spine 1997;22(15):1747–1754.

10. Omokhodion FO, Sanya AO. Risk factors for low back pain among office workers in Ibadan, Southwest Nigeria. Occup Med (Lond) 2003;53(4):287–289.

11. Omokhodion FO. Low back pain in a rural community in South West Nigeria. West Afr J Med 2002;21(2):87–90.

12. Tsuji T, Matsuyama Y, Sato K, Hasegawa Y, Yimin Y, Iwata H. Epidemiology of low back pain in the elderly: correlation with lumbar lordosis. J Orthop Sci 2001;6(4):307–311.

13. Griffin LY, Agel J, Albohm MJ, et al. Noncontact anterior cruciate ligament injuries: risk factors and prevention strategies. J Am Acad Orthop Surg 2000;8(3):141–150.

14. Hill CL, Seo GS, Gale D, Totterman S, Gale ME, Felson DT. Cruciate ligament integrity in osteoarthritis of the knee. Arthritis Rheum 2005;52:3:794–799.

15. Mandelbaum BR, Silvers HJ, Watanabe DS, Knarr JF, Thomas SD, Griffin LY, Kirkendall DT, Garrett W Jr. Effectiveness of a neuromuscular and proprioceptive training program in preventing anterior cruciate ligament injuries in female athletes: 2-year follow-up. Am J Sports Med 2005;33(7):1003–1010.

16. Centers for Disease Control and Prevention. 2006 Jan 31. Physical activity and good nutrition: Essential elements to prevent chronic disease and obesity. <http://www.cdc.gov/nccdphp/publica-tions/aag/dnpa.htm> Accessed 2006 Feb 8.

17. Pedersen BK, Saltin B. Evidence for prescribing exercise as therapy in chronic disease. Scand J Med Sci Sports 2006;16(Suppl 1):3–63.

18. Sherman SE, Agostino RBD, Silbershatz H, Kannel WB. Comparison of past versus recent physical activity in the prevention of premature death and coronary artery disease. Am Heart J 1999;138:900–907.

19. Centers for Disease Control and Prevention. Ambulatory care visits to physician offices, hospital outpatient departments, and emergency departments: United States, 2001–02. Vital Health Stat 13 2006;13(159). <http://www.cdc.gov/nchs/data/series/sr_13/sr13_159.pdf>

20. Bureau of Labor Statistics. 2005 Dec 15. Workplace injuries and illnesses in 2004. News release. <http://www.bls.gov/iif/home.htm> Accessed 2006 Feb 8.

21. Centers for Disease Control and Prevention. Adult ß—United States, 2001 and 2003. MMWR Morb Mortal Wkly Rep 2005;54(47):1208–1212.

22. Barr KP, Griggs M, Cadby T. Lumbar stabilization: core concepts and current literature, Part 1. Am J Phys Med Rehabil 2005;84(6):473–480.

23. Watkins J. Structure and Function of the Musculoskeletal System. Champaign, IL: Human Kinetics, 1999.

24. Jones BH, Cowan DN, Knapik J. Exercise, training, and injuries. Sports Med 1994;18(3):202–214.

25. Hammer WI. Muscle imbalance and postfacilitation stretch. In: Hammer WI (ed). Functional Soft Tissue Examination and Treatment by Manual Methods, 2nd ed. Gaithersburg, MD: Aspen Publishers, 1999.

26. Powers CM. The influence of altered lower-extremity kinematics on patellofemoral joint dysfunc-tion: a theoretical perspective. J Orthop Sports Phys Ther 2003;33(11):639–646.

27. Comerford MJ, Mottram SL. Movement and stability dysfunction—contemporary developments. Man Ther 2001;6(1):15–26.

28. Panjabi MM. The stabilizing system of the spine. Part I: Function, dysfunction, adaptation, and enhancement. J Spinal Disord 1992;5(4):383–389.

29. Paterno MV, Myer GD, Ford KR, Hewett TE. Neuromuscular training improves single-limb stabil-ity in young female athletes. J Orthop Sports Phys Ther 2004;34(6):305–316.

30. Hungerford B; Gilleard W, Hodges P. Evidence of altered lumbopelvic muscle recruitment in the presence of sacroiliac joint pain. Spine 2003;28(14):1593–1600.

31. Edgerton VR, Wolf S, Roy RR. Theoretical basis for patterning EMG amplitudes to assess muscle dysfunction. Med Sci Sports Exerc 1996;28(6)744–751.

32. Williford HN, Olson MS, Gauger S, Duey WJ, Blessing DL. Cardiovascular and metabolic costs of forward, backward, and lateral motion. Med Sci Sports Exerc 1998;30(9):1419–1423.

33. Ogita F, Stam RP, Tazawa HO, Toussaint HM, Hollander AP. Oxygen uptake in one-legged and two-legged exercise. Med Sci Sports Exerc 2000;32(10):1737–1742.

Basic Exercise Science

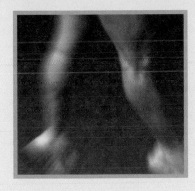

OBJECTIVES

After studying this chapter, you will be able to:

- Define the components of the kinetic chain.
- Explain the structure and function of:
  - The central and peripheral nervous systems
  - Bones
  - Joints
  - Muscles
- Describe how they all relate to human movement.

KEY TERMS

Appendicular skeleton	Kinetic chain	Neurotransmitter
Arthrokinematics	Ligament	Nonsynovial joints
Axial skeleton	Mechanoreceptors	Peripheral nervous system
Bones	Motor (efferent) neurons	Process
Central nervous system	Motor function	Sarcomere
Depression	Motor unit	Sensory (afferent) neurons
Golgi tendon organs	Muscle spindles	Sensory function
Integrative function	Muscular system	Skeletal system
Interneurons	Nervous system	Synovial joints
Joint receptors	Neural activation	Tendons
Joints	Neuron	

INTRODUCTION TO HUMAN MOVEMENT

Structure allows for and provides the basis of function.[1] Therefore, the components that make up a structure have a drastic influence on how that structure ultimately functions. In the human body, the components that make up the human movement system include the nervous system, the skeletal system, and the muscular system. Together, these components are known as the **kinetic chain** and are responsible for human movement (Figure 2-1).[2,3]

> **Kinetic chain:** The combination and interrelation of the nervous, muscular, and skeletal systems.

All systems of the kinetic chain must work together to produce movement. If one system (or component) of the kinetic chain is not working properly, it will affect the other systems and ultimately affect movement.[4-7] Therefore, it is imperative that the health and fitness professional fully understand all components of the kinetic chain and how they work together to construct efficient movement. To gain a complete understanding of the kinetic chain, it is necessary to look at the structure and function of each component.

The Nervous System

OVERVIEW OF THE NERVOUS SYSTEM

> **Nervous system:** The communication network within the body.

The **nervous system** is a conglomeration of billions of cells forming nerves that are specifically designed to provide a communication network within the human body. It is the central command center that allows us to gather information about our internal and external environments, process and interpret the information, and then respond to it.[8-11]

> **Sensory function:** The ability of the nervous system to sense changes in either the internal or external environment.

> **Integrative function:** The ability of the nervous system to analyze and interpret sensory information to allow for proper decision making, which produces the appropriate response.

> **Motor function:** The neuromuscular response to the sensory information.

The three primary functions of the nervous system include sensory, integrative, and motor functions.[8-10] **Sensory function** is the ability of the nervous system to sense changes in either the internal or external environment, such as a stretch placed on a muscle (internal) or the change from walking on the sidewalk to walking on sand (external). **Integrative function** is the ability of the nervous system to analyze and interpret the sensory information to allow for proper decision making, which produces the appropriate response. The **motor function** is the neuromuscular (or nervous and muscular systems') response to the sensory information, such as causing the muscle to initially contract when stretched, or changing our walking pattern when in the sand as opposed to the sidewalk.[8-10]

The key aspect to note here is that all movement is directly dictated by the nervous system. Thus, it becomes important to train the nervous system efficiently to ensure that proper movement patterns are being developed, which enhances performance and decreases the risk of injuries.[8,10,12] This important concept will be discussed throughout the remainder of the text.

Nervous system
+
Skeletal system
+
Muscular system
=
The Kinetic Chain

Figure 2.1   The equation for movement.

ANATOMY OF THE NERVOUS SYSTEM

The Neuron

Neuron: The functional unit of the nervous system.

The functional unit of the nervous system is known as the **neuron** (Figure 2-2).[8] Billions of neurons make up the complex structure of the nervous system and provide it with the ability to communicate internally with itself, as well as externally with the outside environment. Collectively, the merging of many neurons together forms the nerves of the body. Neurons are composed of three main parts: the cell body, axon, and dendrites.[8–10,13]

The cell body (or soma) of a neuron is much like any other cell body in that it contains a nucleus and other organelles such as lysosomes, mitochondria, and a Golgi complex. The axon is a cylindrical projection from the cell body that transmits nervous impulses to other neurons or effector sites (muscles, organs, other neurons). This is the part of the neuron that provides communication from the brain and spinal cord to other parts of the body. The dendrites are responsible for gathering information from other structures back into the neuron.[8–10,13]

Sensory (afferent) neurons: Transmit nerve impulses from effector sites to the brain or spinal cord.

Interneurons: Transmit nerve impulses from one neuron to another.

Motor (efferent) neurons: Transmit nerve impulses from the brain and spinal cord to effector sites.

Essentially, there are three main functional classifications of neurons that are determined by the direction of their nerve impulses. **Sensory (afferent) neurons** transmit nerve impulses from effector sites (such as muscles and organs) via receptors to the brain and spinal cord. **Interneurons** transmit nerve impulses from one neuron to another.[9,13] **Motor (efferent) neurons** transmit nerve impulses from the brain and spinal cord to the effector sites such as muscles or glands.

A demonstration of the way these different neurons work together to produce a given response can be explained through the example of a person touching a hot object. The sensory (afferent) neurons send a signal from the hand to the brain telling the brain that the object is hot. This signal makes its way to the brain by traveling from one neuron to another via the interneurons. Once the signal has made it to the brain, the brain then interprets the information sent from the sensory neurons (the object is hot) and sends the appropriate signals down to the muscles of the hand and arm via the motor neurons, telling the muscles to contract to pull the hand away from the hot object, protecting the hand from injury.

The Central and Peripheral Nervous Systems

Central nervous system: Composed of the brain and spinal cord.

Peripheral nervous system: Cranial and spinal nerves that spread throughout the body.

The nervous system is composed of two interdependent divisions. These include the central nervous system and the peripheral nervous system.[1,8–10,13] The **central nervous system** consists of the brain and the spinal cord (Figure 2-3).[1,8–10,13] The central nervous system serves mainly to interpret information.

The **peripheral nervous system** consists of 12 cranial nerves, 31 pairs of spinal nerves (which branch out from the brain and spinal cord), and sensory receptors (Figure 2-4).[8–10,13]

These peripheral nerves serve two main functions. First, they provide a connection for the nervous system to activate different effector sites, such as muscles (motor function).

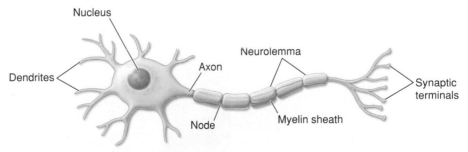

Figure 2.2   The neuron.

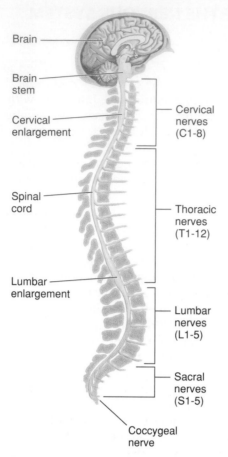

Brain

Brain stem

Cervical enlargement

Spinal cord

Lumbar enlargement

Cervical nerves (C1-8)

Thoracic nerves (T1-12)

Lumbar nerves (L1-5)

Sacral nerves (S1-5)

Coccygeal nerve

Figure 2.3   The central nervous system.

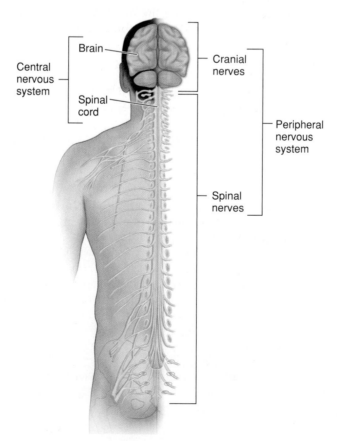

Central nervous system

Brain

Spinal cord

Cranial nerves

Peripheral nervous system

Spinal nerves

Figure 2.4   The peripheral nervous system.

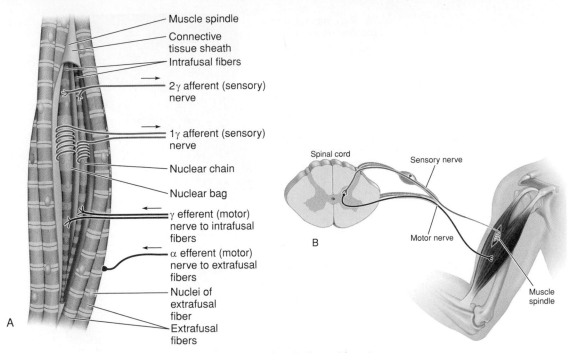

Figure 2.5   Muscle spindle and function.

Second, peripheral nerves relay information from the effector sites back to the brain via sensory receptors (sensory function), thus providing a constant update on the relation between the body and the environment.[8-11,13]

The sensory receptors are specialized structures located throughout the body that are designed to transform environmental stimuli (heat, light, sound, taste, motion) into sensory information that the brain and spinal cord can then interpret to produce a response. These receptors can be subdivided into four major categories. Mechanoreceptors respond to mechanical forces (touch and pressure), nociceptors respond to pain (pain receptors), chemoreceptors respond to chemical interaction (smell and taste), and photoreceptors respond to light (vision).[10,13] For relevance to this text, we will focus attention on the mechanoreceptors.

With respect to the health and fitness professional and human movement, **mechanoreceptors** are specialized structures that are essentially responsible for sensing distortion in tissues.[14-19] This is brought about through stretch, compression, traction, or tension to the tissue and then transmitted to the nervous system. Furthermore, it has been demonstrated that mechanoreceptors are located in muscles, tendons, ligaments, and joint capsules.[17,18,20-24] Mechanoreceptors include muscle spindles, Golgi tendon organs, and joint receptors.

Muscle spindles are the major sensory organs of the muscle and sit parallel to the muscle's fibers (Figure 2-5). Muscle spindles are sensitive to change in length and rate of length change.[1,5-7,10,13,15,18,24] When a muscle is stretched, the spindles of that muscle are also stretched. This information is transmitted to the brain and spinal cord to update the nervous system on the status of the muscle length and the rate at which that muscle is lengthening. When excited, the muscle spindle will cause the muscle to contract. This is to prevent the muscle from stretching too far or too fast, either of which could otherwise cause injury.[1,5-7,10,13,15,18,24]

Golgi tendon organs (GTO) are at the point where the muscle and tendon meet (musculotendinous junction) and are sensitive to changes in muscular tension and rate of the tension change (Figure 2-6).[1,5-7,10,13,15,18,24] When excited, the Golgi tendon organ will cause the muscle to relax. This is to prevent the muscle from being placed under excessive stress and sustaining injury.

Mechanoreceptors: Sensory receptors responsible for sensing distortion in body tissues.

Muscle spindles: Receptors sensitive to change in length of the muscle and the rate of that change.

Golgi tendon organs: Receptors sensitive to change in tension of the muscle and the rate of that change.

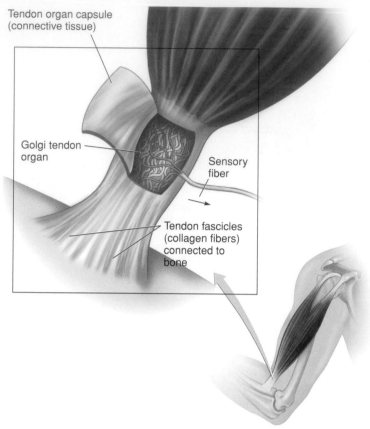

Figure 2.6 Golgi tendon organ.

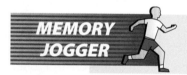

It will be important to understand the function of the muscle spindles and GTO as they play an integral part in flexibility training (Chapter 6).

Joint receptors: Receptors that respond to pressure, acceleration, and deceleration in the joint.

Joint receptors are located in and around the joint capsule. They respond to pressure and to acceleration and deceleration of the joint (Figure 2-7). These receptors act to signal extreme joint positions and thus help to prevent injury. They can also act to initiate a reflexive inhibitory response in the surrounding muscles if

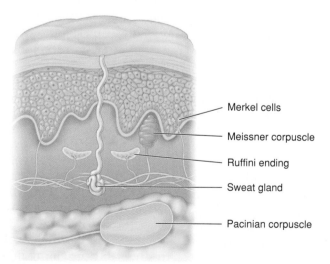

Merkel cells

Meissner corpuscle

Ruffini ending

Sweat gland

Pacinian corpuscle

Figure 2.7 Joint receptors.

there is too much stress placed on that joint.[17,18,25-27] Examples would include Ruffini endings and Pacinian corpuscles.

SUMMARY

The movement system of the human body is called the kinetic chain. The three components of the kinetic chain are the nervous system, the skeletal system, and the muscular system.

The nervous system is composed of billions of neurons that transfer information throughout the body, through two interdependent systems: the central nervous system (brain and spinal cord) and the peripheral nervous system (nerves that branch out from the brain and spinal cord). The system gathers information about our external and internal environments, processes that information, and then responds to it. It has three major functions, which are sensory (recognizes changes), integrative (combines information and interprets it), and motor (produces a neuromuscular response).

The Skeletal System

OVERVIEW OF THE SKELETAL SYSTEM

Skeletal system: The body's framework, composed of bones and joints.

Bones: Provide a resting ground for muscles and protection of vital organs.

Joints: The movable junction where two or more bones meet.

The **skeletal system** is the framework for our structure and movement (Figure 2-8). It helps to determine our stature, as the positioning of our bones will determine our size and shape.[9,28,29] Therefore, it is very important to understand that the growth, maturation, and functionality of the skeletal system are greatly affected by our posture, activity (or lack thereof), and nutrition.[28]

Further, this structure is the resting ground for the muscles of our body. **Bones** form junctions that are connected by muscles and connective tissue. These junctions are known as **joints**.[30] Joints are the sites where movement occurs as a result of muscle contraction.[30,31]

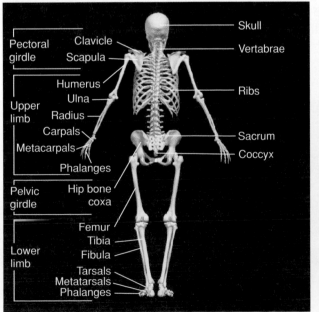
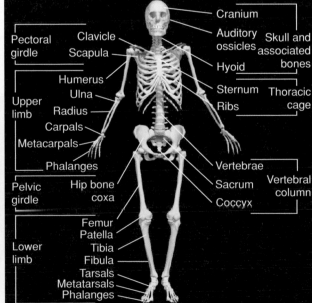

A   B

Figure 2.8 The skeletal system.

DIVISIONS OF THE SKELETAL SYSTEM

The skeletal system is divided into two divisions: the axial and appendicular skeletal systems.[9,30] The **axial skeleton** is made up of the skull, the rib cage, and the vertebral column. In all, there are approximately 80 bones in the axial skeleton.[9] The **appendicular skeleton** is made up of the upper and lower extremities as well as the shoulder and pelvic girdles.[9] (Some authors, however, note that the pelvic girdle could be considered a component of either the axial or appendicular system and that it is actually a link between the two systems.[30]) The appendicular skeleton encompasses approximately 126 bones.

There are roughly 206 bones in the skeletal system with approximately 177 of these being used in voluntary movement.[9,29,30] In all, the bones in the body form more than 300 joints.[29]

With regard to movement, the bones (skeleton) provide two main functions. The first is leverage. The bones act and perform as levers when acted on by muscles.[28,30] The second primary function of bones (skeleton) relative to movement is to provide support.[28] This translates into posture, which is necessary for the efficient distribution of forces acting on the body.[28,31–34]

Bone Markings

The majority of all bones have specific distinguishing structures known as surface markings.[9] These structures are necessary for increasing the stability in joints as well as providing attachment sites for muscles.[9] Some of the more prominent and important ones will be discussed here. These surface markings can be divided into two simple categories: depressions and processes.[9]

DEPRESSIONS

Depressions are simply flattened or indented portions of the bone.[9] One common depression is called a fossa. An example is the supraspinous or infraspinous fossa located on the scapulae (Figure 2-9). These are attachment sites for the supraspinatus and infraspinatus muscles, respectively.[9]

Another form of a depression is known as a sulcus. This is simply a groove in a bone that allows soft tissue (i.e., tendon) to pass through.[9] An example of this is the intertubercular sulcus located between the greater and lesser tubercles of the humerus (Figure 2-10).[9] This is commonly known as the groove for the biceps tendon.

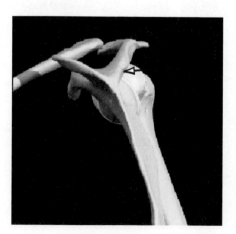

Figure 2.9   Fossa.

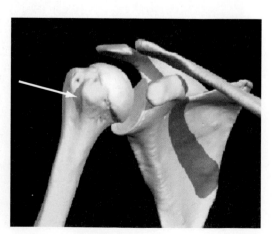

Figure 2.10   Sulcus.

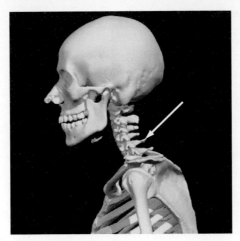

Figure 2.11   Process.

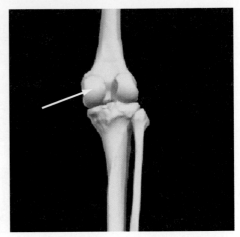

Figure 2.12   Condyle.

PROCESSES

Processes are projections protruding from the bone to which muscles, tendons, and ligaments can attach.[9] Some of the more common processes are called process, condyle, epicondyle, tubercle, and trochanter.[9] Examples of a process include the spinous processes found on the vertebrae and acromion and coracoid process found on the scapula (Figure 2-11).

Condyles are located on the inner and outer portion at the bottom of the femur and top of the tibia to form the knee joint (Figure 2-12).

Epicondyles are located on the inner and outer portion of the humerus to help form the elbow joint (Figure 2-13).

The tubercles are located at the top of the humerus at the glenohumeral joint (Figure 2-14). There are the greater and lesser tubercles, which are attachment sites for shoulder musculature.

Finally, the trochanters are located at the top of the femur and are attachment sites for the hip musculature (Figure 2-15).[9] The greater trochanter is commonly called the hipbone.

Joints

Joints are formed by one bone that articulates with another bone.[9] Joints can be categorized by both their structure and their function (or the way they move).[9,29,31]

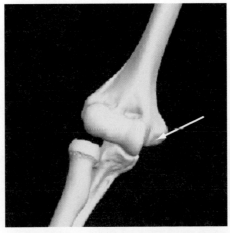

Figure 2.13   Epicondyle.

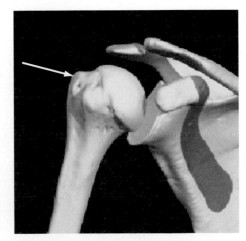

Figure 2.14   Tubercle.

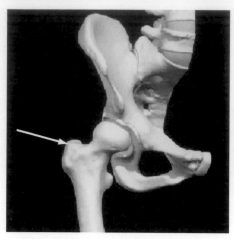

Figure 2.15 Trochanter.

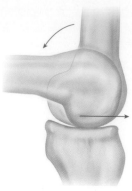

Figure 2.16 Rolling.

Arthrokinematics: Joint motion.

Joint motion is referred to as **arthrokinematics**, with the three major motion types being roll, slide, and spin.[7,31,35] It must be noted that these motions rarely occur, if ever, as an isolated, true motion. As is typically the case with the human body, variations and combinations of these joint motions take place during functional movement.[35]

In a roll movement, one joint rolls across the surface of another much like the tire of a bicycle rolls on the street (Figure 2-16). An example of roll in the body is the femoral condyles moving (rolling) over the tibial condyles during a squat.

In a slide movement, one joint's surface slides across another much like the tire of a bicycle skidding across the street (Figure 2-17). An example of slide in the human body is the tibial condyles moving (sliding) across the femoral condyles during a knee extension.

In a spin movement, one joint surface rotates on another much like twisting the lid off of a jar (Figure 2-18). An example of spin in the human body is the head of the radius rotating on the end of the humerus during pronation and supination of the forearm.

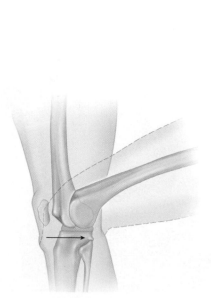

Figure 2.17 Slide.

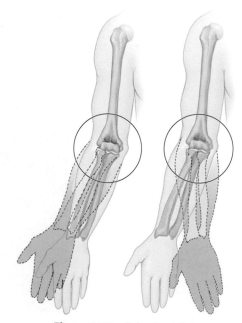

Figure 2.18 Spinning joint.

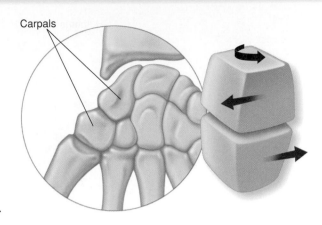

Figure 2.19   Gliding joint.

CLASSIFICATION OF JOINTS

Synovial joints are the joints most associated with movement in the body. They comprise approximately 80% of the joints in the body and have the greatest capacity for motion.[9,28,29,31] The synovial joint is characterized by the absence of fibrous or cartilaginous tissue directly connecting the bones. Rather, they are loosely held together by a joint capsule and ligaments.[9,28,29,31] This gives synovial joints their increased mobility.[31] Synovial joints also have another unique quality in that they produce synovial fluid. Synovial fluid resembles egg whites and works much like engine oil. It is secreted within the joint capsule from the synovial membrane.[9,29,31] Synovial fluid is essential for lubrication of the joint surfaces to reduce excessive wear and to nourish the cartilage cells that line the joint.[9,28,29,31]

There are several types of synovial joints in the body. They include gliding (plane), condyloid (condylar or ellipsoidal), hinge, saddle, pivot, and ball-and-socket.[9,28,29]

A gliding (plane) joint is a nonaxial joint that has the simplest movement of all joints.[9,28] It moves either back and forth or side to side. An example is the joint between the navicular bone and the second and third cuneiform bones in the foot or the carpals of the hand and in the facet joints (Figure 2-19).[9,28,29]

Condyloid (condylar or ellipsoidal) joints are termed so because the condyle of one bone fits into the elliptical cavity of another bone to form the joint.[9] Movement predominantly occurs in one plane (flexion and extension in the sagittal plane) with minimal movement in the others (rotation in the transverse plane; adduction and abduction in the frontal plane). These joints are seen in the wrist between the radius and carpals and in the knee joint (Figure 2-20).[28]

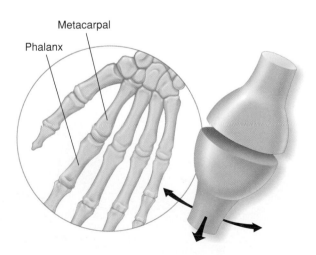

Figure 2.20   Condyloid joint.

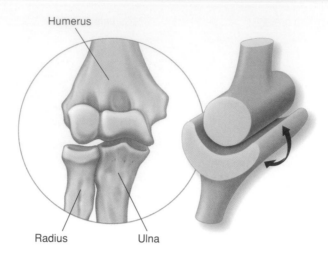

Humerus

Radius   Ulna

Figure 2.21 Hinge joint.

The hinge joint is a uniaxial joint allowing movement predominantly in only one plane of motion, the sagittal plane. Joints such as the elbow, interphalangeal, and ankle are considered hinge joints (Figure 2-21).[9,28]

The saddle joint is named after its appearance. One bone looks like a saddle with the articulating bone straddling it like a rider. This joint is only found in the carpometacarpal joint in the thumb.[9,28] It allows movement predominantly in two planes of motion (flexion and extension in the sagittal plane; adduction and abduction in the frontal plane) with some rotation to produce circumduction (Figure 2-22).[9,28]

Pivot joints allow movement in predominantly one plane of motion (rotation, pronation, and supination in the transverse plane). These joints are found in the atlantoaxial joint at the base of the skull (top of spine) and between the radioulnar joint (Figure 2-23).[9,28]

Ball-and-socket joints are the most mobile of the joints. They allow movement in all three planes. Examples of these joints are the shoulder and hip (Figure 2-24).[9,28]

Nonsynovial joints are named as such because they have no joint cavity, fibrous connective tissue, or cartilage in the uniting structure. They can be structured in either a fibrous or cartilaginous manner. These joints exhibit little to no movement. Examples of this joint type are seen in the sutures of the skull, the distal joint of the tibia and fibula (ankle), and the symphysis pubis (Figure 2-25).[9,31]

Nonsynovial joints: Joints that do not have a joint cavity, connective tissue, or cartilage.

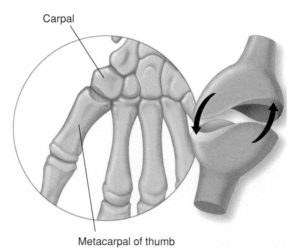

Carpal

Metacarpal of thumb

Figure 2.22 Saddle joint.

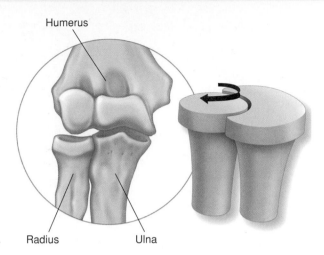

Figure 2.23 Pivot joint.

See Table 2-1 for a full description of the characteristics of these types of joints and examples of each.

Function of Joints

First and foremost, joints provide the bones a means to be manipulated, allowing for movement throughout segments of the body.[30,31] Joints also provide stability, allowing for movement to take place without unwanted movement.

All joints in the human body are linked together. This implies that movement of one joint directly affects the motion of others.[7,31] This is an essential concept for a health and fitness professional to understand because it creates an awareness of how the body functionally operates and is the premise behind kinetic chain movement.[7,31]

This concept is very easy to demonstrate. First, start by standing with both feet firmly on the ground. Next, roll your feet inward and outward. Notice what your knee and hips are doing. Keep your feet stationary and rotate your hips. Notice what your knees and feet are doing. Moving one of these joints will inevitably move the others. If you understand this concept, then you are well on your way to understanding true kinetic chain movement. Moreover, it should be easy to see that if one joint is not working properly, it will affect the other joints it works with.[7]

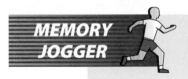

This is an extremely important concept to understand when performing movement assessments, designing programs, and monitoring exercise technique, all of which will be covered in later chapters.

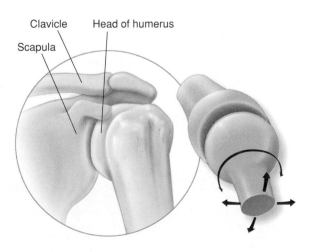

Figure 2.24 Ball-and-socket joint.

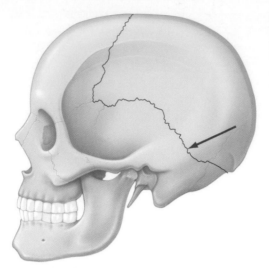

Figure 2.25   Nonsynovial joint.

Figure 2.26   Ligament.

JOINT CONNECTIVE TISSUE

Ligament: Primary connective tissue that connects bones together and provides stability, input to the nervous system, guidance, and the limitation of improper joint movement.

The primary connective tissue for a joint is the **ligament**. Ligaments connect bone to bone and provide static and dynamic stability as well as input to the nervous system (proprioception; Figure 2-26).[36,37] Ligaments are primarily made up of a protein called collagen with varying amounts of a second protein called elastin. Collagen fibers are situated in a more parallel fashion to the forces that are typically placed on the ligament. Thus, they provide the ligament with the ability to withstand tension (tensile strength). Elastin gives a ligament some

Table 2.1

Types of Joints

Joint	Characteristic	Example
Nonsynovial	No joint cavity and fibrous connective tissue; little or no movement	Sutures of the skull
Synovial	Produces synovial fluid, has a joint cavity and fibrous connective tissue	Knee
Gliding (Figure 2-19)	No axis of rotation; moves by sliding side-to-side or back and forth	Carpals of the hand
Condyloid (Figure 2-20)	Formed by the fitting of condyles of one bone into elliptical cavities of another; moves predominantly in one plane	Knee
Hinge (Figure 2-21)	Uniaxial; moves predominantly in one plane of motion (sagittal)	Elbow
Saddle (Figure 2-22)	One bone fits like a saddle on another bone; moves predominantly in two planes (sagittal, frontal)	Only: carpometacarpal joint of thumb
Pivot (Figure 2-23)	Only one axis; moves predominantly in one plane of motion (transverse)	Radioulnar
Ball-and-socket (Figure 2-24)	Most mobile of joints; moves in all three planes of motion	Shoulder

flexibility or elastic recoil to withstand the bending and twisting it may have to endure. Not all ligaments will have the same amount of elastin. For example, the anterior cruciate ligament of the knee contains a very low amount of elastin and is predominantly composed of collagen. Because of this, it is much better suited for resisting strong forces and makes a good stabilizing structure of the knee.[36,37]

Each synovial joint has a joint capsule that is much like a compartment for fluid and tissues that surround the joint. Much of the tissue of the joint capsule is also ligamentous in nature.

Finally, it is important to note that ligaments are characterized by poor vascularity (or blood supply), meaning that ligaments do not heal or repair very well and may be slower to adapt.[36–39]

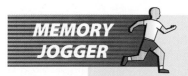

MEMORY JOGGER   The repairing capabilities of ligaments will be important to remember when considering the number of days' rest taken and the structure of your daily exercise programming plan when performing high-intensity exercise. This will be discussed in Chapter 13, Program Design.

SUMMARY

The skeletal system is the body's framework and is made up of bones and joints in two divisions: axial and appendicular. The four main types of bones are long, short, flat, and irregular, which all have markings of depressions or processes. Bones are connected (via ligaments) by either synovial or nonsynovial joints, which both provide movement as well as stability. Joints are interconnected, and movement of one will affect the others.

The Muscular System

OVERVIEW OF THE MUSCULAR SYSTEM

The nervous system is the control center for movement production, and the skeletal system provides the structural framework for our bodies. However, to complete the cycle of movement production, the body must have a device that the nervous system can command to move the skeletal system. This is the **muscular system** (Figure 2-27). Muscles generate internal tension that, under the control of the nervous

Muscular system: Series of muscles that moves the skeleton.

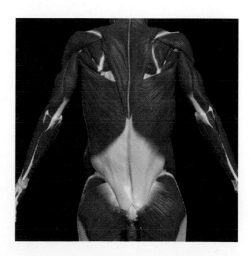

Figure 2.27   Muscular system.

system, manipulates the bones of our body to produce movements. Muscles are the movers and stabilizers of our bodies.

THE STRUCTURE OF SKELETAL MUSCLE

The structure of skeletal muscle is an important piece of this complex system. It provides the health and fitness professional with a foundation of knowledge that will help to illuminate the function of the muscular system as well as the kinetic chain. The following section will discuss the structure of muscle tissue and its connective tissues as well as the microscopic view of the muscle fiber and its contractile elements.

Muscle and Its Connective Tissue

Skeletal muscle is the compilation of many individual muscle fibers that are neatly wrapped together with connective tissue that forms different bundles, much like a cable is made up of bundles of wires encased in an outer covering (Figure 2-28).[30] Breaking the bundles down into layers from outer to innermost, the first bundle is the actual muscle itself wrapped by an outer layer of connective tissue called fascia and an inner layer immediately surrounding the muscle called the epimysium. The fascia and epimysium are also intimately connected with the bone and help to form the muscle's tendon.[8–10,13,15,28–31,36,40] The next bundle of muscle fiber is called a fascicle. Each fascicle is wrapped by connective tissue called perimysium. Each fascicle is in turn made up of many individual muscle fibers that are wrapped by connective tissue called endomysium (Figure 2-28).[8–10,13,15,28–31,36,40]

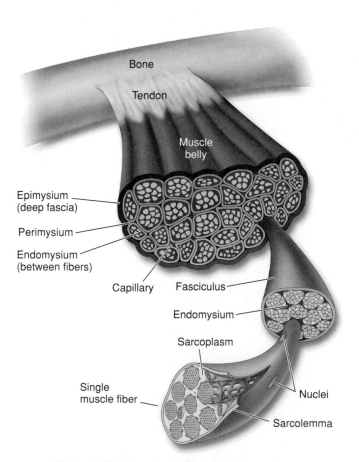

Figure 2.28 Structure of the skeletal muscle.

The connective tissues within the muscle play a vital role in movement. They allow the forces generated by the muscle to be transmitted from the contractile components of the muscle (discussed next) to the bones, creating motion. Each layer of connective tissue extends the length of the muscle, helping to form the tendon.

Tendons are the structures that attach muscles to bone and provide the anchor from which the muscle can exert force and control the bone and joint.[8-10,13,15,28-31,36,40] They are very similar to ligaments in that they have poor vascularity (blood supply), which leaves them susceptible to slower repair and adaptation.[38,31]

Tendons: Connective tissues that attach muscle to bone and provide an anchor for muscles to produce force.

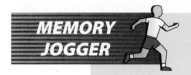

MEMORY JOGGER

As with ligaments, the tendon's poor vascularity will be important to remember when considering the number of days' rest taken and the structure of your daily exercise programming plan when performing high-intensity exercise to ensure one does not develop overuse injuries.

Muscle Fibers and Their Contractile Elements

Muscle fibers are encased by a plasma membrane known as the sarcolemma and contain typical cell components like cellular plasma called sarcoplasm (which contains glycogen, fats, minerals, and oxygen-binding myoglobin), nuclei, and mitochondria (which transform energy from food into energy for the cell). However, unlike typical cells they also have structures called myofibrils. Myofibrils contain myofilaments that are the actual contractile components of muscle tissue. These myofilaments are known as actin (thin stringlike filaments) and myosin (thick filaments).

The actin (thin) and myosin (thick) filaments form a number of repeating sections within a myofibril. Each one of these particular sections is known as a **sarcomere** (Figure 2-29). A sarcomere is the functional unit of the muscle, much like the neuron is for the nervous system. It lies in the space between two Z lines. Each Z line denotes another sarcomere along the myofibril.[8-10,13,15,28-31,36,40]

Two protein structures that are also important to muscle contraction are tropomyosin and troponin. Tropomyosin is located on the actin filament and blocks myosin binding sites located on the actin filament, keeping myosin from attaching to actin while the muscle is in a relaxed state. Troponin, also located on the actin

Sarcomere: The functional unit of muscle that produces muscular contraction and consists of repeating sections of actin and myosin.

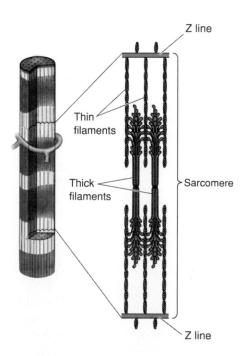

Figure 2.29   Sarcomere.

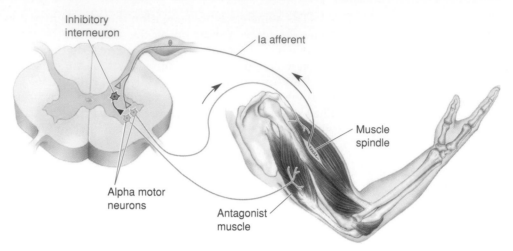

Figure 2.30 Neural activation.

filament, plays a role in muscle contraction by providing binding sites for both calcium and tropomyosin when a muscle needs to contract. (For further information, see the excitation-contraction coupling section of this chapter.)

Generating Force in a Muscle

Muscles generate force through a variety of methods. These methods, which include neural activation, the sliding filament theory, and excitation-contraction-coupling mechanism, will be reviewed. Muscle fiber types, recruitment and firing rate, will also be discussed as they relate to force production.

NEURAL ACTIVATION

Neural activation: The contraction of a muscle generated by neural stimulation.

Motor unit: A motor neuron and all of the muscle fibers it innervates.

Neurotransmitter: Chemical messengers that cross synapses to transmit electrical impulses from the nerve to the muscle.

Neural activation is essential for a muscle to contract, for movement and stabilization. This activation is generated by the communication between the nervous system and the muscular system. The motor neurons of the body are connected to the muscle fibers. A motor neuron and the muscle fibers with which it connects (innervates) is known as a **motor unit**. The point at which the neuron meets an individual muscle fiber is called the neuromuscular junction (nerve to muscle). This junction is actually a small gap between the nerve and muscle fiber often called a synapse (Figure 2-30).

Electrical impulses (also known as action potentials) are transported from the central nervous system down the axon of the neuron. When the impulse reaches the end of the axon (axon terminal), chemicals called **neurotransmitters** are released.

Neurotransmitters are chemical messengers that cross the synapse between the neuron and muscle fiber, transporting the electrical impulse from the nerve to the muscle (much like a boat carries people from one side of a river to the other). The neurotransmitters fall into receptor sites on the muscle fiber, specifically designed for their attachment, much like a square peg fits into a square hole. The neurotransmitter used by the neuromuscular system is termed acetylcholine (ACh). Once attached, ACh stimulates the muscle fibers to go through a series of steps that produce muscle contractions.[8–10,13,15,28–31,36,40]

SLIDING FILAMENT THEORY

The sliding filament theory is the proposed process of how the contraction of the filaments within the sarcomere takes place, after a muscle has been given the order to contract via neural activation (Table 2-2; Figure 2-31).

Table 2.2

Sliding Filament Theory

Steps in the sliding filament theory are summarized as follows:[8,10,13,40]

1. A sarcomere shortens as a result of the Z lines moving closer together.
2. The Z lines converge as the result of myosin heads attaching to the actin filament and asynchronously pulling (power strokes) the actin filament across the myosin, resulting in shortening of the muscle fiber.

EXCITATION-CONTRACTION COUPLING: PUTTING IT ALL TOGETHER

Excitation-contraction coupling is the process of neural stimulation creating a muscle contraction. It involves a series of steps that start with the initiation of a neural message (neural activation) and end up with a muscle contraction (sliding filament theory; Figure 2-32).

Muscle Fiber Types

Muscle fiber types vary in their chemical and mechanical properties. Essentially they have been delineated into two main categories, type I and type II fibers (Table 2-3).[8–10,13,15,28–31,36,40]

Type I (slow twitch) muscle fibers contain a higher number of capillaries, mitochondria (which transform energy from food into ATP, or cellular energy), and myoglobin, which allows for improved delivery of oxygen. Myoglobin is similar to hemoglobin, the red pigment found in red blood cells, and therefore type I muscle fibers are often referred to as *red fibers*.[8,10,13,40]

Type II (fast twitch) muscle fibers are subdivided into type IIa and type IIb based again on their chemical and mechanical properties. They generally contain fewer capillaries, mitochondria, and myoglobin. Type II muscle fibers are often referred to as white fibers. Type IIb muscle fibers have a low oxidative capacity (ability to use oxygen) and fatigue quickly. Type IIa muscle fibers have a higher oxidative capacity and fatigue more slowly than type IIb.[8,10,13,15,40]

Looking at the whole picture, slow twitch type I muscle fibers are smaller in size (diameter), slower to produce maximal tension, and more resistant to fatigue.[42–45] These fibers are important for muscles producing long-term contractions necessary for stabilization and postural control. An example would include sitting upright, while maintaining ideal posture against gravity, for an extended period of time.

Fast twitch type II muscle fibers are larger in size, quick to produce maximal tension, and fatigue more quickly than type I fibers. These fibers are important for muscles producing movements requiring force and power such as performing a sprint.

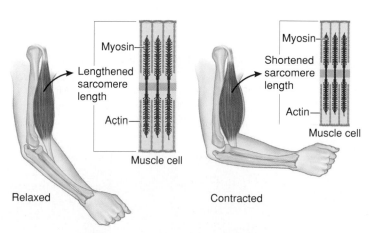

Figure 2.31 Sliding filament theory.

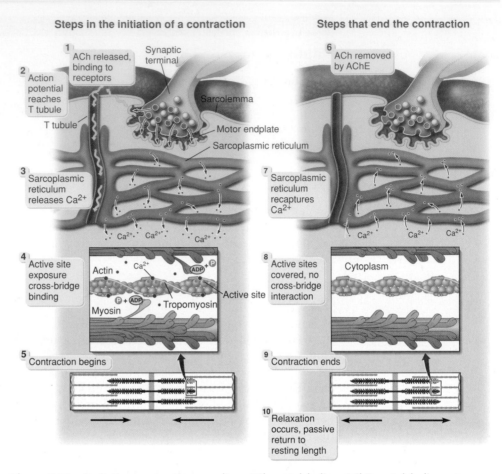

Figure 2.32 Excitation-contraction coupling. *ACh,* acetylcholine; *AChE,* acetylcholine esterase.

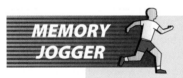

When designing a program, it becomes very important for the health and fitness professional to incorporate specific training parameters to fulfill specific muscular requirements (stabilization, strength, and power). This is demonstrated in the OPT™ model and discussed in Chapter 13.

Table 2.3

Muscle Fiber Types

Type	Characteristic
Type I *(Slow twitch)*	More capillaries, mitochondria, and myoglobin Increased oxygen delivery Smaller in size Less force produced Slow to fatigue Long-term contractions (stabilization) Slow twitch
Type II *(Fast twitch)*	Fewer capillaries, mitochondria, and myoglobin Decreased oxygen delivery Larger in size More force produced Quick to fatigue Short-term contractions (force and power) Fast twitch

Table 2.4

Muscles as Movers

Muscle Type	Muscle Function	Exercise	Muscle(s) Used
Agonist	Prime mover	Chest press Overhead press Row Squat	Pectoralis major Deltoid Latissimus dorsi Gluteus maximus, quadriceps
Synergist	Assist prime mover	Chest press Overhead press Row Squat	Anterior deltoid, triceps Triceps Posterior deltoid, biceps Hamstrings

Stabilizer	Stabilize while prime
	  mover and synergist
	  work
		Chest press
		Overhead press
		Row
		Squat
			Rotator cuff
			Rotator cuff
			Rotator cuff
			Transversus abdominis

Antagonist	Oppose prime mover	Chest press Overhead press Row Squat	Posterior deltoid Latissimus dorsi Pectoralis major Psoas

It is important to note that all muscles have a combination of slow and fast twitch fibers that will vary depending on the function of the muscle.[8,10,13,15,40] For example, it has been shown that the human anterior tibialis muscle (muscle on the shin) has approximately 73% slow twitch type I muscle fibers whereas the lateral head of the gastrocnemius (superficial calf muscle) has approximately 49% slow twitch type I muscle fibers.[46,47]

Muscles as Movers

Muscles provide the human body with a variety of functions that allow for the manipulation of forces placed on the body and to produce and slow down movement. These muscle functions categorize the muscle as an agonist, synergist, stabilizer, or antagonist (Table 2-4).[7,28]

Agonist muscles are muscles that act as prime movers, or, in other words, they are the muscles most responsible for a particular movement. For example, the gluteus maximus is an agonist for hip extension.

Synergist muscles assist prime movers during movement. For example, the hamstring and the erector spinae are synergistic with the gluteus maximus during hip extension.

Stabilizer muscles support or stabilize the body while the prime movers and the synergists perform the movement patterns. For example, the transversus abdominis, internal oblique, and multifidus (deep muscles in the low back) stabilize the low back, pelvis, and hips (lumbo-pelvic-hip complex) during hip extension.

Antagonist muscles perform the opposite action of the prime mover. For example, the psoas (a deep hip flexor) is antagonistic to the gluteus maximus during hip extension.

Please refer to Chapter 4, Human Movement Science, for a more detailed description of all major muscles of the muscular system.

SUMMARY

The muscular system is made up of many individual fibers and attaches to bones by way of tendons. There are different muscle fiber types and arrangements of them that affect how they move. Muscles generate force, through neural activation, sliding filament theory, and excitation-contraction coupling.

The nervous system receives and delivers information throughout the body, by way of neurons. The stimulation of the nervous system activates sarcomeres, which generates tension in the muscles. This tension is transferred through tendons to the bones, and this produces motion.

Review Questions

1 *Match up the mechanoreceptors to their functions:*

a. Muscle spindles   i. *Sense tension and rate of tension developed and cause relaxation.*

b. Golgi tendon organs   ii. *Sense pressure, acceleration, and deceleration at a joint.*

c. Joint receptors   iii. *Sense length and rate of length change, causing contraction.*

2 *Match the synovial joint with an example.*

a. Gliding joint   i. *Carpals of the hand*

b. Hinge joint   ii. *Shoulder*

c. Saddle joint   iii. *Elbow*

d. Ball-and-socket joint   iv. *Carpometacarpal joint of thumb*

3 *Match up the muscle with its appropriate action during hip extension.*

a. Gluteus maximus   i. *Synergist*

b. Hamstrings   ii. *Stabilizer*

c. Transversus abdominis   iii. *Antagonist*

d. Psoas   iv. *Agonist*

4 *Which kind of muscle fibers are "fast twitch"?*

a. Type I

b. Type II

5 *All movement is directly dictated by the nervous system.*

a. True

b. False

REFERENCES

1. Cohen H. Neuroscience for Rehabilitation, 2nd ed. Philadelphia: Lippincott Williams & Wilkins, 1999.
2. Panjabi MM. The stabilizing system of the spine. Part 1. Function, dysfunction, adaptation, and enhancement. J Spinal Disord 1992;5:383–389.
3. Liebenson CL. Active muscle relaxation techniques. Part II. Clinical application. J Manipulative Physiol Ther 1990;13(1):2–6.

4. Edgerton VR, Wolf S, Roy RR. Theoretical basis for patterning EMG amplitudes to assess muscle dysfunction. Med Sci Sports Exerc 1996;28(6):744–751.
5. Liebenson C. Active rehabilitation protocols. In: Liebenson C (ed). Rehabilitation of the Spine. Baltimore: Williams & Wilkins, 1996.
6. Chaitow L. Muscle Energy Techniques. New York: Churchill Livingstone, 1997.
7. Clark MA. Integrated Training for the New Millennium. Thousand Oaks, CA: National Academy of Sports Medicine, 2001.
8. Milner-Brown A. Neuromuscular Physiology. Thousand Oaks, CA: National Academy of Sports Medicine, 2001.
9. Tortora GJ. Principles of Human Anatomy, 7th ed. New York: Harper Collins College Publishers, 1995.
10. Fox SI. Human Physiology, 5th ed. Dubuque, IA: Wm C. Brown Publishers, 1996.
11. Brooks GA, Fahey TD, White TP. Exercise Physiology: Human Bioenergetics and Its Application, 2nd ed. Moutain View, CA: Mayfield Publishing Company, 1996.
12. Drury DG. Strength and proprioception. Ortho Phys Ther Clin 2000;9(4):549–561.
13. Vander A, Sherman J, Luciano D. Human Physiology: The Mechanisms of Body Function, 8th ed. New York: McGraw-Hill, 2001.
14. Biedert RM. Contribution of the three levels of nervous system motor control: spinal cord, lower brain, cerebral cortex. In: Lephart SM, Fu FH (eds.) Proprioception and Neuromuscular Control in Joint Stability. Champaign, IL: Human Kinetics, 2000.
15. Enoka RM. Neuromechanical Basis of Kinesiology, 2nd ed. Champaign, IL: Human Kinetics, 1994.
16. Rose DJ. A Multi Level Approach to the Study of Motor Control and Learning. Needham Heights, MA: Allyn & Bacon, 1997.
17. Barrack RL, Lund PJ, Skinner HB. Knee proprioception revisited. J Sport Rehab 1994;3:18–42.
18. Grigg P. Peripheral neural mechanisms in proprioception. J Sport Rehab 1994;3:2–17.
19. Wilkerson GB, Nitz AJ. Dynamic ankle stability: mechanical and neuromuscular interrelationships. J Sport Rehab 1994;3:43–57.
20. Boyd IA. The histological structure of the receptors in the knee joint of the cat correlated with their physiological response. J Physiol (Lond) 1954;124:476–488.
21. Edin B. Quantitative analysis of static strain sensitivity in human mechanoreceptors from hairy skin. J Neurophysiol 1992;67:1105–1113.
22. Edin B, Abbs JH. Finger movement responses of cutaneous mechanoreceptors in the dorsal skin of the human hand. J Neurophysiol 1991;65:657–670.
23. Gandevia SC, McClosky DI, Burke D. Kinesthetic signals and muscle contraction. Trends Neurosci 1992;15:62–65.
24. McClosky DJ. Kinesthetic sensibility. Physiol Rev 1978;58:763–820.
25. Lephart SM, Rieman BL, Fu FH. Introduction to the sensorimotor system. In: Lephart SM, Fu FH (eds). Proprioception and Neuromuscular Control in Joint Stability. Champaign, IL: Human Kinetics, 2000.
26. Lephart SM, Pincivero D, Giraldo J, Fu F. The role of proprioception in the management and rehabilitation of athletic injuries. Am J Sports Med 1997;25:130–137.
27. Proske U, Schaible HG, Schmidt RF. Joint receptors and kinaesthesia. Exp Brain Res 1988;72:219–224.
28. Hamill J, Knutzen JM. Biomechanical Basis of Human Movement. Baltimore, MD: Williams & Wilkins, 1995.
29. Watkins J. Structure and Function of the Musculoskeletal System. Champaign, IL: Human Kinetics, 1999.
30. Luttgens K, Hamilton N. Kinesiology: Scientific Basis of Human Motion, 9th ed. Dubuque, IA: Brown & Benchmark Publishers, 1997.
31. Norkin CC, Levangie PK. Joint Structure and Function: A Comprehensive Analysis, 2nd ed. Philadelphia: FA Davis Company, 1992.
32. Chaffin DB, Andersson GJ, Martin BJ. Occupational Biomechanics. New York: Wiley-Interscience, 1999.
33. Whiting WC, Zernicke RF. Biomechanics of Musculoskeletal Injury. Champaign, IL: Human Kinetics, 1998.
34. Bogduk N. Clinical Anatomy of the Lumbar Spine and Sacrum, 3rd ed. New York: Churchill Livingstone, 1997.
35. Hertling D, Kessler RM. Management of Common Musculoskeletal Disorders. Philadelphia: Lippincott Williams & Wilkins, 1996.
36. Alter MJ. Science of Flexibility, 2nd ed. Champaign, IL: Human Kinetics, 1996.
37. Gross J, Fetto J, Rosen E. Musculoskeletal Examination. Malden, MA: Blackwell Sciences, 1996.
38. Nordin M, Lorenz T, Campello M. Biomechanics of tendons and ligaments. In: Nordin M, Frankel VH (eds). Basic Biomechanics of the Musculoskeletal System, 3rd ed. Philadelphia: Lippincott Williams & Wilkins, 2001.
39. Solomonow M, Baratta R, Zhou BH, Shoji H, Bose W, Beck C, D'Ambrosia R. The synergistic action of the anterior cruciate ligament and thigh muscles in maintaining joint stability. Am J Sports Med 1987;15:207–213.
40. McComas AJ. Skeletal Muscle: Form and Function. Champaign, IL: Human Kinetics, 1996.

41. Kannus P. Structure of the tendon connective tissue. Scand J Med Sci Sports 2000;10(6):312–320.
42. Al-Amood WS, Buller AJ, Pope R. Long-term stimulation of cat fast twitch skeletal muscle. Nature 1973;244:225–227.
43. Buller AJ, Eccles JC, Eccles RM. Interaction between motorneurons and muscles in respect of the characteristic speeds of their responses. J Physiol (Lond) 1960;150:139–417.
44. Dubowitz V. Cross-innervated mammalian skeletal muscle: histochemical, phyusiological and biomechanical observations. J Physiol (Lond) 1967;193:481–496.
45. Hennig R, Lomo T. Effects of chronic stimulation on the size and speed of long-term denervated and innervated rat fast and slow skeletal muscles. Acta Physiol Scand 1987;130:115–131.
46. Johnson MA, Polgar J, Weightman D, Appleton D. Data on the distribution of fiber types in thirty-six human muscles. J Neurol Sci 1973;18:111–129.
47. Green HJ, Daub B, Houston ME, Thomson JA, Fraser I, Ranney D. Human vastus lateralis and gastrocnemius muscles. A comparative histochemical analysis. J Neurol Sci 1981;52:200–201.

3

The Cardiorespiratory System

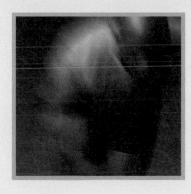

KEY TERMS

Adenosine triphosphate	Blood	Inspiration
Aerobic	Blood vessel	Mediastinum
Anaerobic	Capillaries	Respiratory system
Arteries	Cardiorespiratory system	Veins
Arterioles	Cardiovascular system	Ventricle
Atrium	Expiration	Venules
Bioenergetics	Heart	

INTRODUCTION TO THE CARDIORESPIRATORY SYSTEM

It has been established that the kinetic chain is the primary system for movement production, under the direct control of the nervous system. To maintain a constant state of efficient operation, however, it needs to have support systems. One such support system is known as the cardiorespiratory system. The **cardiorespiratory system** is composed of the cardiovascular and respiratory systems. Together they provide the tissues of the kinetic chain with oxygen (O_2), nutrients, protective agents, and a means to remove waste by-products.[1-5] This ensures optimal cellular function within the kinetic chain. This chapter will focus on the structure and function of the cardiovascular and respiratory systems.

Cardiorespiratory system: A system of the body composed of the cardiovascular and respiratory systems.

The Cardiovascular System

Cardiovascular system: A system of the body composed of the heart, blood, and blood vessels.

The **cardiovascular system** is composed of the heart, the blood it pumps, and the blood vessels that transport the blood from the heart to the tissues of the body (Figure 3-1). A basic understanding of the structure and function of the cardiovascular system is necessary to understand the kinetic chain.

THE HEART

Heart: A hollow muscular organ that pumps a circulation of blood through the body by means of rhythmic contraction.

The **heart** is a muscular pump that rhythmically contracts to push blood throughout the body. It is positioned obliquely in the center of the chest (or thoracic cavity), lying anteriorly to the spine and posteriorly to the sternum.[4] It is flanked laterally by the lungs.[4] This area is called the **mediastinum**.[6] The adult heart is approximately the size of a typical adult fist and weighs roughly 300 g (approximately 10 ounces).[4,6]

Mediastinum: The space in the chest between the lungs that contains all the internal organs of the chest, except the lungs.

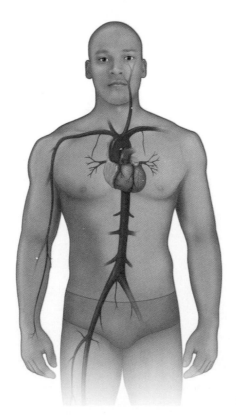

Figure 3.1   The cardiovascular system.

Heart muscle is termed cardiac muscle and has similar characteristics to skeletal muscle. It is made up of myofibrils containing actin and myosin that form crossbridges to cause contractions and is surrounded by a sarcolemma.[1-3,6] Cardiac muscle is for the most part considered an involuntary muscle, meaning that it cannot typically be consciously controlled.

Cardiac Muscle Contraction

Cardiac muscle fibers are shorter and more tightly connected than skeletal muscle, thus enabling the contraction of one fiber to stimulate the others to contract synchronously.[1-3] The conduction system (or means by which the muscle fibers are activated) is much different than in skeletal muscle. All cardiac muscle fibers have a built-in contraction rhythm, and the fibers with the highest rhythm determine the heartbeat or heart rate.[1-3] The typical discharge rate, and thus heart rate, is between 70 and 80 beats per minute.[3,4,6,7]

The specialized conduction system of cardiac muscle that provides the rhythm for heart rate includes several items (Figure 3-2).[1-4,6,7] The sinoatrial (SA) node, which is located in the right atrium, is termed the pacemaker for the heart because it initiates the heartbeat. Internodal pathways transfer the impulse from the SA node to the atrioventricular (AV) node. The AV node delays the impulse before moving on to the ventricles. The AV bundle passes the impulse to the ventricles for contraction via the left and right bundle branches of the Purkinje fibers.

Structure of the Heart

The heart is composed of four hollow chambers that are delineated into two interdependent (but separate) pumps on either side. These two pumps are separated by the interatrial septum (separates the atria) and interventricular septum (separates the ventricles).[4-6] Each side of the heart has two chambers: an atrium and a ventricle (Figure 3-3).[1-4,6,7]

The **atria** are smaller chambers, located superiorly on either side of the heart. They essentially gather blood coming to the heart, much like a reservoir. The right atrium gathers deoxygenated blood returning to the heart from the entire body, whereas the left atrium gathers reoxygenated blood coming to the heart from the lungs.

Atrium: The superior chamber of the heart that receives blood from the veins and forces it into the ventricles.

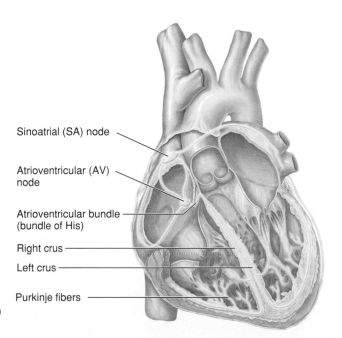

Sinoatrial (SA) node

Atrioventricular (AV) node

Atrioventricular bundle (bundle of His)

Right crus

Left crus

Purkinje fibers

Figure 3.2   Conduction system of the heart.

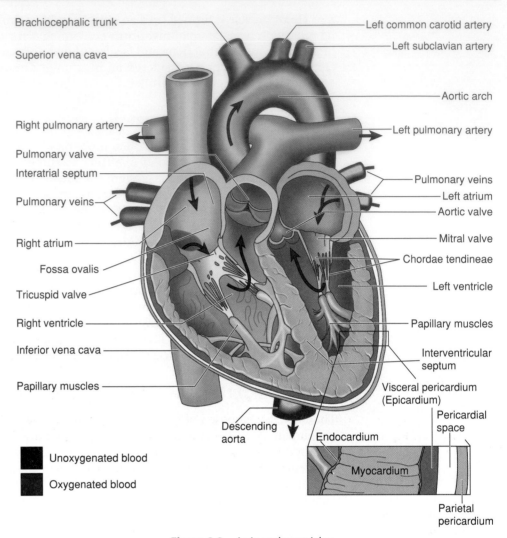

Figure 3.3   Atria and ventricles.

Ventricle: The inferior chamber of the heart that receives blood from its corresponding atrium and, in turn, forces blood into the arteries.

The **ventricles** are larger chambers located inferiorly on either side of the heart. They are the main pumps in the heart, as they pump blood out to the rest of the body. The right ventricle receives the deoxygenated blood from the right atrium and then pumps it to the lungs to be saturated with incoming oxygen. The left ventricle receives the reoxygenated blood from the left atrium and proceeds to pump it to the entire body.

Each chamber of the heart is separated from one another and major veins and arteries via valves to prevent a backflow or spillage of blood back into the chambers. These valves include the atrioventricular valves (tricuspid and mitral valves) and the semilunar valves (pulmonary and aortic valves).

Function of the Heart

As previously mentioned, the heart is a hollowed mass of muscle that encompasses two separate pumps (left and right ventricles), each of which distributes blood to specific parts of the body.[1-4,6,7]

Each contraction of a ventricle pushes blood from the heart into the body. The amount of blood that is pumped out with each contraction of a ventricle is the stroke volume (SV). The stroke volume of a typical adult is approximately 75 to 80 mL per beat.[1-3,5]

Table 3.1

Functions of the Heart

Terminology	Action	Average Measurement
Stroke volume	The amount of blood that is pumped out with each contraction of a ventricle	For a typical adult, approximately 75–80 mL/beat
Heart rate	The rate with which the heart pumps	For a typical adult, approximately 70–80 bpm
Cardiac output	The combination of how many times the heart beats per minute and how much blood is being pumped out with each beat	

The rate with which the heart pumps is referred to as the heart rate (HR). The heart rate of the typical person is approximately 70 to 80 beats per minute (bpm).[1-3,5]

Together, the heart rate and the stroke volume make up the overall performance of the heart and are collectively termed cardiac output (Q̇). Cardiac output is the combination of how many times the heart beats per minute and how much blood is being pumped out with each beat (Table 3-1).

Although it is next to impossible for a health and fitness professional to gauge the stroke volume of a client, it is relatively easy to determine the heart rate. Monitoring heart rate during exercise provides a good gauge as to the amount of work the heart is doing at any given time.[3,8] The proper procedure for manually monitoring the heart rate can be seen in Figure 3-4. Another procedure commonly used is the heart rate monitor, which is worn on the body and automatically derives the beats per minute.

BLOOD

Blood: Fluid that circulates in the heart, arteries, capillaries, and veins, which carries nutrients and oxygen to all parts of the body and also rids the body of waste products.

A properly functioning heart transports **blood** efficiently throughout the body. Blood acts as a medium to deliver and collect essential products to and from the tissues of the body.[1,2,5] Blood is thicker and heavier than water and constitutes approximately 8% of total body weight.[1,2,5] The average person holds about 5 L (roughly 1.5 gallons) of blood in his or her body at any given time.[1,2,5] Blood is a vital support mechanism, which provides an internal transportation, regulation, and protection system for the kinetic chain (Table 3-2).

Table 3.2

Support Mechanisms of Blood

Mechanism	Function
Transportation	Transports oxygen and nutrients to tissues Transports waste products from tissues Transports hormones to organs and tissues Carries heat throughout the body
Regulation	Regulates body temperature and acid balance in the body
Protection	Protects the body from excessive bleeding by clotting Contains specialized immune cells to help fight disease and sickness

How To Manually Monitor Heart Rate

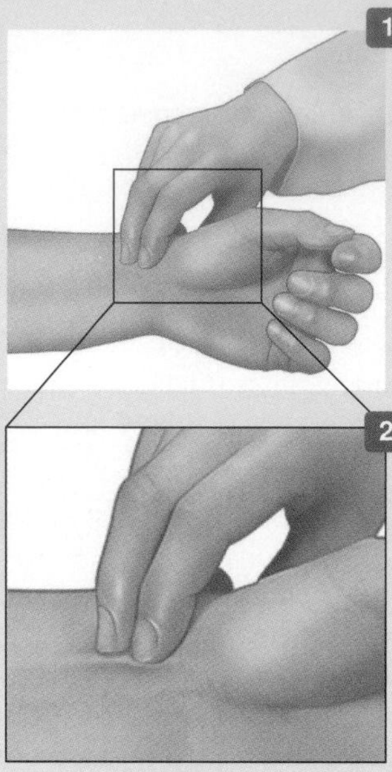

1 Place index and middle fingers around the palm side of the wrist (about one inch from the top of wrist, on the thumb side).

Although some people use the carotid artery in the neck, NASM does not recommend this location for measuring pulse rate. Pressure on this artery reduces blood flow to the brain, which can cause dizziness or an inaccurate measurement.

2 Locate the artery by feeling for a pulse with the index and middle fingers. Apply light pressure to feel the pulse. Do not apply excessive pressure as it may distort results.

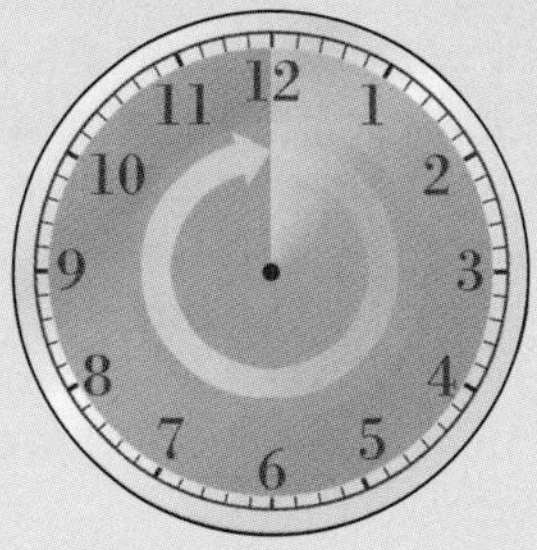

3 When measuring the pulse during rest, count the number of beats in 60 seconds.

There are some factors that may affect resting heart rate, including digestion, mental activity, environmental temperature, biological rhythms, body position, and cardiorespiratory fitness. Because of this, resting heart rate should be measured on waking (or at the very least, after you have had 5 minutes of complete rest).

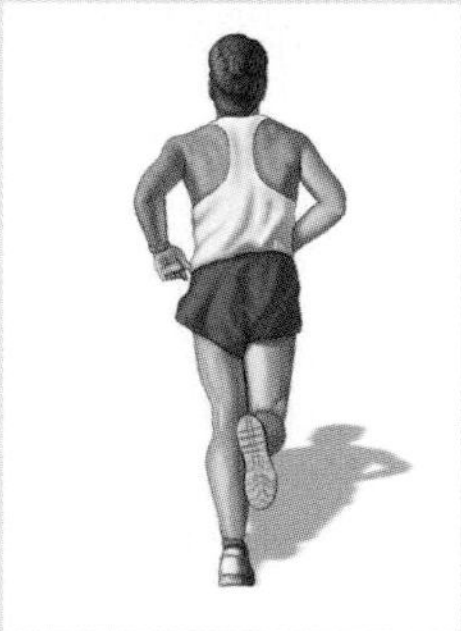

4 When measuring the pulse during exercise, count the number of beats in 6 seconds and add a zero to that number. Adding the zero will provide an estimate of the number of beats in 60 seconds. Or one can simply multiply the number by 10 and that will provide the health and fitness professional with the same number.

Example: Number of beats in 6 seconds = 17. Adding a zero = 170. This gives a pulse rate of 170 bpm or, 17 x 10 = 170

Figure 3.4   How to manually monitor heart rate.

Transportation

Blood transports life-giving oxygen to and collects waste products from all tissues. It also transports hormones that act as chemical messengers to various organs and tissues in the body. Nutrients from the gastrointestinal tract are delivered to specific tissues by way of the bloodstream as well. Blood also conducts heat throughout the body.[1,2,5]

Regulation

Blood provides a means to regulate body temperature, as a result of the properties of its water content and its path of flow. As blood travels close to the skin it can give off heat or can be cooled depending on the environment.[1-3,6] Blood is essential in the regulation of the pH levels (acid balance) in the body as well as water content of bodily cells.[6]

Protection

Blood provides protection from excessive blood loss through its clotting mechanism, which seals off damaged tissue.[1,2,5] It also provides specialized immune cells to fight against foreign toxins within the body, decreasing disease and sickness.[1-3,5] Ironically, however, by this same mechanism, blood can also spread diseases and sickness.[5]

BLOOD VESSELS

With each pump of each ventricle, blood is dispersed throughout the body. Concurrently, blood is also reentering the heart. To circulate blood properly throughout the body and back to the heart, it must have a network through which it can travel. This network is composed of **blood vessels**.[1,2,4-7]

Blood vessels form a closed circuit of hollow tubes that allow blood to be transported to and from the heart (Figure 3-5). Vessels that transport blood away from the heart are termed **arteries**. Vessels that transport blood back to the heart are termed **veins**.[1,2,4-7]

Blood vessels: Network of hollow tubes that circulates blood throughout the body.

Arteries: Vessels that carry blood away from the heart.

Veins: Vessels that carry blood from the capillaries toward the heart.

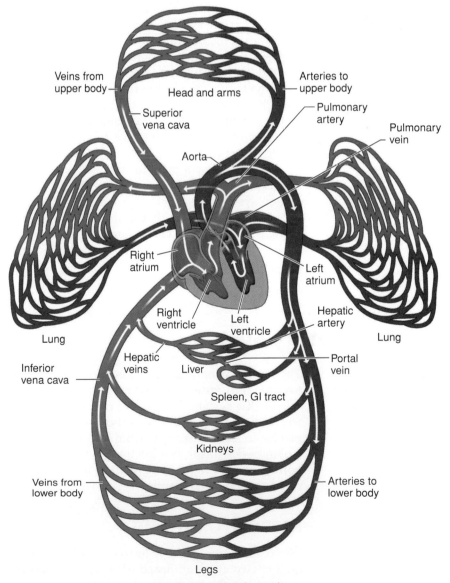

Figure 3.5 Blood vessels.

Arteries

Arteries leaving the heart are initially large and elastic.[4,6] These large arteries then branch out into medium-sized muscular arteries that extend to various areas throughout the body.[1,2,4-6] The medium-sized arteries further divide into smaller arteries that are called **arterioles**.[1,2,4-7] In turn, arterioles branch out into a multitude of microscopic vessels known as **capillaries**.[1,2,4-7] It is here in the capillaries that substances such as oxygen, nutrients, hormones, and waste products are exchanged between tissues.[1,2,4-7]

Arterioles: Small terminal branches of an artery, which end in capillaries.

Capillaries: The smallest blood vessels, which connect venules with arterioles.

Venules: The very small veins that connect capillaries to the larger veins.

Veins

Once substances are exchanged in the capillaries and waste products are gathered, they must then be transported to the proper area for cleaning and eventually back to the heart. The vessels that collect blood from the capillaries to perform this duty are called **venules**.[1,2,4-7] Venules progressively merge with other venules and form veins. Veins then transport all of the blood from the body back to the heart.[1,2,4-7]

SUMMARY

The cardiorespiratory system is composed of the cardiovascular system and the respiratory system. Together, they provide the body with oxygen, nutrients, protective agents, and a means to remove waste products.

The cardiovascular system is composed of the heart, blood, and blood vessels. The heart is located in the mediastinum and is made up of involuntary cardiac muscle, which contracts according to a built-in rhythm to regularly pump blood throughout the body. It is divided into four chambers: two atria (which gather blood from the body) and two ventricles (which pump blood out to the body) on each side.

The heart rate and the stroke volume make up the overall performance of the heart. Cardiac output is the combination of how many times the heart beats per minute and how much blood is being pumped out with each beat. Heart rate can be monitored manually.

Blood acts as a medium to deliver and collect essential products to and from the tissues of the body, providing an internal transportation, regulation, and protection system.

The blood vessels that transport blood away from the heart are called arteries (which have smaller components called arterioles). The vessels that bring blood back to the heart are called veins (which have smaller components called venules). Capillaries are the smallest blood vessels and connect venules with arterioles.

The Respiratory System

Respiratory system: A system of organs (the lungs and respiratory passageways) that collects oxygen from the external environment and transports it to the bloodstream.

The second functional component of the cardiorespiratory system is the **respiratory system**, often referred to as the pulmonary system (Figure 3-6). The primary role of this system is to ensure proper cellular function.[9,10] The respiratory system works intimately with the cardiovascular system to accomplish this by providing a means to collect oxygen from the environment and transport it to the bloodstream.[10] For this to be effectively accomplished, there must be an integrated functioning of the respiratory pump to move air in and out of the body and respiratory passageways to channel the air (Table 3-3).[10]

RESPIRATORY PUMP

The respiratory pump is located in the thorax or the thoracic (chest and abdominal) cavity. It is composed of skeletal structures (bones) and soft tissue (muscles

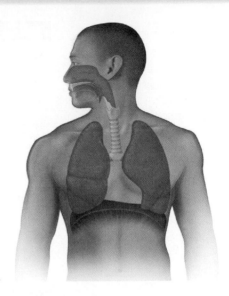

Figure 3.6   The respiratory system.

Inspiration: The process of actively contracting inspiratory muscles to move air into the body.

Expiration: The process of actively or passively relaxing inspiratory muscles to move air out of the body.

and pleural membranes). These systems, together with the nervous system, must work synergistically to allow for proper respiratory mechanics to occur much the same way as these systems work together to produce everyday functional movements. The skeletal structures provide the framework for the muscles to attach to as well as protection for the organs within the thorax (Table 3-3). Although they are strong enough to provide support, they are also flexible enough to allow for the expansion and compression needed for proper breathing.[1,2,5,6,10]

Breathing (or ventilation) is the actual process of moving air in and out of the body. It is divided into two phases: **inspiration** (or inhalation) and **expiration** (exhalation). Inspiratory ventilation is active. This means that it requires active contraction of inspiratory muscles to increase the thoracic cavity volume, which decreases the intrapulmonary pressure (or pressure within the thoracic cavity) (Table 3-3). When the intrapulmonary pressure decreases below that of the atmospheric pressure (or the everyday pressure in the air), air is drawn into the lungs.[1-3,10,11]

Inspiratory ventilation occurs in two forms: normal resting state (quiet) breathing and heavy (deep, forced) breathing. Normal breathing requires the use of the primary respiratory muscles (i.e., diaphragm, external intercostals) whereas heavy breathing requires the additional use of the secondary respiratory muscles. (scalenes, pectoralls minor)[1,2,5,6,10,12]

Table 3.3	
Structures of the Respiratory Pump	
Bones	Sternum Ribs Vertebrae
Muscles Inspiration	Diaphragm External intercostals Scalenes Sternocleidomastoid Pectoralis minor
Expiration	Internal intercostals Abdominals

Table 3.4	
Structures of the Respiratory Passageways	
Conduction	Nasal cavity Oral cavity Pharynx Larynx Trachea Right and left pulmonary bronchi Bronchioles
Respiratory	Alveoli Alveolar sacs

Expiratory ventilation can be both active and passive. During normal breathing, expiratory ventilation is passive as it results from the relaxation of the contracting inspiratory muscles. During heavy or forced breathing, the expiratory ventilation relies on the activity of expiratory muscles to compress the thoracic cavity and force air out.[1,2,5,6,10,13]

RESPIRATORY PASSAGEWAYS

The purpose of ventilation is to move air in and out of the body. However, the air must have passageways to funnel it in and out of the lungs for proper utilization. These respiratory passageways are divided into two categories, the conduction passageway and the respiratory passageway.

The conduction passageway consists of all the structures that air travels through before entering the respiratory passageway (Table 3-4). The nasal and oral cavities, mouth, pharynx, larynx, trachea, and bronchioles provide a gathering station for air and oxygen to be funneled into the body (Figure 3-7). These structures also allow the incoming air to be purified, humidified (or moisture added), and warmed or cooled to match body temperature.[1-3,5,7,9,10]

The respiratory passageway collects the channeled air coming from the conducting passageway.[1,2,5,6,9] At the end of the bronchioles sit the alveoli, which are made up of clusters of alveolar sacs (Figure 3-7).[1,2,5,6,9] It is here, in the alveolar sacs, that gases such as oxygen and carbon dioxide (CO_2) are transported in and out of the bloodstream through a process known as diffusion.[1-3,6,9] This is how oxygen gets from the outside environment to the tissues of the body.

SUMMARY

The respiratory system collects oxygen from the environment and transports it to the bloodstream. The respiratory pump moves air in and out of the body and respiratory passageways to channel the air.

Breathing is divided into the inspiratory phase (or inhalation) and expiratory phase (or exhalation). Inspiratory ventilation is active, whereas expiratory ventilation can be both active and passive (as during normal breathing, when it results from the relaxation of the contracting inspiratory muscles).

There are two respiratory passageways. The first is the conduction passageway, which consists of all the structures that air travels through before entering the respiratory passageway. These structures purify, humidify, and warm or cool air to match body temperature. The second passageway is the respiratory passageway, which collects the channeled air coming from the conduction passageway and allows gases such as oxygen and carbon dioxide to be transported in and out of the bloodstream.

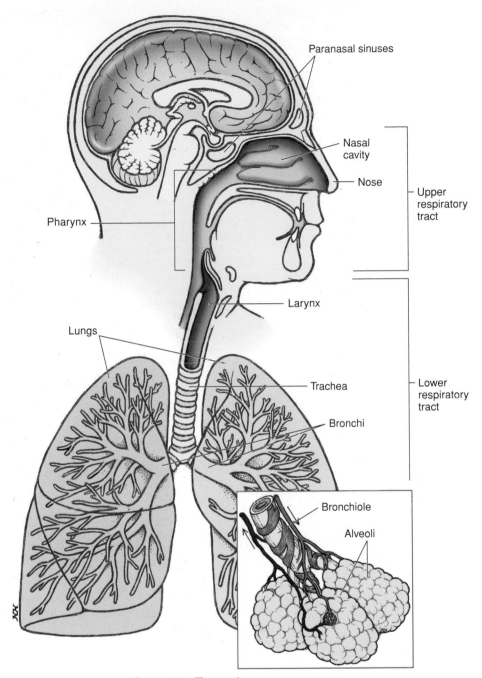

Figure 3.7 The respiratory passageways.

Cardiorespiratory System Function

Together, the cardiovascular and respiratory systems make up the cardiorespiratory system. They form a vital support system to provide the kinetic chain with many essential elements (such as oxygen), while removing waste products that can cause dysfunction in the body.

The primary element for proper body function is oxygen.[3] The respiratory system provides the means to gather oxygen from the environment and transfer it into our bodies. It is inhaled through the nose and mouth, and conducted through the trachea, and then down through the bronchi, where it eventually reaches the lungs

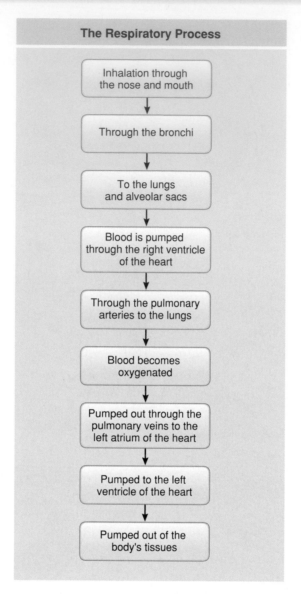

Figure 3.8   The respiratory process.

and alveolar sacs.[1–3,5,6,9] Deoxygenated blood is pumped from the right ventricle to the lungs through the pulmonary arteries. Pulmonary capillaries surround the alveolar sacs, and as oxygen fills the sacs it diffuses across the capillary membranes and into the blood.[3] The oxygenated blood then returns to the left atrium through the pulmonary veins where it is pumped into the left ventricle and out to the tissues of the body (Figure 3-8).

Concurrently, as the cells of the body are using oxygen, they produce an oxygen waste by-product known as carbon dioxide.[1–3,5,6,9] Carbon dioxide is transported from the tissues back to the heart and eventually to the lungs in the deoxygenated blood. In the alveolar sacs, it diffuses into the pulmonary capillaries and is released through exhalation.[1–3,5,6,9] In a simplistic overview, oxygen and carbon dioxide trade places in the tissues of the body, blood, and lungs. As one is coming in, the other is going out.

OXYGEN CONSUMPTION

The cardiovascular and respiratory systems work together to transport oxygen to the tissues of the body. Our capacity to efficiently use oxygen is dependent on the respiratory system's ability to collect oxygen and the cardiovascular system's ability to absorb and transport it to the tissues of the body.[14] The usage of oxygen by the body is known as oxygen uptake (or oxygen consumption).[1–3,5,6,9,10]

At rest, oxygen consumption ($\dot{V}O_2$) is estimated to be approximately 3.5 mL of oxygen per kilogram of bodyweight per minute (3.5 mL $\cdot$ kg^{-1} $\cdot$ min^{-1}), typically termed 1 metabolic equivalent or 1 MET.[3,5,7,10,14–16] It is calculated as:

$$\dot{V}O_2 = \dot{Q} \times a - v\,O_2 \text{ difference}$$

In the equation, $\dot{V}O_2$ is oxygen consumption, $\dot{Q}$ is cardiac output (HR $\times$ SV), and $a - v\,O_2$ difference is the difference in the O_2 content between the blood in the arteries and the blood in the veins.

From this equation, it is very easy to see how influential the cardiovascular system is on the body's ability to consume oxygen, and that heart rate plays a major factor in $\dot{V}O_2$.

Maximal oxygen consumption ($\dot{V}O_2$ max) is generally accepted as the best means of gauging cardiorespiratory fitness.[3,5,7,15] Essentially, $\dot{V}O_2$ max is the highest rate of oxygen transport and utilization achieved at maximal physical exertion.[10,14,15] $\dot{V}O_2$ max values can range anywhere from 40 to 80 mL $\cdot$ kg^{-1} $\cdot$ min^{-1}, or approximately 11 to 23 METs.[7,15]

Maximal testing, however, is not very practical for most clientele, and, as such, many submaximal testing procedures have been established to estimate $\dot{V}O_2$ max.[14,16] These include the Rockport Walk Test, the Step Test, and field protocols.[14,16] Although these protocols deliver a good generalization of a client's overall cardiorespiratory fitness level, they are based on several assumptions that are rarely met and can contribute to estimate errors.[14,16] However, given repeatedly during a period of weeks or months they may show a cardiorespiratory trend.

OXYGEN AND ENERGY

Oxygen is the necessary catalyst for sustaining many bodily functions when activity is prolonged for periods of greater than 30 seconds.[3,5,16,17] In these situations, activity is said to be **aerobic**, meaning it requires oxygen.[3,17,18] Many activities, however, last for only a few seconds and are not dependent on oxygen for proper execution. These activities are described as **anaerobic**, meaning they do not require oxygen.[3,17,18] To generate either form of activity, however, the body must still produce sufficient amounts of energy.

Energy is essentially the capacity to do work.[3,18] The study of energy in the human body, known as **bioenergetics**, looks at how chemical energy (food) is converted into mechanical energy (work).[3,18,19] During this conversion process, chemical bonds are broken, and this releases energy that is used to produce work (muscle contractions). This process is termed energy-yielding, as it produces energy much like a fruit tree yields fruit.[3,18,19] This energy can only be productive, however, if it can be captured and transferred to a place where it can be used. When the energy is used it is termed an energy-utilizing reaction.[3,18,19] In other words, energy is gathered from an energy-yielding source (the breakdown of food) by some storage unit and then transferred to a site that can use this energy (muscle contraction). Typically, the storage and transfer unit within the cells of the body is **adenosine triphosphate** (ATP).[3,18,19]

ATP is structurally composed of a nitrogen-based compound, adenine, a five-carbon sugar called ribose, and three phosphates. ATP has the ability to store large amounts of energy in the chemical bonds of the phosphates. Essentially, this is the energy needed for muscle contraction, which performs physical activity. The supply of ATP in each cell is limited, however, and therefore cells must have a means of producing more. There are three main bioenergetic pathways that produce ATP.[3,15,18] These include the ATP-CP and the glycolysis pathways, which are categorized as anaerobic (without oxygen) systems, and the oxidative (oxygen) pathway, classified as an aerobic (with oxygen) system. Collectively, these systems are known as the bioenergetic continuum (Table 3-5).[20]

Aerobic: Requires oxygen.

Anaerobic: Does not require oxygen.

Bioenergetics: The biology of energy transformations and exchanges within the body, and between it and the environment.

Adenosine triphosphate (ATP): A cellular structure that supplies energy for many biochemical cellular processes by undergoing enzymatic hydrolysis.

Table 3.5			
The Bioenergetic Continuum			
Pathway	**System**	**Use**	**Time**
ATP-CP	Anaerobic	High-intensity, short-duration activity such as heavy weight training	Up to approximately 10 seconds of activity
Glycolysis	Anaerobic	Moderate- to high-intensity, moderate-duration activities such as a typical set of 8–12 repetitions	30–50 seconds of activity
Oxidative	Aerobic	Lower intensity, longer duration activities such as walking on the treadmill for 20–30 minutes	Activities greater than 2 minutes

ATP-CP Pathway

Together, ATP and CP (creatine phosphate) are called phosphagens and therefore, this system is sometimes referred to as the phosphagen system.[18] The ATP-CP system provides energy for primarily high-intensity, short-duration bouts of exercise or activity. This would be seen in power and strength forms of training in which heavy loads are used with only a few repetitions, or during short sprinting events. However, this system is activated at the onset of activity, regardless of intensity, because of its ability to produce energy very rapidly in comparison with the other systems.[3,18,21]

This bioenergetic system provides energy through the interactions of ATP and CP with enzymes (chemical catalysts that cause a change) such as myosin-ATPase and creatine kinase.

The enzyme myosin ATPase causes the breaking off of one of the phosphate bonds from ATP. This results in ADP (adenosine diphosphate, meaning that there are now two phosphates instead of three). By breaking one of the high-energy phosphate bonds, energy is released.[3,18,21] This system is limited in its capacity to sustain energy production (approximately 10 seconds) because it must rely on the minimal storage of ATP and CP within the cells.[3,18,21]

Glycolysis

Glycolysis (anaerobic system) uses the breakdown of carbohydrates (glucose) to rapidly produce ATP.[3,18,21]

Here, one glucose molecule will produce 2 ATP through anaerobic glycolysis. One of the by-products of this process is pyruvate. If pyruvate cannot be used fast enough by the muscle cell, a buildup of lactic acid will occur. Excess lactic acid causes an increase in the acidity of the muscle cell and will interfere with muscle contractions.[3,18,21]

Although this system can produce a significantly greater amount of energy than the ATP-CP system, it too is limited to approximately 30 to 50 seconds of duration.[3,18,21] Most fitness workouts will place a greater stress on this system than the other systems because a typical repetition range of 8 to 12 repetitions falls within this time frame.

Oxidative

The oxidative system relies primarily on carbohydrates and fats for the production of ATP. This system is the slowest producing of the three systems because it requires increased amounts of oxygen to match the muscular requirement of the exercise. Oxygen must be supplied through respiration, and it takes a while to elevate the respiration rate to consume appropriate amounts of oxygen. Needless to say, this system results in a greater amount of ATP. The oxidative system uses a somewhat similar process to anaerobic glycolysis. Glucose supplied from the glycogen stores within the body is broken down in the presence of oxygen. With the presence of oxygen, pyruvate is not converted to lactic acid and becomes a usable substrate for ATP production.[3,18,21]

Here, one glucose molecule will produce 36 ATP. Depending on the specific substrates and pathways, it is possible for one glucose molecule to produce 38 ATP.[3,18,21] This system becomes more involved in activities of longer than 30 seconds and is the predominant system in activities of more than 2 minutes.[3]

DYSFUNCTIONAL BREATHING

The importance of all systems in the body working synergistically can be further demonstrated in the intimacy between the cardiorespiratory system and the kinetic chain. The cardiorespiratory system is a major support system for the kinetic chain. However, it is also the kinetic chain that provides essential support for the cardiorespiratory system. Muscles, bones, and the nervous system are all essential components of the cardiorespiratory system that enable it to function optimally. Thus, if there is a dysfunction in the cardiorespiratory system, this can directly impact the components of the kinetic chain and perpetuate further dysfunction. Alterations in breathing patterns are a prime example of this relationship.

Breathing dysfunction is a very common predecessor to kinetic chain dysfunction.[22] It often results from breathing associated with high stress or anxiety. As a result of this altered breathing pattern, the follow scenarios can occur:[23]

- The breathing pattern becomes more shallow, using the secondary respiratory muscles more predominantly than the diaphragm. This shallow, upper-chest breathing pattern becomes habitual, causing overuse to the secondary respiratory muscles such as the scalenes, sternocleidomastoid, levator scapulae, and upper trapezius.
- These muscles also play a major postural role in the kinetic chain, all connecting directly to the cervical and cranial portions of the body. Their increased activity and excessive tension often result in headaches, light-headedness, and dizziness.
- Excessive breathing (short, shallow breaths) can lead to altered carbon dioxide and oxygen blood content that stimulates various sensors.
- This can lead to feelings of anxiety that further initiate an excessive breathing response.
- Inadequate oxygen and retention of metabolic waste within muscles can create fatigued stiff muscles.
- Inadequate joint motion of the spine and rib cage, as a result of improper breathing, causes joints to become restricted and stiff.

All of these situations can lead to a decreased functional capacity that may result in headaches, feelings of anxiety, fatigue, and poor sleep patterns, as well as poor circulation. As a health and fitness professional, it is not your job to try to diagnose these problems. If a client presents any of these scenarios, refer them immediately to a medical professional for assistance.

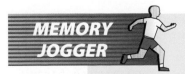

MEMORY JOGGER

Teaching your client to breathe diaphragmatically (through the stomach) can be a way to help avoid these symptoms. Assessing one's breathing pattern ("chest breather") can also help determine potential muscle imbalances.

SUMMARY

The respiratory system gathers oxygen from the environment, and processes it to be delivered to the tissues of the body. As cells use oxygen, they produce carbon dioxide, which is transported back to the heart and lungs in the deoxygenated blood, to be released through exhalation.

The usage of oxygen by the body is known as oxygen consumption. Maximal oxygen consumption ($\dot{V}O_2$ max) is the highest rate of oxygen transport and utilization achieved at maximal physical exertion. It is generally accepted as the best means of gauging cardiorespiratory fitness. Values can range anywhere from 11 to 23 METs.

Oxygen is the necessary catalyst for aerobic activity prolonged for periods of greater than 30 seconds. Anaerobic activities that last for only a few seconds are not dependent on oxygen for proper execution. To generate either form of activity, however, the body must still produce sufficient energy.

The study of how chemical energy (food) is converted into mechanical energy (work) is known as bioenergetics. Typically, energy is gathered by adenosine triphosphate (ATP) and is transferred to a site that can use this energy (muscle contraction).

ATP has the ability to store the large amounts of energy needed for muscle contraction to perform physical activity. However, the supply of ATP in each cell is limited, and cells must produce more through the bioenergetic continuum, which consists of ATP-CP and the glycolysis pathways (anaerobic systems), and the oxidative pathway (an aerobic system).

The ATP-CP system provides energy for high-intensity, short bouts of activity. This system relies on the minimal storage of ATP and CP (creatine phosphate) within the cells and thus is limited to energy production of approximately 10 seconds. Glycolysis uses the breakdown of carbohydrates to rapidly produce ATP. This system is limited to 30 to 50 seconds of duration. The oxidative system relies primarily on carbohydrates and fats, results in a higher production of ATP, allowing for activities longer than 30 seconds, and is the predominant system in activities longer than 2 minutes.

Alterations in breathing patterns can directly impact the components of the kinetic chain and lead to further dysfunction. If the breathing patterns become more shallow, the body uses secondary respiratory muscles more than the diaphragm, which can negatively impact posture. This may create excessive muscular tension, resulting in headaches, lightheadedness, and dizziness. Short, shallow breaths can also lead to altered carbon dioxide and oxygen blood content, which causes feelings of anxiety. Inadequate oxygen and retention of metabolic waste within muscles can create stiff muscles and joints. If a client complains of headaches, feelings of anxiety, fatigue, poor sleep patterns, or poor circulation, refer them immediately to a medical professional for assistance.

Review Questions

1 *What are the three components of the cardiovascular system?*

2 *Which system(s) of the bioenergetic continuum is (are) aerobic?*

  a. ATP-CP

  b. Glycolysis

  c. Oxidative

3 *Which pathway of the bioenergetic continuum would most likely be used during heavy weight training?*

4 *The <u>right / left</u> atrium gathers deoxygenated blood returning to the heart from the entire body, whereas the <u>right / left</u> atrium gathers reoxygenated blood coming to the heart from the lungs.*

REFERENCES

1. Fox SI. Human Physiology, 5th ed. Dubuque, IA: Wm C. Brown Publishers, 1996.
2. Vander A, Sherman J, Luciano D. Human Physiology: The Mechanisms of Body Function, 8th ed. New York: McGraw-Hill, 2001.
3. Brooks GA, Fahey TD, White TP. Exercise Physiology: Human Bioenergetics and Its Application, 2nd ed. Moutain View, CA: Mayfield Publishing Company, 1996.
4. Murray TD, Murray JM. Cardiovascular anatomy. In: American College of Sports Medicine (ed). ACSM's Resource Manual for Guidelines for Exercise Testing and Prescription, 3rd ed. Baltimore, MD: Williams & Wilkins, 1998.
5. Hicks GH. Cardiopulmonary Anatomy and Physiology. Philadelphia: WB Saunders, 2000.
6. Tortora GJ. Principles of Human Anatomy, 7th ed. New York: Harper Collins College Publishers, 1995.
7. Williams MA. Cardiovascular and respiratory anatomy and physiology: responses to exercise. In: Baechle TR (ed). Essentials of Strength Training and Conditioning. Champaign, IL: Human Kinetics, 1994.
8. Holly RG, Shaffrath JD. Cardiorespiratory endurance. In: American College of Sports Medicine (ed). ACSM's Resource Manual for Guidelines for Exercise Testing and Prescription, 3rd ed. Baltimore, MD: Williams & Wilkins, 1998.
9. Mahler DA. Respiratory anatomy. In: American College of Sports Medicine (ed). ACSM's Resource Manual for Guidelines for Exercise Testing and Prescription, 3rd ed. Baltimore, MD: Williams & Wilkins, 1998.
10. Brown DD. Pulmonary responses to exercise and training. In: Garrett WE, Kirkendall DT (eds). Exercise and Sport Science. Philadelphia: Lippincott Williams & Wilkins, 2000.
11. Leech JA, Ghezzo H, Stevens D, Becklake MR. Respiratory pressures and function in young adults. Am Rev Respir Dis 1983;128:17–23.
12. Farkas GA, Decramer M, Rochester DF, De Troyer A. Contractile properties of intercostal muscles and their functional significance, J Appl Physiol 1985;59:528–535.
13. Sharp T, Goldberg NB, Druz WF, Danon J. Relative contributions of rib cage and abdomen to breathing in normal subjects. J Appl Physiol 1975;39:601.
14. McConnell TR. Cardiorespiratory assessment of apparently healthy populations. In: American College of Sports Medicine (ed). ACSM's Resource Manual for Guidelines for Exercise Testing and Prescription, 3rd ed. Baltimore, MD: Williams & Wilkins, 1998.
15. Franklin BA. Cardiovascular responses to exercise and training. In: Garrett WE, Kirkendall DT (eds). Exercise and Sport Science. Philadelphia: Lippincott Williams & Wilkins, 2000.
16. American College of Sports Medicine. ACSM's Guidelines for Exercise Testing and Prescription, 5th ed. Philadelphia: Williams & Wilkins, 1995.
17. Greenhaff PL, Timmons JA. Interaction between aerobic and anaerobic metabolism during intense muscle contraction. In: Holsey JO (ed). Exercise and Sport Science Reviews, vol 26. Baltimore: Williams & Wilkins, 1998:1–30.
18. Stone MH, Conley MS. Bioenergetics. In: Baechle TR (ed). Essentials of Strength Training and Conditioning. Champaign, IL: Human Kinetics, 1994.
19. Volek JS. Enhancing exercise performance: nutritional implications. In: Garrett WE, Kirkendall DT (eds). Exercise and Sport Science. Philadelphia: Lippincott Williams & Wilkins, 2000.
20. Clark MA. Integrated Training for The New Millennium. Thousand Oaks, CA: National Academy of Sports Medicine, 2001.
21. Billeter R, Hoppeler H. Muscular basis of strength. In: Komi PV (ed). Strength and Power in Sport. London: Blackwell Scientific Publications, 1992.
22. Chaitow L. Cranial Manipulation Theory and Practice: Osseous and Soft Tissue Approaches. London: Churchill Livingstone, 1999.
23. Timmons B. Behavioral and Psychological Approaches to Breathing Disorders. New York: Plenum Press, 1994.

4

Human Movement Science

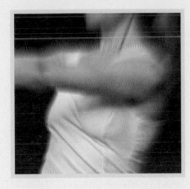

OBJECTIVES

After completing this chapter, you will be able to:

- Understand the concepts and theories of motor behavior.
- Explain, in terms of training:
  - Why sensory information is important to human movement
  - What internal and external feedbacks are
- Describe how muscle actions and outside forces relate to human movement.
- Define the three stages of motor learning as well as basic biomechanical terminology.

KEY TERMS

Abduction	Force	Motor learning
Adduction	Force couple relationships	Posterior (or dorsal)
Anterior (or ventral)	Frontal plane	Proprioception
Biomechanics	Inferior	Proximal
Concentric contraction	Internal feedback	Rotary motion
Contralateral	Internal rotation	Sagittal plane
Distal	Ipsilateral	Sensorimotor integration
Eccentric contraction	Isometric contraction	Superior
Extension	Lateral	Synergies
External feedback	Length tension relationships	Torque
External rotation	Medial	Transverse plane
Feedback	Motor behavior	
Flexion	Motor control	

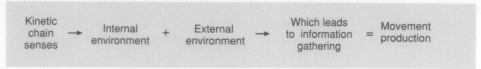

Figure 4.1　The process of movement.

INTRODUCTION TO HUMAN MOVEMENT SCIENCE

The components and structures of the kinetic chain have now been reviewed. Although they seem separate, each system and their components must collaborate with the others to form interdependent links that create a functional chain. In turn, this entire chain must be aware of its relationship to internal and external environments, gather necessary information about them, and produce the appropriate movement patterns (Figure 4-1). This process ensures optimum functioning of the kinetic chain and, thus, optimum human movement (Figure 4-2).

With this in mind, the following chapter will focus on how the kinetic chain works interdependently to learn, form, and produce efficient movement. In doing so, we will discuss motor behavior and fundamental biomechanics.

Biomechanics

BIOMECHANICS

Biomechanics: A study that uses principles of physics to quantitatively study how forces interact within a living body.

Biomechanics is a study that uses principles of physics to quantitatively study how forces interact within a living body. Specifically, this text focuses on the motions that the kinetic chain produces and the forces that act on it.[1,2] This includes basic anatomic terminology, planes of motion, joint motions, muscle action, force couples, leverage, forces, and the force-velocity relationship.

Terminology

All industries have language that is specific to their needs. Because health and fitness professionals deal with human motion and the human body, it is necessary that they understand the basic anatomic terminology to allow for effective com-

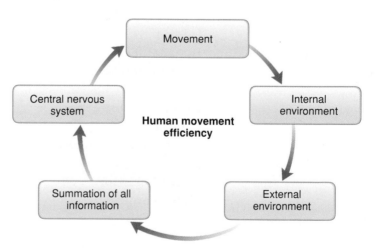

Figure 4.2　Human movement efficiency.

munication among one another. This section will include anatomic locations, planes of motion, and joint motions.

ANATOMIC LOCATIONS

Superior: Positioned above a point of reference.

Inferior: Positioned below a point of reference.

Proximal: Positioned nearest the center of the body, or point of reference.

Distal: Positioned farthest from the center of the body, or point of reference.

Anterior (or ventral): On the front of the body.

Posterior (or dorsal): On the back of the body.

Anatomic location refers to terms that describe locations on the body (Figure 4-3). These include medial, lateral, contralateral, ipsilateral, anterior, posterior, proximal, distal, inferior, and superior.

Superior refers to a position above a reference point. The femur is superior to the tibia. The pectoralis major is superior to the rectus abdominis.

Inferior refers to a position below a reference point. The calcaneus is inferior to the talus. The gastrocnemius is inferior to the hamstrings.

Proximal refers to a position nearest the center of the body or point of reference. The knee is more proximal to the hip than the ankle. The lumbar spine is more proximal to the sacrum than the sternum.

Distal refers to a position farthest from the center of the body or point of reference. The ankle is more distal to the hip than the knee. The sternum is more distal to the sacrum than the lumbar spine.

Anterior refers to a position on the front or toward the front of the body. The quadriceps are located on the anterior aspect of the thigh.

Posterior refers to a position on the back or toward the back of the body. The hamstrings are located on the posterior aspect of the thigh.

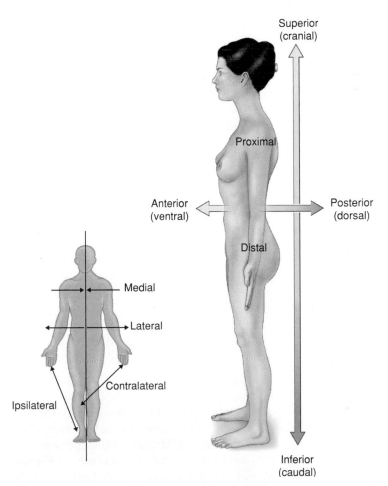

Figure 4.3   Anatomic locations.

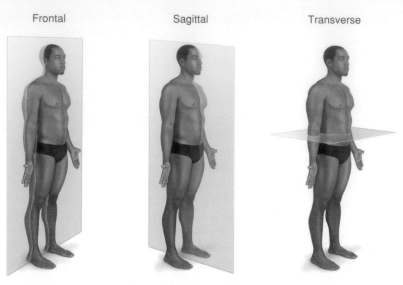

Frontal   Sagittal   Transverse

Figure 4.4 Planes of motion.

Medial: Positioned near the middle of the body.

Lateral: Toward the outside of the body

Contralateral: Positioned on the opposite side of the body.

Ipsilateral: Positioned on the same side of the body.

Medial refers to a position relatively closer to the midline of the body. The adductors are on the medial side of the thigh, because they are on the side of the limb closest to the midline of the body. The sternum is more medial than the shoulder.

Lateral refers to a position relatively farther away from the midline of the body or toward the outside of the body. The ears are on the lateral side of the head because they are farther away from the midline of the body.

Contralateral refers to a position on the opposite side of the body. The right foot is contralateral to the left hand.

Ipsilateral refers to a position on the same side of the body. The right foot is ipsilateral to the right hand.

PLANES OF MOTION, AXES, AND JOINT MOTIONS

The universally used method of describing human movements in three dimensions is based on a system of planes and axes (Figure 4-4). Three imaginary planes are positioned through the body at right angles so they intersect at the center of mass of the body. They include the sagittal, frontal, and transverse planes. Movement is said to occur more predominantly in a specific plane if it is actually along the plane or parallel to it. Although movements can be one-plane dominant, no motion occurs strictly in one plane of motion. Movement in a plane occurs on an axis running perpendicular to that plane, much like the axle that a car wheel revolves around. This is known as *joint motion*. Joint motions are termed for their action in each of the three planes of motion (Table 4-1).

Sagittal plane: An imaginary bisector that divides the body into left and right halves.

Flexion: The bending of a joint, causing the angle to the joint to decrease.

Extension: The straightening of a joint, causing the angle to the joint to increase.

The Sagittal Plane. The **sagittal plane** bisects the body into right and left halves. Sagittal plane motion occurs around a coronal axis.[1,2,3] Movements in the sagittal plane include flexion and extension. **Flexion** is a bending movement in which the relative angle between two adjacent segments decreases.[2,8] **Extension** is a straightening movement in which the relative angle between two adjacent segments increases.[2,4] Flexion and extension occur in many joints in the body including vertebral, shoulder, elbow, wrist, hip, knee, foot, and hand (Figure 4-5). At the ankle, flexion is referred to as dorsiflexion and exten-

Table 4.1

Examples of Planes, Motions, and Axes

Plane	Motion	Axis	Example
Sagittal	Flexion/extension	Coronal	Biceps curl Triceps pushdown Squat Front lunge Calf raise Walking Running Vertical jumping Climbing stairs
Frontal	Adduction/abduction Lateral flexion Eversion/inversion	Anterior-posterior	Side lateral raise Side lunge Side shuffle
Transverse	Internal rotation External rotation Left/right rotation Horizontal adduction Horizontal abduction	Longitudinal	Trunk rotation Throwing Golfing Swinging a bat

sion is plantarflexion (Figure 4-6).[1,2,4] Examples of predominantly sagittal plane movements include biceps curls, triceps pushdowns, squats, front lunges, calf raises, walking, running, vertical jump, climbing stairs, and shooting a basketball.

Frontal plane: An imaginary bisector that divides the body into front and back halves.

Abduction: Movement of a body part away from the middle of the body.

Adduction: Movement of a body part toward the middle of the body.

Transverse plane: An imaginary bisector that divides the body into top and bottom halves.

Internal rotation: Rotation of a joint toward the middle of the body.

External rotation: Rotation of a joint away from the middle of the body

The Frontal Plane. The **frontal plane** bisects the body to create front and back halves. Frontal plane motion occurs around an anterior-posterior axis.[1,2,3] Movements in the frontal plane include abduction and adduction in the limbs (relative to the trunk), lateral flexion in the spine, and eversion and inversion at the foot and ankle complex.[1,2,3,4] **Abduction** is a movement away from the midline of the body or, similar to extension, it is an increase in the angle between two adjoining segments, but in the frontal plane (Figure 4-7).[1,2,3,4] **Adduction** is a movement of the segment toward the midline of the body or, like flexion, it is a decrease in the angle between two adjoining segments, but in the frontal plane (Figure 4-8).[1,2,3,4] Lateral flexion is the bending of the spine (cervical, thoracic, or lumbar) from side to side or simply side-bending.[1,2,3,4] Eversion and inversion follow the same principle, but relate more specifically to the movement of the calcaneus and tarsals in the frontal plane.[1,2,3,4] Examples of frontal plane movements include side lateral raises, side lunges, and side shuffling.

The Transverse Plane. The **transverse plane** bisects the body to create upper and lower halves. Transverse plane motion occurs around a longitudinal or vertical axis.[1,2,3] Movements in the transverse plane include **internal rotation** and **external rotation** for the limbs, right and left rotation for the head and trunk, and radioulnar pronation and supination (Figures 4-9 and 4-10).[1,2,3] The foot, because it is a unique entity, has transverse plane motion termed abduction (toes pointing outward, externally rotated) and adduction (toes pointing inward, internally rotated).[2] Examples of transverse plane movements include trunk rotation, turning lunges, throwing a ball, throwing a Frisbee, golfing, and swinging a bat.

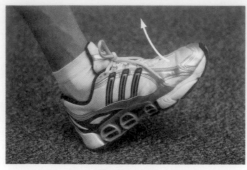

Dorsiflexion

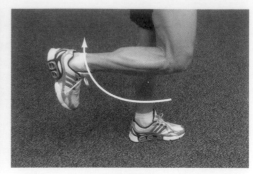

Knee flexion

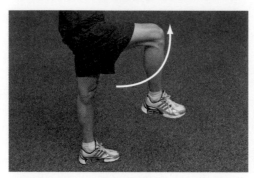

Hip flexion

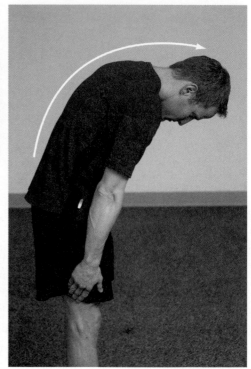

Spinal flexion

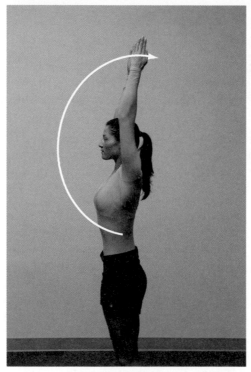

Shoulder flexion

Figure 4.5 Flexion.

Muscle Actions

Muscles produce a variety of actions to effectively manipulate gravity, ground reaction forces, momentum, and external resistance. There are three different actions that muscles produce:

- Eccentric
- Isometric
- Concentric

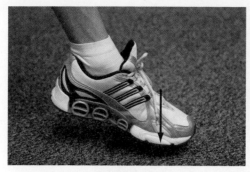

Plantarflexion

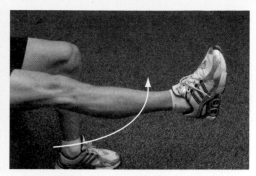

Knee extension

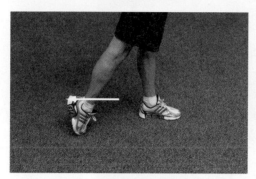

Hip extension

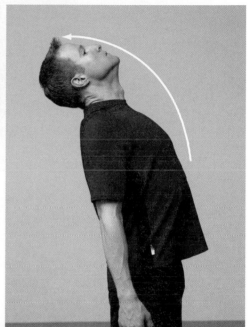

Spinal extension

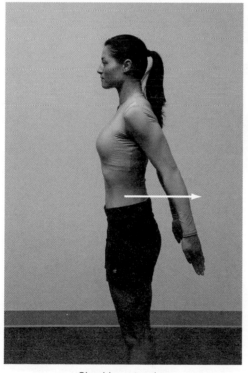

Shoulder extension

Figure 4.6 Extension.

This range of muscle action is known as the muscle action spectrum and is necessary to produce efficient movement (Table 4-2).

ECCENTRIC

Eccentric contraction: The lengthening of a muscle.

When a muscle contracts **eccentrically**, it is exerting less force than is being placed on it. This results in a lengthening of the muscle. As the muscle lengthens, the actin and myosin crossbridges are pulled apart and reattach, allowing the muscle to

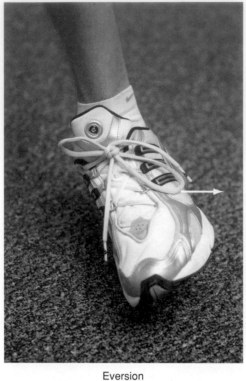

Eversion

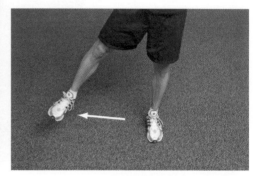

Hip abduction

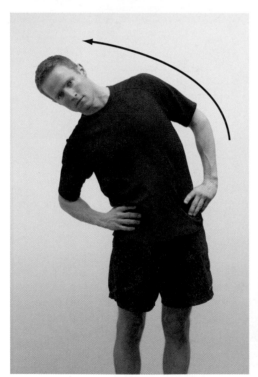

Lateral flexion

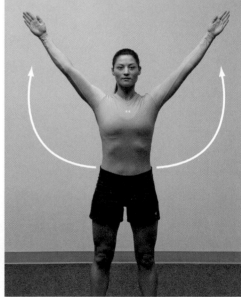

Shoulder abduction

Figure 4.7

lengthen.[2,4] In actuality, the lengthening of the muscle usually refers to its return to a resting length and not actually increasing in its length as if it were being stretched.[4]

Eccentric muscle action is also known as "a negative" in the health and fitness industry. The term "negative" was derived from the fact that in eccentric movement,

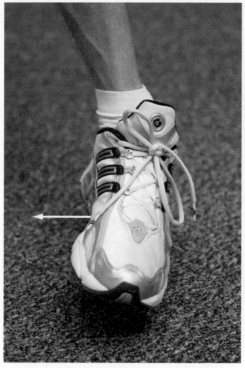

Inversion

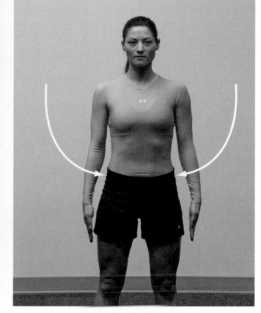

Shoulder adduction

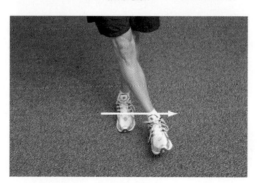

Hip adduction   **Figure 4.8**

work is actually being done on the muscle (because forces move the muscle) rather than the muscle doing the work (or the muscle moving the forces).[2,4] This is owing to the fact that eccentric motion moves in the same direction as the resistance is moving (known as direction of resistance).[1,2,4]

In functional activities, such as daily movements and sports, muscles work as much eccentrically as they do concentrically or isometrically.[5] Eccentrically, the muscles must decelerate or reduce the forces acting on the body (or force reduction). This is seen in all forms of resistance exercise. Whether walking on a treadmill or bench pressing, the weight of either the body or the bar must be decelerated and then stabilized to be properly accelerated (Table 4-2).

ISOMETRIC

Isometric contraction: A muscle maintaining a certain length.

When a muscle contracts **isometrically**, it is exerting force equal to that placed on it. This results in no appreciable change in the muscle length.[2,4]

In functional activities such as daily movements and sports, isometric actions are used to dynamically stabilize the body. This can be seen in stabilizers that are isometrically stabilizing a limb from moving in an unwanted direction. For example,

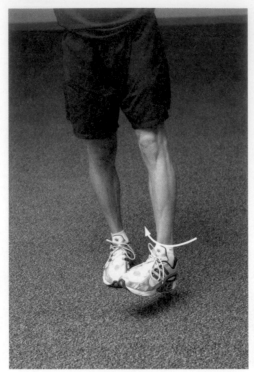

Hip internal rotation

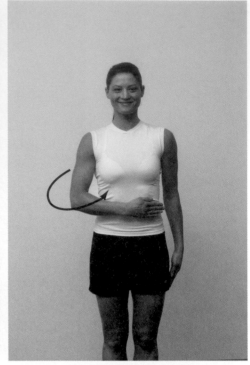

Shoulder internal rotation

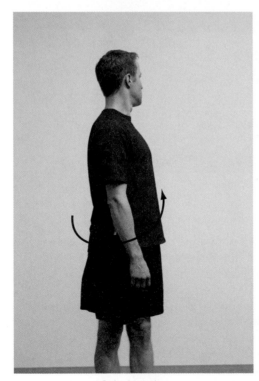

Spinal rotation

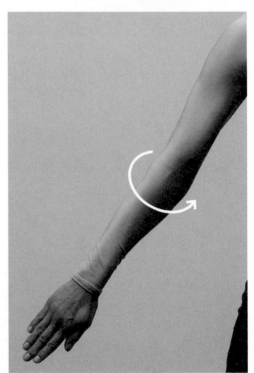

Pronation

Figure 4.9

the adductors and abductors of the thigh during a squat will dynamically stabilize the leg from moving too much in the frontal and transverse planes.[4,5] During a ball crunch, the transversus abdominis and multifidus muscles stabilize the lumbar spine. During a dumbbell bench press, the rotator cuff musculature dynamically stabilizes the shoulder joint. When performing a push-up, the deep cervical flexors

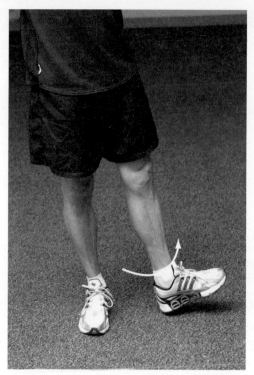

Hip external rotation

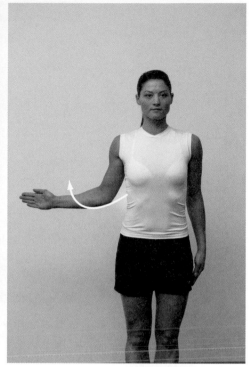

Shoulder external rotation

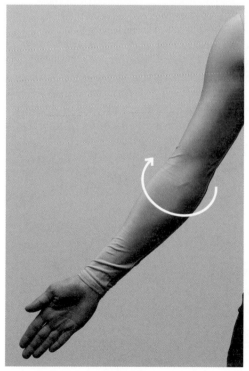

Supination

Figure 4.10

Table 4.2	
Muscle Action Spectrum	
Action	**Performance**
Eccentric	Moving in the same direction as the resistance Decelerates or reduces force
Isometric	No visible movement with or against resistance Dynamically stabilizes force
Concentric	Moving in opposite direction of force Accelerates or produces force

(longus coli, longus capitus) stabilize the cervical spine and head, keeping the head from migrating toward the ground.

CONCENTRIC

Concentric contraction: The shortening of a muscle.

When a muscle contracts **concentrically**, it is exerting more force than is being placed on it. This results in a shortening of the muscle. As the muscle shortens, the actin and myosin crossbridges move together (known as sliding-filament theory), allowing the muscle to shorten.[2,4]

Functional Anatomy

The traditional perception of muscles is that they work concentrically and predominantly in one plane of motion. However, to more effectively understand motion and design efficient training, reconditioning, and rehabilitation programs, it is imperative to view muscles functioning in all planes of motion and through the entire muscle contraction spectrum (eccentrically, stabilization, and concentrically). The following section describes the isolated and integrated functions of the major muscles of the kinetic chain.[6–8]

LEG MUSCULATURE
Lower Leg Complex

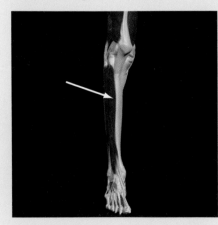

ANTERIOR TIBIALIS

ORIGIN
- Lateral condyle and proximal two thirds of the lateral surface of the tibia

INSERTION
- Medial and plantar aspects of the medial cuneiform and the base of the first metatarsal

ISOLATED FUNCTION
- Concentrically accelerates dorsiflexion and inversion

INTEGRATED FUNCTION
- Eccentrically decelerates plantarflexion and eversion
- Isometrically stabilizes the arch of the foot

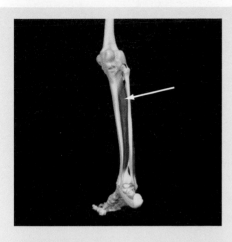

POSTERIOR TIBIALIS

ORIGIN
- Proximal two thirds of posterior surface of the tibia and fibula

INSERTION
- Every tarsal bone (naviular, cuneiform, cuboid) but the talus plus the bases of the second through the fourth metatarsal bones. The main insertion is on the navicular tuberosity and the medial cuneiform bone

ISOLATED FUNCTION
- Concentrically accelerates plantarflexion and inversion of the foot

INTEGRATED FUNCTION
- Eccentrically decelerates the dorsiflexion and eversion of the foot
- Isometrically stabilizes the arch of the foot

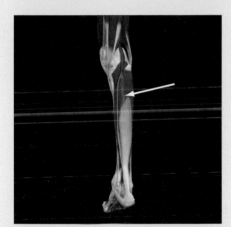

SOLEUS

ORIGIN
- Posterior surface of the fibular head and proximal one third of its shaft and from the posterior side of the tibia

INSERTION
- Calcaneus via the Achilles tendon

ISOLATED FUNCTION
- Concentrically accelerates plantarflexion

INTEGRATED FUNCTION
- Decelerates ankle dorsiflexion
- Isometrically stabilizes the foot and ankle complex

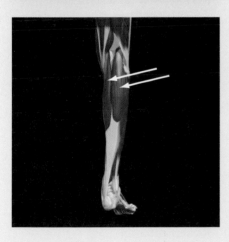

GASTROCNEMIUS

ORIGIN
- Posterior aspect of the lateral and medial femoral condyles

INSERTION
- Calcaneus via the Achilles tendon

ISOLATED FUNCTION
- Concentrically accelerates plantarflexion

INTEGRATED FUNCTION
- Decelerates ankle dorsiflexion
- Isometrically stabilizes the foot and ankle complex

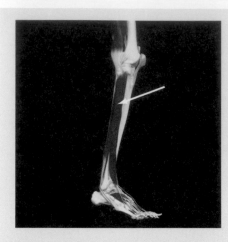

PERONEUS LONGUS

ORIGIN
- Lateral condyle of tibia, head, and proximal two thirds of the lateral surface of the fibula

INSERTION
- Lateral surface of the medial cuneiform and lateral side of the base of the first metatarsal

ISOLATED FUNCTION
- Concentrically plantarflexes and everts the foot

INTEGRATED FUNCTION
- Decelerates ankle dorsiflexion
- Isometrically stabilizes the foot and ankle complex

Hamstring Complex

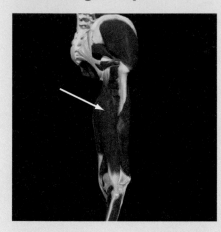

BICEPS FEMORIS—LONG HEAD

ORIGIN
- Ischial tuberosity of the pelvis, part of the sacrotuberous ligament

INSERTION
- Head of the fibula

ISOLATED FUNCTION
- Concentrically accelerates knee flexion and hip extension
- Tibial external rotation

INTEGRATED FUNCTION
- Eccentrically decelerates knee extension
- Eccentrically decelerates hip flexion
- Eccentrically decelerates tibial internal rotation at mid-stance of the gait cycle
- Isometrically stabilizes the lumbo-pelvic-hip complex and knee

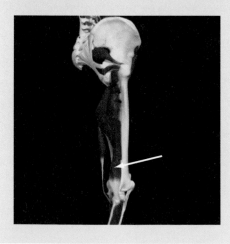

BICEPS FEMORIS—SHORT HEAD

ORIGIN
- Lower one third of the posterior aspect of the femur

INSERTION
- Head of the fibula

ISOLATED FUNCTION
- Concentrically accelerates knee flexion and tibial external rotation

INTEGRATED FUNCTION
- Eccentrically decelerates knee extension
- Eccentrically decelerates tibial internal rotation
- Isometrically stabilizes the knee

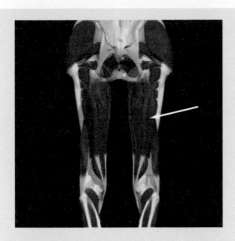

SEMIMEMBRANOSUS

ORIGIN
- Ischial tuberosity of the pelvis

INSERTION
- Posterior aspect of the medial tibial condyle of the tibia

ISOLATED FUNCTION
- Concentrically accelerates knee flexion, hip extension, and tibial internal rotation

INTEGRATED FUNCTION
- Eccentrically decelerates knee extension
- Eccentrically decelerates hip flexion
- Eccentrically decelerates tibial external rotation
- Isometrically stabilizes the lumbo-pelvic-hip complex and knee

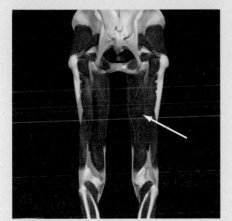

SEMITENDINOSUS

ORIGIN
- Ischial tuberosity of the pelvis and part of the sacrotuberous ligament

INSERTION
- Proximal aspect of the medial tibial condyle of the tibia (pes anserine)

ISOLATED FUNCTION
- Concentrically accelerates knee flexion, hip extension, and tibial internal rotation

INTEGRATED FUNCTION
- Eccentrically decelerates knee extension
- Eccentrically decelerates hip flexion
- Eccentrically decelerates tibial external rotation
- Isometrically stabilizes the lumbo-pelvic-hip complex and knee

Quadriceps Complex

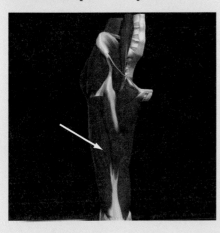

VASTUS LATERALIS

ORIGIN
- Anterior and inferior border of the greater trochanter, lateral region of the gluteal tuberosity, lateral lip of the linea aspera of the femur

INSERTION
- Base of patella and tibial tuberosity of the tibia

ISOLATED FUNCTION
- Concentrically accelerates knee extension

INTEGRATED FUNCTION
- Eccentrically decelerates knee flexion, adduction, and internal rotation
- Isometrically stabilizes the knee

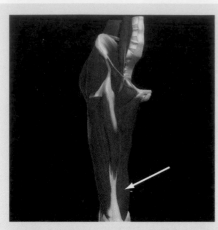

VASTUS MEDIALIS

ORIGIN
- Lower region of intertrochanteric line, medial lip of linea aspera, proximal medial supracondylar line of the femur

INSERTION
- Base of patella, tibial tuberosity of the tibia

ISOLATED FUNCTION
- Concentrically accelerates knee extension

INTEGRATED FUNCTION
- Eccentrically decelerates knee flexion, adduction, and internal rotation
- Isometrically stabilizes the knee

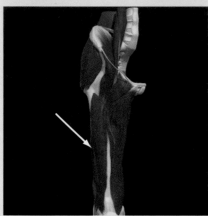

VASTUS INTERMEDIUS

ORIGIN
- Anterior-lateral regions of the upper two thirds of the femur

INSERTION
- Base of patella, tibial tuberosity of the tibia

ISOLATED FUNCTION
- Concentrically accelerates knee extension

INTEGRATED FUNCTION
- Eccentrically decelerates knee flexion, adduction, and internal rotation
- Isometrically stabilizes the knee

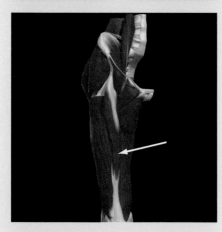

RECTUS FEMORIS

ORIGIN
- Anterior-inferior iliac spine of the pelvis

INSERTION
- Base of patella, tibial tuberosity of the tibia

ISOLATED FUNCTION
- Concentrically accelerates knee extension and hip flexion

INTEGRATED FUNCTION
- Eccentrically decelerates knee flexion, adduction, and internal rotation
- Decelerates hip extension
- Isometrically stabilizes the lumbo-pelvic-hip complex and knee

Hip Musculature
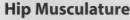

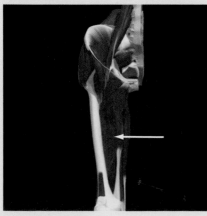

ADDUCTOR LONGUS

ORIGIN
- Anterior surface of the inferior pubic ramus of the pelvis

INSERTION
- Proximal one third of the linea aspera of the femur

ISOLATED FUNCTION
- Concentrically accelerates hip adduction, flexion, and internal rotation

INTEGRATED FUNCTION
- Eccentrically decelerates hip abduction, extension, and external rotation
- Isometrically stabilizes the lumbo-pelvic-hip complex

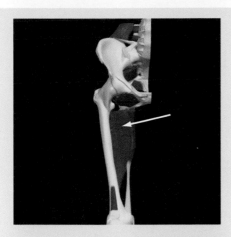

ADDUCTOR MAGNUS—ANTERIOR FIBERS

ORIGIN
- Ischial ramus of the pelvis

INSERTION
- Linea aspera of the femur

ISOLATED FUNCTION
- Concentrically accelerates hip adduction, flexion, and internal rotation

INTEGRATED FUNCTION
- Eccentrically decelerates hip abduction, extension, and external rotation
- Dynamically stabilizes the lumbo-pelvic-hip complex

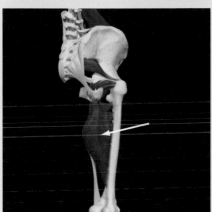

ADDUCTOR MAGNUS—POSTERIOR FIBERS

ORIGIN
- Ischial tuberosity of the pelvis

INSERTION
- Adductor tubercle on femur

ISOLATED FUNCTION
- Concentrically accelerates hip adduction, extension, and external rotation

INTEGRATED FUNCTION
- Eccentrically decelerates hip abduction, flexion, and internal rotation
- Isometrically stabilizes the lumbo-pelvic-hip complex

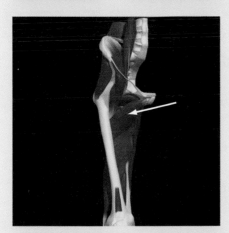

ADDUCTOR BREVIS

ORIGIN
- Anterior surface of the inferior pubic ramus of the pelvis

INSERTION
- Proximal one third of the linea aspera of the femur

ISOLATED FUNCTION
- Concentrically accelerates hip adduction, flexion, and internal rotation

INTEGRATED FUNCTION
- Eccentrically decelerates hip abduction, extension, and external rotation
- Isometrically stabilizes the lumbo-pelvic-hip complex

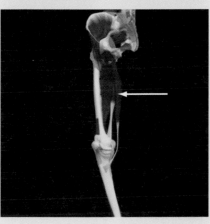

GRACILIS

ORIGIN
- Anterior aspect of lower body of pubis

INSERTION
- Proximal medial surface of the tibia (pes anserine)

ISOLATED FUNCTION
- Concentrically accelerates hip adduction, flexion, and internal rotation
- Assists in tibial internal rotation

INTEGRATED FUNCTION
- Eccentrically decelerates hip abduction, extension, and external rotation
- Isometrically stabilizes the lumbo-pelvic-hip complex and knee

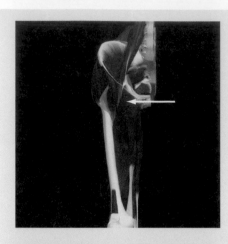

PECTINEUS

ORIGIN
- Pectineal line on the superior pubic ramus of the pelvis

INSERTION
- Pectineal line on the posterior surface of the upper femur

ISOLATED FUNCTION
- Concentrically accelerates hip adduction, flexion, and internal rotation

INTEGRATED FUNCTION
- Eccentrically decelerates hip abduction, extension, and external rotation
- Isometrically stabilizes the lumbo-pelvic-hip complex

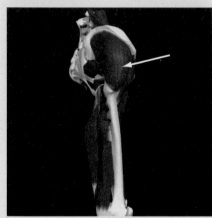

GLUTEUS MEDIUS—ANTERIOR FIBERS

ORIGIN
- Outer surface of the ilium of the pelvis

INSERTION
- Lateral surface of the greater trochanter on the femur

ISOLATED FUNCTION
- Concentrically accelerates hip abduction and internal rotation

INTEGRATED FUNCTION
- Eccentrically decelerates hip adduction and external rotation
- Isometrically stabilizes the lumbo-pelvic-hip complex

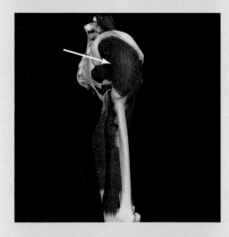

GLUTEUS MEDIUS—POSTERIOR FIBERS

ORIGIN
- Outer surface of the ilium of the pelvis

INSERTION
- Lateral surface of the greater trochanter on the femur

ISOLATED FUNCTION
- Concentrically accelerates hip abduction and external rotation

INTEGRATED FUNCTION
- Eccentrically decelerates hip adduction and internal rotation
- Isometrically stabilizes the lumbo-pelvic-hip complex

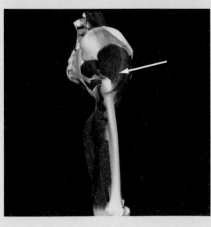

GLUTEUS MINIMUS

ORIGIN
- Ilium of the pelvis between the anterior and inferior gluteal line

INSERTION
- Greater trochanter of the femur

ISOLATED FUNCTION
- Concentrically accelerates hip abduction and internal rotation

INTEGRATED FUNCTION
- Eccentrically decelerates hip adduction and external rotation
- Isometrically stabilizes the lumbo-pelvic-hip complex

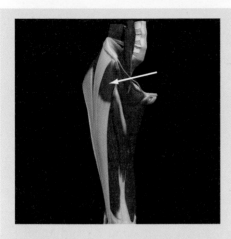

TENSOR FASCIA LATAE (TFL)

ORIGIN
- Outer surface of the iliac crest just posterior to the anterior-superior iliac spine of the pelvis

INSERTION
- Proximal one third of the iliotibial band

ISOLATED FUNCTION
- Concentrically accelerates hip flexion, abduction, and internal rotation

INTEGRATED FUNCTION
- Eccentrically decelerates hip extension, adduction, and external rotation
- Isometrically stabilizes the lumbo-pelvic-hip complex

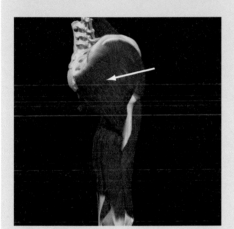

GLUTEUS MAXIMUS

ORIGIN
- Outer ilium of the pelvis, posterior side of sacrum and coccyx, and part of the sacrotuberous and posterior sacroiliac ligament

INSERTION
- Gluteal tuberosity of the femur and iliotibial tract

ISOLATED FUNCTION
- Concentrically accelerates hip extension and external rotation

INTEGRATED FUNCTION
- Eccentrically decelerates hip flexion and internal rotation
- Decelerates tibial internal rotation via the iliotibial band
- Isometrically stabilizes the lumbo-pelvic-hip complex

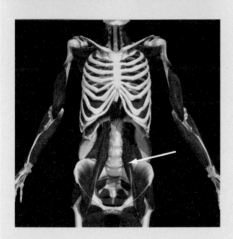

PSOAS

ORIGIN
- Transverse processes and lateral bodies of the last thoracic and all lumbar vertebrae including intervetebral disks

INSERTION
- Lesser trochanter of the femur

ISOLATED FUNCTION
- Concentrically accelerates hip flexion and external rotation
- Concentrically extends and rotates lumbar spine

INTEGRATED FUNCTION
- Eccentrically decelerates hip internal rotation
- Eccentrically decelerates hip extension
- Isometrically stabilizes the lumbo-pelvic-hip complex

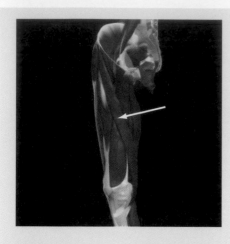

SARTORIUS

ORIGIN
- Anterior-superior iliac spine of the pelvis

INSERTION
- Proximal medial surface of the tibia

ISOLATED FUNCTION
- Concentrically accelerates hip flexion, external rotation, and abduction
- Concentrically accelerates knee flexion and internal rotation

INTEGRATED FUNCTION
- Eccentrically decelerates hip extension and internal rotation
- Eccentrically decelerates knee extension and external rotation
- Isometrically stabilizes the lumbo-pelvic-hip complex and knee

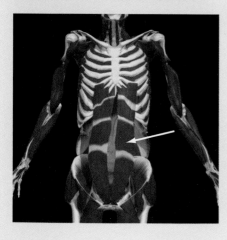

PIRIFORMIS

ORIGIN
- Anterior side of the sacrum

INSERTION
- The greater trochanter of the femur

ISOLATED FUNCTION
- Concentrically accelerates hip external rotation, abduction, and extension

INTEGRATED FUNCTION
- Eccentrically decelerates hip internal rotation, adduction, and flexion
- Isometrically stabilizes the hip and sacroiliac joints

Abdominal Musculature

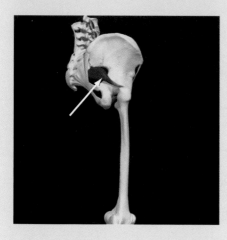

RECTUS ABDOMINIS

ORIGIN
- Pubic symphysis of the pelvis

INSERTION
- Ribs 5–7
- Xiphoid process of the sternum

ISOLATED FUNCTION
- Concentrically accelerates spinal flexion, lateral flexion, and rotation

INTEGRATED FUNCTION
- Eccentrically decelerates spinal extension, lateral flexion, and rotation
- Isometrically stabilizes the lumbo-pelvic-hip complex

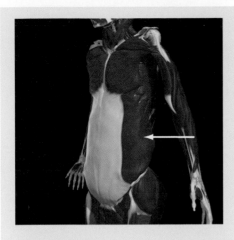

EXTERNAL OBLIQUE

ORIGIN
- External surface of ribs 4–12

INSERTION
- Anterior iliac crest of the pelvis, linea alba, and contralateral rectus sheaths

ISOLATED FUNCTION
- Concentrically accelerates spinal flexion, lateral flexion, and contralateral rotation

INTEGRATED FUNCTION
- Eccentrically decelerates spinal extension, lateral flexion, and rotation
- Isometrically stabilizes the lumbo-pelvic-hip complex

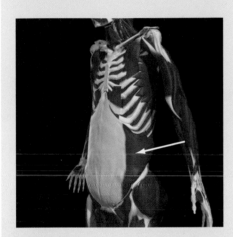

INTERNAL OBLIQUE

ORIGIN
- Anterior two thirds of the iliac crest of the pelvis and thoracolumbar fascia

INSERTION
- Ribs 9–12, linea alba, and contralateral rectus sheaths

ISOLATED FUNCTION
- Concentrically accelerates spinal flexion, lateral flexion, and ipsilateral rotation

INTEGRATED FUNCTION
- Eccentrically decelerates spinal extension, rotation, and lateral flexion
- Isometrically stabilizes the lumbo-pelvic-hip complex

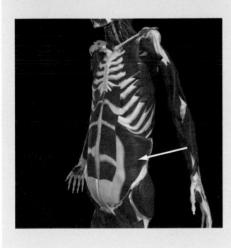

TRANSVERSUS ABDOMINIS

ORIGIN
- Ribs 7–12, anterior two thirds of the iliac crest of the pelvis, and thoracolumbar fascia

INSERTION
- Lineae alba and contralateral rectus sheaths

ISOLATED FUNCTION
- Increases intra-abdominal pressure
- Supports the abdominal viscera

INTEGRATED FUNCTION
- Isometrically stabilizes the lumbo-pelvic-hip complex

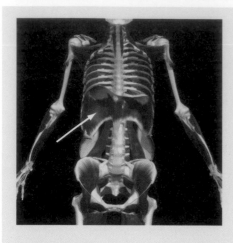

DIAPHRAGM

ORIGIN
- Costal part: inner surfaces of the cartilages and adjacent bony regions of ribs 6–12
- Sternal part: posterior side of the xiphoid process
- Crural (lumbar) part: (1) two aponeurotic arches covering the external surfaces of the quadratus lumborum and psoas major; (2) right and left crus, originating from the bodies of L1–L3 and their intervertebral disks

INSERTION
- Central tendon

ISOLATED FUNCTION
- Concentrically pulls the central tendon inferiorly, increasing the volume in the thoracic cavity

INTEGRATED FUNCTION
- Stabilizes the lumbo-pelvic-hip complex

Back Musculature

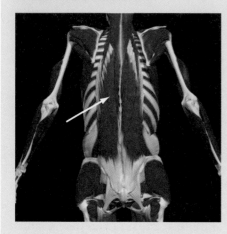

SUPERFICIAL ERECTOR SPINAE: ILIOCOSTALIS, LONGISSIMUS, AND SPINALIS

DIVISION IN THE GROUP
- Lumborum (lumbar)
- Thoracis (thoracic)
- Cervicis (cervical)

COMMON ORIGIN
- Iliac crest of the pelvis
- Sacrum
- Spinous and transverse process of T11–L5

INSERTION

ILIOCOSTALIS
- Lumborum: Inferior border of ribs 7–12
- Thoracis: Superior border of ribs 1–6
- Cervicis: Transverse process of C4–C6

LONGISSIMUS
- Thoracis: Transverse process T1–T12; ribs 2–12
- Cervicis: Transverse process of C6–C2
- Capitis: Mastoid process of the skull

SPINALIS
- Thoracis: Spinous process of T7–T4
- Cervicis: Spinous process of C3–C2
- Capitis: Between the superior and inferior nuchal lines on occipital bone of the skull

ISOLATED FUNCTION
- Concentrically accelerates spinal extension, rotation, and lateral flexion

INTEGRATED FUNCTION
- Eccentrically decelerates spinal flexion, rotation, and lateral flexion
- Dynamically stabilizes the spine during functional movements

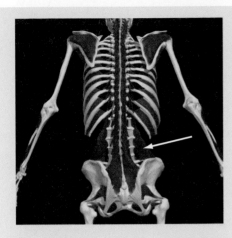

QUADRATUS LUMBORUM

ORIGIN
* Iliac crest of the pelvis

INSERTION
* 12th rib
* Transverse process L2–L5

ISOLATED FUNCTION
* Spinal lateral flexion

INTEGRATED FUNCTION
* Eccentrically decelerates contralateral later spinal flexion
* Isometrically stabilizes the lumbo-pelvic-hip complex

Transversospinalis Complex

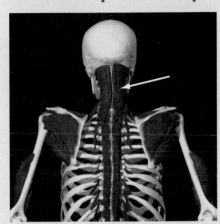

SEMISPINALIS: THORACIS, CERVICIS, CAPITIS

ORIGIN
* Thoracis: Transverse process T12–T7
* Cervicis: Transverse process T6–C4
* Capitis: Transverse process T6–C7
    Articular process C6–C4

INSERTION
* Thoracis: Spinous process T4–C6
* Cervicis: Spinous process C5–C2
* Capitis: Nuchal line of occipital bone of the skull

ISOLATED FUNCTION
* Concentrically produces spinal extension and lateral flexion
* Concentrically produces extension and contralateral rotation of the head

INTEGRATED FUNCTION
* Eccentrically decelerates lateral flexion of the spine
* Eccentrically decelerates flexion and contralateral rotation of the head
* Isometrically stabilizes the spine

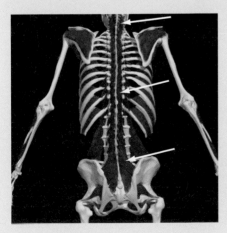

MULTIFIDUS

ORIGIN
* Posterior aspect of the sacrum
* Processes of the lumbar, thoracic, and cervical spine

INSERTION
* Spinous processes one to four segments above the origin

ISOLATED FUNCTION
* Concentrically accelerates spinal extension and contralateral rotation

INTEGRATED FUNCTION
* Eccentrically decelerates spinal flexion and rotation
* Isometrically stabilizes the spine

Shoulder Musculature

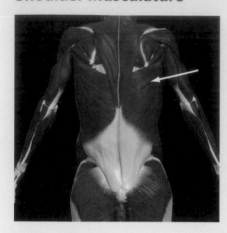

LATISSIMUS DORSI

ORIGIN
- Spinous processes of T7–T12
- Iliac crest of the pelvis
- Thoracolumbar fascia
- Ribs 9–12

INSERTION
- Inferior angle of the scapula
- Intertubercular groove of the humerus

ISOLATED FUNCTION
- Concentrically accelerates shoulder extension, adduction, and internal rotation

INTEGRATED FUNCTION
- Eccentrically decelerates shoulder flexion, abduction, and external rotation
- Eccentrically decelerates spinal flexion
- Isometrically stabilizes the lumbo-pelvic-hip complex and shoulder

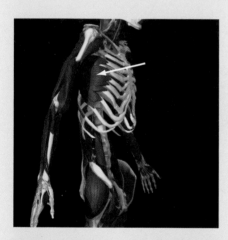

SERRATUS ANTERIOR

ORIGIN
- Ribs 4–12

INSERTION
- Medial border of the scapula

ISOLATED FUNCTION
- Concentrically accelerates scapular protraction

INTEGRATED FUNCTION
- Eccentrically decelerates dynamic scapular retraction
- Isometrically stabilizes the scapula

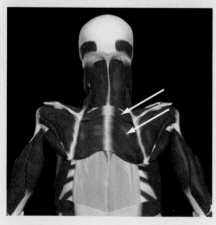

RHOMBOIDS

ORIGIN
- Spinous processes C7–T5

INSERTION
- Medial border of the scapula

ISOLATED FUNCTION
- Concentrically produces scapular retraction and downward rotation

INTEGRATED FUNCTION
- Eccentrically decelerates scapular protraction and upward rotation
- Isometrically stabilizes the scapula

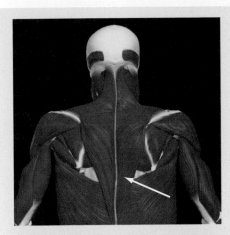

LOWER TRAPEZIUS

ORIGIN
- Spinous processes of T6–T12

INSERTION
- Spine of the scapula

ISOLATED FUNCTION
- Concentrically accelerates scapular depression

INTEGRATED FUNCTION
- Eccentrically decelerates scapular elevation
- Isometrically stabilizes the scapula

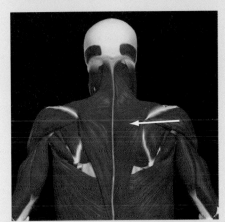

MIDDLE TRAPEZIUS

ORIGIN
- Spinous processes of T1–T5

INSERTION
- Acromion process of the scapula
- Superior aspect of the spine of the scapula

ISOLATED FUNCTION
- Concentrically accelerates scapular retraction

INTEGRATED FUNCTION
- Eccentrically decelerates scapular elevation
- Isometrically stabilizes the scapula

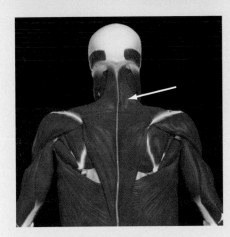

UPPER TRAPEZIUS

ORIGIN
- External occipital protuberance of the skull
- Spinous process of C7

INSERTION
- Lateral third of the clavicle
- Acromion process of the scapula

ISOLATED FUNCTION
- Concentrically accelerates cervical extension, lateral flexion, and rotation
- Concentrically accelerates scapular elevation

INTEGRATED FUNCTION
- Eccentrically decelerates cervical flexion, lateral flexion, and rotation
- Eccentrically decelerates scapular depression
- Isometrically stabilizes the cervical spine and scapula

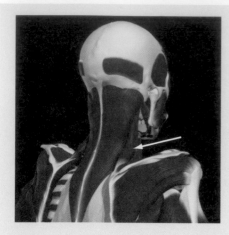

LEVATOR SCAPULAE

ORIGIN
- Transverse processes of C1–C4

INSERTION
- Superior vertebral border of the scapulae

ISOLATED FUNCTION
- Concentrically accelerates cervical extension, lateral flexion, and ipsilateral rotation when the scapulae is anchored
- Assists in elevation and downward rotation of the scapulae

INTEGRATED FUNCTION
- Eccentrically decelerates cervical flexion and contralateral cervical rotation and lateral flexion
- Eccentrically decelerates scapular depression and upward rotation when the neck is stabilized
- Stabilizes the cervical spine and scapulae

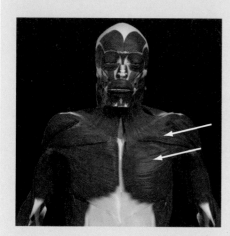

PECTORALIS MAJOR

ORIGIN
- Clavicular: Anterior surface of the clavicle
- Sternocostal: Anterior surface of the sternum, cartilage of ribs 1–7

INSERTION
- Greater tubercle of the humerus

ISOLATED FUNCTION
- Concentrically accelerates shoulder flexion (clavicular fibers), horizontal adduction, and internal rotation

INTEGRATED FUNCTION
- Eccentrically decelerates shoulder extension, horizontal abduction, and external rotation
- Isometrically stabilizes the shoulder girdle

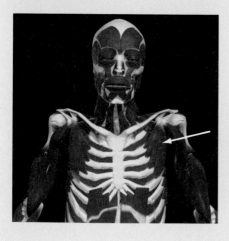

PECTORALIS MINOR

ORIGIN
- Ribs 3–5

INSERTION
- Coracoid process of the scapula

ISOLATED FUNCTION
- Concentrically protracts the scapula

INTEGRATED FUNCTION
- Eccentrically decelerates scapular retraction
- Isometrically stabilizes the shoulder girdle

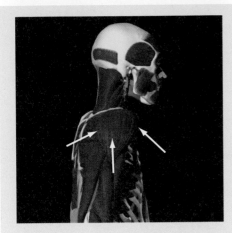

DELTOID—ANTERIOR, MIDDLE, AND POSTERIOR

ORIGIN
- Anterior: Lateral third of the clavicle
- Middle: Acromion process of the scapula
- Posterior: Spine of the scapula

INSERTION
- Deltoid tuberosity of the humerus

ISOLATED FUNCTION
- Anterior: Concentrically accelerates shoulder flexion and internal rotation
- Middle: Concentrically accelerates shoulder abduction
- Posterior: Concentrically accelerates shoulder extension and external rotation

INTEGRATED FUNCTION
- Anterior: Eccentrically decelerates shoulder extension and external rotation, isometrically stabilizes the shoulder girdle
- Middle: Eccentrically decelerates shoulder adduction, isometrically stabilizes the shoulder girdle
- Posterior: Eccentrically decelerates shoulder flexion and internal rotation, isometrically stabilizes the shoulder girdle

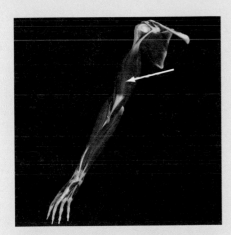

BICEPS BRACHII

ORIGIN
- Short head: Coracoid process of the scapula
- Long head: Tubercle above glenoid cavity on the humerus

INSERTION
- Radial tuberosity of the radius

ISOLATED FUNCTION
- Concentrically accelerates elbow flexion, supination of the radioulnar joint, and shoulder flexion

INTEGRATED FUNCTION
- Eccentrically decelerates elbow extension, pronation of the radioulnar joint, and shoulder extension
- Isometrically stabilizes the elbow and shoulder girdle

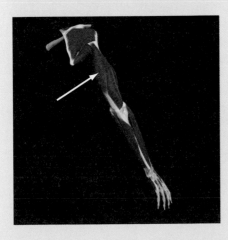

TRICEPS

ORIGIN
- Long head: Infraglenoid tubercle of the scapula
- Short head: Posterior humerus
- Medial head: Posterior humerus

INSERTION
- Olecranon process of the ulna

ISOLATED FUNCTION
- Concentrically accelerates elbow extension and shoulder extension

INTEGRATED FUNCTION
- Eccentrically decelerates elbow flexion and shoulder flexion
- Isometrically stabilizes the elbow and shoulder girdle

Rotator Cuff

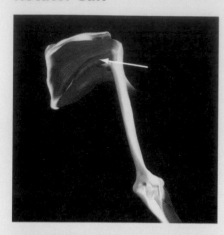

TERES MINOR

ORIGIN
- Lateral border of the scapula

INSERTION
- Greater tubercle of the humerus

ISOLATED FUNCTION
- Concentrically accelerates shoulder external rotation

INTEGRATED FUNCTION
- Eccentrically decelerates shoulder internal rotation
- Isometrically stabilizes the shoulder girdle

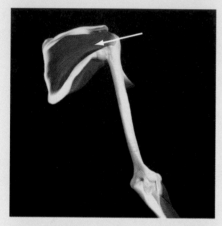

INFRASPINATUS

ORIGIN
- Infraspinous fossa of the scapula

INSERTION
- Middle facet of the greater tubercle of the humerus

ISOLATED FUNCTION
- Concentrically accelerates shoulder external rotation

INTEGRATED FUNCTION
- Eccentrically decelerates shoulder internal rotation
- Isometrically stabilizes the shoulder girdle

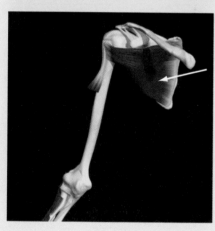

SUBSCAPULARIS

ORIGIN
- Subscapular fossa of the scapula

INSERTION
- Lesser tubercle of the humerus

ISOLATED FUNCTION
- Concentrically accelerates shoulder internal rotation

INTEGRATED FUNCTION
- Eccentrically decelerates shoulder external rotation
- Isometrically stabilizes the shoulder girdle

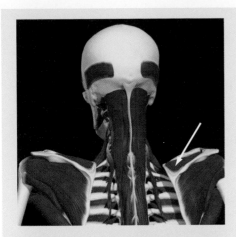

SUPRASPINATUS

ORIGIN
- Supraspinous fossa of the scapula

INSERTION
- Superior facet of the greater tubercle of the humerus

ISOLATED FUNCTION
- Concentrically accelerates abduction of the arm

INTEGRATED FUNCTION
- Eccentrically decelerates adduction of the arm
- Isometrically stabilizes the shoulder girdle

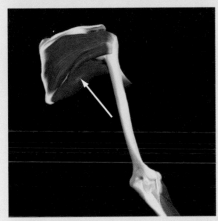

TERES MAJOR

ORIGIN
- Inferior angle of the scapula

INSERTION
- Lesser tubercle of the humerus

ISOLATED FUNCTION
- Concentrically accelerates shoulder internal rotation, adduction, and extension

INTEGRATED FUNCTION
- Eccentrically decelerates shoulder external rotation, abduction, and flexion
- Isometrically stabilizes the shoulder girdle

Neck Musculature

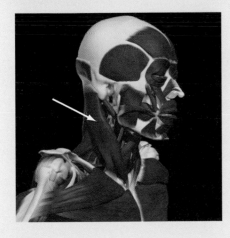

STERNOCLEIDOMASTOID

ORIGIN
- Sternal head: Top of manubrium of the sternum
- Clavicular head: Medial one third of the clavicle

INSERTION
- Mastoid process, lateral superior nuchal line of the occiput of the skull

ISOLATED FUNCTION
- Concentrically accelerates cervical flexion, rotation, and lateral flexion

INTEGRATED FUNCTION
- Eccentrically decelerates cervical extension, rotation, and lateral flexion
- Isometrically stabilizes the cervical spine and acromioclavicular joint

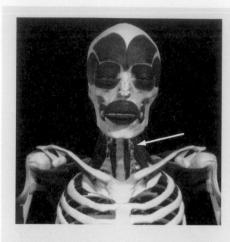

SCALENES

ORIGIN
- Transverse processes of C3–C7

INSERTION
- First and second ribs

ISOLATED FUNCTION
- Concentrically accelerates cervical flexion, rotation, and lateral flexion
- Assists rib elevation during inhalation

INTEGRATED FUNCTION
- Eccentrically decelerates cervical extension, rotation, and lateral flexion
- Isometrically stabilizes the cervical spine

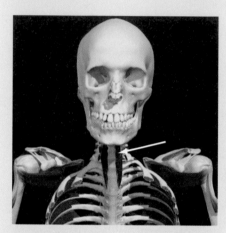

LONGUS COLI

ORIGIN
- Anterior portion of T1–T3

INSERTION
- Anterior and lateral C1

ISOLATED FUNCTION
- Concentrically accelerates cervical flexion, lateral flexion, and ipsilateral rotation

INTEGRATED FUNCTION
- Eccentrically decelerates cervical extension, lateral flexion, and contralateral rotation
- Isometrically stabilizes the cervical spine

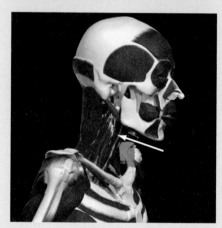

LONGUS CAPITIS

ORIGIN
- Transverse processes of C3–C6

INSERTION
- Inferior occipital bone

ISOLATED FUNCTION
- Concentrically accelerates cervical flexion and lateral flexion

INTEGRATED FUNCTION
- Eccentrically decelerates cervical extension
- Isometrically stabilizes the cervical spine

SUMMARY OF THE FUNCTIONAL ANATOMY OF MUSCLES

This review should make it clear that all muscles function in all three planes of motion (sagittal, frontal, and transverse) and through the entire muscle action spectrum (eccentric, isometric, and concentric). In addition, it is evident that several muscles work synergistically to produce force, stabilize the body, and reduce force.

The more functional anatomy is understood, the more specific exercise prescription can become. A lack of understanding of the synergistic function of the

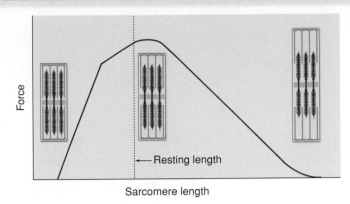

Figure 4.11 Length-tension relationship.

kinetic chain muscles in all three planes of motion commonly leads to a lack of optimum performance and the potential of developing muscle imbalances.

Muscular Force

Force: An influence applied by one object to another, which results in an acceleration or deceleration of the second object.

Force is defined as the interaction between two entities or bodies that result in either the acceleration or deceleration of an object.[1,2,9] Forces are characterized by magnitude (how much) and direction (which way they are moving).[1,2,9] The kinetic chain is designed to manipulate variable forces from a multitude of directions to effectively produce movement. As such, the health and fitness professional must gain an understanding of some of the more pertinent forces that the kinetic chain must deal with and how they affect motion.

Length-Tension Relationships

Length-tension relationship: The length at which a muscle can produce the greatest force.

Length-tension relationship refers to the length at which a muscle can produce the greatest force.[10-16] There is an optimal muscle length at which the actin and myosin filaments in the sarcomere have the greatest degree of overlap (Figure 4-11). This results in the ability of myosin to make a maximal amount of connections with actin and thus results in the potential for maximal force production of that muscle. Lengthening a muscle beyond this optimal length and then stimulating it reduces the amount of actin and myosin overlap, reducing force production (Figure 4-11). Similarly, shortening a muscle too much and then stimulating it places the actin and myosin in a state of maximal overlap and allows for no further movement to occur between the filaments, reducing its force output (Figure 4-11).[10-16]

This concept is vitally important to the health and fitness professional and coincides with the previously discussed concept of joint alignment. Just as the position of one joint can drastically affect other joints, it can also affect the muscles that surround the joint. If muscle lengths are altered as a result of misaligned joints (i.e., poor posture), then they will not be able to generate proper force to allow for efficient movement. This is the beginning of understanding the kinetic chain and how it works. If one component of the kinetic chain (nervous, skeletal, or muscular) is dysfunctional, it will have a direct effect on the others.

Force-Velocity Curve

The force-velocity curve refers to the ability of muscles to produce force with increasing velocity (Figure 4-12). As the velocity of a concentric muscle contraction increases, its ability to produce force decreases. This is thought to be the result of overlapping the actin filament that may interfere with its ability to crossbridge with myosin. Conversely, with eccentric muscle action, as the velocity of muscle action increases the ability to develop force increases. This is believed to be the result of the use of the elastic component of the connective tissue surrounding and within the muscle.[1,4,9,17]

Muscle force
Velocity of contraction

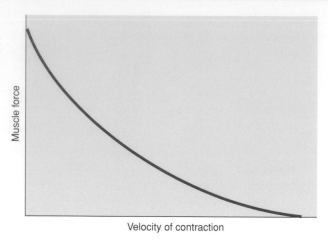

Figure 4.12 The force-velocity curve.

Force-Couple Relationships

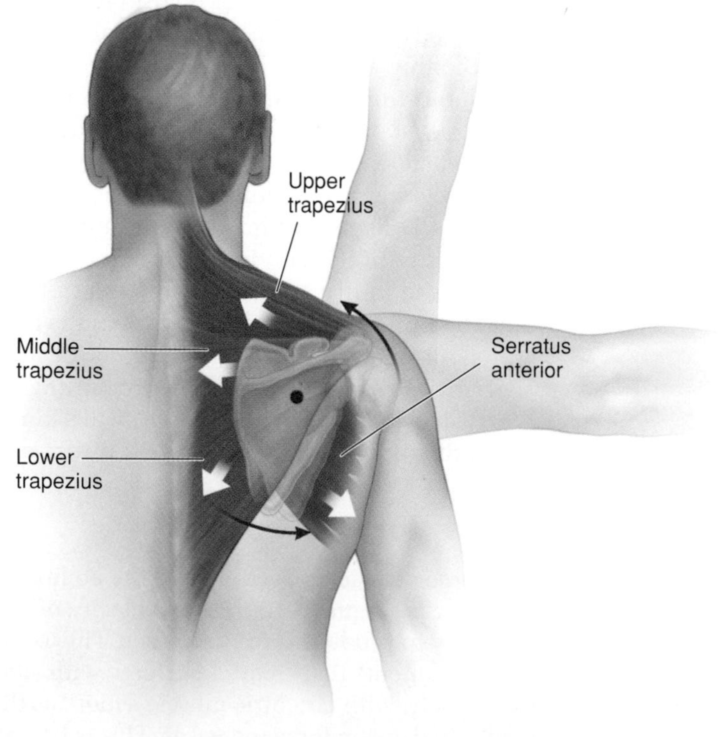

Force-couple: Muscle groups moving together to produce movement around a joint.

Muscles produce a force that is transmitted to bones through their connective tissues (tendons). Because muscles are recruited as groups, many muscles will transmit force onto their respective bones, creating movement at the joints.[6,18-20] This synergistic action of muscles to produce movement around a joint is also known as a **force-couple**.[4,8] Muscles in a force-couple provide divergent pulls on the bone or bones they connect with. This is a result of the fact that each muscle has different attachment sites, pulls at a different angle, and creates a different force on that joint. The motion that results from these forces is dependent on the structure of the joint and the collective pull of each muscle involved (Figure 4-13, Table 4-3).[2,4]

In reality, however, every movement we produce must involve all muscle actions (eccentric, isometric, concentric) and all functions (agonists, synergists,

Upper trapezius
Middle trapezius
Lower trapezius
Serratus anterior

Figure 4.13 Force-couple relationship.

Table 4.3	
Common Force-Couples	
Muscles	**Movement Created**
Internal and external obliques	Trunk rotation
Upper trapezius and the lower portion of the serratus anterior	Upward rotation of the scapula
Gluteus maximus, quadriceps, and calf muscles	Produce hip and knee extension during walking, running, stair climbing, etc.
Gastrocnemius, peroneus longus, and tibialis posterior	Performing plantarflexion at the foot and ankle complex
Deltoid and rotator cuff	Performing shoulder abduction

stabilizers, and antagonists) to ensure proper joint motion as well as to eliminate unwanted motion. Therefore, all muscles working together for the production of proper movement are said to be working in a force-couple.[2] To ensure that the kinetic chain moves in the right manner, it must exhibit proper force-couple relationships. This can only happen if the muscles are at the right length-tension relationships and the joints have proper arthrokinematics (or joint motion). Collectively, proper length-tension relationships, force-couple relationships, and arthrokinematics allow for proper sensorimotor integration and ultimately proper and efficient movement.[2]

Muscular Leverage and Arthrokinematics

The amount of force that the kinetic chain can produce is not only dependent on motor unit recruitment and muscle size, but also on the leverage of the muscles and bones.[1,2,4] In the kinetic chain, the bones act as levers that are moved by the force of the muscles. These levers are moved around different axes, which are our joints. This movement around an axis can be termed **rotary motion** and implies that the levers (bones) rotate around the axis (joints).[1,2,4] This "turning" effect of the joint is often referred to as **torque** (Figure 4-14).[1,2,4]

In resistance training, bones provide the means by which we can attach forces (or torque) to our joints. These joints must be reduced eccentrically, stabilized (or held) isometrically, or overcome concentrically by the muscles. Because the neuromuscular system is ultimately responsible for manipulating force, the amount of leverage the kinetic chain will have (for any given movement) depends

Rotary motion: Movement of the bones around the joints.

Torque: A force that produces rotation.

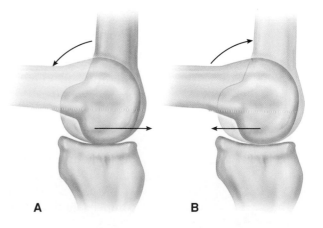

Figure 4.14 Torque.   **A**   **B**

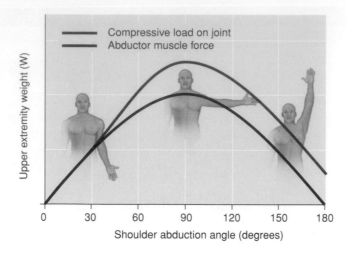

Figure 4.15 Weight distance and torque relationship.

on the leverage of the muscles in relation to the resistance. The difference between the distance that the weight is from the center of the joint and the muscle's attachment and line of pull (direction that the tendon pulls) is from the joint will determine the efficiency with which the muscles will be able to manipulate the movement.[1,2,4] Because we cannot alter the attachment sites or the line of pull of our muscles, the easiest way to alter the amount of torque generated at a joint is to move the resistance. In other words, the closer the weight is to the joint, the less torque it creates. The farther away the weight is from the joint, the more torque it creates (Figure 4-15).

For example, to hold a dumbbell straight out to the side at arm's length (shoulder abduction), the weight may be approximately 24 inches from the center of the shoulder joint. The prime mover for shoulder abduction is the deltoid muscle. Let's say its attachment is approximately 2 inches from the joint center. That is a disparity of 22 inches (or roughly 12 times the difference). However, if the weight is moved closer to the joint center, let's say to the elbow, the resistance is only approximately 12 inches from the joint center. Now the difference is only 10 inches or 5 times greater. Essentially, the weight was reduced by half. Many people performing side lateral raises with dumbbells (raising dumbbells out to your side) do this inadvertently by bending their elbow and bringing the weight closer to the shoulder joint.

Health and fitness professionals can use this principle as a regression to exercises that are too demanding by reducing the torque placed on the kinetic chain, or as a progression to increase the torque and place a greater demand on the kinetic chain.

SUMMARY

The study of biomechanics looks at how internal and external forces affect the way the body moves. To understand the body and communicate about it effectively, a trainer must know the terminology for the various anatomic locations. It is also important to know how the body moves in the sagittal, frontal, and transverse planes as well as the joint motions in each of these planes.

Muscles move in one of three ways: eccentrically (to decelerate force), isometrically (to stabilize), or concentrically (to accelerate force). All muscles have isolated and integrated functions to create these various actions. Each muscle should be studied at length to examine its functions as well as how it moves synergistically with others.

Muscles are influenced by outside forces from a multitude of directions. To compensate they produce corresponding forces in groups to move bones and joints, in force-couple actions. However, the amount of force that can be produced is dependent on leverage (or how far a weight being moved is from the joint). This leverage directly affects rotary motion and torque.

Motor Behavior

Motor behavior: The process of the body responding to internal and external stimuli.

Motor behavior is the kinetic chain's response to environmental stimuli (internal and external). To study it, we must examine the manner with which the nervous, skeletal, and muscular systems interact to produce movement via sensory information from internal and external environments. In this text, the study of motor behavior consists of the studies of motor control (or how the kinetic chain creates movement) and motor learning (or how the kinetic chain learns those movements).[2]

MOTOR CONTROL

Motor control: The study of posture and movements and the involved structures and mechanisms that the central nervous system uses to assimilate and integrate sensory information with previous experiences.

For the kinetic chain to move in an organized and efficient manner, it must exhibit precise control over its segments. This segmental control is an integrated process involving all components of the kinetic chain (neural, skeletal, and muscular) to produce appropriate motor responses. This process (and the study of these movements) is known as **motor control**. More specifically, it looks at the involved structures and mechanisms that the nervous system uses to gather all sensory information (internal and external) and integrates it all with previous experiences to produce a motor response.[2,6,18-21] Essentially, motor control is concerned with those neural structures that are involved with motor behavior and how they produce movement.[19]

Muscles Synergies

Synergies: Groups of muscles that are recruited by the central nervous system to provide movement.

One of the most important concepts in motor control is that muscles are recruited by the central nervous system as groups (or **synergies**).[6,18-20] This simplifies movement by allowing muscles and joints to operate as a functional unit.[11] Through practice of proper movement patterns (proper exercise technique), these synergies become more fluent and automated (Table 4-4).

Proprioception

Proprioception: The cumulative sensory input to the central nervous system from all mechanoreceptors that sense position and limb movements.

The mechanoreceptors, discussed in the previous chapter, collectively feed the nervous system with a form of sensory information known as **proprioception**. Proprioception uses information from the mechanoreceptors (muscle spindle, Golgi tendon organ, and joint receptors) to provide information about body position, movement, and sensation, as it pertains to muscle and joint force.[19] Proprioception is a vital source of information that the nervous system uses to gather information about the environment to produce the most efficient movement.[22] Research has demonstrated that proprioception is altered after injury. This becomes relevant to the health fitness professional as 85% of the adult population experiences low back pain, and an estimated 80,000 to 100,000 anterior cruciate ligament (ACL) injuries occur annually as well as more than 2 million ankle sprains. This means that many of today's health club members may have altered proprioception as a result of past injuries. This provides a rationale for core and balance training to enhance one's proprioceptive capabilities, increasing postural control and decreasing tissue overload.

Sensorimotor Integration

Sensorimotor integration: The cooperation of the nervous and muscular system in gathering information, interpreting, and executing movement.

Sensorimotor integration is the ability of the nervous system to gather and interpret sensory information and to select and execute the proper motor response.[2,18,22-28]

Table 4.4

Common Muscle Synergies

Exercise	Muscle Synergies
Squat 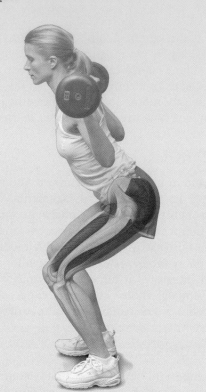	Quadriceps, hamstrings, gluteus maximus
Shoulder press 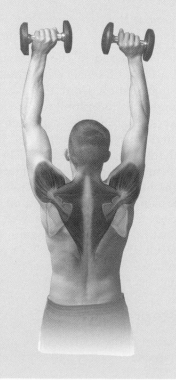	Deltoid, rotator cuff, trapezius

The definition tells us that the nervous system ultimately dictates movement. Sensorimotor integration is only as effective as the quality of incoming sensory information.[2,25-27] If individuals train with improper form, improper sensory information will be delivered to the central nervous system, leading to movement compensations and potential injury. Thus, it is important to design proper programs and train with correct technique. For example, if an individual consistently performs a chest press while rounding and elevating their shoulders, this can lead to altered length-tension relationships of muscles (decreased force production), altered force-couple relationships (improper recruitment pattern of muscles), and altered arthrokinematics (improper joint motion). This can ultimately lead to shoulder impingement.

MOTOR LEARNING

Motor learning: Repeated practice of motor control processes, which lead to a change in the ability to produce complex movements.

Motor learning is the integration of these motor control processes, with practice and experience, leading to a relatively permanent change in the capacity to produce skilled movements.[2,18,29] Essentially, the study of motor learning looks at how movements are learned and retained for future use. Examples would include riding a bike, throwing a baseball, playing the piano, or even performing a squat. In each of these instances, proper practice and experience will lead to a permanent change in one's ability to perform the movement efficiently. For this to occur, the utilization of feedback will be necessary to ensure optimal development of these skilled movements.

Feedback

Feedback: The use of sensory information and sensorimotor integration to help the kinetic chain in motor learning.

Feedback is the utilization of sensory information and sensorimotor integration to aid the kinetic chain in the development of permanent neural representations of motor patterns. This allows for efficient movement. This is achieved through two different forms of feedback. These are internal (or sensory) feedback and external (or augmented) feedback.

INTERNAL FEEDBACK

Internal feedback: The process whereby sensory information is used by the body to reactively monitor movement and the environment.

Internal feedback (or sensory feedback) is the process whereby sensory information is used by the body via length-tension relationships (posture), force-couple relationships, and arthrokinematics to reactively monitor movement and the environment. Essentially, internal (sensory) feedback acts as a guide, steering the kinetic chain to the proper force, speed, and amplitude of movement patterns. Thus, it is important to have proper form when exercising to ensure that the incoming sensory feedback is correct information, allowing for optimal sensorimotor integration and ideal structural and functional efficiency.

EXTERNAL FEEDBACK

External feedback: Information provided by some external source, such as a health and fitness professional, videotape, mirror, or heart rate monitor to supplement the internal environment.

External feedback is simply information provided by some external source, such as a health and fitness professional, videotape, mirror, or heart rate monitor. It is used to supplement internal feedback.[18,30] External feedback provides the client with another source of information that allows him or her to associate whether the achieved movement pattern was "good" or "bad" with what he or she is feeling internally.

Two major forms of external feedback are knowledge of results and knowledge of performance (Figure 4-16).[18,28-31] *Knowledge of results* are used after the completion of a movement to help inform the client about the outcome of their performance. This should come from the health and fitness professional as well as from the client. An example of this is the fitness professional telling a client that their squats were "good" and asking the client if they could "feel" or "see" their form. By getting the client to become involved with the knowledge of results, they increase their awareness and augment the other forms of sensory feedback. This can be done after each repetition, after a few repetitions, or after the set is completed. As

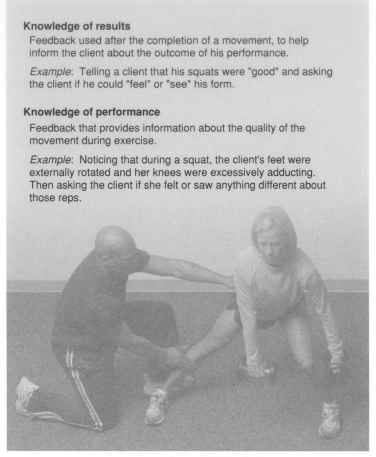

Knowledge of results

Feedback used after the completion of a movement, to help inform the client about the outcome of his performance.

Example: Telling a client that his squats were "good" and asking the client if he could "feel" or "see" his form.

Knowledge of performance

Feedback that provides information about the quality of the movement during exercise.

Example: Noticing that during a squat, the client's feet were externally rotated and her knees were excessively adducting. Then asking the client if she felt or saw anything different about those reps.

Figure 4.16 Forms of external feedback.

the client becomes more familiar with the desired technique of a movement (exercise), knowledge of results from the health and fitness professional should be given less frequently. This improves neuromuscular efficiency.[30]

Knowledge of performance provides information about the quality of the movement during an exercise. An example of this would be noticing that during a squat, the client's feet were externally rotated and the knees were excessively adducting and then, asking the client whether her or she felt or saw anything different about those reps. Again, this gets the client involved in his or her own sensory process. It should be given less frequently as the client becomes more proficient.[30]

These forms of external feedback allow for the identification of performance errors. They are also an important component in motivation. Furthermore, they give the client supplemental sensory input to help create an awareness of the desired action.[18,29-31] However, it is important to state that a client must not become dependent on external feedback, especially from the health and fitness professional, as this may detract from his or her responsiveness to internal sensory input.[18,29-31] This could alter sensorimotor integration and affect the client's motor learning and, ultimately, movement patterns (especially in the absence of a health and fitness professional).

SUMMARY

Each system of the kinetic chain is interdependent. The entire chain must work together to gather information from internal and external environments to create and learn movements (or motor behavior). The body uses proprioception, sensorimotor integration, and muscle synergies to create efficient movement (motor control). Then, repeated practice, as well as internal and external feedback, allows this efficient movement to be reproduced (motor learning).

Review Questions

1 *Abduction and adduction occur in which plane of motion?*

2 *Lowering a barbell down toward the chest during a bench press is an example of which kind of muscle contraction?*

   a. Eccentric

   b. Concentric

   c. Isometric

3 *Which is considered internal feedback used by the body to monitor movement?*

   a. Length-tension relationships

   b. Force-couple relationships

   c. Arthrokinematics

   d. All of the above

4 *Sensorimotor integration requires proprioception.*

   a. True

   b. False

5 *A heart rate monitor is an example of which type of feedback?*

   a. Internal

   b. External

REFERENCES

1. Hamill J, Knutzen JM. Biomechanical Basis of Human Movement. Baltimore: Williams & Wilkins, 1995.
2. Norkin CC, Levangie PK. Joint Structure and Function: A Comprehensive Analysis, 2nd ed. Philadelphia: FA Davis Company, 1992.
3. Kendall FP, McCreary EK, Provance PG. Muscles Testing and Function, 4th ed. Baltimore: Lippincott Williams & Wilkins, 1993.
4. Luttgens K, Hamilton N. Kinesiology: Scientific Basis of Human Motion, 9th ed. Dubuque, IA: Brown & Benchmark Publishers, 1997.
5. Gray GW. Chain Reaction Festival. Adrian, MI: Wynn Marketing, 1996.
6. Brooks VB. The neural basis of motor control. New York: Oxford University Press, 1986.
7. Gel'fand IM, Gurfinkel VS, Tsetlin ML, Shik ML. Some problems in the analysis of movements. In: Gel'fand IM, Gurfinkel VS, Formin SV, Tsetlin ML (eds). Models of the Structural-Functional Organization of Certain Biological Systems. Cambridge, MA: MIT Press, 1971.
8. Gambetta V. Everything in balance. Train Cond 1996;1(2)15–21.
9. Enoka RM. Neuromechanical Basis of Kinesiology, 2nd ed. Champaign, IL: Human Kinetics, 1994.
10. Milner-Brown A. Neuromuscular Physiology. Thousand Oaks, CA: National Academy of Sports Medicine, 2001.
11. Fox SI. Human Physiology, 5th ed. Dubuque, IA: Wm C Brown Publishers, 1996.
12. Vander A, Sherman J, Luciano D. Human Physiology: The Mechanisms of Body Function, 8th ed. New York: McGraw-Hill, 2001.
13. Hamill J, Knutzen JM. Biomechanical Basis of Human Movement. Baltimore: Williams & Wilkins, 1995.
14. Watkins J. Structure and Function of the Musculoskeletal System. Champaign, IL: Human Kinetics, 1999.
15. Luttgens K, Hamilton N. Kinesiology: Scientific Basis of Human Motion, 9th ed. Dubuque, IA: Brown & Benchmark Publishers, 1997.

16. Norkin CC, Levangie PK. Joint Structure and Function: A Comprehensive Analysis, 2nd ed. Philadelphia: FA Davis Company, 1992.

17. Fleck SJ, Kraemer WJ. Designing Resistance Training Programs, 2nd ed. Champaign, IL: Human Kinetics, 1997.

18. Rose DJ. A Multi Level Approach to the Study Of Motor Control and Learning. Needham Heights, MA: Allyn & Bacon, 1997.

19. Newton RA. Neural systems underlying motor control. In: Montgomery PC, Connoly BH (eds). Motor Control and Physical Therapy: Theoretical Framework and Practical Applications. Hixson, TN: Chattanooga Group, Inc, 1991.

20. Kelso JAS. Dynamic Patterns. The Self-Organization of Brain and Behavior. Cambridge, MA: The MIT Press, 1995.

21. Gurfinkel VS, Cordo PJ. The scientific legacy of Nikolai Berstein. In: Latash ML (ed). Progress in Motor Control, Vol 1. Berstein's Traditions in Movement Studies. Champaign, IL: Human Kinetics, 1998.

22. Ghez C. The control of movement. In: Kandel E, Schwartz J, Jessel T (eds). Principles of Neuroscience. New York: Elsevier Science, 1991.

23. Biedert RM. Contribution of the three levels of nervous system motor control: spinal cord, lower brain, cerebral cortex. In: Lephart SM, Fu FH (eds). Proprioception and Neuromuscular Control in Joint Stability. Champaign, IL: Human Kinetics, 2000.

24. Boucher JP. Training and exercise science. In: Liebension C (ed). Rehabilitation of the Spine. Baltimore: Williams & Wilkins, 1996.

25. Janda V, Va Vrova M. Sensory motor stimulation. In: Liebension C (ed). Rehabilitation of the Spine. Baltimore: Williams & Wilkins, 1996.

26. Gagey PM, Gentez R. Postural disorders of the body axis. In: Liebension C (ed). Rehabilitation of the Spine. Baltimore: Williams & Wilkins, 1996.

27. Drury DG. Strength and proprioception. Ortho Phys Ther Clin 2000;9(4):549–561.

28. Grigg P. Peripheral neural mechanisms in proprioception. J Sport Rehab 1994;3:2–17.

29. Schmidt RA, Lee TD. Motor Control and Learning: A Behavioral Emphasis, 3rd ed. Champaign, IL: Human Kinetics, 1999.

30. Swinnen SP. Information feedback for motor skill learning: a review. In: Zelaznik HN (ed). Advances in Motor Learning and Control. Champaign, IL: Human Kinetics, 1996.

31. Schmidt RA, Wrisberg CA. Motor Learning and Performance, 2nd ed. Champaign, IL: Human Kinetics, 2000.

PART 2

ASSESSMENTS, TRAINING CONCEPTS, AND PROGRAM DESIGN

POWER

STRENGTH

STABILIZATION

Phase 1 STABILIZATION ENDURANCE

Phase 2 STRENGTH ENDURANCE

HYPERTROPHY

MAXIMAL STRENGTH

Fitness Assessment

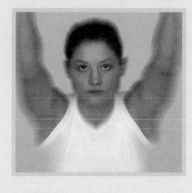

OBJECTIVES

After completing this chapter, you will be able to:

- Explain the components and function of an integrated fitness assessment.
- Ask appropriate general and medical questions to gather subjective information from clients.
- Understand the importance of posture and how it relates to movement observation.
- Perform a systematic assessment to obtain objective information about clients.

KEY TERMS

Functional strength	Objective information	Posture
Integrated fitness assessment	Postural distortion patterns	Skin-fold calipers
Neuromuscular efficiency	Postural equilibrium	Subjective information

OVERVIEW OF FITNESS ASSESSMENTS

Designing an individualized, systematic, integrated fitness assessment can only be properly accomplished by having an understanding of a client's goals, needs, and abilities. This entails knowing what a client wants to gain from a training program, what a client needs from their program to successfully accomplish their goal(s), and how capable they are (structurally and functionally) of performing the required tasks within an integrated program. The information necessary to create the right program for a specific individual (or group of individuals) comes through a proper fitness assessment. The remainder of this chapter will focus on a fitness assessment for the health and fitness professional.

Definition

A fitness assessment is a systematic problem-solving method that provides the health and fitness professional with a basis for making educated decisions about exercise and acute variable selection. Assessments provide an ongoing gathering of information, allowing the health and fitness professional to modify and progress a client through an integrated training program. Fitness assessments allow the health and fitness professional to continually monitor a client's needs, functional capabilities, and physiologic effects of exercise, enabling the client to realize the full benefit of an individualized training program.

It is important that the health and fitness professional understand that a fitness assessment is not designed to diagnose any condition, but rather to observe each client's individual structural and functional status. Furthermore, the fitness assessment presented by NASM is not intended to replace a medical examination. If a client exhibits extreme difficulty or pain with any observation or exercise, the health and fitness professional should refer the client to his or her physician or qualified health-care provider to identify any underlying cause (Table 5-1).

WHAT INFORMATION DOES A FITNESS ASSESSMENT PROVIDE?

A fitness assessment provides the health and fitness professional with a three-dimensional representation of the client. It gives insight into the client's past, present, and perhaps their future. The assessment covers information regarding habits, hobbies, movement abilities, and past and present medical history. Essentially, a fitness assessment allows the health and fitness professional to see the current structure and function of a client.

By gathering information through the fitness assessment, a fundamental representation of a client's goals, needs, and status can be created. This enables proper construction of an integrated training program that is individualized specifically for each client. When conducting a fitness assessment, it is essential to use a variety of observation methods to obtain a balanced overview of a client (Figure 5-1).

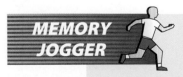

MEMORY JOGGER

Keep in mind that the program you design for your client is only as good as your assessment! The more information you know about your client, the more individualized the program. This ensures the safety and effectiveness of the program, thus creating greater value in the health and fitness professional.

Table 5.1

Guidelines for Health and Fitness Professionals

Do Not	Do
Diagnose medical conditions.	Obtain exercise or health guidelines from a physician, physical therapist, or registered dietitian. Follow national consensus guidelines of exercise prescription for medical disorders. Screen clients for exercise limitations. Identify potential risk factors for clients through screening procedures. Refer clients who experience difficulty or pain or exhibit other symptoms to a qualified medical practitioner.
Prescribe treatment.	Design individualized, systematic progressive exercise programs. Refer clients to a qualified medical practitioner for medical exercise prescription.
Prescribe diets or recommend specific supplements.	Provide clients with general information on healthy eating, according to the food pyramid. Refer clients to a qualified dietitian or nutritionist for specific diet plans.
Provide treatment of any kind for injury or disease.	Refer clients to a qualified medical practitioner for treatment of injury or disease. Use exercise to help clients improve overall health. Assist clients in following the medical advice of a physician or therapist.
Provide rehabilitation services for clients.	Design exercise programs for clients after they are released from rehabilitation. Provide postrehabilitation services.
Provide counseling services for clients.	Act as a coach for clients. Provide general information. Refer clients to a qualified counselor or therapist.

Components of a Fitness Assessment

Subjective Information
General and medical history:
Occupation, Lifestyle, Medical, and Personal Information

Objective Information
Physiologic assessments
Body composition testing
Cardiorespiratory assessments
Static and dynamic postural assessments
Performance assessments

Figure 5.1 Components of a fitness assessment.

SUMMARY

A health and fitness professional's primary responsibility is to safely and effectively guide clients to successful attainment of their goals. To do so requires a comprehensive understanding of clients' personal and professional backgrounds as well as their physical capabilities and desires. The fitness assessment is a comprehensive tool to systematically gather subjective and objective information about clients and use the information appropriately. It is *not* designed to diagnose any condition or replace a medical examination. Health and fitness professionals should refer clients to qualified health-care providers whenever necessary.

Subjective Information Provided in the Fitness Assessment

TYPES OF SUBJECTIVE INFORMATION

Subjective information is gathered from a prospective client to give the health and fitness professional feedback regarding personal history such as occupation, lifestyle, and medical background.

General and Medical History

Gathering personal background information about a client can be very valuable. It can help a health and fitness professional to understand a client's physical condition and can also provide insight to what types of imbalances they may exhibit. One of the easiest forms of gathering this information is through a questionnaire (Figure 5-2).[1] The Physical Activity Readiness Questionnaire (PAR-Q) is a questionnaire that has been designed to help qualify a person for low to moderate to high activity levels.[1,2] Furthermore, it aids in identifying people for whom certain activities may not be appropriate or who may need further medical attention.

The PAR-Q is directed toward detecting any possible cardiorespiratory dysfunction, such as coronary heart disease. It is a good beginning point for gathering personal background information concerning a prospective client's cardiorespiratory function. However, it is only one component of a thorough fitness assessment. Although this information is extremely important for a health and fitness professional, asking other questions can provide additional information about a client. This includes questions about a client's general and medical history.

	Questions	Yes	No
1	Has your doctor ever said that you have a heart condition and that you should only perform physical activity recommended by a doctor?		
2	Do you feel pain in your chest when you perform physical activity?		
3	In the past month, have you had chest pain when you are not performing any physical activity?		
4	Do you lose your balance because of dizziness or do you ever lose consciousness?		
5	Do you have a bone or joint problem that could be made worse by a change in your physical activity?		
6	Is your doctor currently prescribing any medication for your blood pressure or for a heart condition?		
7	Do you know of *any* other reason why you should not engage in physical activity?		

If you have answered "Yes" to one or more of the above questions, consult your physician before engaging in physical activity. Tell your physician which questions you answered "Yes" to. After a medical evaluation, seek advice from your physician on what type of activity is suitable for your current condition.

Figure 5.2 Sample Physical Activity Readiness Questionnaire (PAR-Q).

GENERAL HISTORY

Asking some very basic questions about a client's history and personal background can provide a wealth of information. Two important areas to start with are occupation and lifestyle.

Occupation

Knowing a client's occupation can provide the health and fitness professional with insight into what his or her movement capacity is and what kinds of movement patterns are performed throughout the day. Examples of typical questions are shown in Figure 5-3.

By obtaining this information, a health and fitness professional can begin to recognize important clues about the structure and, ultimately, the function of a client. Each question provides relevant information.

EXTENDED PERIODS OF SITTING

This is a very important question that provides a lot of information. First, if a client is sitting a large portion of the day, the client's hips are flexed for prolonged periods of time. This, in turn, can lead to tight hip flexors that can cause postural imbalances within the kinetic chain. Second, if a client is sitting for prolonged periods of time, especially at a computer, there is a tendency for the shoulders and head to fatigue under the constant influence of gravity. This often leads to a postural imbalance of rounding of the shoulders and head.

REPETITIVE MOVEMENTS

Repetitive movements can create a pattern overload to muscles and joints, which may lead to tissue trauma and eventually kinetic chain dysfunction.[3] This can be seen in jobs that require a lot of overhead work such as construction or painting. Working with the arms overhead for long periods of time may lead to shoulder soreness that could be the result of tightness in the latissimus dorsi and weakness in the rotator cuff. This imbalance does not allow for proper shoulder motion or stabilization during activity.

DRESS SHOES

Wearing shoes with a heel puts the ankle complex in a plantarflexion position for extended periods of time. This can lead to tightness in the gastrocnemius and

	Questions	Yes	No
1	What is your current occupation?		
2	Does your occupation require extended periods of sitting?		
3	Does your occupation require extended periods of repetitive movements? (If yes, please explain.)		
4	Does your occupation require you to wear shoes with a heel (dress shoes)?		
5	Does your occupation cause you anxiety (mental stress)?		

Figure 5.3 Sample questions: client occupation.

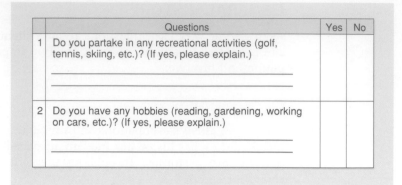

Figure 5.4 Sample questions: client lifestyle.

soleus, causing postural imbalance, such as overpronation at the foot and ankle complex (flattening of the arch of the foot).

MENTAL STRESS

Mental stress or anxiety can lead to a dysfunctional breathing pattern that can further lead to postural distortion and kinetic chain dysfunction.[4,5] Please refer to Chapter 3 (Dysfunctional Breathing) for details.

Lifestyle

Questions pertaining to a client's lifestyle will reflect what a client does in his or her free time. This is generally known as their recreation and hobbies. Examples of typical questions are shown in Figure 5-4.

As discussed earlier, each of the questions above provides relevant information.

RECREATION

Recreation, in the context of assessment, refers to a client's physical activities outside of the work environment. By finding out what recreational activities a client performs, a health and fitness professional can better design a program to fit these needs.

For example, many clients like to golf, ski, play tennis, or perform a variety of other sporting activities in their spare time. Proper forms of training must be incorporated to ensure that clients are trained in a manner that optimizes the efficiency of the kinetic chain, without predisposing it to injury.

HOBBIES

Hobbies, in the context of assessment, refer to activities that a client may partake in regularly, but are not necessarily athletic in nature. Examples include gardening, working on cars, playing cards, reading, watching television, or playing video games. In many of these cases, the client does not receive a lot of physical stimulation.

In instances in which clients have hobbies that require little physical activity, it is still necessary to take lifestyle choices into account to create a properly planned integrated training program. It should be noted, however, that these clients probably will not be at the same level of training as someone who plays a lot of tennis.

MEDICAL HISTORY

Finding out a client's medical history (Figure 5-5) is absolutely crucial. Most importantly, it provides the health and fitness professional with information about any

	Questions	Yes	No
1	Have you ever had any pain or injuries (ankle, knee, hip, back, shoulder, etc.)? (If yes, please explain.)		
2	Have you ever had any surgeries? (If yes, please explain.)		
3	Has a medical doctor ever diagnosed you with a chronic disease, such as coronary heart disease, coronary artery disease, hypertension (high blood pressure), high cholesterol, or diabetes? (If yes, please explain.)		
4	Are you currently taking any medication? (If yes, please list.)		

Figure 5.5   Sample questions: client medical history.

life-threatening chronic diseases (such as coronary heart disease, high blood pressure, or diabetes).[1] Furthermore, it provides information about the structure and function of the client. Some important areas to cover include past injuries, surgeries, and chronic conditions.

Past Injuries

Inquiring about a client's past injuries can illuminate possible dysfunctions. There is a vast array of research that has demonstrated that past injuries affect the functioning of the kinetic chain. This is especially true of the following injuries:

1. Ankle sprains: Ankle sprains have been shown to decrease the neural control to the gluteus medius and gluteus maximus muscles. This, in turn, can lead to poor control of the lower extremities during many functional activities, which can eventually lead to injury.[6-15]

2. Knee injuries involving ligaments: Knee injury can cause a decrease in the neural control to muscles that stabilize the patella (kneecap) and lead to further injury. Knee injuries that are not the result of contact (noncontact injuries) are often the result of ankle or hip dysfunctions, such as the result of an ankle sprain. The knee is caught between the ankle and the hip. If the ankle or hip joint begins to function improperly, this results in altered movement and force distribution of the knee. Over time, this can lead to further injury.[16-31]

3. Low back injuries: Low back injuries can cause decreased neural control to stabilizing muscles of the core, resulting in poor stabilization of the spine. This can further lead to dysfunction in upper and lower extremities.[32-42]

4. Shoulder injuries: Shoulder injuries cause altered neural control of the rotator cuff muscles, which can lead to instability of the shoulder joint during functional activities.[43-47]

5. Other injuries: Injuries that result from kinetic chain imbalances include repetitive hamstring strains, groin strains, patellar tendonitis (jumper's

knee), plantar fasciitis (pain in the arch of the foot), posterior tibialis tendonitis (shin splints), biceps tendonitis (shoulder pain), and headaches.

All of the aforementioned past injuries should be taken into consideration while assessing clients, as the mentioned imbalances will manifest over time unless proper care has been given.

Past Surgeries

Surgical procedures create trauma for the body and may have similar effects to those of an injury. They can create dysfunction, unless properly rehabilitated. Some common surgical procedures include:

- Foot and ankle surgery
- Knee surgery
- Back surgery
- Shoulder surgery
- Cesarean section for birth (cutting through the abdominal wall to deliver a baby)
- Appendectomy (cutting through the abdominal wall to remove the appendix)

In each case, surgery will cause pain and inflammation that can alter neural control to the affected muscles and joints if not rehabilitated properly.[48,49]

Chronic Conditions

It is estimated that more than 75% of the American adult population does not partake, on a daily basis, in 30 minutes of low-to-moderate physical activity.[50] The risk of chronic disease goes up significantly in individuals who are not as physically active as this minimal standard.[51,52] Some chronic diseases include:[50,53]

- Cardiovascular disease, coronary heart disease, coronary artery disease, or congestive heart failure
- Hypertension (high blood pressure)
- High cholesterol
- Stroke
- Lung or breathing problems
- Obesity
- Diabetes mellitus

Medications

Many clients coming into the fitness industry will be under the care of a medical professional and may be required to use any one of a variety of medications. It is *not* the role of any health and fitness professional to administer, prescribe, or educate on the usage and effects of any of these medications.

Always consult with the clients' medical professionals for their health information and any medication they may be using.

The purpose of this section is to briefly outline some of the primary classes of drugs and their proposed physiologic effects (Table 5-2). The table is merely intended to present a simplistic overview of medications. It is *not* intended to serve as conclusive evidence regarding the medications or their effects. For more complete

Table 5.2	
Common Medications By Classification	
Medication	**Basic Function**
Beta-blockers (β-blockers)	Generally used as antihypertensive (high blood pressure), may also be prescribed for arrhythmias (irregular heart rate)
Calcium-channel blockers	Generally prescribed for hypertension and angina (chest pain)
Nitrates	Generally prescribed for hypertension, congestive heart failure
Diuretics	Generally prescribed for hypertension, congestive heart failure, and peripheral edema
Bronchodilators	Generally prescribed to correct or prevent bronchial smooth muscle constriction in individuals with asthma and other pulmonary diseases
Vasodilators	Used in the treatment of hypertension and congestive heart failure
Antidepressants	Used in the treatment of various psychiatric and emotional disorders

information regarding medications, contact a medical professional or refer to the *Physician's Desk Reference* (PDR).

SUMMARY

A health and fitness professional can gather essential information that provides insight to a client's daily physical activity by gathering subjective information about a client's personal history, including occupation, lifestyle, and medical background. Asking questions can provide important clues about the structure and function of a client. It provides information about movement capacity and what kinds of movement patterns are performed throughout the day. The Physical Activity Readiness Questionnaire (PAR-Q) qualifies clients for low to moderate to high activity levels and aids in identifying people who may need medical attention.

Questions about recreation and hobbies will reflect what a client does in his or her free time. Proper forms of training for specific activities must be incorporated to increase the efficiency of the kinetic chain, while avoiding injury. Clients with sedentary hobbies will probably not be at the same level of training as those who participate in recreational sports.

Finding out a client's medical history is crucial. Past injuries affect the functioning of the kinetic chain and are important to ask about to discover possible dysfunctions. Surgical procedures have similar effects as injuries because they cause pain and inflammation that can alter neural control to the affected muscles and joints, if not rehabilitated properly. It is also important to ask about chronic conditions, which are likely to occur in individuals who are not physically active. Finally, many clients use medications. It is important to know some of their basic effects (Table 5-3); however, health and fitness professionals should *not* administer, prescribe, or educate on the usage and effects of any of these medications. Be sure to consult with the clients' medical professionals if they use medication.

Table 5.3		
Effects of Medication on Heart Rate and Blood Pressure		
Medication	**Heart Rate**	**Blood Pressure**
Beta-blockers (β-blockers)	↓	↓
Calcium-channel blockers	↑ ↔ or ↓	↓
Nitrates	↑ ↔	↔ ↓
Diuretics	↔	↔ ↓
Bronchodilators	↔	↔
Vasodilators	↑ ↔ or ↓	↓
Antidepressants	↑ or ↔	↔ or ↓

↑, increase; ↔, no effect; ↓, decrease.

Objective Information Provided in the Fitness Assessment

TYPES OF OBJECTIVE INFORMATION

Objective information:
Measurable data about a client's physical state such as body composition, movement, and cardiovascular ability.

Objective information is gathered to provide the health and fitness professional with forms of measurable data. This information can be used to compare beginning numbers with those measured weeks, months, or years later, denoting improvements in the client, as well as the effectiveness of the training program. Categories of objective information include:

- Physiologic assessments
- Body-composition assessments
- Cardiorespiratory assessments
- Movement assessments (posture)
- Performance assessments

PHYSIOLOGIC ASSESSMENTS

Physiologic assessments provide the health and fitness professional with valuable information regarding the status of the client's health. By assessing and reassessing a client's *resting heart rate* and *blood pressure*, health and fitness professionals gather valuable information in designing a client's conditioning program. In addition, the following tests can be used as motivational tools assisting in client retention.

Heart Rate

The resting heart rate can be taken on the inside of the wrist (radial pulse; preferred) or on the neck to the side of the windpipe (carotid pulse; use with caution). To gather an accurate recording, it is best to teach clients how to test their resting heart rate on rising in the morning. Instruct them to test their resting heart rate three mornings in a row and average the three readings.

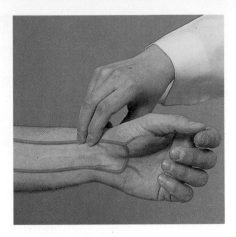

Figure 5.6   Radial pulse.

Radial Pulse

To find the radial pulse, lightly place two fingers along the arm in line and just above the thumb (Figure 5-6). Once a pulse is identified, count the pulses for 60 seconds. Record the 60-second pulse rate and average over the course of 3 days. Points to consider:

- The touch should be gentle.
- The test must be taken when the client is calm.
- All three tests must be taken at the same time to ensure accuracy.

Carotid Pulse

To find the carotid pulse, lightly place two fingers on the neck, just to the side of the larynx (Figure 5-7). Once a pulse is identified, count the pulses for 60 seconds. Record the 60-second pulse rate and average over the course of 3 days. Points to consider:

- The touch should be gentle.
- Excessive pressure can decrease heart rate and blood pressure, leading to an inaccurate reading, possible dizziness, and fainting.[1]
- The test must be taken when the client is calm.
- All three tests should be taken at the same time to ensure accuracy.

Resting heart rates can vary. However, on average, the resting heart rate for a male is 70 beats per minute and 75 beats per minute for a female.[1]

The health and fitness professional can also calculate the training heart rate zone in which a client should perform cardiorespiratory exercise (Table 5-4). There

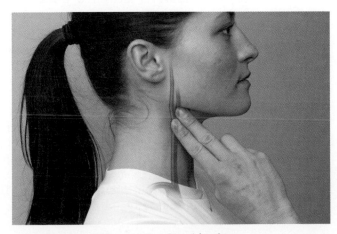

Figure 5.7   Carotid pulse.

Table 5.4

Heart Rate Training Zones

Training Zone	Purpose
One	Builds aerobic base and aids in recovery
Two	Increases endurance and trains the anaerobic threshold
Three	Builds high-end work capacity

are many ways to determine heart rate zones. Create heart rate zones by first determining the client's estimated maximum heart rate by subtracting the client's age from the number 220 (220 – age). Second, multiply the estimated maximum heart rate by the appropriate intensity (65–90%) at which the client should work while performing cardiorespiratory exercise.[1]

Zone one	Maximum heart rate $\times$ 0.65
	Maximum heart rate $\times$ 0.75
Zone two	Maximum heart rate $\times$ 0.80
	Maximum heart rate $\times$ 0.85
Zone three	Maximum heart rate $\times$ 0.86
	Maximum heart rate $\times$ 0.90

The heart rate zone numbers should be combined with the various cardiorespiratory assessments (discussed later in this chapter) to establish which heart rate zone a client will start in. This calculation is a crude average that will most likely have to be modified. Intensity levels may need to be lowered (40–55%) depending on the client's physical condition.

Blood Pressure

Blood pressure measurements consist of systolic and diastolic readings. The systolic reading (top number) reflects the pressure produced by the heart as it pumps blood to the body. Normal systolic pressure ranges from 120 millimeters of mercury (mm Hg) to 130 mm Hg. The diastolic blood pressure (lower number) signifies the minimum pressure within the arteries through a full cardiac cycle. Normal diastolic pressure ranges from 80 to 85 mm Hg.[1]

Blood Pressure Testing

Blood pressure is measured using a sphygmomanometer, which consists of an inflatable cuff, a pressure meter, and a bulb with a valve, and a stethoscope. To record blood pressure, instruct the client to assume a comfortable seated position and place the appropriate size cuff on the client, just above the elbow (Figure 5-8). Next, rest the arm on a supported chair (or support the arm using your own arm) and place the stethoscope over the brachial artery, using a minimal amount of pressure. Continue by rapidly inflating the cuff to 20 to 30 mm Hg above the point when the pulse can no longer be felt at the wrist. Next, release the pressure at a rate of about 2 mm Hg per second, listening for a pulse. To determine the systolic pressure, listen for the first observation of the pulse. Diastolic pressure is determined when the pulse fades away. For greater reliability, repeat procedure on the opposite arm.[1]

It is important for the health and fitness professional to go through formal training in taking blood pressure before assessing blood pressure on health club members.

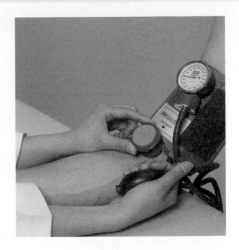

Figure 5.8   Proper sphygmomanometer placement.

BODY COMPOSITION

Gathering body-composition statistics about a client provides the health and fitness professional with a measure of a client's starting point. Using body fat, circumference measurements, hip-to-waist ratio, or body mass index to assess and then reassess can be motivating for a client. In addition, it is a good indication of how well the training program has been designed.

Body Fat Measurements

One of the most important pieces of information that can be obtained by a health and fitness professional is the client's starting body fat percentage. Body fat reduction is often the primary goal of many clients. As such, its analysis can be a powerful tool to use when discussing progress. Other methods would include asking a client how his or her clothes are fitting, using before and after pictures, and getting comments from friends.

Body fat can be measured in a variety of ways. Depending on the tools available, the most common methods are discussed below.

1. Skin-fold calipers measure a client's amount of subcutaneous fat (or fat beneath the skin) by calculating the size of skin folds.

2. Bioelectrical impedance uses a portable instrument to conduct an electrical current through the body to measure fat. This form of assessment is based on the hypothesis that tissues that are high in water content conduct electrical currents with less resistance than those with little water (such as adipose tissue).

3. Underwater weighing is a method of determining the proportion of fat to lean tissue. This difference is determined by weighing a person through normal methods and then weighing the person under water. Because lean tissue is denser than fat, the more lean a person is, the more he or she will weigh underwater. The results of underwater weighing indicate a person's overall density (compared with the water) and, as such, are a composite of body weight to body volume.

SKIN-FOLD CALIPER MEASUREMENTS

Most health and fitness professionals do not have an exercise physiology laboratory at their disposal, so the skin-fold caliper method will be the method emphasized in this text. When using caliper measurements, health and fitness professionals must be consistent with the exact areas of skin folds measured, as well as the conditions of administering the assessment. For example, if a skin-fold measurement is taken before a client's workout, this agenda should remain consistent in future assessments.

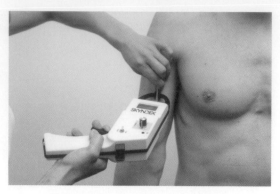

Figure 5.9 Biceps measurement.

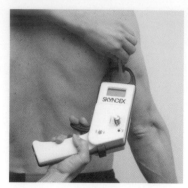

Figure 5.10 Triceps measurement.

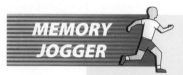
MEMORY JOGGER

Assessing one's body fat using skin-fold calipers can be a sensitive situation, particularly for very overweight individuals. The accuracy of the skin-fold measurements in these situations typically decrease; thus, it would be more appropriate to not use this method for assessing body fat. Instead, use bioelectrical impedance (if available), circumference measurements, scale weight, or even how clothes fit to evaluate one's weight loss and body fat reduction progress.

CALCULATING BODY FAT PERCENTAGES

The National Academy of Sports Medicine utilizes the Durnin formula (sometimes known as the Durnin–Womersley formula) to calculate a client's percentage of body fat.[54] This formula was chosen for its simple four-site upper body measurement process. The Durnin formula's four sites of skin-fold measurement are as follows:

1. Biceps: A vertical fold on the front of the arm over the biceps muscle, halfway between the shoulder and the elbow (Figure 5-9).
2. Triceps: A vertical fold on the back of the upper arm, with the arm relaxed and held freely at the side. This skin fold should also be taken halfway between the shoulder and the elbow (Figure 5-10).
3. Subscapular: A 45-degree angle fold of 1 to 2 cm, below the inferior angle of the scapula (Figure 5-11).
4. Iliac crest: A 45-degree angle fold, taken just above the iliac crest and medial to the axillary line (Figure 5-12).

When taking these measurements, all should be taken on the right side of the body (unless otherwise noted on the assessment form) for standardization purposes.

After the four sites have been measured, add the totals of the four sites (this should be done in millimeters). Then, find the appropriate sex and age categories for the body composition on the Durnin–Womersley body fat percentage calculation table (Table 5-5).

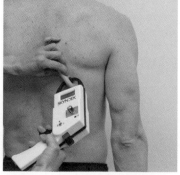

Figure 5.11 Subscapular measurement.

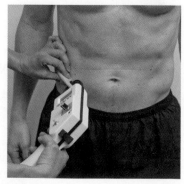

Figure 5.12 Iliac crest measurement.

Table 5.5

Durnin–Womersley Body Fat Percentage Calculation

Sum of Folds	Males					Females				
	<19	20–29	30–39	40–49	>50	<19	20–29	30–39	40–49	>50
5	−7.23	−7.61	−1.70	−5.28	−6.87	−2.69	−3.97	0.77	3.91	4.84
10	0.41	0.04	5.05	3.30	2.63	5.72	4.88	8.72	11.71	13.10
15	5.00	4.64	9.09	8.47	8.38	10.78	10.22	13.50	16.40	18.07
20	8.32	7.96	12.00	12.22	12.55	14.44	14.08	16.95	19.78	21.67
25	10.92	10.57	14.29	15.16	15.84	17.33	17.13	19.66	22.44	24.49
30	13.07	12.73	16.17	17.60	18.56	19.71	19.64	21.90	24.64	26.83
35	14.91	14.56	17.77	19.68	20.88	21.74	21.79	23.81	26.51	28.82
40	16.51	16.17	19.17	21.49	22.92	23.51	23.67	25.48	28.14	30.56
45	17.93	17.59	20.41	23.11	24.72	25.09	25.34	26.96	29.59	32.10
50	19.21	18.87	21.53	24.56	26.35	26.51	26.84	28.30	30.90	33.49
55	20.37	20.04	22.54	25.88	27.83	27.80	28.21	29.51	32.09	34.75
60	21.44	21.11	23.47	27.09	29.20	28.98	29.46	30.62	33.17	35.91
65	22.42	22.09	24.33	28.22	30.45	30.08	30.62	31.65	34.18	36.99
70	23.34	23.01	25.13	29.26	31.63	31.10	31.70	32.60	35.11	37.98
75	24.20	23.87	25.87	30.23	32.72	32.05	32.71	33.49	35.99	38.91
80	25.00	24.67	26.57	31.15	33.75	32.94	33.66	34.33	36.81	39.79
85	25.76	25.43	27.23	32.01	34.72	33.78	34.55	35.12	37.58	40.61
90	26.47	26.15	27.85	32.83	35.64	34.58	35.40	35.87	38.31	41.39
95	27.15	26.83	28.44	33.61	36.52	35.34	36.20	36.58	39.00	42.13
100	27.80	27.48	29.00	34.34	37.35	36.06	36.97	37.25	39.66	42.84
105	28.42	28.09	29.54	35.05	38.14	36.74	37.69	37.90	40.29	43.51
110	29.00	28.68	30.05	35.72	38.90	37.40	38.39	38.51	40.89	44.15
115	29.57	29.25	30.54	36.37	39.63	38.03	39.06	39.10	41.47	44.76
120	30.11	29.79	31.01	36.99	40.33	38.63	39.70	39.66	42.02	45.36
125	30.63	30.31	31.46	37.58	41.00	39.21	40.32	40.21	42.55	45.92
130	31.13	30.82	31.89	38.15	41.65	39.77	40.91	40.73	43.06	46.47
135	31.62	31.30	32.31	38.71	42.27	40.31	41.48	41.24	43.56	47.00
140	32.08	31.77	32.71	39.24	42.87	40.83	42.04	41.72	44.03	47.51
145	32.53	32.22	33.11	39.76	43.46	41.34	42.57	42.19	44.49	48.00
150	32.97	32.66	33.48	40.26	44.02	41.82	43.09	42.65	44.94	48.47
155	33.39	33.08	33.85	40.74	44.57	42.29	43.59	43.09	45.37	48.93
160	33.80	33.49	34.20	41.21	45.10	42.75	44.08	43.52	45.79	49.38
165	34.20	33.89	34.55	41.67	45.62	43.20	44.55	43.94	46.20	49.82
170	34.59	34.28	34.88	42.11	46.12	43.63	45.01	44.34	46.59	50.24
175	34.97	34.66	35.21	42.54	46.61	44.05	45.46	44.73	46.97	50.65
180	35.33	35.02	35.53	42.96	47.08	44.46	45.89	45.12	47.35	51.05
185	35.69	35.38	35.83	43.37	47.54	44.86	46.32	45.49	47.71	51.44
190	36.04	35.73	36.13	43.77	48.00	45.25	46.73	45.85	48.07	51.82
195	36.38	36.07	36.43	44.16	48.44	45.63	47.14	46.21	48.41	52.19
200	36.71	36.40	36.71	44.54	48.87	46.00	47.53	46.55	48.75	52.55

For example, a 40-year-old female client with the sum of the skin folds being 40 has a body fat percentage of 28.14 (or round down to 28%).

Another benefit to assessing one's body fat is the ability to determine approximately how much of an individual's scale weight comes from body fat and how much from lean body mass (everything but fat). This becomes very useful when it comes time to reassess the individual as it allows the health and fitness professional to determine how much fat mass one has lost and how much lean body mass was gained, maintained, or even lost. The formula below outlines how to calculate one's fat mass and lean body mass:

1. Body fat % × scale weight = fat mass
2. Scale weight − fat mass = lean body mass

For example, if the above 40-year-old female client weighted 130 pounds, her fat mass and lean body mass would be calculated as such:

1. 0.28 (body fat %) × 130 (scale weight) = 36 pounds of body fat
2. 130 (scale weight) − 36 (pounds of body fat) = 94 pounds of lean body mass

Circumference Measurements

Circumference measurements can also be another source of feedback used with clients who have the goal of altering body composition. They are designed to assess girth changes in the body. The most important factor to consider when taking circumference measurements is consistency. Remember when taking measurements to make sure the tape measure is taut and level around the area that is being measured.

1. Neck: Across the Adam's apple (Figure 5-13)
2. Chest: Across the nipple line (Figure 5-14)
3. Waist: Measure at the narrowest point of the waist, below the rib cage and just above the top of the hipbones. If there is no apparent narrowing of the waist, measure at the navel (Figure 5-15).
4. Hips: With feet together, measure circumference at the widest portion of the buttocks (Figure 5-16).
5. Thighs: Measure 10 inches above the top of the patella for standardization (Figure 5-17).
6. Calves: At the maximal circumference between the ankle and the knee, measure the calves (Figure 5-18).
7. Biceps: At the maximal circumference of the biceps, measure with arm extended, palm facing forward (Figure 5-19).

Circumference measurements can also be used to calculate body fat percentage. This is an important method to have available particularly when skin-fold measurements are not an option. (Refer to the conversion tables in the Appendix for proper calculations.)

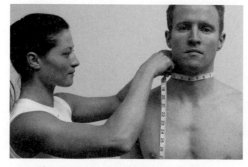

Figure 5.13 Neck measurement.

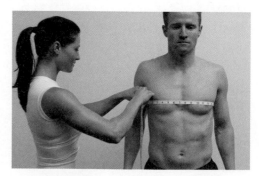

Figure 5.14 Chest measurement.

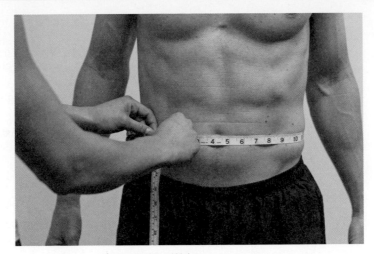

Figure 5.15   Waist measurement.

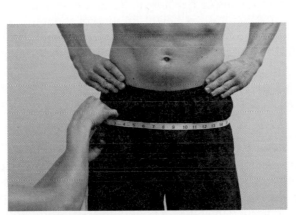

Figure 5.16   Hips measurement.

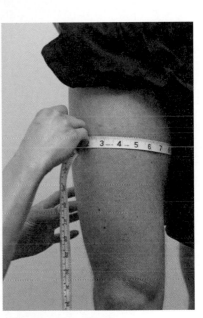

Figure 5.17   Thigh measurement.

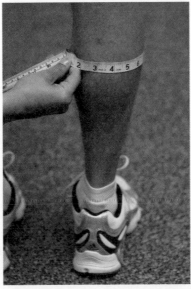

Figure 5.18   Calves measurement.

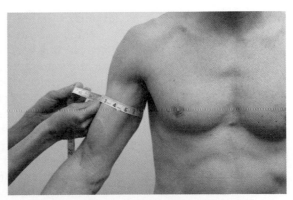

Figure 5.19   Biceps measurement.

Waist-to-Hip Ratio

The waist-to-hip ratio is one of the most used clinical applications of girth measurements. This assessment is important because there is a correlation between chronic diseases and fat stored in the midsection.[1]

The waist-to-hip ratio can be computed by dividing the waist measurement by the hip measurement, by doing the following:[1]

1. Measure the smallest part of the client's waist, without instructing the client to draw in the stomach.
2. Measure the largest part of the client's hips.
3. Compute the waist-to-hip ratio by dividing the waist measurement by the hip measurement.
4. For example, if a client's waist measures 30 inches and his or her hips measure 40 inches, divide 30 by 40 for a waist-to-hip ratio of 0.75.

A ratio above 0.80 for women and above 0.95 for men may put these individuals at risk for a number of diseases.

Body Mass Index (BMI)

Although this assessment is not designed to assess body fat, the body mass index (BMI) is a quick and easy method for determining whether your client's weight is appropriate for his or her height. To assess weight relative to height, divide body weight (in kilograms) by height (in meters squared) or, kg/m^2.[53]

It has been shown that obesity-related health problems increase when a person's BMI exceeds 25. The obesity classifications using BMI are the following:[1]

- Mild   = 25–30
- Moderate   = 30–35
- Severe   > 35

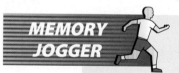

MEMORY JOGGER

Keep in mind that a BMI and hip-to-waist measurement does not take into account percent body fat or lean body mass. Thus, one may possess a high BMI or hip-to-waist ratio score but have a low percentage of body fat and a high percentage of lean body mass, indicating their risk for obesity-related health problems may not be as high as their results may show.

SUMMARY

Objective information (such as body composition, movement observation, and cardiovascular assessment) provides measurable data that track changes in a client. It can be motivating for a client to assess and reassess body fat, circumference measurements, hip-to-waist ratio, or body mass index.

Many clients want to lose body fat, and, as such, it is important to be able to determine starting body fat percentage. Skin-fold calipers are one of the easiest ways to do this in a gym setting. Consistency (in location and administration) is vital when measuring skin folds. Calculate a client's percentage of body fat by measuring four sites with the calipers, adding the totals of all four sites, and then finding the appropriate sex and age categories on the Durnin–Wormersley body fat percentage calculation table.

Circumference measurements and waist-to-hip ratio are other sources of feedback that assess girth changes in the body. Again, consistency in measurements is key. A waist-to-hip ratio above 0.80 for women and above 0.95 for men may put these individuals at risk for a number of diseases.

Finally, the body mass index (BMI) is a good way to determine whether a client's weight is appropriate for his or her height. The chances of having obesity-related health problems potentially increases when a person's BMI exceeds 25.

Cardiorespiratory Assessments

Cardiorespiratory assessments provide the health and fitness professional with valuable information regarding cardiorespiratory efficiency and overall condition. They can also provide health and fitness professionals with a starting point for determining in which zone their client should begin cardiorespiratory exercise (specific to that person's physical condition and goals). Two common forms of assessing cardiorespiratory efficiency are the 3-minute step test and the Rockport walk test.

Three-Minute Step Test

This test is designed to estimate a cardiovascular starting point.[55] The starting point is then modified, based on ability level. Once determined, refer to the Cardiorespiratory Training Concepts chapter of the text for specific programming strategies.

Step one: Determine the client's maximum heart rate by subtracting the client's age from the number 220 (220 – age). Then, take the maximum heart rate and multiply it by the following figures to determine the heart rate ranges for each zone.

Zone one	Maximum heart rate × 0.65
	Maximum heart rate × 0.75
Zone two	Maximum heart rate × 0.80
	Maximum heart rate × 0.85
Zone three	Maximum heart rate × 0.86
	Maximum heart rate × 0.90

Step two: Perform a 3-minute step test by having a client do 24 steps per minute on an 18-inch step (may need to be lowered depending on client's physical capabilities), for a total of 3 minutes (roughly 72 steps total). Have the client rest for 1 minute. Then, measure the client's pulse for 30 seconds and record the number as the recovery pulse. Determine fitness level by:

$$\frac{\text{Duration of exercise (sec)} \times 100}{\text{Recovery pulse} \times 5.6} = \text{cardiovascular efficiency}$$

Step three: Locate the final number in one of the following categories:

28–38	Poor
39–48	Fair
49–59	Average
60–70	Good
71–100	Very good

Step four: Determine the appropriate starting program using the appropriate category:

Poor	Zone one
Fair	Zone one
Average	Zone two
Good	Zone two
Very good	Zone three

Please refer to Chapter 7 (Cardiorespiratory Training Concepts) for proper use of these zones through specific-stage training programs.

Rockport Walk Test

This test is also designed to estimate a cardiovascular starting point. The starting point is then modified, based on ability level. Once determined, refer to the Cardiorespiratory Training Concepts chapter of the text for specific programming strategies.

Step one: Determine the client's maximum heart rate by subtracting the client's age from the number 220 (220 – age). Then, take the maximum heart rate and multiply it by the following figures to determine the heart rate ranges for each zone.

Zone one   Maximum heart rate × 0.65
             Maximum heart rate × 0.75
Zone two   Maximum heart rate × 0.80
             Maximum heart rate × 0.85
Zone three   Maximum heart rate × 0.86
             Maximum heart rate × 0.90

Step two: First, record the client's weight. Have the client walk 1 mile, as fast as he or she can control, on a treadmill. Record the time it takes the client to complete the walk. Immediately record the client's heart rate (beats per minute) at the 1-mile mark. Use the following formula to determine the oxygen consumption ($\dot{V}O_2$) score:[56]

$132.853 - (0.0769 \times \text{weight}) - (0.3877 \times \text{age}) + (6.315 \times 1)$ for men or $+ (6.315 \times 0)$ for women $- (3.2649 \times \text{time}) - (0.1565 \times \text{heart rate}) = \dot{V}O_2$ score

Step three: Locate the $\dot{V}O_2$ score in one of the following categories:

Males

Age	Heart Rate Zone				
	Poor	Fair	Average	Good	Very Good
20–24	32–37	38–43	44–50	51–56	57–62
25–29	31–35	32–36	43–48	49–53	54–59
30–34	29–34	35–40	41–45	46–51	52–56
35–39	28–32	33–38	39–43	44–48	49–54
40–44	26–31	32–35	36–41	42–46	47–51
45–49	25–29	30–34	35–39	40–43	44–48
50–54	24–27	28–32	33–36	37–41	42–46
55–59	22–26	27–30	31–34	35–39	40–43
60–65	21–24	25–28	29–32	33–36	37–40

Females

Age	Heart Rate Zone				
	Poor	Fair	Average	Good	Very Good
20–24	27–31	32–36	37–41	42–46	47–51
25–29	26–30	31–35	36–40	41–44	45–49
30–34	25–29	30–33	34–37	38–42	43–46
35–39	24–27	28–31	32–35	36–40	41–44
40–44	22–25	26–29	30–33	34–37	38–41
45–49	21–23	24–27	28–31	32–35	36–38
50–54	19–22	23–25	26–29	30–32	33–36
55–59	18–20	21–23	24–27	28–30	31–33
60–65	16–18	19–21	22–24	25–27	28–30

Step four: Determine the appropriate starting program using the appropriate category:

Poor   Zone one
Fair   Zone one

Average   Zone two
Good   Zone two
Very good   Zone three

Please refer to Chapter 7 (Cardiorespiratory Training Concepts) for proper use of these zones through specific-stage training programs.

SUMMARY

There are many ways to determine heart rate zones, based on cardiovascular assessments. Once the ability level is determined, special programs can be chosen. Two popular cardiorespiratory assessments that can be used to determine one's starting point include the 3-minute step test and the Rockport walk test.

Posture and Movement Assessments

GENERAL STATIC AND MOVEMENT OBSERVATION

Posture: The alignment and function of all components of the kinetic chain at any given moment.

Every movement needs a base from which to generate (and accept) force. This is better known as posture. **Posture** is the alignment and function of all components of the kinetic chain at any given moment. It is under the control of the central nervous system.[57-59]

Posture

Structural efficiency: The alignment of the musculoskeletal system that allows our center of gravity to be maintained over our base of support.

Posture is often viewed as being static (or without movement). However, everyday posture is constantly changing to meet the demands placed on the kinetic chain. The main purpose of proper posture is to maintain enough **structural efficiency** to overcome constant forces placed on the body (i.e., gravity).[58,60] Structural efficiency is defined as the alignment of the musculoskeletal system, which allows our center of gravity to be maintained over a base of support.

Functional efficiency: The ability of the neuromuscular system to monitor and manipulate movement during functional tasks using the least amount of energy, creating the least amount of stress on the kinetic chain.

Any deviation from proper postural alignment can cause a change in the body's center of gravity, which affects the **functional efficiency** of the kinetic chain.[57,61] Functional efficiency is defined as the ability of the neuromuscular system to monitor and manipulate movement during functional tasks using the least amount of energy, creating the least amount of stress on the kinetic chain.

Postural equilibrium: Maintaining a state of balance in the alignment of the kinetic chain.

The ability to efficiently maintain balance is termed **postural equilibrium**.[62] The kinetic chain exhibits some type of posture and requires maintenance of that posture at all times. Therefore, it can be said that posture is the position from which all movement begins and ends.[63]

Neuromuscular efficiency: The ability of the nervous system to communicate effectively with the muscular system.

IMPORTANCE OF POSTURE

Proper postural alignment allows optimum **neuromuscular efficiency** (Figure 5-20).[3,32,57,64-67] This is particularly true with respect to the neuromuscular system. Proper posture ensures that the muscles of the body are optimally aligned at the proper length-tension relationships necessary for efficient functioning of force-couples.[3,32,57,64-66] This allows for proper joint mechanics (or arthrokinematics) and effective absorption and distribution of forces throughout the kinetic chain, alleviating excess stress on joints.[3,32,57,64-67]

Functional strength: The ability of the neuromuscular system to contract eccentrically, isometrically, and concentrically in all three planes of motion.

Proper postural alignment allows the kinetic chain to produce high levels of functional strength with optimal neuromuscular efficiency. **Functional strength** is the ability of the neuromuscular system to perform dynamic eccentric, isometric, and concentric muscle actions in all three planes of motion.

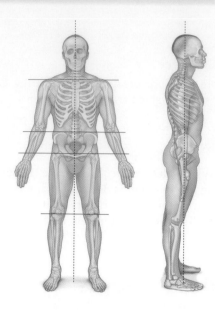

Figure 5.20 Proper postural alignment.

All muscles must be activated with precise timing to work in complete synergy. Think of the muscles in the body as an orchestra. The conductor (nervous system) must bring the wind, percussion, and string sections (various muscles) into the musical piece at the right time for the music to have a perfect melody (functional strength). The same holds true for the kinetic chain.

Without proper postural alignment, we set the body up for degeneration.[3,57,65–68] Altered movement patterns result from muscle imbalances, which can place unusual stresses on the joints.[57,65] This affects other joints and muscles in the kinetic chain, which can cause tissue stress throughout the body. These traumas are known as **postural distortion patterns**, which are simply predictable patterns of muscle imbalance.[3,57,65–68] Causes of muscle imbalances and strategies in improving these imbalances will be discussed in Chapter 6 (Flexibility Training Concepts).

Postural distortion patterns: Predictable occurrences of muscle imbalances caused by altered movement patterns.

Observing Dynamic Posture

Dynamic postural observations (looking at movements) are often the quickest way to gain an overall impression of a client's functional status. Because posture is a dynamic quality, these observations show postural distortion and potential overactive and underactive muscles in its naturally dynamic setting.

Movement observations should relate to basic functions such as squatting, pushing, pulling, and balancing, in addition to providing crucial information about muscle and joint interplay. The observation process should search for any imbalances in anatomy, physiology, or biomechanics that may decrease a client's results and possibly lead to injury (both in and out of the fitness environment). With the limited time that most health and fitness professionals have for observation, incorporating a systematic assessment sequence is essential. (At the end of this chapter, different assessment scenarios are provided to aid in time efficiency.)

There are various assessment techniques that will be described below and can be incorporated as a first workout for your client. Each assessment described also contains key kinetic chain checkpoints to observe. These checkpoints include the feet, knees, lumbo-pelvic-hip complex, shoulders, and head.

DYNAMIC POSTURAL ASSESSMENTS

Overhead Squat Assessment

This observation is designed to assess dynamic flexibility on both sides of the body as well as integrated total body strength.

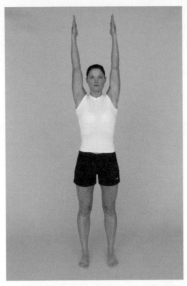

Figure 5.21 Overhead squat assessment, anterior view.

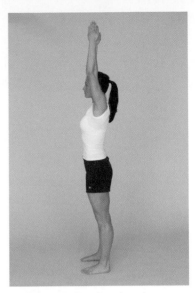

Figure 5.22 Overhead squat assessment, lateral view.

Position

1. Client stands with feet shoulder-width apart and pointed straight ahead. The foot and ankle complex should be in a neutral position.
2. Have client raise his or her arms overhead, with elbow fully extended. The upper arm should bisect the torso (Figures 5-21 and 5-22).

Movement

3. Instruct client to squat to roughly the height of a chair and return to the start position.
4. Have the client repeat the movement five repetitions in each position (anterior, and lateral).

Views

5. View feet, ankles, and knees from the front (Figure 5-23; Table 5-4).
6. View the lumbo-pelvic-hip complex, shoulder, and cervical complex from the side (Figure 5-24; Table 5-4).

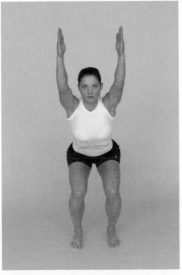

Figure 5.23 Overhead squat assessment observation, anterior view.

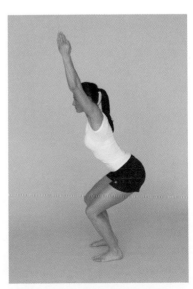

Figure 5.24 Overhead squat assessment observation, lateral view.

Follow the kinetic chain checkpoints in Figure 5-25 for each view. When doing an observation, record all findings in writing. Figure 5-25 shows what each compensation looks like and the associated overactive muscles (red) and underactive muscles (purple). Figure 5-25 also lists each compensation and potential overactive and underactive muscles.

View	Kinetic chain checkpoints	Movement observation	Yes
Anterior	1. Feet	Turns out	
	2. Knees	Moves inward	
Lateral	3-4. Lumbo pelvic hip complex	Excessive forward lean	
		Low back arches	
	5. Shoulder complex	Arms fall forward	

Normal

1.

2.

3.

Figure 5.25   Observational findings, overhead squat assessment.

4. Normal

5.

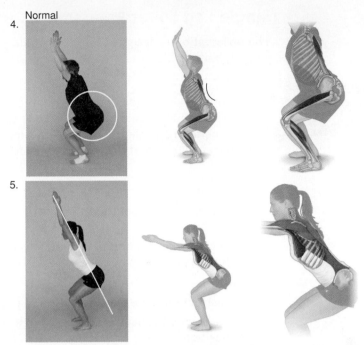

View	Checkpoint	Compensation	Probably overactive muscles	Probably underactive muscles
Anterior	Feet	Turns out	Soleus Lat. Gastrocnemius Biceps femoris (short head)	Med. Gastrocnemius Med. Hamstring Gracilis Sartorius Popliteus
	Knees	Move inward	Adductor complex Biceps femoris (short head) TFL Vastus lateralis	Gluteus medius/maxlmus Vastus medialis oblique (VMO)

View	Checkpoint	Compensation	Probably overactive muscles	Probably underactive muscles
Lateral	LPHC	Excessive forward lean	Soleus Lat. Gastrocnemius Hip flexor complex Abdominal complex	Anterior tibialis Gluteus Maximus Erector Spinae
		Low back arches	Hip flexor complex Erector Spinae	Gluteus Maximus Hamstrings Intrinsic core stabalizers (transverse abdominis, multifidis, transverso- spinalis, internal oblique pelvic floor muscles)
	Upper body	Arms fall forward	Latissimus dorsi Teres major Pectoralis major/ minor	Mid/lower trapezius Rhomboids Rotator cuff

Figure 5.25

Single-Leg Squat Assessment

The observation is designed to assess ankle proprioception, core strength, and hip joint stability.

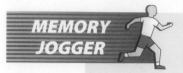
MEMORY JOGGER

For some individuals, the single-leg squat assessment may be too difficult to perform (e.g., elderly client). Other options include using outside support for assistance or simply perform a single-leg balance assessment to assess movement compensation and their ability to control themselves in a relatively unstable environment.

Position

1. Client should stand with hands on the hips and eyes focused on an object straight ahead.
2. Feet should be pointed straight ahead, and the foot, ankle, and knee and the lumbo-pelvic-hip complex should be in a neutral position (Figure 5-26).

Movement

3. Instruct client to raise one leg and place it parallel to the stance leg.
4. Have client squat to a comfortable level (Figure 5-27) and return to the start position.
5. Perform up to five repetitions before switching sides.

Views

6. View the knee from the front.

Follow the kinetic chain checkpoints in Figure 5-28. When doing an observation, record all findings in writing. Figure 5-28 shows what each compensation looks like and the associated overactive muscles and underactive muscles. Figure 5-28 also lists each compensation and potential overactive and underactive muscles.

Pushing Assessment

Position

1. Instruct client to stand with abdomen drawn inward, feet in a split stance, and toes pointing forward (Figure 5-29).

Movement

2. Instruct client to press handles forward and return slowly (Figure 5-30).

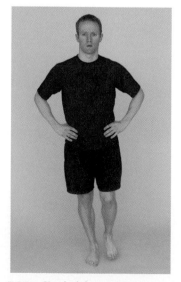
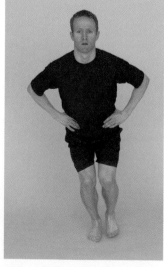

Figure 5.26 Single-leg squat assessment, start. **Figure 5.27** Single-leg squat assessment, finish.

View	Kinetic chain checkpoints	Movement observation	Right	Left
Anterior	Knee	Moves inward		

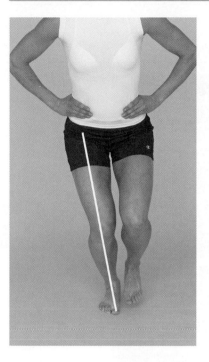
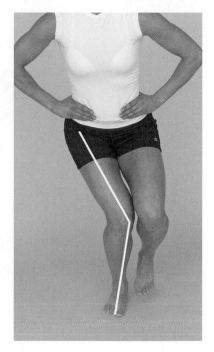

View	Checkpoint	Compensation	Probably overactive muscles	Probably underactive muscles
Anterior	Knee	Move inward	Adductor complex Biceps femoris (short head) TFL Vastus lateralis	Gluteus medius/maximus Vastus medialis oblique (VMO)

Figure 5.28 Observational findings, single-leg squat assessment.

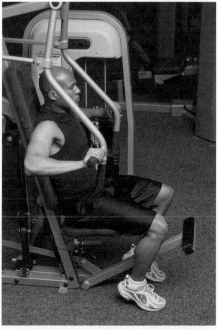
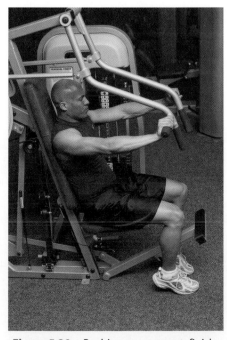

Figure 5.29 Pushing assessment, start.

Figure 5.30 Pushing assessment, finish.

Kinetic chain checkpoints	Movement observation	Yes
1. Lumbo-pelvic hip complex	Low back arches	
2. Shoulder complex	Shoulders elevate	
3. Head	Head protrudes while pushing	

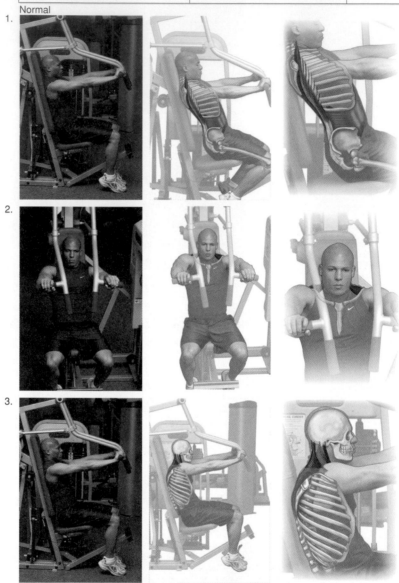

Checkpoint	Compensation	Probably overactive muscles	Probably underactive muscles
LPHC	Low back arches	Hip flexors Erector spinae	Intrinsic core stabalizers
Shoulder complex	Shoulder elevation	Upper trapezius Sternocleidomastoid Levator scapulae	Mid and lower trapezius
Head	Head protrudes forward	Upper trapezius Sternocleidomastoid Levator scapulae	Deep cervical flexors

Figure 5.31   Observational findings, pushing assessment.

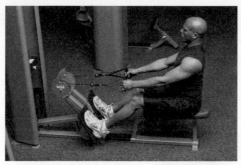

Figure 5.32   Pulling assessment, start.

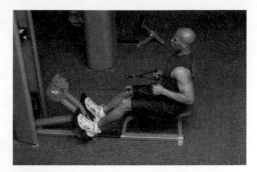

Figure 5.33   Pulling assessment, finish.

3. Perform up to 20 repetitions in a controlled fashion (2/0/2).

4. Use the checklist below to record movement faults (Figure 5-31).

Pulling Assessment

Position

1. Instruct client to stand with abdomen drawn inward, feet shoulder-width apart, and toes pointing forward (Figure 5-32).

Movement:

2. Instruct client to pull handles toward their body and return slowly (Figure 5-33).

3. Perform 20 repetitions in a controlled fashion (2/0/2).

4. Use the checklist in Figure 5-34 to record movement faults.

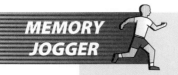

MEMORY JOGGER

Performing this assessment in a standing position places more of a demand on the core and can provide the health and fitness professional with more information on total body movement efficiency. This position, however, may be too demanding for some individuals and can be performed in a more stable environment (machine).

SUMMARY

Posture is the alignment and function of all parts of the kinetic chain. Its main purpose is to overcome constant forces placed on the body by maintaining structural efficiency. The kinetic chain requires constant postural equilibrium.

Proper postural alignment puts the body in a state of optimum neuromuscular efficiency, allowing for proper joint mechanics and effective distribution of force throughout the kinetic chain. It lets the body produce high levels of functional strength. Without it, the body may degenerate or experience postural distortion patterns.

A dynamic postural observation examines basic movements and provides crucial information about how muscles and joints interact. It searches for any imbalances in anatomy, physiology, or biomechanics.

Kinetic chain checkpoints	Movement observation	Yes
1. Lumbo-pelvic hip complext	Low back arches	
2. Shoulder complex	Shoulders elevate	
3. Head	Head protrudes while pulling	

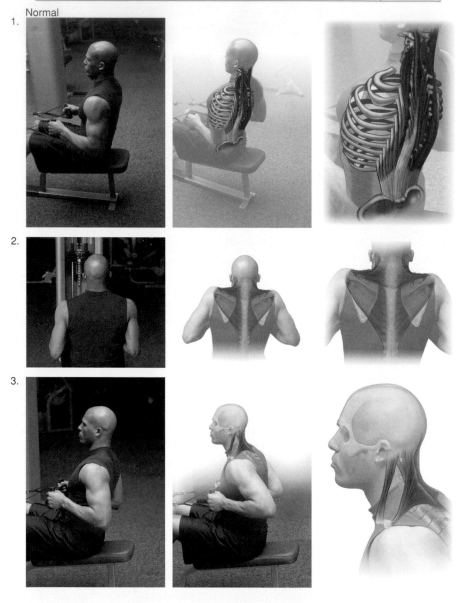

Checkpoint	Compensation	Probably overactive muscles	Probably underactive muscles
LPHC	Low back arches	Hip flexors Erector spinae	Intrinsic core stabalizers
Shoulder complex	Shoulder elevation	Upper trapezius Sternocleidomastoid Levator scapulae	Mid and lower trapezius
Head	Head protrudes forward	Upper trapezius Sternocleidomastoid Levator scapulae	Deep cervical flexors

Figure 5.34 Observational findings, pulling assessment.

OVERVIEW

Performance assessments can be incorporated into the assessment process for clients looking to improve athletic performance. Short descriptions of the purpose of each test follow:

- Davies: Assesses upper extremity stability.
- Shark skill: Assesses overall athletic ability.
- Upper extremity strength: Advanced assessment that estimates one-rep maximum and upper extremity strength.
- Lower extremity strength: Advanced assessment that estimates one-rep maximum and lower extremity strength.

There are various dynamic postural assessment techniques. Short descriptions of the purpose of each follow:

- Overhead squat: Assesses dynamic flexibility and integrated total body strength.
- Single-leg squat: Assesses ankle proprioception, core strength, and hip joint stability.
- Pushing and pulling: Assesses upper extremity neuromuscular efficiency.

Basic Performance Assessments

Performance assessments can be used for clients trying to improve athletic performance. These assessments will measure upper extremity stability, lower extremity agility, and overall strength. Basic performance assessments include the Davies test, shark skill test, bench press strength assessment, and leg press strength assessment.

Davies Test

This observation is designed to assess upper extremity agility and stabilization. This assessment may not be suitable for individuals who lack shoulder stability.

Position

1. Place two pieces of tape on the floor, 36 inches apart.
2. Have client assume a push-up position, with one hand on each piece of tape (Figure 5-35).

Movement

3. Instruct client to quickly move his or her right hand to touch the left hand (Figure 5-36).
4. Perform alternating touching on each side for 15 seconds.
5. Repeat for three trials.
6. Reassess in the future to measure improvement of number of touches.
7. Record the number of lines touched by both hands in Figure 5-38.

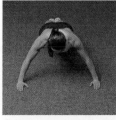 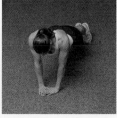 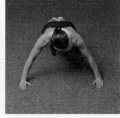 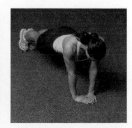

Figure 5.35 Davies test, start.

Figure 5.36 Davies test, movement.

Figure 5.37 Davies test, start.

Figure 5.38 Davies test, movement.

Distance of points	Trial number	Time	Repetitions performed
36 inches	One	15 sec.	
36 inches	Two	15 sec.	
36 inches	Three	15 sec.	

Figure 5.39 Observational findings, Davies assessment.

Shark Skill Test

The observation is designed to assess lower extremity agility and neuromuscular control. It should be viewed as a progression from the single-leg squat and, as such, may not be suitable for all individuals.

Position

1. Position client in the center box of a grid, with hands on hips and standing on one leg (Figure 5-40).

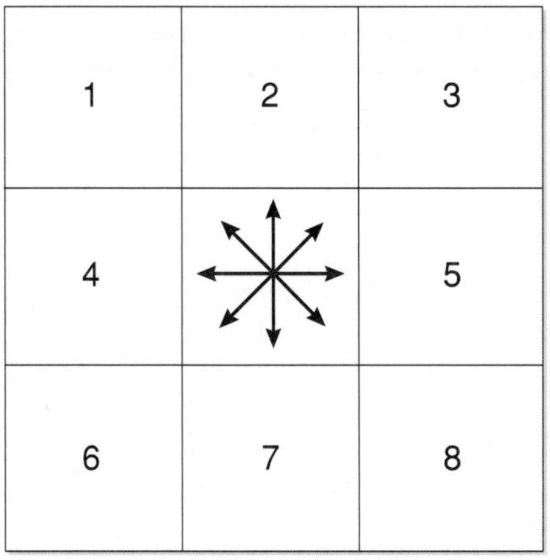

Figure 5.40 Shark skill test, start.

Movement

2. Instruct client to hop to each box in a designated pattern, always returning to the center box. Be consistent with the patterns.
3. Perform one practice run through the boxes with each foot.
4. Perform test twice with each foot (four times total). Keep track of time.
5. Record the times in Figure 5-41.
6. Add 0.10 seconds for each of the following faults:

   Nonhopping leg touches ground.

   Hands come off hips.

   Foot goes into wrong square.

   Foot does not return to center square.

Trial	Side	Time (seconds)	Deduction tally	Total deduction (# faults X 0.1)	Final total (Time - total ded.)
Practice	Right				
	Left				
One	Right				
	Left				
Two	Right				
	Left				

Figure 5.41   Observational findings, Shark skill test.

Upper Extremity Strength Assessment: Bench Press

This observation is designed to estimate the one-rep maximum, for training intensity purposes. This is considered an advanced assessment (for strength-specific goals) and, as such, may not be suitable for many clients.

Position

1. Position client on a bench, lying on his or her back. Feet should be pointed straight ahead. The low back should be in a neutral position (Figure 5-42).

Movement

2. Instruct the client to warm up with a light resistance that can be easily performed for 8 to 10 repetitions.
3. Take a 1-minute rest.
4. Add 10 to 20 pounds (5–10%) and perform 3 to 5 repetitions.
5. Take a 2-minute rest.
6. Repeat steps 4 and 5 until the individual fails at 3 to 5 repetitions.
7. Use the one-rep maximum estimation chart in the appendix to calculate one-repetition max.

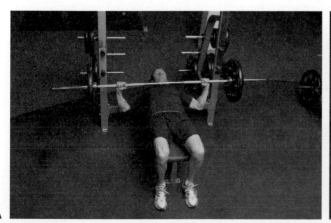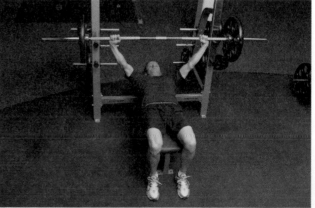

A   B

Figure 5.42   (A) Upper extremity strength assessment: bench press, start. (B) Upper extremity strength assessment: bench press, finish.

Lower Extremity Strength Assessment: Squat

This observation is designed to estimate the one-rep squat maximum, for training intensity purposes. This is considered an advanced assessment (for strength-specific goals) and, as such, may not be suitable for many clients.

Position

1. Feet should be shoulder-width apart, pointed straight ahead, and with knees in line with the toes. The low back should be in a neutral position (Figure 5-43).

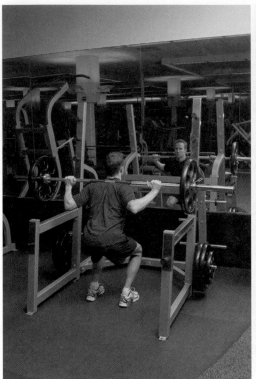 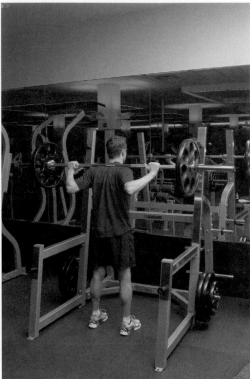

A · B

Figure 5.43   (A) Lower extremity strength assessment. (B) Lower extremity strength assessment.

Movement

2. Instruct the client to warm up with a light resistance that can be easily performed for 8 to 10 repetitions.
3. Take a 1-minute rest.
4. Add 30 to 40 pounds (10–20%) and perform 3 to 5 repetitions.
5. Take a 2-minute rest.
6. Repeat steps 4 and 5 until the individual fails at 3 to 5 repetitions.
7. Use the one-rep maximum estimation chart in the appendix to calculate one-repetition max.

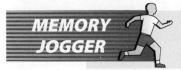

MEMORY JOGGER   Make sure in both the bench press and squat assessments that the individual performs the exercises with minimal movement compensations!

Implementing the Fitness Assessment

ASSESSMENT PARAMETERS

The fitness assessment builds the foundation for the entire template. It enables the health and fitness professional to decide the appropriate selection of flexibility, cardiovascular, core, balance, power, and strength training exercises. Listed below are several sample clients, along with the pertinent subjective information that would have been obtained in their first session. From this information, it will also list the appropriate objective assessments that a health and fitness professional would want to include to ensure that the program is individualized to these clients' specific goals and needs.

Client 1: Lita

General Information

Age:	38
Occupation:	Secretary. She spends a lot of time sitting behind a computer and on the phone. Lita is required to wear business attire.
Lifestyle:	Has two children (ages 6 and 9). Enjoys hiking, gardening, and playing sports with her kids.
Medical history:	Has had low back pain in the past (approximately 2 months ago), but does not currently experience any pain. She also, at times, experiences a feeling of "tension" through her neck when working on the computer. Lita had a C-section with her second child. She is in good overall health and is not taking any medications.
Goals:	Decrease body fat and "tone up." Become less "tense" to be able to continue her recreational activities and be simply "overall healthy."

Recommended Objective Assessments for Lita

- Body fat measurement
- Circumference measurement
- Resting heart rate
- Blood pressure
- Step test or Rockport walk test
- Movement assessment
- Overhead squat
- Single-leg squat or single-leg balance
- Pushing assessment (time permitting)
- Pulling assessment (time permitting)

Client 2: Ron

General Information

Age:	72
Occupation:	Retired business executive
Lifestyle:	Enjoys traveling, long walks with his wife, golf, carpentry, and playing with his seven grandkids.

Medical history: Had a triple bypass surgery (10 years ago). Takes medication for high cholesterol. Has lower back and shoulder pain after he plays golf.

Goals: Ron weighs 170 pounds and is not concerned with altering his body composition. He wants to be healthy, increase some overall strength, and decrease his back and shoulder pain to play golf and with his grandkids more easily.

Recommended Objective Assessments for Ron

- Obtain a medical release from Ron's physician
- Resting heart rate
- Blood pressure
- Three-minute step test or Rockport walk test
- Movement assessment
- Overhead squat
- Assisted single-leg squat or single-leg balance
- Pushing assessment (time permitting)
- Pulling assessment (time permitting)

Client 3: Brian

General Information

Age: 24

Occupation: Semiprofessional soccer player

Lifestyle: He travels often, competing in various soccer tournaments. He likes to work out with weights three to four times per week, practices 5 days per week, and plays in an organized game at least two times per week.

Medical history: Had surgery for a torn anterior cruciate ligament in his left knee 3 years ago and has sprained his left ankle two times since his knee surgery. Went through physical therapy for his last ankle sprain 6 months ago and was cleared to work out and play again. For the most part, his knee and ankle have not been giving him any trouble, other than some occasional soreness after games and practice. He has recently gone through a physical to begin playing again, and his physician gave him a clean bill of health.

Goals: He wants to increase his overall performance by enhancing his flexibility, speed, cardiorespiratory efficiency, and leg strength. He also wants to decrease his risk of incurring other injuries. After being out of soccer because of the injury, he increased his body fat percentage and would like to lower it.

Recommended Objective Assessments for Brian

- Body fat measurement
- Three-minute step test or Rockport walk test
- Movement assessment
- Overhead squat
- Single-leg squat

- Performance assessments
- Davies test
- Shark skill test
- Leg press strength assessment

FILLING IN THE TEMPLATE

The name should obviously be filled in, to keep proper records of the correct client. The date is necessary to follow a client's progression with time and keep track of what workouts occurred on what dates (Figure 5-44).

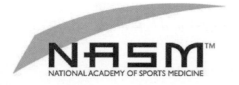

OPT For Fitness

Name: John Smith	Month: 1
Date: 08/10/06	Week: 1
Professional: Scott Lucett	Day: 1

Program Goal: Fat Loss

STEP 1		
A. Foam Roll		
Foam Roll	Sets	Duration
B. Stretch		
Exercise	Sets	Duration
C. Cardiovascular		

STEP 2				
A. Core				
Exercise	Sets	Reps	Tempo	Rest
B. Balance				
Exercise	Sets	Reps	Tempo	Rest
C. Reactive				
Exercise	Sets	Reps	Tempo	Rest

Resistance Training Program						
	Body Part Exercise	Sets	Reps	Intensity	Tempo	Rest
STEP 3	Total Body					
	Chest					
	Back					
	Shoulder					
	Legs					

Cool-Down
STEP 4
Repeat Steps 1A and 1B

Figure 5.44 Filled out assessment section of the template.

The phase signifies where in the OPT™ model the client is. This can also act as a reminder about the acute variables significant to this phase. (This will be discussed in detail later in the text.)

Review Questions

1 *If a client spends a lot of time sitting at his or her job, it can lead to tightness in the:*

   a. Lower trapezius

   b. Latissimus dorsi

   c. Hip flexors

2 *Which four sites of the body are used to determine a sum for the Durnin–Womersley formula?*

   a. Thighs

   b. Calves

   c. Biceps

   d. Triceps

   e. Iliac crest

   f. Hips

   g. Subscapular

3 <u>*Static/dynamic*</u> *postural observations should relate to movements such as squatting, bending, pulling, pushing, and balancing.*

4 *What heart rate zone should a 50-year-old male client be in if he achieved a recovery pulse of 90 after performing the 3-minute step test?*

   $$\frac{180 \ (seconds) \times 100 = 36}{90 \times 5.6} \qquad Poor$$

5 *When performing the Shark skill test, how much time do you add to the completion time for each fault?*

   a. 0.05 seconds

   b. 0.10 seconds

   c. 0.15 seconds

REFERENCES

1. American College of Sports Medicine. ACSM's Guidelines for Exercise Testing and Prescription, 5th ed. Philadelphia: Williams & Wilkins, 1995.
2. Thomas S, Reading J, Shephard RJ. Revision of the Physical Activity Readiness Questionnaire (PAR-Q). Can J Sports Sci 1992;17:338–345.
3. Bachrach RM. The relationship of low back pain to psoas insufficiency. J Orthop Med 1991;13:34–40.
4. Janda V. In: Grant R (ed). Physical Therapy of the Cervical and Thoracic Spine. Edinburgh: Churchill Livingstone, 1988.
5. Leahy PM. Active release techniques: logical soft tissue treatment. In: Hammer WI (ed). Functional Soft Tissue Examination and Treatment by Manual Methods. Gaithersburg, MD: Aspen Publishers, 1999.

6. Lewitt K. Manipulation in Rehabilitation of the Locomotor System. London: Butterworth, 1993.
7. Chaitow L. Cranial Manipulation Theory and Practice: Osseous and Soft Tissue Approaches. London: Churchill Livingstone, 1999.
8. Timmons B. Behavioral and Psychological Approaches to Breathing Disorders. New York: Plenum Press, 1994.
9. Bullock-Saxton JE. Local sensation changes and altered hip muscle function following severe ankle sprain. Phys Ther 1994;74(1):17–23.
10. Freeman MAR, Wyke B. Articular reflexes at the ankle joint: an EMG study of normal and abnormal influences of ankle joint mechanoreceptors upon reflex activity in the leg muscles. Br J Surg 1967;54:990–1001.
11. Cornwall M, Murrell P. Postural sway following inversion sprain of the ankle. J Am Pod Med Assoc 1991;81:243–247.
12. Feurbach JW, Grabiner MD. Effect of the Aircast on unilateral postural control: amplitude and frequency variables. J Orthop Sports Phys Ther 1993;7:149–154.
13. Forkin DM, Koczur C, Battle R, Newton RA. Evaluation of kinesthetic deficits indicative of balance control in gymnasts with unilateral chronic ankle sprains. J Orthop Sports Phys Ther 1996;23(4): 245–250.
14. Freeman MAR, Dean MRE, Hanham IWF. The etiology and prevention of functional instability of the foot. J Bone Joint Surg 1965;47B:678–685.
15. Freeman MAR, Wyke B. Articular contributions to limb muscle reflexes. Br J Surg 1966;53:61–69.
16. Guskiewicz KM, Perrin DM. Effect of orthotics on postural sway following inversion ankle sprain. J Orthop Sports Phys Ther 1996;23(5):326–331.
17. Nitz AJ, Dobner JJ, Kersey D. Nerve injury and grades II and III ankle sprains. Am J Sports Med 1985;13:177–182.
18. Wilkerson GB, Nitz AJ. Dynamic ankle stability: mechanical and neuromuscular interrelationships. J Sport Rehabil 1994;3:43–57.
19. Barrack RL, Lund PJ, Skinner HB. Knee proprioception revisited. J Sport Rehab 1994;3:18–42.
20. Beard DJ, Kyberd PJ, O'Connor JJ, Fergusson CM. Reflex hamstring contraction latency in ACL deficiency. J Orthop Res 1994;12(2):219–228.
21. Boyd IA. The histological structure of the receptors in the knee joint of the cat correlated with their physiological response. J Physiol (Lond) 1954;124:476–488.
22. Ciccotti MG, Perry J, Kerian RK, Pink M. An EMG analysis of the normal, the rehabilitated ACL deficient, and the ACL reconstructed patient during functional activities. Abstract presented at AOSSM Society's Specialty Day Meeting, San Fransisco, CA, 1993.
23. Corrigan JP, Cashman WF, Brady MP. Proprioception in the cruciate deficient knee. J Bone Joint Surg 1992;74B:247–250.
24. DeCarlo M, Klootwyk T, Shelbourne K. ACL surgery and accelerated rehabilitation. J Sports Rehabil 1997;6(2):144–156.
25. Ekholm J, Eklund G, Skoglund S. On the reflex effects from knee joint of the cat. Acta Physiol Scand 1960;50:167–174.
26. Feagin JA. The syndrome of a torn ACL. Orthop Clin North Am 1979;10:81–90.
27. Irrgang J, Whitney S, Cox E. Balance and proprioceptive training for rehabilitation of the lower extremity. J Sport Rehabil 1994;3:68–83.
28. Irrgang J, Harner C. Recent advances in ACL rehabilitation: clinical factors. J Sport Rehab 1997;6(2):111–124.
29. Johansson H, Sjolander P. Receptors in the knee joint ligaments and their role in the biomechanics of the joint. Crit Rev Biomed Eng 1988;18(5):341–368.
30. Johansson H. Role of knee ligaments in proprioception and regulation of muscle stiffness. J Electomyogr Kinesiol 1991;1(3):158–179.
31. Johansson H, Sjolander P, Sojka P. A sensory role for the cruciate ligaments. Clin Orthop 1991;268: 161–178.
32. Noyes F, Barber S, Mangine R. Abnormal lower limb symmetry determined by functional hop test after ACL rupture. Am J Sports Med 1991;19(5):516–518.
33. Raunst J, Sager M, Burgner E. Proprioceptive mechanisms in the cruciate ligaments: An EMG study on reflex activity in thigh muscles. J Trauma 1996;41(3):488–493.
34. Solomonow M, Barratta R, Zhou BH. The synergistic action of the ACL and thigh muscles in maintaining joint stability. Am J Sports Med 1987;15:207–213.
35. Janda V. Muscle weakness and inhibition in back pain syndromes. In: Grieve GP (ed). Modern Manual Therapy of the Vertebral Column. New York: Churchill Livingstone, 1986.
36. Lewit K. Muscular and articular factors in movement restriction. Man Med 1985;1:83–85.
37. Hodges PW, Richardson CA. Neuromotor dysfunction of the trunk musculature in low back pain patients. In: Proceedings of the International Congress of the World Confederation of Physical Therapists, Washington, DC, 1995.
38. Hodges PW, Richardson CA. Inefficient muscular stabilization of the lumbar spine associated with low back pain. Spine 1996;21(22):2640–2650.
39. Bullock-Saxton JE, Janda V, Bullock M. Reflex activation of gluteal muscles in walking: an approach to restoration of muscle function for patients with low back pain. Spine 1993;18(6):704–708.
40. Hodges PW, Richardson CA. Contraction of the abdominal muscles associated with movement of the lower limb. Phys Ther 1997;77:132–144.

41. Hodges PW, Richardson CA, Jull G. Evaluation of the relationship between laboratory and clinical tests of transverse abdominis function. Physiother Res Int 1996;1:30–40.

42. Richardson CA, Jull G, Toppenberg R, Comerford M. Techniques for active lumbar stabilization for spinal protection. Austr J Physiother 1992;38:105–112.

43. O'Sullivan PE, Twomey L, Allison G, Sinclair J, Miller K, Knox J. Altered patterns of abdominal muscle activation in patients with chronic low back pain. Austr J Physiother 1997;43(2):91–98.

44. Jull G, Richardson CA, Comerford M. Strategies for the initial activation of dynamic lumbar stabilization. Proceedings of Manipulative Physiotherapists Association of Australia. New South Wales, 1991.

45. Jull G, Richardson CA, Hamilton C, Hodges PW, Ng J. Towards the validation of a clinical test for the deep abdominal muscles in back pain patients. Manipulative Physiotherapists Association of Australia. Gold Coast, Queensland, 1995.

46. Glousman R, Jobe F, Tibone JE, Moynes D, Antonelli D, Perry J. Dynamic electromyographic analysis of the throwing shoulder with glenohumeral instability. J Bone Joint Surg 1988;70(2):220–226.

47. Broström L-Å, Kronberg M, Nemeth G. Muscle activity during shoulder dislocation. Acta Orthop Scand 1989;60:639–641.

48. Howell SM, Kraft TA. The role of the supraspinatus and infraspinatus muscles in glenohumeral kinematics of anterior shoulder instability. Clin Orthop 1991;263:128–134.

49. Kronberg M, Broström L-Å, Nemeth G. Differences in shoulder muscle activity between patients with generalized joint laxity and normal controls. Clin Orthop 1991;269:181–192.

50. Glousman R. Electromyographic analysis and its role in the athletic shoulder. Clin Orthop 1993; 288:27–34.

51. Mense S, Simons DG. Muscle Pain. Understanding its Nature, Diagnosis, and Treatment. Philadelphia: Lippincott Williams & Wilkins, 2001.

52. Trott PH, Grant R. Manipulative physical therapy in the management of selected low lumbar syndromes. In: Twomey LT, Taylor JR (eds). Physical Therapy of the Low Back, 3rd ed. New York: Churchill Livingstone, 2000.

53. Whaley MA, Kaminsky LA. Epidemiology of physical activity, physical fitness, and selected chronic diseases. In: American College of Sports Medicine (ed). ACSM's Resource Manual for Guidelines for Exercise Testing and Prescription, 3rd ed. Baltimore: Williams & Wilkins, 1998.

54. Prate RR, Pratt MM, Blair SN, Haskell WL, Macera CA, Bouchard C, Buchner D, Ettinger W, Heath GW, King AC. Physical activity and public health: a recommendation from the Centers for Disease Control and Prevention and the American College of Sports Medicine. JAMA 1995; 273:402–407.

55. Lambert EV, Bohlmann I, Cowling K. Physical activity for health: understanding the epidemiological evidence for risk benefits. Int Sport Med J 2001;1(5):1–15.

56. American College of Sports Medicine. ACSM's Resource Manual for Guidelines for Exercise Testing and Prescription, 3rd ed. Baltimore: Williams & Wilkins, 1998.

57. Durnin JVGA, Womersley J. Body fat assessed from total body density and its estimation from skinfold thickness measurements on 481 men and women aged 16–72 years. Br J Nutr 1974;32:77–97.

58. Ehrman JK, Gordon PM, Visich PS, Keteyian SJ. Clinical Exercise Physiology. Champaign, IL: Human Kinetics, 2003.

59. McArdle WD, Katch FI, Katch VL. Exercise Physiology: Energy, Nutrition and Human Performance. Philadelphia: Williams & Wilkins, 1996.

60. Kendall FP, McCreary EK, Provance PG. Muscles Testing and Function, 4th ed. Baltimore: Lippincott Williams & Wilkins, 1993.

61. Norkin CC, Levangie PK. Joint Structure and Function, 2nd ed. Philadelphia: FA Davis, 1992.

62. Soderberg GL. Kinesiology, 2nd ed. Baltimore: Williams & Wilkins, 1997.

63. Rash PJ, Burke RK. Kinesiology and Applied Anatomy. Philadelphia; Lea & Febiger, 1971.

64. Gross J, Fetto J, Rosen E. Musculoskeletal Examination. Malden, MA: Blackwell Sciences, 1996.

65. Hansen PD, Woollacott MH, Debu B. Postural responses to changing task conditions. Exp Brain Res 1988;73:627–636.

66. Dietz V. Human neuronal control of automatic functional movements: interactions between central programs and afferent input. Physiol Rev 1992;72:33–69.

67. Liebension C. Integrating rehabilitation into chiropractic practice (blending active and passive care). In: Liebenson C (ed). Rehabilitation of the Spine. Baltimore: Williams & Wilkins, 1996.

68. Janda V. Muscle strength in relation to muscle length, pain and muscle imbalance. In: Harms-Rindahl K (ed). Muscle Strength. New York: Churchill Livingstone, 1993.

Flexibility Training Concepts

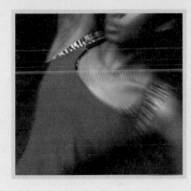

OBJECTIVES

After studying this chapter, you will be able to:

- Explain the effects of muscle imbalances on the kinetic chain.
- Provide a scientific rationale for the use of an integrated flexibility training program.
- Differentiate between the types of flexibility techniques.
- Perform and instruct appropriate flexibility techniques for given situations.

KEY TERMS

Active-isolated stretching
Altered reciprocal inhibition
Arthrokinematics
Arthrokinetic dysfunction
Autogenic inhibition
Davis's law
Dynamic functional flexibility

Dynamic range of motion
Dynamic stretching
Extensibility
Flexibility
Muscle imbalance
Neuromuscular efficiency
Pattern overload

Postural distortion patterns
Relative flexibility
Self-myofascial release
Static stretching
Synergistic dominance

INTRODUCTION TO FLEXIBILITY TRAINING

With the completion of the assessment section, all pertinent information needed to fill out the remainder of the programming template has been gathered. The focus can now be shifted toward designing the program. The next portion of the Optimum Performance Training (OPT™) programming template that needs to be filled out is the warm-up section (Step 1). In designing the warm-up program, the components of flexibility and cardiorespiratory training need to be reviewed. Most clients require flexibility training to properly perform any type of cardiorespiratory work, so that is a good place to start.

Current Concepts in Flexibility Training

WHY IS FLEXIBILITY TRAINING IMPORTANT?

Today's society is plagued by postural imbalances, primarily owing to sedentary lifestyles caused by advancements in technology. More people today are spending time in office-related jobs, which require individuals to sit for long hours. More than ever before, flexibility training has become a key component in developing neuromuscular efficiency and decreasing these dysfunctions. Flexibility training may decrease the occurrences of muscle imbalances, joint dysfunctions, and overuse injuries. Without optimum levels of flexibility, it may not be possible for clients to achieve their goals without getting injured.[1-4] (see Stretch Your Knowledge: Lack of flexibility and the risk of injury?) It is critical for fitness professionals to learn about flexibility training to properly design an integrated training program.[1-3]

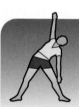

Stretch Your Knowledge

Lack of Flexibility and the Risk of Injury?

- Witvrouw et al. (2003) in a prospective study with 146 male soccer players found that soccer players with increased muscle tightness in the quadriceps and hamstrings were found to have a statistically greater risk for injury compared with the uninjured group.[1]

- Witvrouw et al. (2001) in a prospective study found that decreased flexibility of the hamstrings and quadriceps significantly contributes to the development of patellar tendonitis in the athletic population.[2]

- Cibulka et al. (1998) in a cross-sectional study of 100 patients with unspecified low back pain demonstrated unilateral hip rotation asymmetry.[3]

- Knapik et al. (1991) reported that strength and flexibility imbalances in female collegiate athletes were associated with lower extremity injuries.[4]

1. Witvrouw E, Danneels L, Asselman P, D'Have T, Cambier D. Muscle flexibility as a risk factor for developing muscle injuries in male professional soccer players. A prospective study. Am J Sports Med 2003;31(1):41–46.
2. Witvrouw E, Bellemans J, Lysens R, Danneels L, Cambier D. Intrinsic risk factors for the development of patellar tendinitis in an athletic population. A two-year prospective study. Am J Sports Med 2001;29(2):190–195.
3. Cibulka MT, Sinacore DR, Cromer GS, Delitto A. Unilateral hip rotation range of motion asymmetry in patients with sacroiliac joint regional pain. Spine 1998;23(9):1009–1015.
4. Knapik JJ, Bauman CL, Jones BH, Harris JM, Vaughan L. Preseason strength and flexibility imbalances associated with athletic injuries in female collegiate athletes. Am J Sports Med 1991;19(1):76–81.

WHAT IS FLEXIBILITY?

Flexibility: The normal extensibility of all soft tissues that allow the full range of motion of a joint.

Extensibility: Capability to be elongated or stretched.

Dynamic range of motion: The combination of flexibility and the nervous system's ability to control this range of motion efficiently.

Neuromuscular efficiency: The ability of the neuromuscular system to allow agonists, antagonists, and stabilizers to work synergistically to produce, reduce, and dynamically stabilize the entire kinetic chain in all three planes of motion.

Dynamic functional flexibility: Multiplanar soft tissue extensibility with optimal neuromuscular efficiency throughout the full range of motion.

Flexibility is the normal **extensibility** of all soft tissues that allow the full range of motion of a joint.[1] However, for soft tissue to achieve efficient extensibility, there must be optimum control throughout the entire range of motion.[5] More specifically, this optimum control can be referred to as **dynamic range of motion**. This is the combination of flexibility and the nervous system's ability to control this range of motion efficiently (or neuromuscular efficiency).

Neuromuscular efficiency is the ability of the nervous system to properly recruit the correct muscles (agonists, antagonists, synergists, and stabilizers) to produce force (concentrically), reduce force (eccentrically), and dynamically stabilize (isometrically) the body's structure in all three planes of motion.

For example, when performing a lat pull-down, the latissimus dorsi (agonist) must be able to concentrically accelerate shoulder extension, adduction, and internal rotation while the middle and lower trapezius and rhomboids (synergists) perform downward rotation of the scapulae. At the same time, the rotator cuff musculature (stabilizers) must dynamically stabilize the glenohumeral joint throughout the motion. If these muscles (force-couples) do not work in tandem efficiently, compensations may ensue, leading to muscle imbalances, altered joint motion, and possible injury.

To allow for optimal neuromuscular efficiency, individuals must have proper flexibility in all three planes of motion. This allows for the movement needed to perform everyday activities effectively, such as bending over to tie shoes or reaching in the top cupboard for dishes (Table 6-1).

In review, flexibility requires extensibility, which requires dynamic range of motion, which requires neuromuscular efficiency. This entire chain is referred to as **dynamic functional flexibility** and is achieved by taking an integrated approach toward flexibility training.

Flexibility training must be a multifaceted approach, which integrates various flexibility techniques to achieve optimum soft tissue extensibility in all planes of motion (Table 6-1).

Table 6.1

Multiplanar Flexibility

Muscle	Plane of Motion	Movement
Latissimus dorsi	SAGITTAL	Must have proper extensibility to allow for proper shoulder flexion
	FRONTAL	Must have proper extensibility to allow for proper shoulder abduction
	TRANSVERSE	Must have proper extensibility to allow for proper external humerus rotation
Biceps femoris	SAGITTAL	Must have proper extensibility to allow for proper hip flexion; knee extension
	FRONTAL	Must have proper extensibility to allow for proper hip adduction
	TRANSVERSE	Must have proper extensibility to allow for proper hip and knee internal rotation
Gastrocnemius	SAGITTAL	Must have proper extensibility to allow for proper dorsiflexion of ankle
	FRONTAL	Must have proper extensibility to allow for proper inversion of calcaneus
	TRANSVERSE	Must have proper extensibility to allow for proper internal rotation of femur

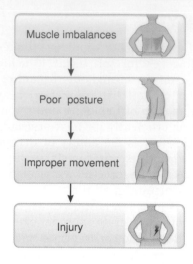

Figure 6.1   Postural distortion patterns.

To better understand integrated flexibility, a few important concepts must first be reviewed. These include the kinetic chain, muscle imbalances, and neuromuscular control (efficiency).

REVIEW OF THE KINETIC CHAIN

The kinetic chain comprises the muscular, skeletal, and nervous systems. Optimum alignment and function of each component of the kinetic chain is the cornerstone of a sound training program. If one segment of the kinetic chain is misaligned and not functioning properly, predictable patterns of dysfunction develop.[5-8] These predictable patterns of dysfunction are referred to as **postural distortion patterns** and lead to decreased neuromuscular efficiency and tissue overload (Figure 6-1).[5]

Postural distortion patterns (movement compensations) are represented by a lack of structural integrity, resulting from decreased functioning of one (or more) components of the kinetic chain.[5-7] This lack of structural integrity comes in the form of altered length-tension relationships, force-couple relationships, and arthrokinematics. There are several postural distortions about which the fitness professional must be aware of, all of which are reviewed in Chapter 5.

Maximum neuromuscular efficiency of the kinetic chain can only exist if all kinetic chain components (muscular, skeletal, and neural) function optimally and interdependently. The ultimate goal of the kinetic chain is to maintain homeostasis (or dynamic postural equilibrium).

Poor flexibility may lead to the development of **relative flexibility**, which is the process in which the kinetic chain seeks the path of least resistance, during functional movement patterns.[9] A prime example of relative flexibility is seen in people who squat with their feet externally rotated (Figure 6-2). As most people today have tightness in their calf muscles, they lack the proper amount of dorsiflexion at the ankle to perform a squat with proper mechanics. By widening their stance and externally rotating their feet, they are able to decrease the amount of dorsiflexion required at the ankle to squat and, thus, compensate for this lack of flexibility. A second example is seen when people perform an overhead shoulder press with excessive lumbar extension (Figure 6-3). Individuals who possess a tight latissimus dorsi will have decreased sagittal-plane shoulder flexion. As a result, they must compensate for this lack of range of motion at the shoulder in the lumbar spine to allow for them to press the load completely above their head.

Muscle Imbalance

Muscle imbalances caused by abnormal structural and functional efficiency of the kinetic chain (altered length-tension relationships, force-couple relationships, and arthrokinematics) are alterations in the lengths of muscles surrounding a given

Postural distortion patterns: Predictable patterns of muscle imbalances.

Relative flexibility: The tendency of the body to seek the path of least resistance during functional movement patterns.

Muscle imbalance: Alteration of muscle length surrounding a joint.

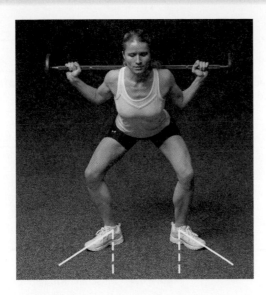

Figure 6.2 Squat with externally rotated feet.

joint, in which some are overactive (forcing compensation to occur) and others may be underactive (allowing for the compensation to occur).[5,7] Examples of such imbalances come in the forms of the movement compensations discussed in Chapter 5.

Muscle imbalance can be caused by a variety of mechanisms.[1,9] These causes may include:

- Postural stress
- Emotional duress
- Repetitive movement

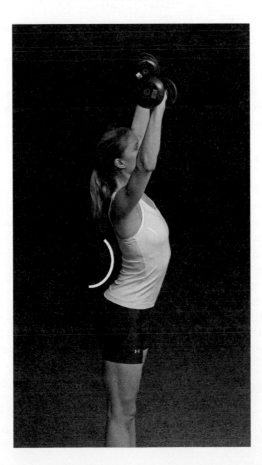

Figure 6.3 Overhead shoulder press with lumbar extension.

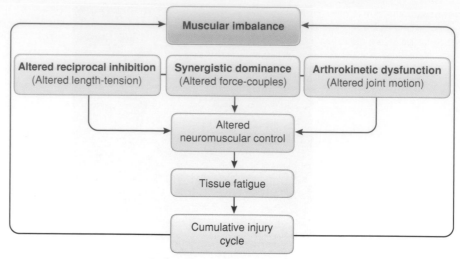

Figure 6.4   Muscular imbalance.

- Cumulative trauma
- Poor training technique
- Lack of core strength
- Lack of neuromuscular control (efficiency)

Muscle imbalances result from altered reciprocal inhibition, synergistic dominance, arthrokinetic dysfunction, and overall decreased neuromuscular control (Figure 6-4). These concepts are reviewed below.

Altered Reciprocal Inhibition

Altered reciprocal inhibition: The concept of muscle inhibition, caused by a tight agonist, which inhibits its functional antagonist.

Altered reciprocal inhibition is the concept of muscle inhibition caused by a tight agonist, which decreases neural drive of its functional antagonist.[1,5–7,10–16] For example, a tight psoas (hip flexor) would decrease neural drive of the gluteus maximus (hip extensor). This results in muscle imbalances, which alter length-tension relationships and force-couple relationships, produce synergistic dominance, and lead to the development of faulty movement patterns, poor neuromuscular control, and arthrokinetic dysfunction.

Synergistic Dominance

Synergistic dominance: The neuromuscular phenomenon that occurs when inappropriate muscles take over the function of a weak or inhibited prime mover.

Synergistic dominance is the neuromuscular phenomenon that occurs when synergists take over function for a weak or inhibited prime mover.[7] Think of this as your body's substitution system. When the starting player on a sports team gets tired, the coach puts in the backup player. The backup player can perform the tasks necessary to play, but not quite as well as the starter. The nervous system reacts in the same manner. For example, when the psoas is tight, it leads to reciprocal inhibition of the gluteus maximus. The result is increased force output of the synergists for hip extension (hamstrings, adductor magnus, and erector spinae) to compensate for the weakened gluteus maximus. This causes faulty movement patterns, leading to arthrokinetic (joint) dysfunction and altered force-couple relationships, decreasing neuromuscular efficiency, and eventually leading to injury.

Arthrokinetic Dysfunction

Arthrokinematics: The motions of joints in the body.

The term **arthrokinematics** refers to the motion of the joints. **Arthrokinetic dysfunction** is a biomechanical and neuromuscular dysfunction leading to

Arthrokinetic dysfunction: Altered forces at the joint that result in abnormal muscular activity and impaired neuromuscular communication at the joint.

altered joint motion.[5-8] Altered joint motion causes altered length-tension relationships and force-couple relationships. This affects the joint and causes poor movement efficiency. For example, externally rotating the feet when squatting forces the tibia and femur to also externally rotate. This alters length-tension relationships of the muscles at the knee and hips, putting the gluteus maximus (agonist) in a shortened position and decreasing its ability to generate force. This causes the biceps femoris and piriformis (synergists) to become synergistically dominant, altering force-couple relationships (recruitment patterns), altering arthrokinematics (joint motion), and increasing stress to the knees and low back.[17] Over time, this stress can lead to pain, which can further alter muscle recruitment and joint mechanics.[5-7]

Neuromuscular Efficiency

As mentioned earlier, neuromuscular efficiency is the ability of the neuromuscular system to properly recruit muscles to produce force (concentrically), reduce force (eccentrically), and dynamically stabilize (isometrically) the entire kinetic chain in all three planes of motion. Because the nervous system is the controlling factor behind this principle, it is important to mention that *mechanoreceptors* (or sensory receptors) located in the muscles and tendons help to determine muscle balance or imbalance. These mechanoreceptors include the muscle spindles and Golgi tendon organ.

MUSCLE SPINDLES

As mentioned in Chapter 2, muscle spindles are the major sensory organ of the muscle and are composed of microscopic fibers that lie parallel to the muscle fiber. Remember that muscle spindles are sensitive to change in length and rate of length change.[5,18-25] When a muscle on one side of a joint is lengthened (owing to a shortened muscle on the other side), the spindles of the lengthened muscle are stretched. This information is transmitted to the brain and spinal cord, exciting the muscle spindle, causing the muscle fibers to contract. This often results in muscle spasms or a feeling of tightness.[1,5,6]

The hamstring is a prime example of this response when the pelvis is rotated anteriorly (forward) (Figure 6-5). This means that the anterior superior iliac spines (front of the pelvis) move downward (inferiorly) and the ischium (bottom posterior portion of pelvis, where the hamstrings originate) moves upward (superiorly). If the attachment of the hamstrings is moved superiorly, it increases the distance between the two attachment sites and lengthens the muscle. In this case, the hamstrings do not need to be statically stretched because they are already in a stretched position. When a lengthened muscle is stretched, it

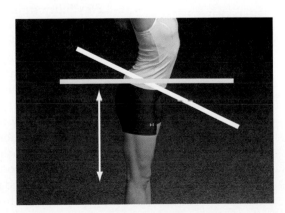

Figure 6.5 Effect of the hamstring with an anteriorly rotated pelvis.

increases the excitement of the muscle spindles and further creates a contraction (spasm) response. With this scenario, the shortened hip flexors are helping to create the anterior pelvic rotation that is causing the lengthening of the hamstrings. Instead, the hip flexors need to be stretched.[17] (This will be reviewed later in the chapter.)

Another example includes an individual whose knees adduct and internally rotate during an overhead squat. The underactive muscle is the gluteus medius (hip abductor and external rotator). Thus, one would not need to stretch the gluteus medius, but instead stretch the adductor complex, which in this case is overactive, pulling the femur into excessive adduction and internal rotation. Individuals with protracted (rounded) shoulders need not stretch the rhomboids and the middle and lower trapezius (underactive), but rather stretch the overactive muscles, pulling them into this position (pectoralis major, pectoralis minor, and latissimus dorsi).

GOLGI TENDON ORGANS

As also mentioned in Chapter 2, Golgi tendon organs are located within the *musculotendinous junction* (or the point where the muscle and the tendon meet) and are sensitive to changes in muscular tension and rate of the tension change.[5,18–25] When excited, the Golgi tendon organ causes the muscle to relax. This prevents the muscle from being placed under excessive stress, which could result in injury.

Prolonged Golgi tendon organ stimulation provides an inhibitory action to muscle spindles (located within the same muscle). This neuromuscular phenomenon is called **autogenic inhibition** and occurs when the neural impulses sensing tension are greater than the impulses causing muscle contraction.[14] The phenomenon is termed "autogenic" because the contracting muscle is being inhibited by its own receptors.

Autogenic inhibition: The process when neural impulses that sense tension is greater than the impulses that cause muscles to contract, providing an inhibitory effect to the muscle spindles.

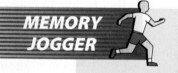

MEMORY JOGGER

Autogenic inhibition is one of the main principles used in flexibility training, particularly with static stretching when one holds a stretch for a prolonged period of time (20–30 seconds). Holding a stretch creates tension in the muscle. This tension stimulates the Golgi tendon organ, which overrides muscle spindle activity in the muscle being stretched, causing relaxation in the overactive muscle and allowing for optimal lengthening of the tissue.

SUMMARY

Flexibility training may decrease the chance of muscle imbalances, joint dysfunctions, and overuse injuries. It is important to have proper range of motion in all three planes. This can be achieved by implementing an integrated approach toward flexibility training.

All segments of the kinetic chain must be properly aligned to avoid postural distortion patterns, decreased neuromuscular efficiency, and tissue overload. The adaptive potential of the kinetic chain is decreased by limited flexibility. This forces the body to move in an altered fashion, leading to relative flexibility.

Muscle imbalances result from altered length-tension relationships, force-couple relationships, and arthrokinematics. These imbalances can be caused by poor posture, poor training technique, or previous injury. These muscle imbalances result in altered reciprocal inhibition, synergistic dominance, and arthrokinetic dysfunction, which in turn lead to decreased neuromuscular control.

Scientific Rationale for Flexibility Training

BENEFITS OF FLEXIBILITY TRAINING

Flexibility training is a key component for all training programs.[1,5] It is used for a variety of reasons, including:

- Correcting muscle imbalances
- Increasing joint range of motion
- Decreasing the excessive tension of muscles
- Relieving joint stress
- Improving the extensibility of the musculotendinous junction
- Maintaining the normal functional length of all muscles
- Improving optimum neuromuscular efficiency
- Improving function

PATTERN OVERLOAD

Pattern overload:
Consistently repeating the same pattern of motion, which may place abnormal stresses on the body.

Significant numbers of people in today's society have muscular imbalances that are a result of **pattern overload**. Pattern overload is consistently repeating the same pattern of motion. There are gym members who train with the same routine repetitively. This may lead to pattern overload and place abnormal stresses on the body.

Pattern overload may not necessarily be directly related to exercise. Consider the person who has a particularly repetitive occupation such as a loading-dock employee lifting and loading packages all day. He or she, too, will experience a pattern overload from moving his or her body in repetitive ways on a daily basis. Even sitting at a computer is a repetitive stress.

CUMULATIVE INJURY CYCLE

Poor posture and repetitive movements create dysfunction within the connective tissue of the kinetic chain.[1,5,26-28] This dysfunction is treated by the body as an injury, and as a result, the body will initiate a repair process termed the cumulative injury cycle (Figure 6-6).[5,28]

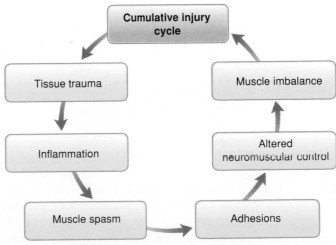

Figure 6.6   Cumulative injury cycle.

Any trauma to the tissue of the body (such as resistance training) creates inflammation. Inflammation, in turn, activates the body's pain receptors and initiates a protective mechanism, increasing muscle tension or causing muscle spasm. Heightened activity of muscle spindles in particular areas of the muscle create a microspasm. As a result of the spasm, adhesions (or knots) begin to form in the soft tissue. These adhesions form a weak, inelastic matrix (unable to stretch) that decreases normal elasticity of the soft tissue.[1,5,28] The result is altered length-tension relationships (leading to altered reciprocal inhibition), altered force-couple relationships (leading to synergistic dominance), and arthrokinetic dysfunction (leading to altered joint motion). Left unchecked, these adhesions can begin to form permanent structural changes in the soft tissue that is evident by Davis's law.

Davis's law: States that soft tissue models along the lines of stress.

Davis's law states that soft tissue models along the lines of stress.[1,5,29] Soft tissue remodels (or rebuilds) itself with an inelastic collagen matrix that forms in a random fashion. This simply means that it usually does not run in the same direction as the muscle fibers. If the muscle fibers are lengthened, these inelastic connective tissue fibers act as roadblocks, preventing the muscle fibers from moving properly. This creates alterations in normal tissue extensibility and causes relative flexibility.[9]

For example, if a muscle is in a constant shortened state (such as the hip flexor musculature when sitting for prolonged periods every day), it will demonstrate poor neuromuscular efficiency (as a result of altered length-tension and force-couple relationships). In turn, this will affect joint motion (ankle, knee, hip, and lumbar spine) and alter movement patterns (leading to synergistic dominance). An inelastic collagen matrix will form along the same lines of stress created by the altered muscle movements. Because the muscle is consistently short and moves in a pattern different from its intended function, the newly formed inelastic connective tissue forms along this altered pattern, reducing the ability of the muscle to extend and move in its proper manner. This is why it is imperative that an integrated flexibility training program be used to restore the normal extensibility of the entire soft tissue complex.[30,31]

It is essential for health and fitness professionals to address their clients' muscular imbalances through an integrated fitness assessment and flexibility training program. By neglecting these phases of programming and simply moving clients right into a resistance training program, it will add additional loads to joints and muscles that have improper mechanics and faulty recruitment patterns.

SUMMARY

Flexibility training has the benefits of improving muscle imbalances, increasing joint range of motion and extensibility, relieving excessive tension of muscles and joint stress, and improving neuromuscular efficiency and function.

People who physically train in a repetitive fashion (or have jobs that require moving their bodies in repetitive ways) may experience pattern overload, which places stress on the body.

Poor posture and repetitive movements may create dysfunctions in connective tissue, initiating the cumulative injury cycle. Tissue trauma creates inflammation, which leads to microspasms and decreases normal elasticity of the soft tissue.

Soft tissue rebuilds itself in a random fashion with an inelastic collagen matrix that usually does not run in the same direction as the muscle fibers. If the muscle fibers are lengthened, these inelastic connective tissue fibers act as roadblocks, creating alterations in normal tissue extensibility and causing relative flexibility. It is essential for fitness professionals to address muscular imbalances through fitness assessment and flexibility training to restore the normal extensibility of the entire soft tissue complex.

The Flexibility Continuum

To fully appreciate the principles of flexibility training, health and fitness professionals must understand the different types. Flexibility, like any other form of training, should follow a systematic progression. This is known as the flexibility continuum. There are three phases of flexibility training: corrective, active, and functional (Figure 6-7).[1,10,14,32,33]

CORRECTIVE FLEXIBILITY

Corrective flexibility is designed to improve muscle imbalances and altered joint motion. It uses the principles of autogenic inhibition. It includes self-myofascial release (foam roll) techniques and static stretching. This form of flexibility is appropriate at the stabilization level (Phase 1) of the OPT™ model.

ACTIVE FLEXIBILITY

Active flexibility is designed to improve the extensibility of soft tissue and increase neuromuscular efficiency by using reciprocal inhibition. Active flexibility allows for agonists and synergist muscles to move a limb through a full range of motion while the functional antagonists are being stretched.[14,34,35] For example, a supine straight leg raise uses the hip flexor and quadriceps to raise the leg and hold it unsupported, while the antagonist hamstring group is stretched. Active flexibility uses self-myofascial release and active-isolated stretching techniques. This form of flexibility would be appropriate at the Strength Level (Phases 2, 3, and 4) of the OPT™ model.

FUNCTIONAL FLEXIBILITY

Functional flexibility is integrated, multiplanar soft tissue extensibility, with optimum neuromuscular control, through the full range of motion.[14] Essentially, it is movement without compensations. Therefore, if a client is compensating during training then he or she needs to be regressed to corrective and active flexibility. Functional flexibility uses self-myofascial release techniques and dynamic flexibility. This form of flexibility would be appropriate at the Power Level (Phase 5) of the OPT™ model.

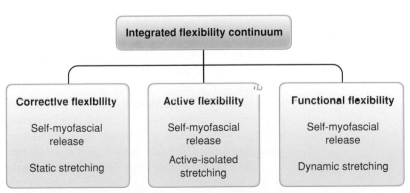

Figure 6.7 Integrated flexibility continuum.

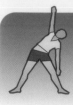

Stretch Your Knowledge

Which Type of Stretching Should be Used? All of Them, in a Progressive, Integrated Fashion.

Static Stretching

- Porter et al. (2002) in a randomized controlled trial with 94 subjects demonstrated that both sustained (3 minutes, 3 times daily) and intermittent stretching (5 sets of 20-second holds, 2 times daily) for the Achilles tendon increased flexibility and decreased pain.[1]

- Hanten et al. (2000) in a randomized clinical trial of 40 subjects found that a home exercise program of ischemic pressure followed by static stretching was effective for decreasing trigger point sensitivity and increasing range of motion.[2]

Active Stretching

- Maddig and Harmer (2002) in a randomized controlled trial with 30 recreational athletes found that active isolated stretching is effective for increasing hamstring range of motion.[3]

Dynamic Stretching

- Sherry and Best (2004) in a prospective randomized comparison study of two rehabilitation programs with 24 athletes demonstrated improved functional outcomes with patients using dynamic functional movements (progressive agility and trunk stabilization) that require stabilization, proprioception, and muscle lengthening to occur simultaneously.[4]

---

1. Porter D, Barrill E, Oneacre K, May BD. The effects of duration and frequency of Achilles tendon stretching on dorsiflexion and outcome in painful heel syndrome. Foot Ankle Int 2002;23(7):619–624.
2. Hanten WP, Olson SL, Butts NL, Nowicki AL. Effectiveness of a home program of ischemic pressure followed by sustained stretch for treatment of myofascial trigger points. Phys Ther 2000;80:997–1003.
3. Maddig TR, Harmer P. Active-isolated stretching is not more effective than static stretching for increased hamstring ROM. Med Sci Sports Exerc 2002;34(5 Suppl 1).
4. Sherry MA, Best TM. A comparison of 2 rehabilitation programs in the treatment of acute hamstring strains. J Orthop Sports Phys Ther 2004;34(3):116–125.

Remember that all functional movements occur in all three planes of motion and that injuries most often occur in the transverse plane. If the appropriate soft tissue is not extensible through the full range of movement, the risk of injury dramatically increases.[2,36] Exercises that increase multiplanar soft tissue extensibility and have high levels of neuromuscular demand are preferred.

SUMMARY

Flexibility training should be progressive, systematic, and based on an assessment. There are three phases of flexibility training: corrective, active, and functional.

Corrective flexibility improves muscle imbalances and altered joint motion by using self-myofascial release and static stretching. Active flexibility improves the extensibility of soft tissue and increases neuromuscular efficiency by using self-myofascial release and active-isolated stretching. Functional flexibility improves the extensibility of soft tissue and increases neuromuscular efficiency by using integrated, multiplanar techniques that move through the full range of motion.

Injuries most often occur in the transverse plane. If the appropriate soft tissue is not extensible through the full range of movement, the risk of injury dramatically increases. Health and fitness professionals should emphasize exercises that

Table 6.2		
Examples of Stretching Within the Flexibility Continuum		
Flexibility Type	**Type of Stretching**	**Examples**
Corrective Flexibility	Self-myofascial release Static	Foam roll Static adductor stretch
Active Flexibility	Self-myofascial release Active-isolated	Foam roll Active adductor stretch
Functional Flexibility	Self-myofascial release Dynamic	Foam roll Side lunge

increase multiplanar soft tissue extensibility and have high levels of neuromuscular demand.

STRETCHING TECHNIQUES

Proper stretching is one way to enhance flexibility and can also be viewed as a continuum. The flexibility continuum consists of specific forms of stretching. For example, corrective flexibility uses self-myofascial release and static stretching; active flexibility uses self-myofascial release and active-isolated stretching; and functional flexibility uses self-myofascial release and dynamic stretching (Table 6-2). Each form of stretching manipulates the receptors and the nervous system, which in turn allows for alteration of muscle extensibility.

Self-Myofascial Release

Self-myofascial release is another stretching technique that focuses on the neural system and fascial system in the body (or, the fibrous tissue that surrounds and separates muscle tissue). By applying gentle force to an adhesion or "knot," the elastic muscle fibers are altered from a bundled position (that causes the adhesion) into a straighter alignment with the direction of the muscle or fascia. The gentle pressure (applied with implements such as a foam roll) will stimulate the Golgi tendon organ and create autogenic inhibition, decreasing muscle spindle excitation and releasing the hypertonicity of the underlying musculature.

It is crucial to note that when a person is using self-myofascial release he or she must find a tender spot (which indicates the presence of muscle hypertonicity) and sustain pressure on that spot for a minimum of 20 to 30 seconds. This will increase the Golgi tendon organ activity and decrease muscle spindle activity, thus the autogenic inhibition response. It may take longer, depending on the client's ability to consciously relax.

This process will help restore the body back to its optimal level of function by resetting the proprioceptive mechanisms of the soft tissue.[37] Self-myofascial release is suggested before static stretching for postural distortion patterns or before activity. In addition, it can be used during the cool-down process.

Gastrocnemius/Soleus

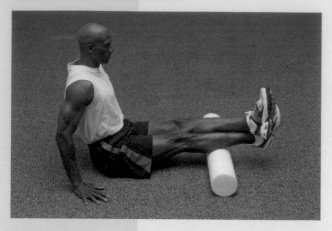

PREPARATION

1. Place foam roll under mid-calf.
2. Cross left leg over right leg to increase pressure (optional).

MOVEMENT

3. Slowly roll calf area to find the most tender spot.
4. Once identified, hold tender spot until the discomfort is reduced.

TFL/IT Band

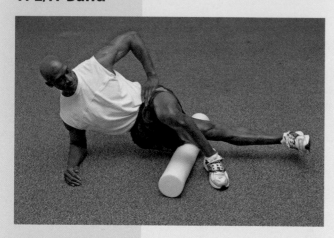

PREPARATION

1. Lie on one side, the foam roll just in front of the hip. Cross the top leg over lower leg, with foot touching the floor and the bottom leg raised slightly off floor.
2. Maintain optimal head alignment (ears in line with shoulders).

MOVEMENT

3. Slowly roll from hip joint to lateral knee to find the most tender spot.
4. Once identified, hold tender spot until the discomfort is reduced.

Adductors

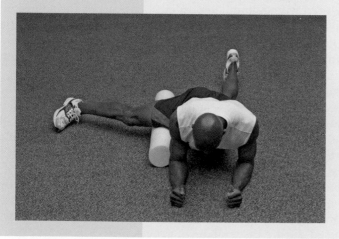

PREPARATION

1. Lie prone with one thigh flexed and abducted and the foam roll in the groin region, inside the upper thigh.

MOVEMENT

2. Slowly roll the medial thigh area to find the most tender spot.
3. Once identified, hold tender spot until the discomfort is reduced.

Piriformis

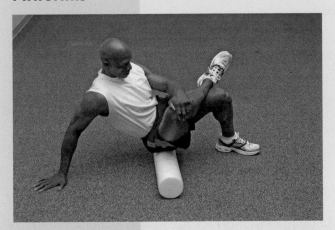

PREPARATION

1. Sit on top of the foam roll, positioned on the back of the hip. Cross one foot to the opposite knee.

MOVEMENT

2. Lean into the hip of the crossed leg. Slowly roll on the posterior hip area to find the most tender spot.
3. Once identified, hold tender spot until the discomfort is reduced.

Latissimus Dorsi

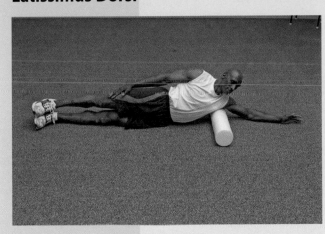

PREPARATION

1. Lie on the floor on one side with the arm closest to the floor outstretched and thumb facing upward.
2. Place the foam roll under the arm (axillary region).

MOVEMENT

3. Slowly move back and forth to find the most tender spot.
4. Once identified, hold tender spot until the discomfort is reduced.

STATIC STRETCHING

Static stretching: The process of passively taking a muscle to the point of tension and holding the stretch for a minimum of 20 seconds.

Static stretching is the process of passively taking a muscle to the point of tension and holding the stretch for a minimum of 20 seconds.[1,2,11] This is the traditional form of stretching that is most often seen in fitness today. It combines low force with longer duration.[14,38]

The proposed mechanism for this type of stretching is autogenic inhibition. By holding the muscle in a stretched position for a prolonged period of time, the Golgi tendon organ is stimulated and produces an inhibitory effect on the muscle spindle (autogenic inhibition). This allows the muscle to relax and provides for better elongation of the muscle (Table 6-3).[5,39] In addition, contracting the antagonistic musculature while holding the stretch can reciprocally inhibit the muscle being stretched, allowing it to relax and enhancing the stretch. For example, when performing the kneeling hip flexor stretch, one should (if possible) contract the hip extender (gluteus maximus) to reciprocally inhibit the hip flexors (psoas, rectus femoris), allowing for greater lengthening of these muscles.

Table 6.3

Static Stretching Summary

Type of Stretch	Mechanism of Action	Acute Variables	Examples
Static stretch	Autogenic inhibition	1–3 sets Hold each stretch 20–30 seconds	Gastrocnemius stretch Kneeling hip flexor stretch Standing adductor stretch Pectoral wall stretch

Static stretching should be used to decrease the muscle spindle activity of a tight muscle before and after activity. Detailed explanations of various static stretching techniques are described below.

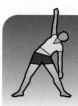

Stretch Your Knowledge

Effects of Static Stretching

- Bandy et al. (1998) demonstrated that both static and active stretching (dynamic range of motion [DROM]) produced significant improvements in hamstring extensibility and that static stretching increased range of motion (ROM) by more than twice that of DROM.[1]

- Davis et al. (2005) compared static stretching with both a self-stretch technique (actively held static stretching) and proprioceptive neuromuscular facilitation (PNF) stretching (often termed contract-relax or neuromuscular stretching) relative to hamstring flexibility. The results showed that although all three groups increased ROM for the hamstring muscles, only the static stretching group significantly increased ROM compared with the control group.[2]

- Shrier (2004) indicated that whereas acute bouts of static stretching may not immediately improve performance, regular long-term static stretching improves force production, jump height, and speed.[3]

---

1. Bandy WD, Irion JM, Briggler M. The effect of static stretch and dynamic range of motion training on the flexibility of hamstring muscles. J Orthop Sports Phys Ther 1998;27(4):295–300.
2. Davis DS, Ashby PE, McCale KL, McQuain JA, Wine JM. The effectiveness of 3 stretching techniques on hamstring flexibility using consistent stretching parameters. J Strength Cond Res 2005;19(1):27–32.
3. Shrier I. Does stretching improve performance? A systematic and critical review of the literature. Clin J Sport Med 2004;14(5):267–273.

Static Gastrocnemius Stretch

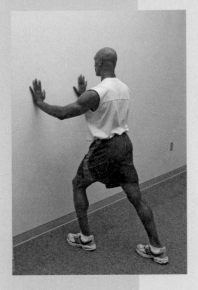

PREPARATION

1. Stand facing a wall or stable object.
2. Extend one leg back, keeping the knee and foot straight and the back heel on the floor.

MOVEMENT

3. Draw belly button inward.
4. Keep rear foot flat, with foot pointed straight ahead. Do not allow the rear foot to flatten.
5. Bend arms and lean forward toward the wall. Keep the gluteal muscles and quadriceps tight and the heel on the ground.
6. Hold for 20–30 seconds.

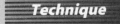 **Technique**   Make sure the gluteals and quadriceps are activated to keep the knee in full extension. This will enhance the stretch to the gastrocnemius.

Static Standing Psoas Stretch

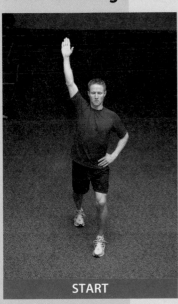
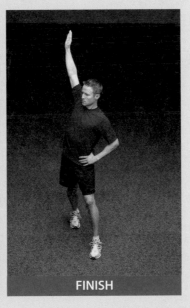

START   FINISH

PREPARATION

1. Stand with one leg bent and slightly forward.
2. Internally rotate back leg.

MOVEMENT

3. Draw navel inward.
4. Squeeze buttocks, while rotating pelvis posteriorly.
5. Slowly, move body forward until a mild tension is achieved in the front of the hip being stretched.
6. As a progression, raise the arm (on the same side as the back leg) up and over to the opposite side, while maintaining pelvis position.
7. Hold side bend position and slowly rotate posteriorly.
8. Hold for 20–30 seconds.
9. Switch sides and repeat.

Technique   Make sure the gluteal musculature is contracted during the stretch. This will reciprocally inhibit the psoas, allowing for greater lengthening of the psoas.

Static Kneeling Hip Flexor Stretch

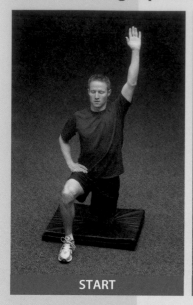

START

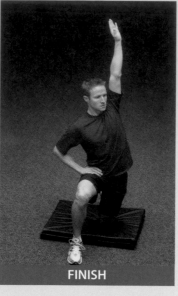

FINISH

PREPARATION

1. Kneel with front and back leg bent at a 90-degree angle.
2. Internally rotate back hip.

MOVEMENT

3. Draw navel inward.
4. Squeeze buttocks of the side being stretched, while rotating pelvis posteriorly.
5. Slowly, move body forward until a mild tension is achieved in the front of the hip being stretched.
6. As a progression raise arm, side bend to opposite side and rotate posteriorly.
7. Hold for 20–30 seconds.

Technique Performing this stretch in a kneeling position will place more of an emphasis on the rectus femoris as it crosses both the knee and hip joints.

Static Standing Adductor Stretch

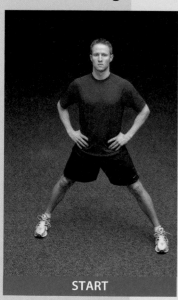

START

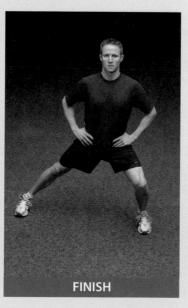

FINISH

PREPARATION

1. Stand in a straddled stance with the feet beyond shoulder width apart. Extend one leg back until the toe of the back leg is in line with the arch of the foot of the other. Both feet should be pointed straight ahead.

MOVEMENT

2. Draw navel inward.
3. Slowly move in a sideways motion (side lunge) until a stretch in the straight leg's groin area is felt.
4. Hold for 20–30 seconds.

Technique Be sure to take a wider than shoulder width apart stance to ensure optimal lengthening.

Static Latissimus Dorsi Ball Stretch

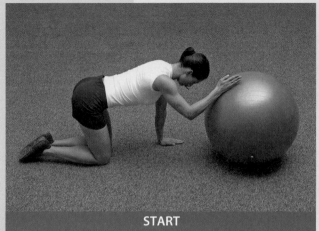
START

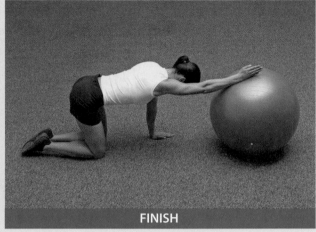
FINISH

PREPARATION

1. Kneel in front of a stability ball.
2. Place one arm on ball, with thumb pointed straight up in the air.

MOVEMENT

3. Draw navel upward.
4. Posteriorly rotate the pelvis.
5. Slowly reach the arm straight out by rolling the ball forward.
6. Hold for 20–30 seconds.

Technique

If this stretch causes any "pinching" in the shoulder, perform the stretch with the palm down on the ball.

Static Pectoral Wall Stretch

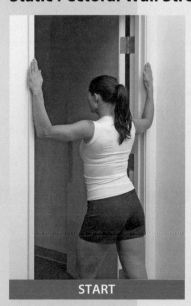
START

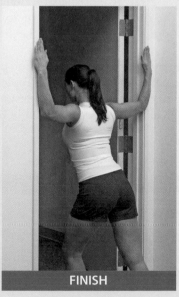
FINISH

PREPARATION

1. Stand against an object and form a 90/90-degree angle with your arms as depicted.

MOVEMENT

2. Draw your navel inward.
3. Slowly lean forward until a slight stretch is felt in the anterior shoulder region.
4. Hold the stretch for 20–30 seconds.

Technique

Make sure the shoulders do not elevate during the stretch. This is an example of relative flexibility and decreases the effectiveness of the stretch.

Static Upper Trapezius/Scalene Stretch

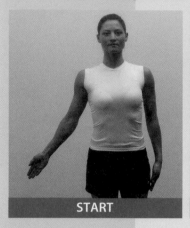
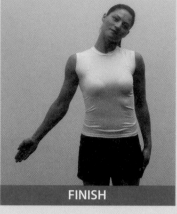

START

FINISH

PREPARATION

1. Stand in optimal posture and place the arm on the side being stretched to the side of the body.

MOVEMENT

2. Draw navel inward.
3. Retract and depress the scapula on the side being stretched.
4. Tuck chin and slowly bring the opposite ear to the opposite shoulder.
5. Hold stretch position for 20–30 seconds.
6. Switch sides and repeat.

Technique

As with the pectoral stretch, keep the shoulder of the side being stretched down by retracting and depressing the scapula on the side being stretched.

ACTIVE-ISOLATED STRETCHING

Active-isolated stretch: The process of using agonists and synergists to dynamically move the joint into a range of motion.

Active-isolated stretching is the process of using agonists and synergists to dynamically move the joint into a range of motion.[14,33] This form of stretching increases motor-neuron excitability, creating reciprocal inhibition of the muscle being stretched.

The active supine biceps femoris stretch is a good example of active stretching.[1,14] The quadriceps extends the knees. This enhances the stretch of the biceps femoris in two ways. First, it increases the length of the biceps femoris. Second, the contraction of the quadriceps causes reciprocal inhibition (decreased neural drive and muscle spindle excitation) of the hamstrings, which allows them to elongate.

Active-isolated stretches are suggested for preactivity warm-up, as long as no postural distortion patterns are present. Typically, 5 to 10 repetitions of each stretch are performed and held for 1 to 2 seconds each. Detailed explanations of various active stretches are given below (Table 6-4).

Table 6.4

Active-Isolated Stretching Summary

Type of Stretch	Mechanism of Action	Acute Variables	Examples
Active-isolated stretch	Reciprocal inhibition	1-2 sets Hold each stretch 1-2 sec. for 5-10 repetitions	Active supine biceps femoris stretch Active kneeling quadriceps stretch Active standing adductor stretch Active pectoral wall stretch

Active Gastrocnemius Stretch With Pronation and Supination

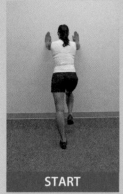

START

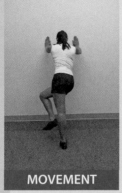

MOVEMENT

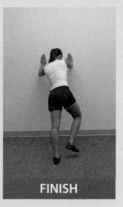

FINISH

PREPARATION

1. Stand near a wall or sturdy object.
2. Bring one leg forward for support. Use upper body and lean against wall.
3. The extended leg should form one straight line and the ankle should be in a neutral position.

MOVEMENT

4. Draw navel inward.
5. Keep rear foot on the ground, with opposite hip flexed.
6. Slowly move through hips, creating controlled supination and pronation through the lower extremity.
7. Hold for 2 seconds and repeat for 5–10 repetitions.

Technique

Make sure when performing the stretch that the majority of the motion is coming from internal and external rotation of the hip, which in turn causes rotation at the knee and eversion and inversion on the foot and ankle.

Active Supine Biceps Femoris Stretch

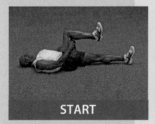

START

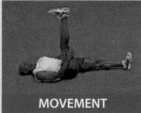

MOVEMENT

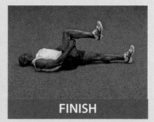

FINISH

PREPARATION

1. Lie supine on floor with legs flat.
2. Flex and adduct the hip of the side being stretched while keeping the knee flexed.
3. Place the opposite hand behind the knee of the leg being stretched.

MOVEMENT

4. Draw navel inward.
5. With hand supporting leg, extend the knee.
6. Hold for 2 seconds and repeat for 5–10 repetitions.

Technique

To place more of an emphasis on the biceps femoris, slightly adduct and internally rotate the hip (while in a hip flexed position) before extending the knee.

Active Standing Psoas Stretch

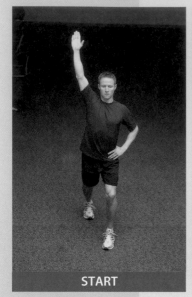
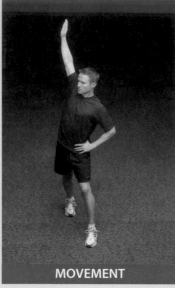
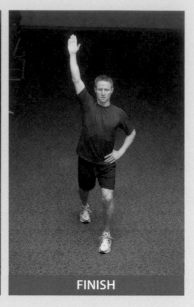

| START | MOVEMENT | FINISH |

PREPARATION

1. Stand with one leg bent and slightly forward.
2. Position the back leg in internal rotation.

MOVEMENT

3. Draw navel inward and raise arm overhead.
4. Squeeze buttocks, while rotating posteriorly.
5. Stride forward, in a controlled manner, until a mild tension is achieved in the front of the hip being stretched. Side bend and rotate posteriorly.
6. Hold for 2 seconds for 5–10 repetitions.

Technique

As with the static stretch make sure the gluteals are contracted when going into the stretch. This will help in enhancing neuromuscular efficiency between the hip flexors and hip extensors.

Active Kneeling Hip Flexor Stretch

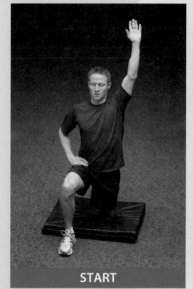

START

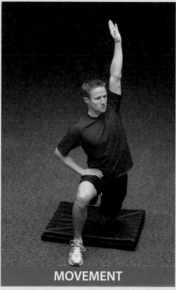

MOVEMENT

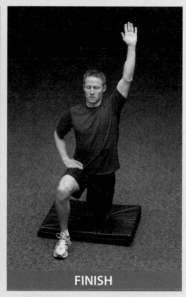

FINISH

PREPARATION

1. Kneel with front and back legs bent at a 90-degree angle.
2. Internally rotate back hip.

MOVEMENT

3. Draw navel inward and raise arm overhead.
4. Squeeze buttocks of the side being stretched, while rotating pelvis posteriorly.
5. Slowly, move body forward until a mild tension is achieved in the front of the hip being stretched. Side bend and rotate posteriorly.
6. Hold for 2 seconds for 5–10 repetitions.

Technique As with any kneeling stretches, make sure the client kneels on a pad or towel for comfort.

Active Standing Adductor Stretch

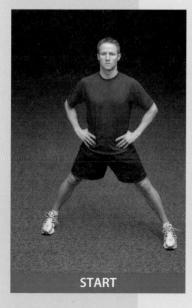

START

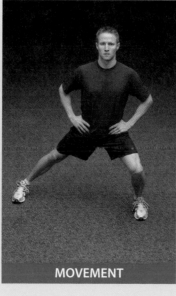

MOVEMENT

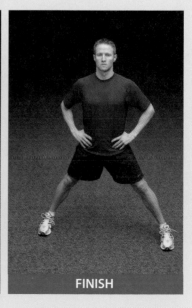

FINISH

PREPARATION

1. Stand in a straddled stance with the feet beyond shoulder width apart. Extend one leg back until the toe of the back leg is in line with the arch of the foot of the other. Both feet should be pointed straight ahead.

MOVEMENT

2. Draw navel inward.
3. Slowly move in a sideways motion (side lunge) until a stretch in the straight leg's groin area is felt.
4. Hold for 2 seconds for 5–10 repetitions.

Technique   Make sure to keep the hips level when going into the stretch.

Active Latissimus Dorsi Ball Stretch

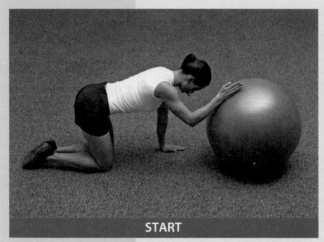

START

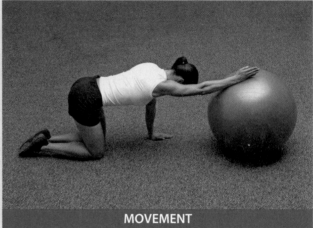

MOVEMENT

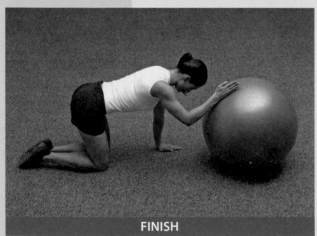

FINISH

PREPARATION

1. Kneel in front of stability ball.
2. Place one arm on ball with thumb straight up in the air.

MOVEMENT

3. Draw navel upward.
4. Maintaining core control, roll ball out until a comfortable stretch is felt.
5. Hold for 2 seconds for 5–10 repetitions.
6. Switch sides and repeat.

Technique   Make sure to initiate the stretch by going into a posterior tilt. This will take the origin and insertion of the latissimus dorsi further apart, enhancing the stretch.

Active Pectoral Wall Stretch

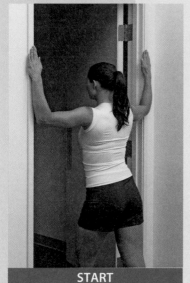 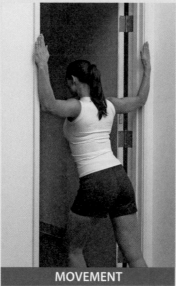 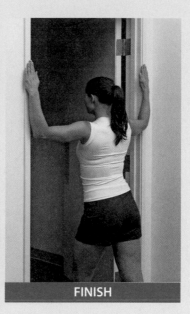

| START | MOVEMENT | FINISH |

PREPARATION

1. Stand against an object and form a 90/90-degree angle with your arms as depicted.

MOVEMENT

2. Draw your navel inward.
3. Slowly lean forward until a slight stretch is felt in the anterior shoulder region.
4. Hold the stretch for 2 seconds and repeat 5–10 repetitions.

Technique Retract the scapulae when going into the stretch. This will reciprocally inhibit the pectoralis major and minor, enhancing the stretch and improving neuromuscular efficiency of the overall shoulder complex.

Active Upper Trapezius/Scalene Stretch

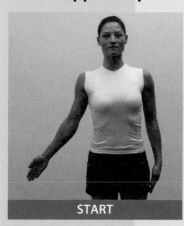 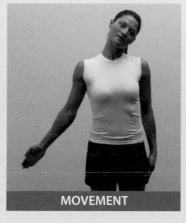 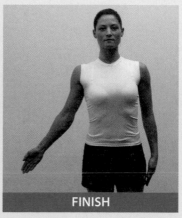

| START | MOVEMENT | FINISH |

PREPARATION

1. Stand with optimal posture.

MOVEMENT

2. Draw navel inward.
3. Tuck chin and laterally flex head (ear to shoulder) in a controlled manner, while retracting and depressing left shoulder complex.
4. Hold for 2 seconds for 5–10 repetitions.

Technique   If tingling is felt down the arm and into the finger, decrease your range of motion of the stretch. This will take stress off of the nerve. Also make sure the head stays in a neutral position during the stretch. Do not allow the head to jut forward.

DYNAMIC STRETCHING

Dynamic stretch: The active extension of a muscle, using force production and momentum, to move the joint through the full available range of motion.

Dynamic stretching uses the force production of a muscle and the body's momentum to take a joint through the full available range of motion (Table 6-5). Dynamic stretching uses the concept of reciprocal inhibition to improve soft tissue extensibility. One can perform one set of 10 repetitions using 3 to 10 dynamic stretches. Medicine ball rotations and walking lunges are a good example of dynamic stretching.[1,14] Dynamic stretching is also suggested as a preactivity warm-up, as long as no postural distortion patterns are present. It is recommended that the client have good levels of tissue extensibility, core stability, and balance capabilities before undertaking an aggressive dynamic stretching program.

Prisoner Squat

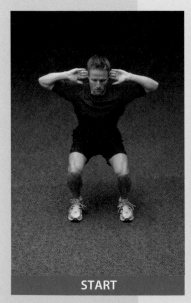
START

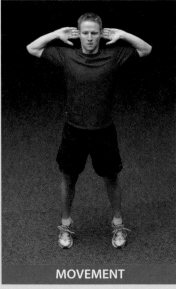
MOVEMENT

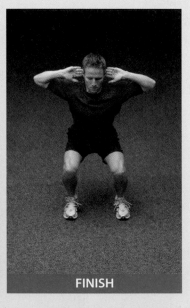
FINISH

PREPARATION

1. Stand in proper alignment, with the hands behind the head.

MOVEMENT

2. Draw navel inward.
3. Lower to a squat position, under control and without compensation (toes straight ahead, knees in line with the toes).

Table 6.5

Dynamic Stretching Summary

Type of Stretch	Mechanism of Action	Acute Variables	Examples
Dynamic stretch	Reciprocal inhibition	1 set 10 repetitions 3–10 exercises	• Prisoner squats • Multiplanar lunges • Single-leg squat touchdowns • Tube walking • Medicine ball chop/lift

4. Extend hips, knees, and ankles (raise onto toes) and repeat.
5. Perform 10 repetitions.

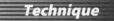 **Technique**   As with all squatting motions, keep the toes straight ahead and the knees in line with the toes.

Multiplanar Lunge

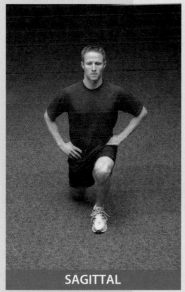 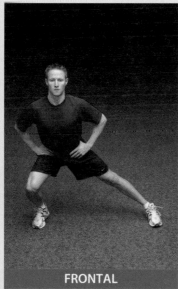 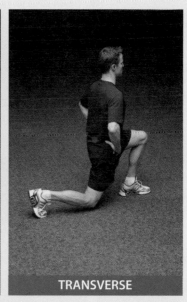

| SAGITTAL | FRONTAL | TRANSVERSE |

PREPARATION

1. Stand in proper alignment with hands on hips and feet straight ahead.

MOVEMENT

2. Draw navel inward.
3. While maintaining total body alignment, step forward (sagittal plane), descending slowly by bending at the hips, knees, and ankles.
4. Use hip and thigh muscles to push up and back to the start position.
5. Perform 10 repetitions.
6. Repeat on opposite leg.
7. Progress to side lunges (frontal plane), followed by turning lunges (transverse plane).

Single-Leg Squat Touchdown

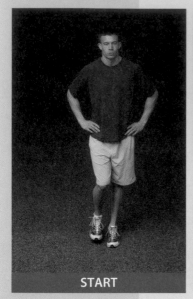

START

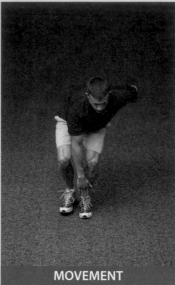

MOVEMENT

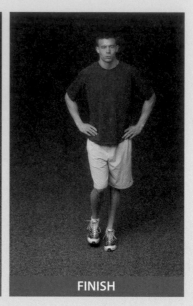

FINISH

PREPARATION

1. Stand on one leg in optimal posture, keeping raised leg parallel to the standing leg.

MOVEMENT

2. Draw navel inward.
3. Squat, in a controlled manner, bending the ankle, knee, and hip.
4. Touch toe of standing leg with the opposite hand.
5. While maintaining drawn-in maneuver and gluteal activity, return to starting position.
6. Perform 10 repetitions.
7. Repeat on opposite side.

Technique

Make sure the knee is tracking in line with the second and third toes. Do not allow the knee of the squatting leg to move inside the foot.

Tube Walking: Side-to-Side

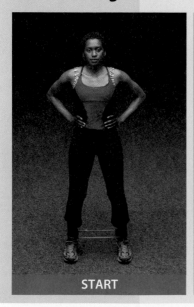

START

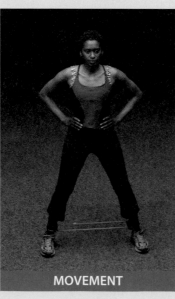

MOVEMENT

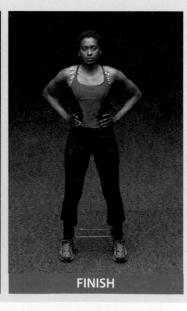

FINISH

PREPARATION

1. Stand with feet hip-width apart, knees slightly bent, and feet straight ahead.
2. Place tubing around mid-lower leg.

MOVEMENT

3. Draw navel inward.
4. Keep feet straight ahead and take 10 small steps sideways, without allowing knees to cave inward.
5. Repeat in the opposite direction.

Technique Make sure the toes stay straight ahead and do not turn the feet out when stepping.

Medicine Ball Chop and Lift

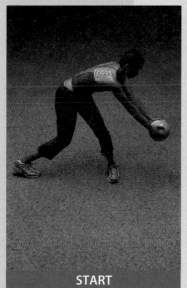

START

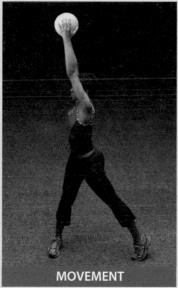

MOVEMENT

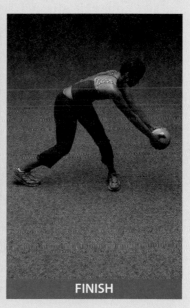

FINISH

PREPARATION

1. Stand with feet hip-width apart, knees slightly bent, and in triple-flexion position.
2. Grasp a medicine ball with both hands and keep elbows fully extended.

MOVEMENT

3. Draw navel inward.
4. Starting from optimal posture, initiate the rotational movement from the trunk outward, lifting the medicine ball from a low position to a high position.
5. Allow the hips to pivot on the back foot as the motion nears end range.
6. Perform 10 repetitions.
7. Repeat on opposite side.

Technique Allow for the hips to rotate during both portions of this exercise (chop/lift). This will improve arthrokinematics through the lumbo-pelvic-hip complex.

SUMMARY

Each type of flexibility training consists of specific stretching techniques. Corrective flexibility uses self-myofascial release and static stretching; active flexibility uses self-myofascial release and active-isolated stretching; and functional flexibility uses self-myofascial release and dynamic stretching.

Self-myofascial release applies gentle pressure on muscle hypertonicity for 20 to 30 seconds. The force applied stimulates the Golgi tendon organ and creates autogenic inhibition, decreasing muscle spindle excitation and releasing the muscle hypertonicity. These techniques are suggested before static stretching or activity, as well as for cool-down.

Static stretching passively takes a muscle to the point of tension and holds it there for a minimum of 20 seconds, thereby creating autogenic inhibition. Also, contracting the antagonistic musculature during the stretch will reciprocally inhibit the muscle being stretched and increases the muscle's ability to lengthen. These should be used before activity and to "reset" soft tissue after activity.

Active-isolated stretches use agonists and synergists to dynamically move joints into their ranges of motion. The reciprocal inhibition of the muscle being stretched allows for greater ranges of motion to be accessed. These are suggested for preactivity warm-up (5 to 10 repetitions, held for 2 seconds each).

Dynamic stretches use force production and momentum to take a joint through the full available range of motion. These are suggested for preactivity warm-up as well.

Practical Application of Flexibility Training

FLEXIBILITY OF MOVEMENT COMPENSATION PATTERNS

As previously mentioned, there are some common movement compensations that must be addressed to ensure the safety and effectiveness of your training program. Proper flexibility is the first step to addressing these problems. Table 6-6 provides the common compensations seen during the assessment process, associated overactive and underactive muscles, and corrective strategies for each (flexibility and strengthening exercises). Further chapters in the text will provide you with proper instruction for the example strengthening exercises that can be implemented to help strengthen the underactive muscles in each of the compensations.

Filling in the Template

After a fitness assessment, the flexibility portion of the template can now be filled in. On the template, select the form of flexibility your client requires. Go to the warm-up section (Step 1). Input the areas to be addressed (Figure 6-8).

For most first-time clients and those requiring correction of postural imbalance, corrective flexibility (self-myofascial release and static stretching) is used before and after training sessions (as well as at home, on off days). Be sure to follow the flexibility guidelines for postural distortion patterns found in this chapter (Table 6-6). Corrective flexibility will be used during the first phase of the OPT™ model.

With a proper progression through the flexibility continuum (and as the client's ability dictates), active (self-myofascial release and active-isolated stretching) and functional (self-myofascial release and dynamic stretching) flexibility can be implemented later in strength and power levels of the OPT™ model.

The use of flexibility techniques can be a great warm-up, but also as a cool-down, especially the self-myofascial release and static stretching. On the template, go to the cool-down section (Step 4) and, as for the warm-up, input the form of stretching to be implemented and the areas to be addressed (Figure 6-8).

Table 6.6

Compensations, Muscle Imbalances, and Corrective Strategies

View	Checkpoint	Compensation	Probable Overactive Muscles	Probable Underactive Muscles	Example of Foam Roll and Static Stretch Techniques	Example of Strengthening Exercises
Anterior	Feet	Turns out	Soleus Lateral gastrocnemius Biceps femoris (short head)	Medial gastrocnemius Medial hamstring Gracilis Sartorius Popliteus	Gastrocnemius/soleus Biceps femoris (short head)	Single-leg balance reach
	Knees	Move inward	Adductor complex Biceps femoris (short head) TFL Vastus lateralis	Gluteus medius/maximus Vastus medialis oblique (VMC)	Adductors TFL/IT band	Tube walking
Lateral	LPHC	Excessive forward lean	Soleus Gastrocnemius Hip flexor complex Abdominal complex	Anterior tibialis Gluteus maximus Erector spinae	Hip flexor complex Piriformis	Ball squats
		Low back arches	Hip flexor complex Erector spinae Latissimus dorsi	Gluteus maximus Hamstrings Intrinsic core stabilizers (transverse abdominis, multifidus, transversospinalis, internal oblique, pelvic floor muscles)	Hip flexor complex Latissimus dorsi Erector spinae	Ball squats
	Upper body	Arms fall forward	Latissimus dorsi Teres major Pectoralis major/minor	Mid/lower trapezius Rhomboids Rotator cuff	Latissimus dorsi Thoracic spine	Squat to row
		Shoulders elevate (pushing/pulling assessment)	Upper trapezius/scalenes Levator scapulae	Mid/lower trapezius Rhomboids Rotator cuff	Upper trapezius/scalene	Ball cobra
		Forward head (pushing/pulling assessment)	Upper trapezius/scalenes Levator scapulae	Deep cervical flexors	Upper trapezius/scalene	Keep head in neutral position during all exercises

LPHC = Lumbo-Pelvic-Hip Complex
TFL = Tensor Fascia Latae
IT = Iliotibial Band

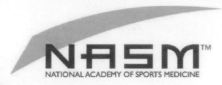

OPT For Fitness

Name: John Smith	Month: 1
Date: 08/10/06	Week: 1
Professional Scott Lucett	Day: 1

Program Goal: Fat Loss

STEP 1

1. Foam Roll

Foam Roll	Sets	Duration
Calves	1	30 sec.
IT Band	1	30 sec.
Adductors	1	30 sec.

2. Stretch

Static Stretching	Sets	Duration
Calves	1	30 sec.
Hip Flexors	1	30 sec.
Adductors	1	30 sec.

3. Cardiovascular

STEP 2

A. Core

Exercise	Sets	Reps	Tempo	Rest

B. Balance

Exercise	Sets	Reps	Tempo	Rest

C. Reactive

Exercise	Sets	Reps	Tempo	Rest

Resistance Training Program

	Body Part Exercise		Sets	Reps	Intensity	Tempo	Rest
STEP 3	Total Body						
	Chest						
	Back						
	Shoulder						

Cool-Down

STEP 4	Repeat Steps 1A and 1B

Figure 6.8 OPT™ template.

Review Questions

1 *The kinetic chain is made up of:*

   a. Nervous system

   b. Muscular system

   c. Skeletal system

   d. All of the above

2 *What is the process in which the body initiates the repair of dysfunction within the connective tissue?*

3 *Active flexibility uses the principle of:*

   a. Reciprocal inhibition

   b. Autogenic inhibition

4 *Which type(s) of stretching stimulates the Golgi tendon organ and produces autogenic inhibition?*

5 *A latissimus dorsi stretch is a good static stretch for which movement compensation during an overhead squat assessment?*

   a. Arms fall forward

   b. Low back rounds

   c. Knees move inward

REFERENCES

1. Alter MJ. Science of Flexibility, 2nd ed. Champaign, IL: Human Kinetics, 1996.
2. Bandy WD, Irion JM, Briggler M. The effect of time and frequency of static stretching on flexibility of the hamstring muscles. Phys Ther Abstract 1997;77(10):1090–1096.
3. Clanton TO, Coupe KJ. Hamstring strains in athletes: diagnosis and treatment. J Am Acad Orthop Surg 1998;6(4):237–248.
4. Condon SA. Soleus muscle electromyographic activity and ankle dorsiflexion range of motion during four stretching procedures. Phys Ther 1987;67:24–30.
5. Chaitow L. Muscle Energy Techniques. New York: Churchill Livingstone, 1997.
6. Janda V. Muscle spasm—a proposed procedure for differential diagnosis. Man Med 199;6136–6139.
7. Liebenson C. Integrating rehabilitation into chiropractic practice (blending active and passive care). In: Liebenson C (ed). Rehabilitation of the Spine. Baltimore: Williams & Wilkins, 1996.
8. Poterfield J, DeRosa C. Mechanical Low Back Pain: Perspectives in Functional Anatomy. Philadelphia: WB Saunders, 1991.
9. Gossman MR, Sahrman SA, Rose SJ. Review of length-associated changes in muscle: experimental evidence and clinical implications. Phys Ther 1982;62:1799–1808.
10. Halbertsma JPK, Van Bulhuis AI, Goeken LNH. Sport stretching: effect on passive muscle stiffness of short hamstrings. Arch Phys Med Rehabil 1996;77(7):688–692.
11. Holcomb WR. Improved stretching with proprioceptive neuromuscular facilitation. J Natl Strength Conditioning Assoc 2000,22(1):59–61.
12. Moore MA, Kukulka CG. Depression of Hoffmann reflexes following voluntary contraction and implications for proprioceptive neuromuscular facilitation therapy. Phys Ther 1991;71(4):321–329.
13. Moore MA. Electromyographic investigation of muscle stretching techniques. Med Sci Sports Exerc 1980;12:322–329.
14. Sady SP, Wortman M, Blanke D. Flexibility training: ballistic, static, or proprioceptive neuromuscular facilitation? Arch Phys Med Rehabil 1982;63(6):261–263.
15. Sherrington C. The Integrative Action of the Nervous System. New Haven, CT: Yale University Press, 1947.
16. Wang RY. Effect of proprioceptive neuromuscular facilitation on the gait of patients with hemiplegia of long and short duration. Phys Ther 1994;74(12):1108–1115.

17. Bachrach RM. Psoas dysfunction/insufficiency, sacroiliac dysfunction and low back pain. In: Vleeming A, Mooney V, Dorman T, Snijders C, Stoeckart R (eds). Movement, Stability and Low Back Pain. London: Churchill Livingstone, 1997.
18. Cohen H. Neuroscience for Rehabilitation, 2nd ed. Philadelphia: Lippincott Williams & Wilkins, 1999.
19. Liebenson C. Active rehabilitation protocols. In: Liebenson C (ed). Rehabilitation of the Spine. Baltimore: Williams & Wilkins, 1996.
20. Milner-Brown A. Neuromuscular Physiology. Thousand Oaks, CA: National Academy of Sports Medicine, 2001.
21. Fox SI. Human Physiology, 5th ed. Dubuque, IA: Wm C Brown Publishers, 1996.
22. Vander A, Sherman J, Luciano D. Human Physiology: the Mechanisms of Body Function, 8th ed. New York: McGraw-Hill, 2001.
23. Enoka RM. Neuromechanical Basis of Kinesiology, 2nd ed. Champaign, IL: Human Kinetics, 1994.
24. McClosky DJ. Kinesthetic sensibility. Physiol Rev 1978;58:763–820.
25. Grigg P. Peripheral neural mechanisms in proprioception. J Sports Rehab 1994;3:2–17.
26. Janda V. In: Grant R (ed). Physical Therapy of the Cervical and Thoracic Spine. Edinburgh: Churchill Livingstone, 1988.
27. Lewitt K. Manipulation in Rehabilitation of the Locomotor System. London: Butterworth, 1993.
28. Leahy PM. Active release techniques: logical soft tissue treatment. In: Hammer WI (ed). Functional Soft Tissue Examination and Treatment by Manual Methods. Gaithersburg, MD: Aspen Publishers, 1999.
29. Spencer AM. Practical Podiatric Orthopedic Procedures. Cleveland: Ohio College of Podiatric Medicine, 1978.
30. Woo SLY, Buckwalter JA. Injury and Repair of the Musculoskeletal Soft Tissues. American Academy of Orthopedic Surgeons, 1987.
31. Zairns B. Soft tissue injury and repair—biomechanical aspects. Int J Sports Med 1982;3:9–11.
32. Beaulieu JA. Developing a stretching program. Physician Sports Med 1981;9:59.
33. Evjenth O, Hamburg J. Muscle Stretching in Manual Therapy—A Clinical Manual. Alfta, Sweden: Alfta Rehab, 1984.
34. Tannigawa M. Comparison of the hold-relax procedure and passive mobilization on increasing muscle length. Phys Ther 1972;52:725.
35. Voss DE, Ionla MK, Meyers BJ. Proprioceptive Neuromuscular Facilitation, 3rd ed. Philadelphia: Harper and Row, 1985.
36. Akeson WH, Woo SLY. The connective tissue response to immobility: biochemical changes in peri-articular connective tissue of the immobilized rabbit knee. Clin Orthop Relat Res 1973;93:356–362.
37. Barnes JF. Myofascial release. In: Hammer WI (ed). Functional Soft Tissue Examination and Treatment by Manual Methods, 2nd ed. Gaithersburg, MD: Aspen Publishers, 1999.
38. Sapega A, Quedenfeld T, Moyer R. Biophysical factors in range of motion exercises. Phys Sports Med 1981;9:57.
39. Etnyre BR, Abraham LD. Gains in range of ankle dorsiflexion using three popular stretching techniques. Am J Phys Med 1986;65:189.

7

Cardiorespiratory Training Concepts

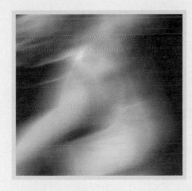

OBJECTIVES

After studying this chapter, you will be able to:

- Define cardiorespiratory training.
- Describe how cardiorespiratory training is used within an integrated training program.
- Provide the guidelines for proper cardiorespiratory training.
- Design cardiorespiratory training programs for a variety of clients.
- Perform and instruct appropriate cardiorespiratory techniques.

KEY TERMS

Enjoyment

Excess postexercise oxygen consumption (EPOC)

Frequency

General warm-up

Integrated cardiorespiratory training

Intensity

Specific warm-up

Time

Type

Current Concepts in Cardiorespiratory Training

Integrated cardiorespiratory training: Training that involves and places a stress on the cardiorespiratory system.

Integrated cardiorespiratory training is simply training that involves and places a stress on the cardiorespiratory system. This means that any form of activity (walking on a treadmill, playing basketball, weight training) can be used as a form of integrated cardiorespiratory training.[1] This is a major concept that can be used to the health and fitness professional's advantage, allowing him or her to maximize the efficiency of the time spent with a client.

WHY IS CARDIORESPIRATORY TRAINING IMPORTANT?

All exercise, regardless of the duration or intensity, must use the cardiorespiratory system to either sustain the activity or recuperate from it.[2,3] Cardiorespiratory exercise in the fitness industry is traditionally viewed as requiring a certain piece of machinery (such as the treadmill, stationary bicycle, or StairClimber). In this case, cardiorespiratory training becomes a separate component of an overall workout program that is used in a few distinct ways. These include:

- Warm-up
- Cool-down
- Workout

The following sections will review each of these forms of cardiorespiratory training, their importance, and examples of traditional as well as integrated approaches.

USES OF CARDIORESPIRATORY TRAINING

Warm-up

General warm-up: Low-intensity exercise consisting of movements that do not necessarily relate to the more intense exercise that is to follow.

Specific warm-up: Low-intensity exercise consisting of movements that mimic those that will be included in the more intense exercise that is to follow.

A warm-up is generally described as preparing the body for physical activity. It can be either general in nature or more specific to the activity.[4,5] A **general warm-up** consists of movements that do not necessarily have any movement specific to the actual activity to be performed. (Examples include warming up by walking on a treadmill or riding a stationary bicycle before weight training.) A **specific warm-up** consists of movements that more closely mimic those of the actual activity. (Examples include performing body-weight squats and push-ups before weight training.) The proposed benefits of a warm-up are outlined in Table 7-1.[2,4-6]

Table 7.1	
Benefits and Effects of a Warm-up	
Benefits	**Effects**
Increased heart and respiratory rate	Increases cardiorespiratory system's capacity to perform work Increases blood flow to active muscle tissue Increases the oxygen exchange capacity
Increased tissue temperature	Increases rate of muscle contraction Increases efficiency of opposing muscle contraction and relaxation Increases metabolic rate Increases the soft tissue extensibility
Increased psychological preparation for bouts of exercise	Increases the mental readiness of an individual

There is speculation as to whether a warm-up is helpful in the prevention of musculoskeletal injury. Although some researchers claim benefits to a warm-up, others show no change between the use of a warm-up before exercise and no warm-up.[7-9] It is proposed, however, that although a warm-up may not be directly associated with injury prevention, it may be beneficial for enhancing overall performance, as indicated by the benefits listed above. In this case, better overall function of the kinetic chain may allow for more efficient and effective movement patterns and thus decrease the chance of future injuries.

Warm-up has been shown to have a possible inhibitory effect on the accumulation of intercellular acidosis during subsequent exercise bouts.[10] Acidosis is the accumulation of excessive hydrogen (H^+) that causes increased acidity (pH) of the blood and muscle that is related to (but, not caused by) lactic acid.[2] Increased acidic levels have been associated with neuromuscular fatigue.[2,11] In turn, neuromuscular fatigue can lead to a decrease in the ability of a muscle to produce sufficient amounts of force.[12,13] The inability of muscles to produce proper levels of force can lead to altered recruitment patterns.[14-17] This can further lead to synergistic dominance and potential injury.[18,19-22] Thus, a warm-up may provide protection from an injury and should be viewed as an important component of a complete workout.

PRACTICAL APPLICATION FOR A WARM-UP

NASM suggests that the cardiorespiratory portion of a warm-up should last up to 10 minutes at a low-to-moderate intensity. However, depending on the client's goals and objectives, this can be altered. Furthermore, the cardiorespiratory portion of a warm-up is usually considered a general warm-up. A complete warm-up should include a general and a specific warm-up. A first-time client, with excessive postural distortion patterns, may initially (the first one to three workouts) spend half of the workout time on the warm-up. Table 7-2 provides examples of suggested warm-ups using flexibility and cardiorespiratory exercise in the stabilization level (Phase 1) of the OPT model.

Table 7.2		
Warm-up for the Stabilization Level Client		
Components	**Examples**	**Time**
Self-myofascial release	Gastrocnemius/soleus Iliotibial band Piriformis Latissimus dorsi	5–10 minutes
Static stretching	Gastrocnemius/soleus Adductors Psoas Latissimus dorsi	5–10 minutes
Cardiorespiratory exercise	Treadmill Stationary bicycle StairClimber Rower Elliptical trainer	5–10 minutes

NOTE: *NASM recommends for individuals who possess musculoskeletal imbalances to first perform self-myofascial release to inhibit overactive muscles and then lengthen the overactive muscles through static stretching. This will help decrease movement compensations when performing the cardiorespiratory portion of the warm-up.*

Once a client has demonstrated an understanding of the techniques necessary for self-myofascial release (foam rolling) and static stretching and operation of the cardiorespiratory equipment, he or she should begin performing this warm-up before time spent with the health and fitness professional. This should take place after the first one to three sessions (or as the health and fitness professional deems appropriate). This will then allow for increased training time in which to focus on other aspects of the training program.

It is very important that the health and fitness professional have a full understanding of the proper cardiorespiratory and flexibility techniques, as his or her demonstration will determine the success of the client. It is imperative to provide clear and concise instructions to the client to allow for proper assimilation of the information.

Table 7-3 provides a sample warm-up for the client who has progressed to the strength level (Phases 2, 3 and 4) of the OPT™ model.

Table 7-4 provides a sample warm-up for the client who has progressed to the power level (Phase 5) of the OPT™ model. Bear in mind that traditional cardiorespiratory exercises may not be necessary in this form of a warm-up because the listed dynamic stretches can be performed in a circuit (performing one exercise after the other), providing an ample cardiorespiratory warm-up.

It should be reemphasized that a warm-up should prepare the body for an activity, not fatigue the body before the activity begins. Again, this can lead to altered muscle recruitment and detract from the purpose of proper training. Keeping the activity to a moderate duration and intensity level will help ensure a proper warm-up.

Cool-down

A cool-down provides the body with a smooth transition from exercise back to a steady state of rest. In essence, a cool-down is the opposite of the warm-up. This portion of a workout is often overlooked and viewed as less important than the other components.[2] However, proper use of a cool-down can have a significant impact on a client's overall health. Sufficient time for a cool-down period is approx-

Table 7.3

Warm-up for the Strength Level Client

Components	Examples	Time
Self-myofascial release	Gastrocnemius/soleus Iliotibial band Glutes/piriformis Latissimus dorsi	5–10 minutes
Active-isolated stretching	Gastrocnemius/soleus Adductors Iliopsoas Latissimus dorsi	3–5 minutes
Cardiorespiratory exercise	Treadmill Stationary bicycle StairClimber Rower Elliptical trainer	5–10 minutes

Table 7.4

Warm-up for the Power Level Client (Dynamic, Functional Warm-up)

Components	Examples	Time
Self-myofascial release	Gastrocnemius/soleus Iliotibial band Glutes/piriformis Latissimus dorsi	5–10 minutes
Dynamic stretching (10 repetitions of each)	Prisoner squats Multiplanar lunge Tube walking Medicine ball lift and chop Single-leg squat touchdown	5–10 minutes

imately 5 to 10 minutes.[23] The proposed benefits of a cool-down are shown in Figure 7-1.[2,4,6,23,24]

PRACTICAL APPLICATION FOR A COOL-DOWN

If an individual is performing cardiorespiratory exercise for an extended period of time, it will be vital that he or she slowly decrease the intensity of the exercise (40 to 50% of maximum heart rate) and work at this lowered intensity for 5 to 10 minutes. This will help in gradually decreasing the heart rate back down to a resting state. It will also ensure that blood does not pool to the lower extremities, leading to dizziness or possible fainting.

Flexibility is also an important component to be used in the cool-down. Because one of the goals of a cool-down is to relax muscles and bring them back to their original resting length after a workout, corrective stretching (self-myofascial release and static stretching) would be the appropriate form of stretching during a cool-down.

The first one to three workouts (or more, if deemed appropriate by the health and fitness professional) should be monitored for completeness and technique with a first-time client. Once the client and the health and fitness professional feel confident that the proper techniques are being used, the cool-down can be performed on the client's own time.

It is important for the client to understand the importance of both the warm-up and the cool-down. This helps to alleviate any anxiety on the part of the client and health and fitness professional that not enough time is being dedicated to the "workout." As the client is capable of a greater workload and requires more time

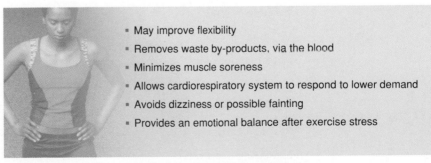

- May improve flexibility
- Removes waste by-products, via the blood
- Minimizes muscle soreness
- Allows cardiorespiratory system to respond to lower demand
- Avoids dizziness or possible fainting
- Provides an emotional balance after exercise stress

Figure 7.1 Benefits of a cool-down.

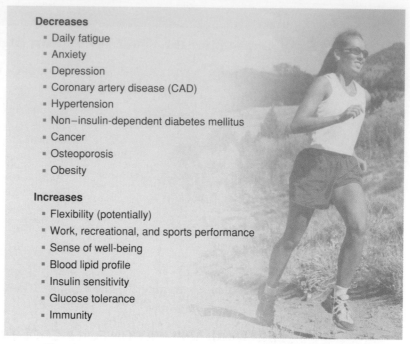

Decreases
- Daily fatigue
- Anxiety
- Depression
- Coronary artery disease (CAD)
- Hypertension
- Non–insulin-dependent diabetes mellitus
- Cancer
- Osteoporosis
- Obesity

Increases
- Flexibility (potentially)
- Work, recreational, and sports performance
- Sense of well-being
- Blood lipid profile
- Insulin sensitivity
- Glucose tolerance
- Immunity

Figure 7.2 Benefits of cardiorespiratory activities or exercise.

for the "workout," the warm-up and cool-down can be performed before and after the workout by the client independently.

Cardiorespiratory Training as a Workout

Most people who perform cardiorespiratory exercise are looking for improvements in their health or fitness levels. However, it has been suggested that there is a difference between the level of activity required for health versus that necessary for increased fitness (excluding cosmetic goals).[25-30] It is viewed that activity levels that may not necessarily produce significant improvements in fitness may have marked effects on health.[30] In either scenario, cardiorespiratory activities or exercise have a profound effect on the overall physical and mental health of a participant as summarized in Figure 7-2.[1,25-33]

These benefits accrue as the result of many physiologic adaptations to cardiorespiratory training. The adaptations are summarized in Table 7-5.

Table 7.5	
Adaptations to Cardiorespiratory Training	
Variable	**Response**
$\dot{V}O_2$ max	Increase
Stroke volume	Increase
Cardiac output	Increase
Oxidative capacity of muscle	Increase
Resting heart rate	Decrease
Exercising heart rate	Decrease

$\dot{V}O_2$ max, maximal oxygen consumption.

SUMMARY

In the fitness industry, cardiorespiratory exercise is typically associated with certain pieces of equipment. However, the cardiorespiratory system is used to either sustain or recover from all physical activity. Integrated cardiorespiratory training is simply training that involves and places a stress on the cardiorespiratory system. Thus, any form of activity can be used as a form of cardiorespiratory training.

Cardiorespiratory training can be used as the warm-up, as the cool-down, or as the workout itself. Regardless of a client's goals, cardiorespiratory training should be incorporated into the program.

A warm-up prepares the body for physical activity and can be either general in nature or more specific to the activity. Typically, the cardiorespiratory portion of a warm-up should last 5 to 10 minutes at a low-to-moderate intensity.

A cool-down of 5 to 10 minutes provides the body with an essential transition from exercise back to a steady state of rest. Flexibility (corrective stretching) is also an important component of the cool-down to bring muscles back to their original resting length after a workout.

Once a client has demonstrated an understanding of proper technique, he or she can begin performing the warm-up and cool-down alone, before and after time spent with the health and fitness professional.

By using a variety of methods to incorporate cardiorespiratory training into one's exercise routine, the health and fitness professional can effectively ensure optimum health in clients, maximize results by minimizing the body's ability to adapt, increase enjoyment of each training session, maximize the personalized aspect of program design, and increase retention and referrals.

General Guidelines for Cardiorespiratory Training

Any form of training must have certain guidelines to allow for the development of a proper program. These guidelines also serve to quantify activity.[1,31] For these purposes, NASM uses the F.I.T.T.E. factors (Figure 7-3).[1,31,34]

FREQUENCY

Frequency: The number of training sessions in a given timeframe.

Frequency refers to the number of training sessions or activity sessions for a given time frame. The time frame usually consists of a week. But, depending on the client and his or her goals, it may be one workout a day, a month, or a year. For general health requirements (Table 7-6), the recommended frequency of activity is preferably every day of the week, for small quantities of time.[25] For improved fitness levels, the frequency is three to five days per week (Table 7-7).[1,31]

INTENSITY

Intensity: The level of demand that a given activity places on the body.

Intensity refers to the level of demand the activity places on the body. This is usually measured by heart rate or maximal oxygen consumption ($\dot{V}O_2$ max).[1,31] For

F Frequency
I Intensity
T Time
T Type
E Enjoyment

Figure 7.3 The F.I.T.T.E. factors.

Table 7.6

General Health Activity Recommendations

Frequency	Intensity	Time	Type	Enjoyment
5–7 days per week	Moderate (enough to increase heart and respiration rates)	30 minutes total per day	General activities Walking Using stairs Gardening Mowing the yard	The greater, the better

general health requirements (Table 7-6), moderate intensity is preferred.[25] This would be perceived as enough demand to increase heart and respiratory rates, but not cause exhaustion or breathlessness.[1,31] For improved fitness levels (Table 7-7), the intensity recommended is 40 to 85% of heart rate reserve (HRR) or 60 to 90% of maximal heart rate (HR max).[1,31]

TIME

Time: The length of time an individual is engaged in a given activity.

Time refers to the length of time engaged in the activity. This is usually measured in minutes. For general health requirements (Table 7-6), approximately 30 total minutes a day is recommended.[25] This could be six 5-minute bouts, three 10-minute bouts, or two 15-minute bouts (or any other combination equaling 30 minutes). For improved fitness levels (Table 7-7), the time recommended is approximately 20 to 60 minutes.[1,31] This will vary, depending on the goal.

TYPE

Type: The type or mode of physical activity that an individual is engaged in.

Type refers to the mode or activity used. This can be virtually any activity. For general health requirements, this may consist of:

- Using stairs (versus elevators)
- Parking farther from the desired location and walking a longer distance
- Mowing the yard with a push mower
- Raking leaves by hand
- Gardening

For improved fitness levels, this may consist of:

- Treadmill, stationary bike, stepper
- Aerobics classes
- Sports
- Weight training

ENJOYMENT

Enjoyment: The amount of pleasure derived from performing a physical activity.

Enjoyment refers to the amount of pleasure derived from the activity by the client. This is often an overlooked component of program design by the health and fitness professional. One of the most important aspects of creating a program is that it fits with a client's personality and interests; however, this does not mean that the client dictates what it is that a health and fitness professional does.

Table 7.7				
Improved Fitness Recommendations				
Frequency	**Intensity**	**Time**	**Type**	**Enjoyment**
3–5 days per week	40–85% $\dot{V}O_2$ max or 60–90% HR max	20–60 minutes per day	Any activity	The greater, the better

One of the most important components of a properly designed training program is that it must be enjoyable. This means that the program and its activities must coincide with the personality, likes, and dislikes of the client. This translates into compliance, and that will equal results. A client is much more apt to continue with a program that is fun and challenging. By complying with a structured program, the client will achieve the desired results. This ultimately allows for a higher level of retention, results, and referrals. For the health and fitness professional, this means having a drastic impact on the life of another human being while building your business.

RECOMMENDATIONS

Exercise parameters used for improved health have been shown to differ from those that are recommended for improved fitness levels (Tables 7-6 and 7-7).[25-31] The benefits from exercise (listed earlier in Table 7-2), however, can be derived from the general health guidelines listed in Table 7-6. This is important for the health and fitness professional to realize, especially for first-time or deconditioned clients. Any activity above what the client is currently involved in will produce some benefit.

The fitness guidelines shown in Table 7-7 may be too extreme for the beginning client. Many clients will not be able to perform the fitness level guidelines for integrated cardiorespiratory training of 20 minutes at 60% of HR max for three to five days per week. However, accumulating a total of 30 minutes of exercise per day during a 5- to 7-day period may be more attainable. It has been shown that performing three 10-minute bouts of exercise is just as effective as one 30-minute continuous bout of the same exercise.[35-37] Also, exercising at lower intensities (40% of $\dot{V}O_2$ max) has been shown to be beneficial for sedentary people, when compared with higher intensities (80% of $\dot{V}O_2$ max) for general health and fitness purposes.[38]

SUMMARY

The F.I.T.T.E. guidelines allow for the development of a proper program and quantify its variables. Recommendations are listed below.

Frequency: Almost every day of the week for short quantities of time.
Intensity: Moderate enough to increase heart and respiratory rates.
Time: 20 to 60 total minutes a day, depending on goals.
Type: Any kind of activity from gardening to weight training.
Enjoyment: The program and its activities should coincide with the personality, likes, and dislikes of the client.

Cardiorespiratory Training and Cosmetic Goals

THE MYTH OF THE "FAT-BURNING" ZONE

Although many clients and health and fitness professionals realize the overall benefits of cardiorespiratory exercise, the primary manner in which it is used is as a workout, to reduce body fat. It is generally assumed that body fat reduction can only result from extended periods of time on a piece of cardio equipment (or in an aerobics class). There is still a popular trend of thinking that suggests there is a magical "fat-burning" zone for exercise. However, body fat reduction can only take place when there is more energy being burned than consumed. This is known as the *law of thermodynamics*.[2] To gain a better insight into effectively using cardiorespiratory training and its role in fat loss, the mystique of the "fat-burning" zone must be eliminated.

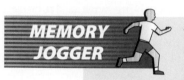

MEMORY JOGGER

The Law of Thermodynamics becomes a very important teaching anchor for the health and fitness professional, particularly when working with a weight loss client. The only way (outside of surgery) one will lose weight or body fat is if one consumes less calories (food and drink) than one expends (activity). If an individual is exercising, but not losing weight, he or she is somehow, some way consuming more calories than he or she is expending.

Cardiorespiratory training, as with any other form of training, falls under the principle of specificity. Typically, the "fat-burning" zone is thought of as the time when the body is mainly using fat as fuel. However, to design appropriate cardiorespiratory training programs, the energy systems used at different generalized heart rate zones must be examined.

Fat and glucose are major sources of fuel for exercise. For them to be used more efficiently, the body must be able to receive enough oxygen (O_2). Oxygen allows fat and glucose to be "burned" as fuel. This, in turn, produces the waste products of carbon dioxide (CO_2) and water. (Think of this like a car burning gasoline, with the body's "exhaust" being CO_2 and water.)

The amount of O_2 and CO_2 exchanged in the lungs normally equals that used and released by body tissues. This allows the body to use these respiratory gasses to estimate caloric expenditure. The method is called *indirect calorimetry*. It can be measured with a metabolic analyzer to detect an individual's respiratory exchange ratio (RER). RER is the ratio of CO_2 produced to the volume of O_2 consumed.[2]

Table 7-8 gives a guide for determining how many of the calories burned come from carbohydrates and fats.[39] To estimate the amount of energy used by the body, first determine the type of energy sources (carbohydrate, fat, or protein) that are being oxidized (or burned for energy). The fact that fat and carbohydrates differ in the amount of oxygen used (in addition to the fact that carbon dioxide is produced during oxidization) can help to determine what kind of fuel is being used.

The body uses the highest percent of its fuel from fat when the body has an RER of 0.71 (Table 7-8). If the body uses a maximal percent of its fuel from fat at 0.71 RER, then why shouldn't an individual exercise at this level all the time? The answer lies in the fact that the only time the body can be at 0.71 RER is when it is at complete rest. This is how the fat-burning zone originated. Although the percentage of fat being burned is maximal, the amount of energy used (calories burned) is minimal and, therefore, not very productive for the goal of weight or fat loss. Remember, it is not how much fat an individual burns that ultimately dictates body fat reduction. Instead, it is how many calories are burned.

Table 7.8

Respiratory Exchange Ratio (RER) and the Percentage of Calories Derived From Fats and Carbohydrates

RER	% From Carbohydrates	% From Fats
0.71	0.0	100.0
0.75	15.6	84.4
0.80	33.4	66.6
0.85	50.7	49.3
0.90	67.5	32.5
0.95	84.0	16.0
1.00	100.0	0.0

RER $= \dot{V}CO_2 \dot{V}O_2$ measured at a steady state of exercise. $\dot{V}CO_2$, carbon dioxide production; $\dot{V}O_2$, oxygen consumption.

EXCESS POSTEXERCISE OXYGEN CONSUMPTION (EPOC)

One of the main objectives of the human body is to expend as little energy as possible. To do so, it must readily adapt to the demands placed on it. Fortunately, the human body is a highly adaptable organism, with the capability to streamline physical and mental demands over time, using minimal energy.[40-44] A health and fitness professional must understand this principle and be able to use it to produce desirable results in the client.

One way a health and fitness professional can combat this is by maximizing the caloric expenditure of a training session. This is made easier by maximizing the O_2 consumption needed for the duration of (as well as the recovery from) the training session. This recovery oxygen consumption is known as **excess postexercise oxygen consumption** (EPOC).

Excess postexercise oxygen consumption (EPOC): Elevation of the body's metabolism after exercise.

EPOC is simply the state in which the body's metabolism is elevated after exercise.[2,45] This means that the body is burning more calories after exercise than before the exercise was initiated. Think of EPOC as a caloric afterburner that is caused by exercise (much like a car engine stays warm for a period of time after it has been driven). After exercise, the body must use increased amounts of oxygen to replenish energy supplies, lower tissue temperature, and return the body to a resting state.[2,45]

Research has indicated that the higher the intensity (percentage of $\dot{V}O_2$ max or percentage of HR max) of the training session, the greater the magnitude of EPOC.[46-48] Furthermore, it has been shown that splitting the training session into multiple sessions (usually two) of equal time has the greatest effect on EPOC.[47-50]

SUMMARY

When the goal is body fat reduction, the key is to focus on burning calories, not burning fat. It is also important to understand that one must expend more calories than is consumed to lower body fat (law of thermodynamics).

The body is designed to expend as little energy as possible. This can be avoided by maximizing the caloric expenditure of a training session and, thus, the excess postexercise oxygen consumption (EPOC). The body will continue to burn more calories after exercise than before exercise was initiated. Increased intensity and splitting training sessions into multiple sessions will both result in higher EPOC.

Cardiorespiratory Training Methodologies

Cardiorespiratory training, as with any other form of training, falls under the general adaptation syndrome and the principle of specificity. This means that the body will adapt to the level of stress placed on it and will then require more or varied amounts of stress to produce a higher level of adaptation carryover. A cardiorespiratory training program for a client who may desire adaptations for weekend sports will probably be different than one for a client who desires general conditioning. The variance of the cardiorespiratory training program will place a different demand on the bioenergetic continuum and will ultimately affect the client's adaptations and goals. There are several methods of incorporating cardiorespiratory exercise into a client's program. As such, stage training and circuit training will be discussed below.

STAGE TRAINING

To ensure continual adaptation, cardiorespiratory training programs must be designed to progress in an organized fashion and to minimize the risk of overtraining and injury.[51] This is the basis behind the stage training system.

Stage training is a three-stage programming system that uses different heart rate training zones based on one's RER. Those zones are organized to maximize cardiorespiratory training benefits. The three different stages of cardiorespiratory training mimic the three stages of training seen in the OPT™ model. Each stage will help to create a strong cardiorespiratory base to build on in subsequent stages.

Translating RER Into Heart Rate Zones

Before discussing each stage, it is essential to know how to translate RER into heart rate zones. The RER numbers seen in Table 7-8 correspond easily with heart rate zones. Table 7-9 demonstrates estimated heart rate numbers that coincide with the RER to give a predictable and usable number to work with. Also shown are the energy systems, energy source, and sample activity. The heart rates are broken up into three heart rate zones that are easily used for program design.

ZONE ONE

Zone one consists of a heart rate of approximately 65 to 75% of a predicted HR max (calculated as 220—client's age). Although this equation is not accurate for

Table 7.9

Respiratory Exchange Ratio (RER) and Heart Rate Zones

Heart Rate Zone	RER	Heart Rate Percentage	Energy System	Energy Source	Activity
Zone one	0.80–0.90	65–75%	Aerobic	Muscle glycogen and fatty acids	Walking or jogging
Zone two	0.95–1.0	80–85%	Aerobic/anaerobic	Muscle glycogen and lactic acid	Group exercise classes
Zone three	1.1	86–90%	Anaerobic	ATP/CP and muscle glycogen	Sprinting

ATP, adenosine triphosphate; CP, creatine phosphate.

everyone, it is a good general tool. This zone is a "recovery zone." It is a great zone to start in and is consistently used for beginners to improve the blood's ability to deliver oxygen throughout the body and remove waste. Regular exercise increases blood volume, which allows more blood to get to the cells. The result is a greater flow of oxygen to a greater number of cells throughout the body, thus helping the cells work to their capacity and allowing the heart to become stronger. This form of training fits very well with the beginning phase of the OPT™ model (stabilization level), in which the goal is to increase blood supply to tissue for recovery. There may be times, however, that even this zone will be too high for some clients. In this case, the general health activity recommendations (Table 7-6) will become very important guidelines to follow.

ZONE TWO

Zone two consists of a heart rate of approximately 80 to 85% of a predicted HR max. This is near the anaerobic threshold. Anaerobic threshold is the point at which the body can no longer produce enough energy for the muscles with normal oxygen intake (aerobic energy system in zone one). As a result, it begins to produce higher levels of lactic acid than can be removed from the body. Training and staying at an aerobic level will result in more calories burned with a higher percentage of those calories coming from fat. Thus, one of the main goals of cardiorespiratory training is to increase the anaerobic threshold. Many people who perform high-intensity workouts every time they use a piece of fitness equipment or attend a group exercise class are usually in this zone, and not truly performing high-intensity training. Zone two would be appropriate for individuals who have progressed to the strength level of the OPT™ model.

ZONE THREE

Zone three consists of a heart rate of approximately 86 to 90% of a predicted HR max. This is a true high-intensity workout and cannot be sustained for long periods of time (more than 10 to 60 seconds). Zone three training should be used in a workout with zones one and two. Staying in zone one or two all the time will also cause clients to hit a plateau. The reason is simple: to improve fitness level or increase metabolism, the body must be overloaded. From the general adaptation syndrome, the same high-intensity level of exercise performed during every workout will exhaust the body and not allow recovery enough to do an overload workout. This will not allow for adaptation and realization of the client's goal. Similarly, doing the same low-intensity level of exercise during every workout will not place enough stress on the body to force an adaptation. The solution is to progress a client to the point that he or she can use all three heart rate zones of training, during the course of each week, varying the intensity for each workout.[52,53] For most clients, going to zone three once a week is enough. Caution must be exercised to not spend too much time in zone three, which can lead to overtraining.[51] Zone three training would be appropriate for the individual who has progressed to the power level of the OPT™ model.

Translating Heart Rate Zones Into Stages

After understanding the different zones and their functions, each of these zones can be applied in a systematic fashion using stage training.

STAGE I (STABILIZATION LEVEL)

This stage is for the beginner who has not been working out and only uses heart rate training zone one (Table 7-9). Just like in weight training, a base needs to be established first. In this stage, clients should start slow and work up to 30 to 60 minutes in zone one (Figure 7-4). A target of 65 to 75% of maximum heart rate

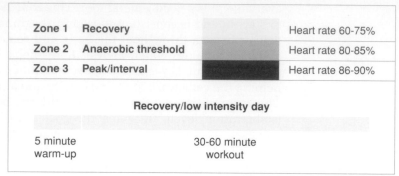

Figure 7.4   Stage I (stabilization level) training parameters.

should be low enough to ensure the client is in an aerobic state. If the client has never worked out before, he or she might start in zone one for only 5 minutes or reduce the heart rate percentage to the general health activity recommendations (Table 7-6). Stage I training also helps a client to better meet the muscular endurance demands of the stabilization level of training in the OPT™ model.

Clients who can maintain zone one heart rate for at least 30 minutes two to three times per week will be ready for stage II. A beginner, however, might take 2 to 3 months to meet this demand. An example might be walking on a treadmill at a speed of 3 miles per hour. The speed may change for each session to stay in zone one, but not the time. During this stage, it will be apparent if the heart rate zones created are good for the client. The progression would be to then slowly add time to the client's light workout.

STAGE II (STRENGTH LEVEL)

This stage is for the intermediate client who has built a good cardiorespiratory base and will use heart rate zones one and two (Figure 7-5). The focus in this stage is on increasing the workload (speed, incline, level) in a way that will help the client alter heart rate in and out of each zone. Remember, it does not matter how hard the equipment is working; what matters is how hard the client is working. This will be determined by heart rate. Some clients can start in this zone if they have been working out for a while with a low intensity and have created the aerobic base. Stage II training helps increase the cardiorespiratory capacity needed for the workout styles in the strength level of the OPT™ model.

Stage II is the introduction to interval training in which intensities are varied throughout the workout. The workout will proceed as follows:

1. Start by warming up in zone one for 5 to 10 minutes.

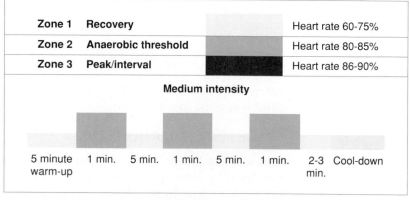

Figure 7.5   Stage II (strength level) training parameters.

2. Move into a 1-minute interval in zone two (Figure 7-5). Gradually increase the workload to raise the heart rate up to zone two within that minute. Once the heart rate reaches 80 to 85% of maximum heart rate, maintain it for the rest of that minute. It might take 45 seconds to reach that heart rate, which means the client will only be at the top end for 15 seconds before reducing the workload (speed, incline, or level), and returning to zone one.

3. After the 1-minute interval, return to zone one for 5 minutes.

4. Repeat this if the client has time and can recover back into the zone one range. The most important part of the interval is to recover back to zone one between the intervals.

During the first workout, adjustments may need to be made. The first thing to look at is the 1-minute push. Did the client get to the zone two heart rate? Was it easy? Could he or she hold that heart rate? (Also, make sure the client was pushing hard enough and didn't progress the workload too slowly.) Based on the answers to these questions, start to create a more accurate, modified training zone for the client.

1. If the client wasn't able to reach the predicted zone two in 1 minute, then use the heart rate he or she was able to reach as their "85%."

2. Take 5% off this number to get the lower end of the client's readjusted zone (85%–5% = 80%).

3. For example, if 150 beats per minute (bpm) was the predicted 85% of HR max, but the client was only able to work up to 145 bpm during the 1-minute push, 145 bpm should now be considered that client's 85% HR max.

4. Take 5% off 145% (5% of 145 is 7 beats; 145 − 7 = 138). So, 138 bpm is the individual's 80% of HR max.

5. If the client got into the readjusted zone two, and then reaching the zones was fine, work slowly to increase the client's time in this zone.

6. If the client's heart rate goes above the predicted zone and he or she still can recover back to zone one at the end, add a couple of beats per minute to the zone and then work on increasing the time.

It is very important to point out that in stage II, it will be important to alternate days of the week with stage I training (Figure 7-6). This means alternating sessions every workout.

Figure 7-6 displays a monthly plan for a 3-days-per-week schedule. Start with stage I on Monday. Then, move to stage II on Wednesday and go back to stage I on Friday. The next week, start with stage II and so on. Rotate the stages to keep workouts balanced. This will become very important in stage III. The monthly plan is only a general guide and may be changed on the basis of the workout (if any) being performed on that day.

STAGE III (POWER LEVEL)

This stage is for the advanced client who has built a very good cardiorespiratory base and will use heart rate zones one, two, and three. It should not be used by

Week	1							2							3							4						
Day	M	T	W	T	F	S	S	M	T	W	T	F	S	S	M	T	W	T	F	S	S	M	T	W	T	F	S	S
Phase 1																												
Phase 2																												
Phase 3																												
Phase 4																												
Phase 5																												
Cardio	S1		S2		S1			S2		S1		S2			S1		S2		S1			S2		S1		S2		
Flexibility	X		X		X			X		X		X			X		X		X			X		X		X		

S1= Stage I   S2= Stage II

Figure 7.6 The monthly plan.

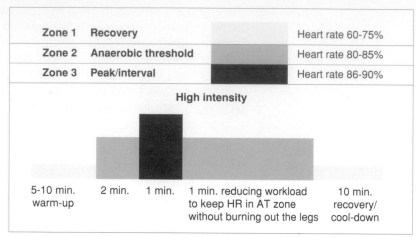

Figure 7.7   Stage III (power level) training parameters. AT, anaerobic threshold; HR, heart rate.

beginning or intermediate clients. Failure to comply with these standards could result in a critical health-related injury to a client. It is imperative that health and fitness professionals follow the proper assessment procedures to avoid legal issues regarding client care.

The focus in this stage is on further increasing the workload (speed, incline, level) in a way that will help the client alter heart rate in and out of each zone (Figure 7-7). Stage III training increases the capacity of the energy systems needed at the power level of the OPT™ model.

The workout will proceed as follows:

1. Warm up in zone one for up to 10 minutes.

2. Then, increase the workload every 60 seconds until reaching zone three. This will require a slow climb through zone two for at least 2 minutes.

3. After pushing for another minute in zone three, decrease the workload. This 1-minute break is an important minute to help gauge improvement.

4. Drop the client's workload down to the level he or she was just working in, before starting the zone three interval. During this minute, the heart rate will drop.

5. As improvements are made during several weeks of training, the heart rate will drop more quickly. The faster the heart rate drops, the stronger the heart is getting.

6. If the client is not able to drop to the appropriate heart rate during the 1-minute break, assume that he or she is tired and about to overtrain. The solution is to stay in zone one or two for the rest of the workout. The bottom line is that the client is not rested enough to do that type of exercise on that day (which may be because of a hard workout the day before, not enough sleep, or poor nutrition). Monitoring heart rate is an excellent tool in avoiding overtraining.

7. If the heart rate does drop to a normal rate, then overload the body again and go to the next zone, zone three, for 1 minute.

8. After this minute, go back to zone one for 10 minutes before starting over.

It is vital when training at this level to rotate all three stages. There will be a low- (stage I), medium- (stage II), and high-intensity day (stage III) to help minimize the risk of overtraining. The monthly plan, shown in Figure 7-8, is only a general

Week	1							2							3							4						
Day	M	T	W	T	F	S	S	M	T	W	T	F	S	S	M	T	W	T	F	S	S	M	T	W	T	F	S	S
Phase 1																												
Phase 2																												
Phase 3																												
Phase 4																												
Phase 5																												
Cardio	S1		S2		S3			S2		S1		S3			S1		S2		S3			S2		S1		S3		
Flexibility	X		X		X			X		X		X			X		X		X			X		X		X		

S1= Stage I S2= Stage II S3= Stage III

Figure 7.8 The monthly plan.

guide and may change based on the workout (if any) that is being performed on that day.

The importance of understanding the three stages of cardiorespiratory training (and using them in an alternating manner) is that EPOC, in and of itself, does not ensure weight loss or increased total caloric expenditure for a given exercise session or its recovery. Rather, it can be a large contributor to the total caloric expenditure, depending on the intensity and duration of the exercise, by increasing the amount of oxygen consumed after exercise.[46-50] Simply increasing the intensity for the same type of training will not produce consistent increases in fitness levels and weight control, as the body will soon adapt.[42] For the intermediate and advanced client, this information becomes crucial to obtaining optimal results. Many clients fail to push themselves to force a new level of fitness and results. That is the purpose of a health and fitness professional. By increasing a client's intensity through the three heart rate zones seen in stage III training, the client can take greater advantage of EPOC and help ensure greater results.

Circuit Training

One of the most beneficial forms of cardiorespiratory training is circuit training. Circuit training allows for comparable fitness results without spending extended periods of time to achieve them. It is a very time-efficient manner in which to train a client and will be thoroughly described as it pertains to cardiorespiratory training.

Circuit training programs consist of a series of resistance training exercises that an individual performs, one after the other, with minimal rest. An example would include:

1. Ball dumbbell chest press
2. Standing cable row
3. Standing overhead dumbbell press
4. Standing dumbbell curl
5. Ball dumbbell triceps extension
6. Step-up
7. Rest

Several recent studies have compared the effects of circuit weight training with traditional endurance forms of exercise (such as treadmills, cross-country skiing, jogging, and bicycling), in relation to energy expenditure, strength, and improving physical fitness.[54-57] It was demonstrated that circuit weight training:

- Was just as beneficial as traditional forms of cardiorespiratory exercise for improving or contributing to improved fitness levels.[53,54]
- Produced greater levels of EPOC and strength.[55,56]

- Produced near-identical caloric expenditure for the same given time span, when compared with walking at a fast pace.[53]

With the assumption that circuit weight training is an effective form of cardiorespiratory training, research has looked at various alterations within a circuit weight training program. When circuit weight training was compared with circuit weight training with a combined 30 seconds of running between each exercise station, no statistical difference was found between the two protocols.[58] Circuit weight training has also been looked at comparing two different rest protocols: 20 seconds and 60 seconds between each exercise.[59] It was found that whereas 20 seconds of rest produced a higher EPOC, 60 seconds of rest produced higher total caloric expenditure. This was attributed to the fact that in the 60-second rest group, the total workout time was greater and used more total energy.[59] However, this is not to be interpreted as advice to take long rest periods and slow a workout down. Much of the benefit derived from shorter rest periods may be lost after 3 minutes of rest.[60]

A prime example of how circuit training can be implemented into one's program (and still use the F.I.T.T.E. principle) can been seen in a client who dislikes traditional cardiorespiratory activity, but loves to weight train. By structuring the client's weight training program in a specific manner (circuit training), a health and fitness professional can accomplish cardiorespiratory work and weight training while keeping the client happy. Circuit training can also incorporate traditional cardiorespiratory exercise into the routine. Some examples may include:

Beginning Client (Stabilization Level)

- 5–10 minutes   Flexibility (self-myofascial release and static stretching)
- 5–10 minutes   Stage I cardiorespiratory training
- 15–20 minutes   Circuit weight training
- 5–10 minutes   Stage I cardiorespiratory training
- 5–10 minutes   Flexibility (self-myofascial release and static stretching)

Intermediate Client (Strength Level)

- 5–10 minutes   Warm-up: flexibility (self-myofascial release and active-isolated stretching)
- 5–10 minutes   Stage II cardiorespiratory training
- 15–20 minutes   Circuit weight training
- 5–10 minutes   Stage II cardiorespiratory training
- 5–10 minutes   Cool-down: flexibility (self-myofascial release and static stretching)

At this level, the warm-up and cool-down may be performed separately by the client, before or after meeting with the health and fitness professional. This will allow for more time to be spent on the cardiorespiratory and circuit training components.

Advanced Client (Power Level)

- 5–10 minutes   Flexibility (self-myofascial release and dynamic stretching)
- 5–10 minutes   Stage III cardiorespiratory training
- 15–20 minutes   Circuit weight training
- 5–10 minutes   Stage II cardiorespiratory training
- 5–10 minutes   Flexibility (self-myofascial release and static stretching)

Again, at this level, the warm-up and cool-down may be performed before or after meeting with the health and fitness professional.

Postural Considerations in Cardiorespiratory Training

As any form of cardiorespiratory training involves movement, it must follow the same kinetic chain technique parameters as flexibility and resistance training exercises. Selecting the appropriate form of cardiorespiratory training is also important for the beginner and should be approached as follows:

CLIENTS WHO POSSESS A ROUNDED SHOULDER OR FORWARD HEAD POSTURE

The health and fitness professional must watch closely for the following kinetic chain deviations:

- During use of stationary bicycles, treadmills, and elliptical trainers, watch for rounding of shoulders and protruding head.
- On steppers and treadmills, watch for the grasping of the handles (with an oversupinated or overpronated hand position), which will cause elevated and protracted shoulders and a protracted head. If possible, this equipment should be used without the assistance of the hands to increase the stabilization component, elevating the caloric expenditure and balance requirements.
- In settings in which a television is present, watch for excessive cervical extension or rotation of the head to view the television.

CLIENTS WHO POSSESS AN ANTERIORLY ROTATED PELVIS (LOW BACK ARCHES)

The health and fitness professional must watch closely for the following kinetic chain deviations:

- Initial use of bicycles or steppers may not be warranted, as the hips are placed in a constant state of flexion, adding to a shortened hip flexor complex. If they are used, emphasize hip flexor stretches before and after use.
- Treadmill speed should be kept to a controllable pace, to avoid overstriding. The hips will not be able to properly extend and will cause the low back to overextend, placing increased stress on the low back. Hip flexor stretches should be emphasized before and after use.

CLIENTS WHOSE FEET TURN OUT AND/OR KNEES MOVE IN

The health and fitness professional must watch closely for the following kinetic chain deviations:

- Use of the all cardio equipment that involves the lower extremities will require proper flexibility of the ankle joint (gastrocnemius and soleus muscles). Emphasize foam rolling for calves, adductors, iliotibial (IT) band, tensor fascia latae (TFL), and latissimus dorsi as well as hip flexor stretches.
- Using the treadmill and steppers that require climbing (or aerobics classes) may initially be too extreme for constant repetition, especially if clients are allowed to hold on to the rails and speed up the pace. If these modalities are used, emphasize the foam roll protocol and keep the pace at a controllable speed.

SUMMARY

Different cardiorespiratory training programs place different demands on the bioenergetic continuum and ultimately affect a client's adaptations and goals. Stage training is a three-stage programming system that uses different heart rate training zones, based on the respiratory exchange ratio (RER). Zone one consists of a heart rate of approximately 65 to 75% of a predicted HR max and is intended for beginners and used as a recovery zone for more advanced clients. Zone two is near the anaerobic threshold, at 80 to 85% of HR max, and is intended for individuals who have progressed to the strength level of the OPT™ model. Zone three is at 86 to 90% of HR max, and is intended for short bouts for individuals who have progressed to the power level of the OPT™ model. These zones can be translated into three stages, which dictate in which zone and for what length of time cardiorespiratory activity should be performed.

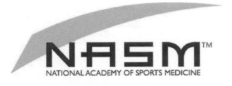

OPT For Fitness

Program Goal: Fat Loss

Name: John Smith	Month: 1
Date: 08/10/06	Week: 1
Professional Scott Lucett	Day: 1 of 12

STEP 1

A. Foam Roll

Foam Roll	Sets	Duration
Calves	1	30 sec.
IT Band	1	30 sec.
Adductors	1	30 sec.

B. Stretch

Static Stretching	Sets	Duration
Calves	1	30 sec.
Hip Flexors	1	30 sec.
Adductors	1	30 sec.

C. Cardiovascular

Treadmill	5-10 min.

STEP 2

A. Core

Exercise	Sets	Reps	Tempo	Rest

B. Balance

Exercise	Sets	Reps	Tempo	Rest

C. Reactive

Exercise	Sets	Reps	Tempo	Rest

STEP 3

Resistance Training Program

Body Part Exercise		Sets	Reps	Intensity	Tempo	Rest
Total Body						
Chest						
Back						
Shoulder						
Legs						

STEP 4

Cool-Down

Repeat Steps 1A and 1B

Figure 7.9 OPT™ template.

Circuit training programs consist of a series of resistance training exercises that an individual performs, one after the other, with minimal rest. Thus, they allow for comparable fitness results in shorter periods of time. It is also a good way to accomplish cardiorespiratory work during weight training.

Because movement is involved, it is vital to monitor kinetic chain checkpoints with clients who are performing cardiorespiratory activity. For clients who have a rounded shoulder or forward head posture, watch for elevated and protracted shoulders and extended cervical spine, particularly on cardio machinery. Individuals with low back arches may hyperextend the low back and minimize hip extension. It may be best to avoid bicycles and steppers for these clients and emphasize hip flexor stretches. Clients whose feet turn out or knees move inward may need to limit the use of cardio machinery and stress foam rolling and static stretching techniques.

FILLING IN THE TEMPLATE

The information in this chapter allows step 1 of the OPT™ template to be completed (Figure 7-9). Here, enter the desired form of cardio that will be used for the warm-up. If a circuit weight training protocol will be used for the workout, the client should still perform some form of warm-up.

Review Questions

1. *One adaptive benefit of cardiorespiratory exercise is that it increases/decreases resting heart rate and increases/decreases exercising heart rate.*

2. *It has been shown that performing three 10-minute bouts of exercise is just as effective as one 30-minute continuous bout of the same exercise.*

    a. *True*

    b. *False*

3. *The Law of Thermodynamics states that body fat reduction can only take place when there is more ____ being burned than consumed.*

4. *Which of the following is/are true about circuit weight training?*

    a. *It is not as beneficial as traditional forms of cardiorespiratory exercise for improving fitness levels.*

    b. *It produces greater levels of EPOC.*

    c. *It produces near-identical caloric expenditure for the same given time span, when compared to walking at a fast pace.*

5. *Clients with an anterior pelvic tilt (low back arches) should use bicycles and steppers to place the hips into flexion.*

    a. *True*

    b. *False*

REFERENCES

1. Holly RG, Shaffrath JD. Cardiorespiratory endurance. In: American College of Sports Medicine (ed). ACSM's Resource Manual for Guidelines for Exercise Testing and Prescription, 3rd ed. Baltimore: Williams & Wilkins, 1998.
2. Brooks GA, Fahey TD, White TP. Exercise Physiology: Human Bioenergetics and Its Application, 2nd ed. Moutain View, CA: Mayfield Publishing Company, 1996.

3. Greenhaff PL, Timmons JA. Interaction between aerobic and anaerobic metabolism during intense muscle contraction. In Holsey JO (ed). Exercise and Sport Science Reviews, Vol 26. Baltimore: Williams & Wilkins, 1998, pp. 1–30.

4. Alter MJ. Science of Flexibility, 2nd ed. Champaign, IL: Human Kinetics, 1996.

5. Kovaleski JE, Gurchiek LR, Spriggs DH. Musculoskeletal injuries: risks, prevention and care. In: American College of Sports Medicine (ed.). ACSM's Resource Manual for Guidelines for Exercise Testing and Prescription. 3rd ed. Baltimore: Williams & Wilkins, 1998.

6. Karvonen J. Importance of warm-up and cool-down on exercise performance. Med Sports Sci 1992;35:182–214.

7. Wilford HN, East JB, Smith FH, Burry LA. Evaluation of warm-up for improved flexibility. Am J Sports Med 1986;14(4):316–319.

8. Walter SD, Hart LE, McIntosh JM, Sutton JR. The Ontario cohort study of running related injuries. Arch Intern Med 1989;149(11):2561–2564.

9. van Mechelen W, Hlobil H, Kemper HCG, Voorn WJ, de Jongh R. Prevention of running injuries by warm-up, cool-down, and stretching exercises. Am J Sports Med 1993;21(5):711–719.

10. Kato Y, Ikata T, Takai H, Takata S, Sairyo K, Iwanaga K. Effects of specific warm-up at various intensities on energy metabolism during subsequent exercise. J Sports Med Phys Fitness 2000;40(2):126–130.

11. Fitts RH. Cellular mechanisms of muscle fatigue. Physiol Rev 1994;74:49.

12. Andrews MA, Godt RE, Nosek TM. Influence of physiological L(+)-lactate concentrations on contractility of skinned striated muscle fibers of rabbit. J Appl Physiol 1996;80(6):2060–2065.

13. Metzger JM, Moss RL. Effects of tension and stiffness due to reduced pH in mammalian fast- and slow-twitch skinned skeletal muscle fibres. J Physiol (Lond) 1990;428:737–750.

14. Dorfman LJ, Howard JE, McGill KC. Triphasic behavioral response of motor units to submaximal fatiguing exercise. Muscle Nerve 1990;13:621–628.

15. Garland SJ, Enoka RM, Serrano LP, Robinson GA. Behavior of motor units in human biceps brachii during submaximal fatiguing contraction. J Appl Physiol 1994;76(6):2411–2419.

16. Grimby L. Single motor unit discharge during voluntary contraction and locomotion. In: Jones NL, McCartney N, McComas AJ (eds). Human Muscle Power. Champaign, IL: Human Kinetics, 1986.

17. Moritani T, Muro M, Nagata A. Intramuscular and surface electromyogram changes during muscle fatigue. J Appl Physiol 1986;60:1179–1185.

18. Edgerton VR, Wolf S, Roy RR. Theoretical basis for patterning EMG amplitudes to assess muscle dysfunction. Med Sci Sports Exerc 1996;28(6):744–751.

19. Janda V. In: Grant R (ed). Physical Therapy of the Cervical and Thoracic Spine. Edinburgh: Churchill Livingstone, 1988.

20. Janda V. Muscle function testing. London: Butterworth, 1983.

21. Liebenson C. Integrating rehabilitation into chiropractic practice (blending active and passive care). In: Liebenson C (ed). Rehabilitation of the Spine. Baltimore: Williams & Wilkins, 1996.

22. Hammer WI. Muscle imbalance and postfacilitation stretch. In: Hammer WI (ed). Functional Soft Tissue Examination and Treatment by Manual Methods, 2nd ed. Gaithersburg, MD: Aspen Publishers, 1999.

23. Carter R 3rd, Watenpaugh DE, Wasmund WL, Wasmund SL, Smith ML. Muscle pump and central command during recovery from exercise in humans. J Appl Physiol 1999;87(4):1463–1469.

24. Raine NM, Cable NT, George KP, Campbell IG. The influence of recovery posture on post-exercise hypotension in normotensive men. Med Sci Sports Exerc 2001;33(3):404–412.

25. Pate RR, Pratt MM, Blair SN, Haskell WL, Macera CA, Bouchard C, Buchner D, Ettinger W, Heath GW, King AC. Physical activity and public health: a recommendation from the Centers for Disease Control and Prevention and the American College of Sports Medicine. JAMA 1995;273:402–407.

26. Lambert EV, Bohlmann I, Cowling K. Physical activity for health: understanding the epidemiological evidence for risk benefits. Int Sport Med J 2001;1(5):1–15.

27. Blair SN, Wei M. Sedentary habits, health, and function in older women and men. Am J Health Promot 2000;15(1):1–8.

28. Blair SN, Kohl HW, Barlow CE, Paffenbarger RS Jr, Gibbons LW, Macera CA. Changes in physical fitness and all-cause mortality. A prospective study of healthy and unhealthy men. JAMA 1995;273(14):1093–1098.

29. Blair SN. Physical inactivity and cardiovascular disease risk in women. Med Sci Sports Exerc 1996;28(1):9–10.

30. Smolander J, Blair SN, Kohl HW 3rd. Work ability, physical activity, and cardiorespiratory fitness: 2-year results from Project Active. J Occup Environ Med 2000;42(9):906–910.

31. American College of Sports Medicine. ACSM's Guidelines for Exercise Testing and Prescription, 5th ed. Philadelphia: Williams & Wilkins, 1995.

32. Wei M, Schwertner HA, Blair SN. The association between physical activity, physical fitness, and type 2 diabetes mellitus. Compr Ther 2000;26(3):176–182.

33. Andreoli A, Monteleone M, Van Loan M, Promenzio L, Tarantino U, De Lorenzo A. Effects of different sports on bone density and muscle mass in highly trained athletes. Med Sci Sports Exerc 2001;33(4):507–511.

34. American College of Sports Medicine. American College of Sports Medicine position stand. The recommended quantity and quality of exercise for developing and maintaining CR and muscular fitness in healthy adults. Med Sci Sports Exerc 1990;22(2):265–274.
35. Murphy MH, Hardman AE. Training effects of short and long bouts of brisk walking in sedentary women. Med Sci Sports Exerc 1998;30(1):152–157.
36. Snyder KA, Donnelly JE, Jabobsen DJ, Hertner G, Jakicic JM. The effects of long-term, moderate intensity, intermittent exercise on aerobic capacity, body composition, blood lipids, insulin, and glucose in overweight females. Int J Obes Relat Metab Disord 1997;21(12):1180–1189.
37. Thomas DQ, Lewis HL, McCaw ST, Adams MJ. The effects of continuous and discontinuous walking on physiological response in college-age subjects. J Strength Cond Res 2001;15(2):264–265.
38. Branch JD, Pate RR, Bourque SP. Moderate intensity exercise training improves cardiorespiratory fitness in women. J Womens Health Gend Based Med 2000;9(1):65–73.
39. Wilmore JH, Costill DL. Physiology of Sport and Exercise. Champaign, IL: Human Kinetics, 1994.
40. Sale DG. Neural adaptation to resistance training. Med Sci Sports Exerc 1988;20(5):S135–145.
41. Enoka RM. Muscle strength and its development. New perspectives. Sports Med 1988;6:146–168.
42. Westerterp KR, Meijer GAL, Janssen GME, Saris WHM, Hoor F. Long-term effect of physical activity on energy balance and body composition. Br J Nutr 1992;68(1):21–30.
43. Conley DL, Krahenbuhl GS. Running economy and distance running performance of highly trained athletes. Med Sci Sports Exerc 1980;12:357.
44. Enoka RM. Neuromechanical Basis of Kinesiology, 2nd ed. Champaign, IL: Human Kinetics, 1994.
45. Gaesser GA, Brooks GA. Metabolic bases of excess post-exercise oxygen consumption: a review. Med Sci Sports Exerc 1984;16:29–43.
46. Bahr R, Ingnes I, Vaage O, Sejersted O, Newsholme E. Effect of duration of exercise on excess post-exercise O_2 consumption. J Appl Physiol 1987;62:485–490.
47. Bahr R, Gronnerod O, Sejersted O. Effect of supramaximal exercise on excess post-exercise O_2 consumption. Med Sci Sports Exerc 1992;24:66–71.
48. Gore C, Whithers R. Effect of exercise intensity and duration on post-exercise metabolism. J Appl Physiol 1990;68:2362–2368.
49. Laforgia J, Whithers RT, Shipp NJ, Gore CJ. Comparison of energy expenditure elevations after submaximal and supramaximal running. J Appl Physiol 1997;82:661–666.
50. Almuzaini KS, Potteiger JA, Green SB. Effects of split exercise sessions on excess postexercise oxygen consumption and resting metabolic rate. Can J Appl Physiol 1998;23(5):433–443.
51. Gerald S, Zavorsky DL, Montgomery DP. Effect of intensity interval workouts on running economy using three recovery durations. Eur J Appl Physiol 1998;77:224–230.
52. Henritze J, Weltman A, Schurrer RL, Barlow K. Effects of training at and above the lactate threshold on the lactate threshold and maximal oxygen uptake. Eur J Appl Physiol 1985;54:84–88.
53. Weltman A, Seip RL, Snead D, Weltman JY, Haskvliz EM, Evans WS, Veldhuis JD, Rogol AD. Exercise training at and above the lactate threshold in previously untrained women. Int J Sports Med 1992;13:257–263.
54. Kaikkonen H, Yrlama M, Siljander E, Byman P, Laukkanen R. The effect of heart rate controlled low resistance circuit weight training and endurance training on maximal aerobic power in sedentary adults. Scand J Med Sci Sports 2000;10(4):211–215.
55. Jurimae T, Jurimae J, Pihl E. Circulatory response to single circuit weight and walking training sessions of similar energy cost in middle-aged overweight females. Clin Physiol 2000;20(2):143–149.
56. Burleson MA, O'Bryant HS, Stone MH, Collins MA, Triplett-McBride T. Effect of weight training exercise and treadmill exercise on post-exercise oxygen consumption. Med Sci Sports Exerc 1998;30(4):518–522.
57. Gillette CA, Bullough RC, Melby CL. Postexercise energy expenditure in response to acute aerobic or resistive exercise. Int J Sport Nutr 1994;4(4):347–360.
58. Gettman LR, Ward P, Hagan RD. A comparison of combined running and weight training with circuit weight training. Med Sci Sports Exerc 1982;14(3):229–234.
59. Haltom RW, Kraemer R, Sloan R, Hebert EP, Frank K, Tryniecki JL. Circuit weight training and its effects on postexercise oxygen consumption. Med Sci Sports Exerc 1999;31(11):1613–1618.
60. Dudley GA, Tesch PA, Harris RT, et al. Influence of eccentric action on the metabolic cost of resistance exercise. Aviat Space Environ Med 1991;62:543–550.

Core-Training Concepts

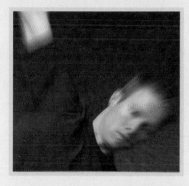

OBJECTIVES

After completing this chapter, you will be able to:

- Understand the importance of the core musculature.
- Differentiate between the stabilization system and the movement system.
- Rationalize the importance of core training.
- Design a core-training program for clients at any level of training.
- Perform, describe, and instruct various core-training exercises.

KEY TERMS

Core	Intermuscular coordination
Drawing-in maneuver	Intramuscular coordination

Concepts in Core Training

This chapter discusses the importance of core training and how to implement this component into a client's program. Successive chapters discuss balance training and reactive training and how these additional components can be incorporated into a training program that will enhance overall functional efficiency.

Core Musculature

Core: The lumbo-pelvic-hip complex and the thoracic and cervical spine, where the body's center of gravity is located.

The **core** has been defined as the lumbo-pelvic-hip complex, and the thoracic and cervical spine.[1,2] The core is where the body's center of gravity is located and where all movement begins.[3-6] An efficient core is necessary for maintaining proper muscle balance throughout the entire kinetic chain (Figure 8-1).

There are 29 muscles that attach to the lumbo-pelvic-hip complex. Optimum lengths (or length-tension relationships), recruitment patterns (or force-couple relationships), and joint motions (or arthrokinematics) in the muscles of the lumbo-pelvic-hip complex establish neuromuscular efficiency throughout the entire kinetic chain. This allows for efficient acceleration, deceleration, and stabilization during dynamic movements, as well as the prevention of possible injuries.[3-12]

The musculature of the core is divided into two categories: the stabilization system and the movement system (Table 8-1). The stabilization system is primarily responsible for stability of the lumbo-pelvic-hip complex, whereas the movement system is responsible for movement of the core.

The core operates as an integrated functional unit, whereby the stabilization system must work in concert with the movement system. When working optimally, each structural component distributes weight, absorbs force, and transfers ground-reaction forces.[1] As such, these interdependent systems must be trained appropriately to allow the kinetic chain to function efficiently during dynamic activities. This means that we must work from the inside (stabilization system) out (movement system). Training the muscles of the movement system before training the muscles of the stabilization system would not make structural, biomechanical, or logical sense. This would be analogous to building a house without a foundation. The foundation must be developed first to provide a stable platform for the remaining components of the house to be built on. One must be stable first to move efficiently.

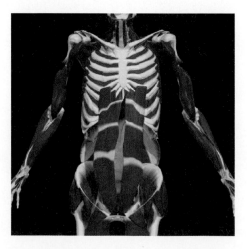

Figure 8.1   Core musculature.

Table 8.1	
Muscles of the Core	
Stabilization Systems	**Movement System**
Transversus abdominis	Latissimus dorsi
Internal oblique	Erector spinae
Lumbar multifidus	Iliopsoas
Pelvic floor muscles	Hamstrings
Diaphragm	Hip adductors
Transversospinalis	Adductor magnus
	Adductor longus
	Adductor brevis
	Gracilis
	Pectineus
	Hip abductors
	Gluteus minimus
	Gluteus medius
	Tensor fascia latae
	Rectus abdominis
	External oblique

Importance of Properly Training the Stabilization System

Many individuals have developed strength, power, neuromuscular control, and muscular endurance in the movement system, which enables them to perform functional activities.[1,9,11] Few people, however, have properly developed the deep stabilization muscles required for lumbo-pelvic-hip complex stabilization.[10-12] The body's stabilization system (core) has to be operating with maximal efficiency to effectively use the strength, power, neuromuscular control, and muscular endurance that has been developed in the prime movers. If the movement system musculature of the core is strong and the stabilization system is weak, the kinetic chain senses imbalance and forces are not transferred or used properly. This leads to compensation, synergistic dominance, and inefficient movements.[1,10-12] Examples include performing a lunge, squat, or overhead press with excessive spinal extension (Figure 8-2).

A weak core is a fundamental problem that causes inefficient movement and can lead to predictable patterns of injury.[10-13] Many people have a strong rectus abdominis, external obliques, and erector spinae, but weak stabilizing muscles. This results in lack of stabilization and unwanted motion of the individual vertebrae, thus increasing forces throughout the lumbo-pelvic-hip complex that may result in low back pain and injury.[14]

SUMMARY

The core is the beginning point for movement and the center of gravity for the body. It consists of the lumbo-pelvic-hip complex and the thoracic and cervical spine. If the core is unstable during movement, it does not allow optimum stabilization, force reduction, production, and transference to occur throughout the kinetic chain.

An efficient core is necessary for maintaining proper muscle balance throughout the entire kinetic chain. Optimum lengths (length-tension relationships), recruitment patterns (force-couple relationships), and joint motions (arthrokinematics) in

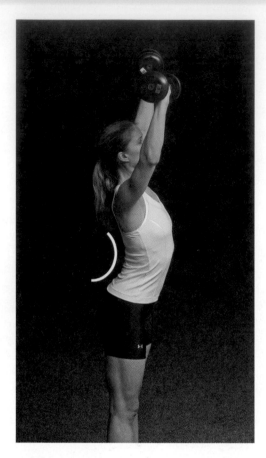

Figure 8.2 Inefficient Core

the muscles of the lumbo-pelvic-hip complex establish neuromuscular efficiency throughout the entire kinetic chain. This allows for efficient acceleration, deceleration, and stabilization during dynamic movements, as well as the prevention of possible injuries.

The musculature of the core is divided into two categories: stabilization and movement systems. The stabilization system is primarily responsible for stability of the lumbo-pelvic-hip complex. The movement system is responsible for movement, force production, and force reduction of the core. Training should begin from the inside (stabilization system) out (movement system). If the core's movement system musculature is strong and the stabilization system is weak, the kinetic chain senses imbalance and forces are not transferred or used properly. This all may result in compensation, synergistic dominance, and inefficient movements.

Scientific Rationale for Core Stabilization Training

SIMILARITIES IN INDIVIDUALS WITH CHRONIC BACK PAIN

Researchers have found that individuals with chronic low back pain (85% of U.S. adults) have decreased activation of certain muscles: transversus abdominis, internal obliques, pelvic floor muscles, multifidus, diaphragm, and deep erector spinae.[10-12,15-17] These individuals also have decreased stabilization endurance.[3,4,18,19]

Performing traditional abdominal exercises without proper lumbo-pelvic-hip stabilization has been shown to increase pressure on the disks and compressive forces in the lumbar spine.[10-12,15,19-22] Furthermore, performing traditional low back hyperextension exercises without proper lumbo-pelvic hip stabilization has been

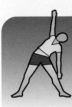

Stretch Your Knowledge

Low Back Pain and an Inefficient Core

- Hungerford et al. (2003) in a cross-sectional study with 14 men with a clinical diagnosis of back pain found delayed onset of the transverse abdominis, internal obliques, multifidus, and gluteus maximus during hip flexion on the support leg, suggesting an alteration in the strategy for lumbo-pelvic-hip stability.[1]

- Hodges and Richardson (1998) reported that slow speed of contraction of the transverse abdominis during arm and leg movements was well correlated with low back pain.[2]

- Hides et al. (1996) demonstrated that recovery from acute back pain did not automatically result in restoration of the normal girth of the multifidus.[3]

- Hides et al. (1994) demonstrated multifidus atrophy in patients with low back pain.[4]

---

1. Hungerford B, Gilleard W, Hodges P. Evidence of altered lumbopelvic muscle recruitment in the presence of sacroiliac joint pain. Spine 2003;28(14):1593–1600.
2. Hodges PW, Richardson CA. Delayed postural contraction of transversus abdominis in low back pain associated with movement of the lower limb. J Spinal Disord 1998;11(1):46–56.
3. Hides JA, Richardson CA, Jull GA. Multifidus muscle recovery is not automatic after resolution of acute, first-episode low back pain. Spine 1996;21(23):2763–2769.
4. Hides JA, Stokes MJ, Saide M, Jull GA, Cooper DH. Evidence of lumbar multifidus wasting ipsilateral to symptoms in subjects with acute/subacute low back pain. Spine1994;19:165–177.

shown to increase pressure on the disks to dangerous levels. These unsupported exercises can cause damage to the ligaments supporting the vertebrae, which may lead to a narrowing of openings in the vertebrae that spinal nerves pass through.[18,20,22]

Therefore, it is crucial for fitness professionals to incorporate a systematic, progressive approach when training the core, ensuring the muscles that stabilize the spine (stabilization system) are strengthened before the musculature that moves the spine (movement system).

Solutions for Stabilization

Drawing-in maneuver: The action of pulling the belly button in toward the spine.

Fortunately, additional research has demonstrated increased electromyogram (EMG) activity and pelvic stabilization when an abdominal **drawing-in maneuver** is performed before core training (Figure 8-3).[18,20,23–30] This maneuver is performed as follows:

1. Pull in the region just below the navel toward the spine (drawing-in maneuver).

Also, maintaining the cervical spine in a neutral position during core training improves posture, muscle balance, and stabilization. If a forward protruding head is noticed during movement, the sternocleidomastoid is preferentially recruited. This increases the compressive forces in the cervical spine. It can also lead to pelvic instability and muscle imbalances as a result of the pelvo-ocular reflex. This reflex is important to maintain the eyes level during movement.[31,32] If the sternocleidomastoid muscle is hyperactive and extends the upper cervical spine, the pelvis rotates anteriorly to realign the eyes. This can lead to muscle imbalances and decreased pelvic stabilization.[31,32]

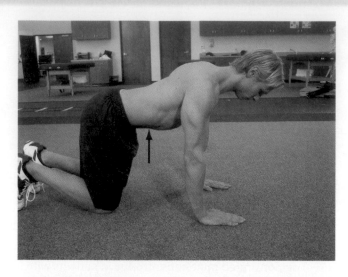

Figure 8.3 Drawing-in maneuver.

REQUIREMENTS FOR CORE TRAINING

The core-stabilization system (transverse abdominis, internal obliques, pelvic floor musculature, diaphragm, transversospinalis, and multifidus) consists primarily of slow-twitch, type I muscle fibers, which respond best to time under tension.[3-6] This means that these muscles need sustained contractions (6 to 20

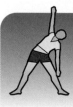

Stretch Your Knowledge

Evidence to Support the Use of Core-Stabilization Training

- Cosio-Lima et al. (2003) in a randomized controlled trial with 30 subjects demonstrated increased abdominal and back extensor strength and single leg balance improvements with a 5-week stability ball training program compared with conventional floor exercises.[1]

- Mills and Taunton (2003) in a randomized controlled trial with 36 subjects demonstrated that agility and balance were improved after a 10-week specific spinal stabilization training program compared with the control group performing an equivalent volume of traditional, nonspecific abdominal exercises.[2]

- Vera-Garcia et al. (2000) in a single-subject design with 8 subjects found that performing abdominal exercises on a labile surface increased activation levels, suggesting increased demand on the motor control system to help stabilize the spine.[3]

- Hahn et al. (1998) in a randomized controlled trial with 35 female subjects demonstrated that traditional floor exercises and stability ball exercises significantly increased core strength during a 10-week training period.[4]

- O'Sullivan et al. (1997) in a randomized clinical trial demonstrated that pain and function improve initially and at 1- and 3-year follow-up in patients with low back pain undergoing specific stabilizing exercises.[5]

1. Cosio-Lima LM, Reynolds KL, Winter C, et al. Effects of physioball and conventional floor exercises on early phase adaptations in back and abdominal core stability and balance in women. J Strength Cond Res 2003;17(4):721–725.
2. Mills JD, Taunton JE. The effect of spinal stabilization training on spinal mobility, vertical jump, agility and balance. Med Sci Sports Exerc 2003;35(5 Suppl).
3. Vera-Garcia FJ, Grenier SG, McGill SM. Abdominal muscle response during curl-ups on both stable and labile surfaces. Phys Ther 2003;80(6):564–594.
4. Hahn S, Stanforth D, Stanforth PR, Philips A. A 10 week training study comparing resistaball and traditional trunk training. Med Sci Sports Exerc 1998;30(5):199.
5. O'Sullivan PB, Twomey L, Allison GT. Evaluation of specific stabilizing exercises in the treatment of chronic low back pain with radiological diagnosis of spondylosis and spondylolisthesis. Spine 1997;22(24):2959–2967.

Intramuscular coordination:
The ability of the neuromuscular system to allow optimal levels of motor unit recruitment and synchronization within a muscle.

Intermuscular coordination:
The ability of the neuromuscular system to allow all muscles to work together with proper activation and timing between them.

seconds) to improve **intramuscular coordination** and motor-unit recruitment within a muscle. This enhances static and dynamic stabilization of the lumbo-pelvic-hip complex.

The core-movement system (rectus abdominis, erector spinae, external obliques, latissimus dorsi, adductors, hamstrings, and iliopsoas) is primarily geared toward movement of the lumbo-pelvic-hip complex. These muscles must work synergistically with the stabilization system to ensure optimal **intermuscular coordination** of the lumbo-pelvic-hip complex.

SUMMARY

Individuals who have chronic low back pain activate their core muscles less and have a lower endurance for stabilization. Performing traditional abdominal and low back exercises without proper pelvic stabilization may cause abnormal forces throughout the lumbo-pelvic-hip complex. These exercises may lead to tissue overload and cause damage. However, the pelvis can be stabilized by using the drawing-in maneuver before core training. In addition, keeping the cervical spine in a neutral position during core training improves posture, muscle balance, and stabilization.

The stabilization system of the core requires sustained contractions of between 6 and 20 seconds to properly stimulate the motor units. These muscles must be trained for prolonged periods to increase endurance and allow for dynamic postural control.

The movement system of the core is primarily geared toward movement of the lumbo-pelvic-hip complex. These muscles must work synergistically with the stabilization system to ensure optimal force production, force reduction, and dynamic stabilization of the lumbo-pelvic-hip complex.

Designing a Core-Training Program

CORE-TRAINING DESIGN PARAMETERS

The core musculature is an integral component of the protective mechanism that relieves the spine of harmful forces that occur during functional activities.[33] A core-training program is designed to help an individual's stabilization, strength, power, muscle endurance, and neuromuscular efficiency in the lumbo-pelvic-hip complex. This integrated approach facilitates balanced muscular functioning of the entire kinetic chain.[1]

Greater neuromuscular control and stabilization strength offers a more biomechanically efficient position for the entire kinetic chain, thereby allowing optimum neuromuscular efficiency.

Thus, a core-training program must be systematic and progressive. Fitness professionals must follow specific program guidelines, proper exercise-selection criteria, and detailed program variables to achieve consistent success with clients (Figure 8-4).

Levels of Core Training

There are three levels of training within the OPT™ model: stabilization, strength, and power (Figure 8-5). A proper core-training program follows the same systematic progression.

Exercise Selection

- Progressive
  - Easy to hard
  - Simple to complex
  - Known to unknown
  - Stable to unstable
- Systematic
  - Stabilization
  - Strength
  - Power
- Activity/Goal-specific
- Integrated
- Proprioceptively challenging
  - Stability ball
  - BOSU ball
  - Reebok core board
  - Half foam roll
  - Airex pad
  - Bodyblade
- Based in current science

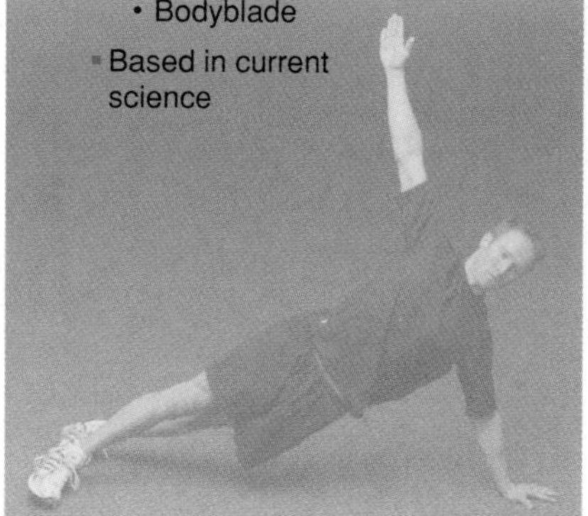

Variables

- Plane of motion
  - Sagittal
  - Frontal
  - Transverse
- Range of motion
  - Full
  - Partial
  - End-range
- Type of resistance
  - Stability ball
  - Cable
  - Tubing
  - Medicine ball
  - Power ball
  - Dumbbells
  - Other
- Body position
  - Supine
  - Prone
  - Side-lying
  - Kneeling
  - Half-kneeling
  - Standing
  - Staggered-stance
  - Standing progression on unstable surface
- Speed of motion
  - Stabilization
  - Strength
  - Power
- Duration
- Frequency
- Amount of feedback
  - Fitness-professional cues
  - Kinesthetic awareness

Figure 8.4 Program-design parameters for core training.

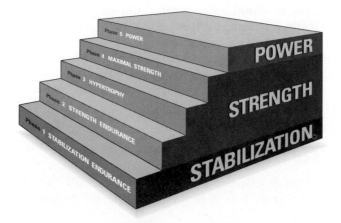

Figure 8.5 OPT™ model.

STABILIZATION

In core stabilization training (phase 1), exercises involve little motion through the spine and pelvis. These exercises are designed to improve the functional capacity of the stabilization system. Sample exercises in this level include:

- Marching
- Floor bridge
- Floor prone cobra
- Prone iso-ab

Marching

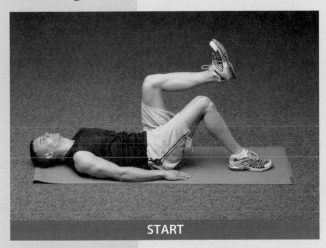

START

PREPARATION

1. Lie supine on floor with knees bent, feet flat, toes pointing straight ahead, and arms by sides.

MOVEMENT

2. Draw navel in.
3. Lift one foot off the floor only as high as can be controlled. Maintain the drawing-in maneuver.
4. Hold for 1 to 2 seconds.
5. Slowly lower.
6. Repeat on the opposite leg.

Technique — Make sure the region just below the navel stays drawn in throughout the duration of the exercise. This ensures the intrinsic core stabilizers are staying activated.

Two-Leg Floor Bridge

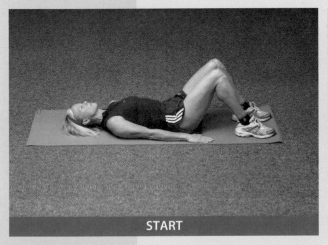

START

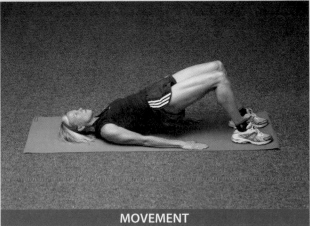

MOVEMENT

PREPARATION

1. Lie supine on the floor with knees bent, feet flat on floor, and toes shoulder-width apart and pointing straight ahead.
2. Place arms to the side, palms down.

MOVEMENT

3. Draw navel in, activate gluteals.
4. Lift pelvis off the floor until the knees, hips, and shoulders are in line.
5. Slowly lower pelvis to the floor.
6. Repeat as instructed.

Safety

When performing a bridge, do not raise the hips too far up off the floor (hyperextending the low back). This places excessive stress to the lumbar spine. Make sure at the end position, the knees, hips, and shoulders are in alignment.

Floor Prone Cobra

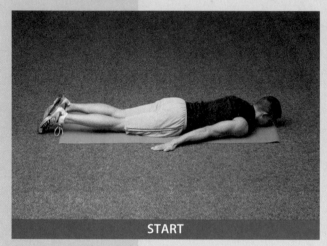
START

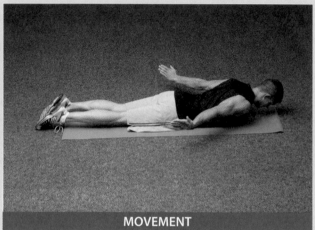
MOVEMENT

PREPARATION

1. Lie prone on the floor with arms to the side of the body, palms facing toward ground.

MOVEMENT

2. Draw navel in, activate gluteals, and pinch shoulder blades together.
3. Lift chest off the floor.
4. Hold for 1 to 2 seconds.
5. Slowly return body to the ground, keeping chin tucked.
6. Repeat as instructed.

Safety

Like the floor bridge, do not come too high off the floor (hyperextending the low back).

Prone Iso-Ab

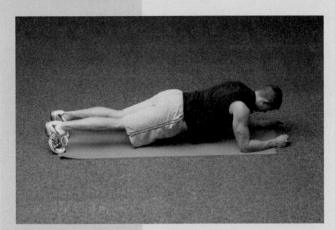

PREPARATION

1. Lie prone on the floor with feet together and fore-arms on ground.

MOVEMENT

2. Draw abs in and activate gluteals.
3. Lift entire body off the ground until it forms a straight line from head to toe, resting on forearms and toes.
4. Hold for 1 to 2 seconds.
5. Slowly return body to the ground, keeping chin tucked and back flat.
6. Repeat as instructed.

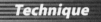

Technique

If this version of the exercise is too difficult for an individual to perform, some regression options include:

- Perform in a standard push-up position.
- Perform in a push-up position with the knees on the floor.
- Perform with the hands on a bench and the feet on the floor.

STRENGTH

In core-strength training (phases 2, 3, and 4), the exercises involve more dynamic eccentric and concentric movements of the spine throughout a full range of motion. The specificity, speed, and neural demand are also progressed in this level. These exercises are designed to improve dynamic stabilization, concentric strength (force production), eccentric strength (force reduction), and neuromuscular efficiency of the entire kinetic chain. Exercises in this level include:

- Ball crunch
- Back extensions
- Reverse crunch
- Cable rotations

Ball Crunch

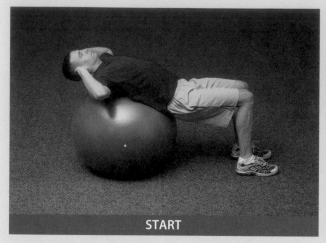

START

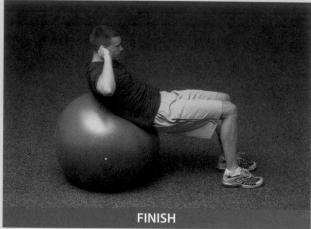

FINISH

PREPARATION

1. Lie supine on a stability ball (ball under low back) with knees bent at a 90-degree angle. Place feet flat on floor with toes shoulder-width apart and pointing straight ahead. Allow back to extend over curve of ball. Cross arms across chest or place hands behind ears.

MOVEMENT

2. Draw navel in and activate gluteals.
3. Slowly crunch upper body forward, raising shoulder blades off the ball and tucking chin to chest.
4. Slowly lower upper body over the ball, maintaining a drawn-in position.
5. Repeat as instructed.
6. To progress, perform as a long-lever exercise.

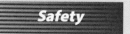

Safety

Make sure to keep the chin tucked while performing the exercise. This will take stress off of the muscles of the cervical spine.

Back Extension

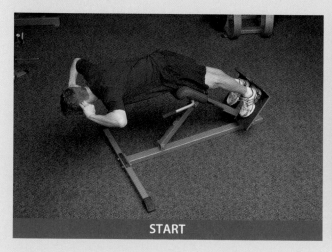

START

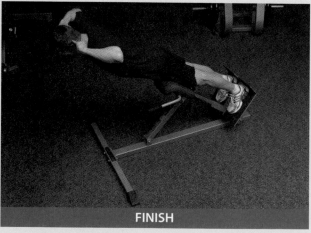

FINISH

PREPARATION

1. Lie prone on a back-extension bench with legs straight and toes shoulder-width apart and pointing straight ahead.
2. Place pads on thighs and cross arms over the chest or hands behind ears.

MOVEMENT

3. Draw navel in, activate gluteals, tuck chin, and retract shoulder blades.
4. Bend forward at waist to end range.
5. Raise upper body to a neutral position, keeping chin tucked and shoulder blades retracted and depressed.
6. Slowly lower upper body toward the ground to end range.
7. Repeat as instructed.

Safety Make sure that at the end position of the exercise, the ankle, knee, hip, shoulders, and ears are all in alignment. Do not hyperextend the low back.

Reverse Crunch

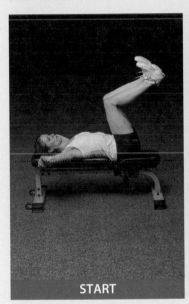

START

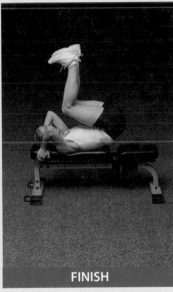

FINISH

PREPARATION

1. Lie supine on a bench with hips and knees bent at a 90-degree angle, feet in the air, and hands gripping a stable object for support.

MOVEMENT

2. Draw navel in.
3. Lift hips off the bench while bringing the knees toward the chest.
4. Slowly lower the hips to the bench.
5. Repeat as instructed.

Technique Do not swing the legs when performing this exercise. Once you have positioned the lower extremities during the setup, they should not move during the execution of the exercise. Swinging the legs increases momentum, increasing the risk of injury and decreasing the effectiveness of the exercise.

Cable Rotation

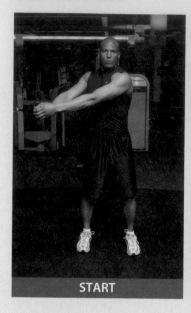

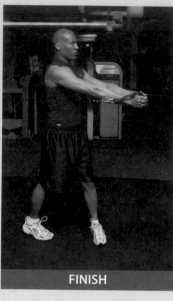

START   FINISH

PREPARATION

1. Stand with feet shoulder width apart, knees slightly flexed, and toes pointing straight ahead.
2. Hold a cable with both hands directly in front of chest, with arms extended and shoulder blades retracted and depressed.

MOVEMENT

3. Draw navel in, activate gluteals, and tuck chin.
4. Rotate body away from the weight stack using abdominals and glutes. Allow back foot to pivot and put back leg into triple extension (hips, knee, ankle).
5. Slowly return to start position.
6. Repeat as instructed.

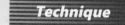

Technique

To decrease stress to the low back, make sure to pivot the back leg into triple extension:

- Hip extension
- Knee extension
- Ankle plantarflexion (extension)

This also ensures proper neuromuscular efficiency of the muscles that extend the lower extremities (gluteus maximus, quadriceps, and gastrocnemius and soleus).

POWER

In core-power training (phase 5), exercises are designed to improve the rate of force production of the core musculature. These forms of exercise prepare an individual to dynamically stabilize and generate force at more functionally applicable speeds. Exercises in this level include:

- Rotation chest pass
- Ball medicine ball (MB) pullover throw
- Front MB oblique throw
- Woodchop throw

Rotation Chest Pass

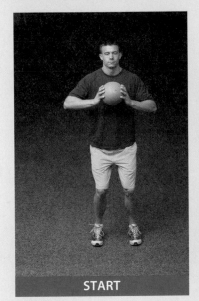

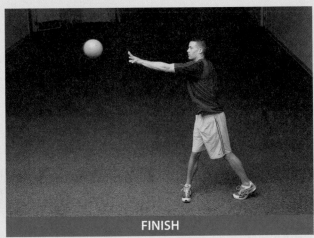

START

FINISH

PREPARATION

1. Stand upright, with body turned at a 90-degree angle to a wall or partner, with feet shoulder width apart and toes pointing straight ahead.
2. Hold a medicine ball (between 5 and 10% of body weight) in hands at chest level.

MOVEMENT

3. Draw navel in and activate gluteals.
4. Use abs and hips to rotate body quickly and explosively to face the wall. As body turns, pivot back leg and allow it to go into triple extension (hips, knee, ankle).
5. Throw medicine ball at wall with the rear arm extending and applying force.
6. Catch and repeat as quickly as can be controlled.

Safety   It is imperative that individuals demonstrate proper stabilization (core-stabilization) and strength (core-strength) before performing core-power exercises. Performing these exercises without proper stabilization and strength will lead to movement compensations, muscle imbalances, and eventually injury.

Ball Medicine Ball Pullover Throw

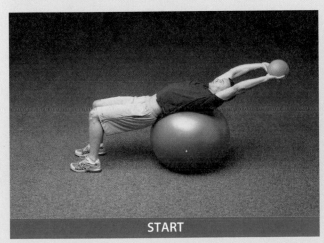

START

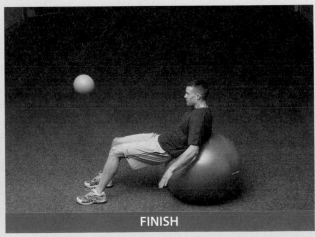

FINISH

PREPARATION

1. Lie on a stability ball (ball under low back) with knees bent at a 90-degree angle, feet flat on floor and toes pointing straight ahead.
2. Hold a medicine ball (between 5 and 10% of body weight) overhead with arms extended.

MOVEMENT

3. Draw navel in, activate gluteals, and tuck chin.
4. Quickly crunch forward, throwing medicine ball against the wall or to a partner.
5. As the ball releases, continue pulling the arms through to the sides of the body.
6. At the end of the follow-through, shoulder blades should be retracted and depressed.
7. Catch ball and repeat.

Safety

It is important that an individual has proper extensibility of the latissimus dorsi before performing this exercise to decrease stress to the low back and shoulders.

Front Medicine Ball Oblique Throw

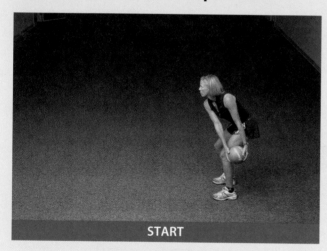

START

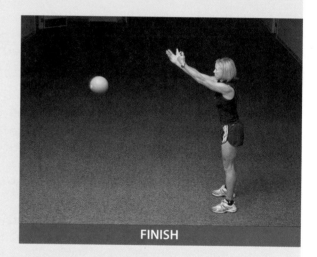

FINISH

PREPARATION

1. Stand facing a wall or partner with feet shoulder width apart, knees slightly bent, and toes pointing straight ahead.
2. Hold a medicine ball (between 5 and 10% of body weight) at waist level.

MOVEMENT

3. Draw navel in and activate gluteals.
4. Use abs, hips, and glutes to quickly rotate body, allowing rear leg to pivot and ready for triple extension (hips, knee, ankle). Avoid arching the back, and keep abdominals drawn in at all times.
5. Toss the ball against the wall or to a partner as body rotates.
6. Use a scooping motion to catch ball.
7. Repeat as quickly as can be controlled.
8. This exercise can be performed continuously to one side or by alternating sides.

Safety

It is important that with all core-power exercises that you go as fast as you can, not as fast as you can't.

Woodchop Throw

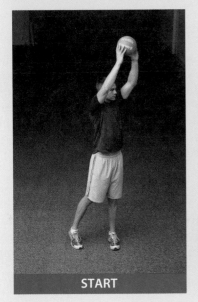

START

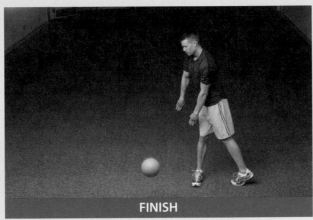

FINISH

PREPARATION

1. Stand facing a wall, with feet pointing straight ahead, shoulder-width apart.
2. Hold a medicine ball (5 to 10% of body weight) overhead.

MOVEMENT

3. Quickly rotate and throw the medicine ball toward the floor, throwing the ball toward the opposite foot (in a woodchopping motion). Keep abdominals drawn in.
4. Repeat.

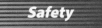

Safety It may be easier to perform this exercise using a D-ball (a medicine ball that does not bounce back) or close to a wall for the medicine ball to bounce off of.

SUMMARY

The core musculature helps protect the spine from harmful forces that occur during functional activities. A core-training program is designed to increase stabilization strength, power, muscle endurance, and neuromuscular control in the lumbo-pelvic-hip complex. Core-training programs must be systematic, progressive, activity- or goal-specific, integrated, and proprioceptively challenging.

A proper core-training program follows the same systematic progression as the OPT™ model: stabilization, strength, and power. In core-stabilization training (phase 1), the emphasis is on stabilization of the lumbo-pelvic-hip complex. It improves the function of the stabilization system. In core-strength training (phases 2, 3, and 4), the spine moves dynamically through a full range of motion, with exercises that require greater specificity, speed, and neural demand. These exercises improve neuromuscular efficiency of the entire kinetic chain. Exercises of core-power training (phase 5) improve the rate of force production in the musculature of the lumbo-pelvic-hip complex (movement system).

Implementing a Core-Training Program

CORE-TRAINING DESIGN PARAMETERS

Implementing a core-training program requires that fitness professionals follow the progression of the OPT™ model (Figure 8-5). For example, if a client is in the stabilization level of training (phase 1), select core-stabilization exercises. For a different client in the strength level of training (phases 2, 3, or 4), the health and fitness professional should select core-strength exercises. For an advanced client in the power level of training (phase 5), select core-power exercises (Table 8-2).

FILLING IN THE TEMPLATE

To fill in the program template (Figure 8-6), go to the section labeled Core (Step 2). You will then refer to Table 8-2 for the appropriate type of core exercise (stabilization, strength, or power), the appropriate number of core exercises, and the appropriate acute variables specific to the phase of training your client will be working in (phases 1–5).

SUMMARY

To choose the proper exercises when designing a program, follow the progression of the OPT™ model. In the stabilization level, choose one to four core stabilization exercises. In the strength level, select zero to four core strength exercises. In the power level, pick zero or two core power exercises.

Table 8.2

Core Training Program Design

Core Systems	OPT™ Level	Phase(s)	Exercise	Number of Exercises	Sets	Reps	Tempo	Rest
Stabilization	Stabilization	1	Core Stabilization	1–4	1–4	12–20	Slow (4/2/1)	0–90 s
Movement	Strength	2 3 4	Core strength	0–4[a]	2–4	8–12	Medium (3/2/1–1/1/1)	0–60 s
Movement	Power	5	Core power	0–2[b]	2–3	8–12	As fast as can be controlled	0–60 s

[a]For the goal of muscle hypertrophy and maximal strength, core training may be optional (although recommended).
[b]Because core exercises are performed in the dynamic warm-up portion of this program and core-power exercises are included in the resistance training portion of the program, separate core training may not be necessary in this phase of training.

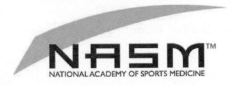

OPT For Fitness

Program Goal: Fat Loss

Name: John Smith	Month: 1
Date: 08/10/06	Week: 1
Professional Scott Lucett	Day: 1

STEP 1

A. Foam Roll

Foam Roll	Sets	Duration
Calves	1	30 sec.
IT Band	1	30 sec.
Adductors	1	30 sec.

B. Stretch

Static Stretching	Sets	Duration
Calves	1	30 sec.
Hip Flexors	1	30 sec.
Adductors	1	30 sec.

C. Cardiovascular

Treadmill	5-10 min.

STEP 2

A. Core

Exercise	Sets	Reps	Tempo	Rest
Floor Bridge	2	12	Slow	0
Floor Prone Cobra	2	12	Slow	90 sec.

B. Balance

Exercise	Sets	Reps	Tempo	Rest

C. Reactive

Exercise	Sets	Reps	Tempo	Rest

Resistance Training Program

	Body Part Exercise		Sets	Reps	Intensity	Tempo	Rest
STEP 3	Total Body						
	Chest						
	Back						
	Shoulder						

Cool-Down

STEP 4	Repeat Steps 1A and 1B

Figure 8.6 OPT template.

Review Questions

1 *The movement system should be trained before the stabilization system.*

   a. True

   b. False

2 *In core stabilization training, exercises involve little motion through the spine and pelvis.*

   a. True

   b. False

3 *Indicate whether the following exercises are stabilization, strength, or power exercises.*

   i. Stabilization

   ii. Strength

   iii. Power

   a. Back extension

   b. Woodchop throw

   c. Floor bridge

   d. Ball crunch

4 *What kind of exercises would you choose for a client in phase 4 (hypertrophy training)?*

   a. Core stabilization

   b. Core strength

   c. Core power

5 *Research shows that individuals who have chronic low back pain display an increased activation of the transversus abdominis, internal oblique, pelvic floor muscles, multifidus, diaphragm, and deep erector spinae.*

   a. True

   b. False

REFERENCES

1. Aaron G. The use of stabilization training in the rehabilitation of the athlete. Sports Physical Therapy Home Study Course. 1996.
2. Dominguez RH. Total Body Training. East Dundee, IL: Moving Force Systems, 1982.
3. Gracovetsky S, Farfan H. The optimum spine. Spine 1986;11:543–573.
4. Gracovetsky S, Farfan H, Heuller C. The abdominal mechanism. Spine 1985;10:317–324.
5. Panjabi MM. The stabilizing system of the spine. Part I: function, dysfunction, adaptation, and enhancement. J Spinal Disord 1992;5:383–389.
6. Panjabi MM, Tech D, White AA. Basic biomechanics of the spine. Neurosurgery 1980;7:76–93.
7. Sahrmann S. Posture and muscle imbalance: faulty lumbo-pelvic alignment and associated musculoskeletal pain syndromes. Orthop Div Rev Can Phys Ther 1992;12:13–20.
8. Sahrmann S. Diagnosis and Treatment of Muscle Imbalances and Musculoskeletal Pain Syndrome. Continuing Education Course. St. Louis: 1997.

9. Dominguez RH. Total Body Training. East Dundee, IL: Moving Force Systems, 1982.
10. Hodges PW, Richardson CA. Neuromotor dysfunction of the trunk musculature in low back pain patients. In: Proceedings of the International Congress of the World Confederation of Physical Therapists. Washington, DC: 1995.
11. Hodges PW, Richardson CA. Inefficient muscular stabilization of the lumbar spine associated with low back pain. Spine 1996;21(22):2640–2650.
12. Hodges PW, Richardson CA. Contraction of the abdominal muscles associated with movement of the lower limb. Phys Ther 1997;77:132–134.
13. Jesse J. Hidden causes of injury, prevention, and correction for running athletes. Pasadena, CA: The Athletic Press, 1977.
14. Janda V. Muscle weakness and inhibition in back pain syndromes. In: Grieve GP (ed). Modern Manual Therapy of the Vertebral Column. New York: Churchill Livingstone, 1986.
15. Hodges PW, Richardson CA, Jull G. Evaluation of the relationship between laboratory and clinical tests of transverse abdominus function. Physiother Res Int 1996;1:30–40.
16. O'Sullivan PE, Twomey L, Allison G, Sinclair J, Miller K, Knox J. Altered patterns of abdominal muscle activation in patients with chronic low back pain. Aus J Physiother 1997;43(2):91–98.
17. Richardson CA, Jull G. Muscle control-pain control. What exercises would you prescribe? Man Med 1995;1:2–10.
18. Beim G, Giraldo JL, Pincivero DM, Borror MJ, Fu FH. Abdominal strengthening exercises: a comparative EMG study. J Sports Rehab 1997;6:11–20.
19 Calliet R. Low Back Pain Syndrome. Oxford, England: Blackwell, 1962.
20. Ashmen KJ, Swanik CB, Lephart SM. Strength and flexibility characteristics of athletes with chronic low back pain. J Sports Rehab 1996;5:275–286.
21. Nachemson A. The load on the lumbar discs in different positions of the body. Clin Orthop 1966;122.
22. Norris CM. Abdominal muscle training in sports. Br J Sports Med 1993;7(1):19–27.
23. Liebenson CL. Active muscle relaxation techniques. Part I. Basic principles and methods. J Manip Physiol Ther 1989;12(6):446–454.
24. Chek P. Scientific Abdominal Training. Correspondence Course. La Jolla, CA: Paul Chek Seminars, 1992.
25. Bittenham D, Brittenham G. Stronger Abs and Back. Champaign, IL: Human Kinetics, 1997.
26. Gustavsen R, Streeck R. Training Therapy; Prophylaxis and Rehabilitation. New York: Thieme Medical Publishers, 1993.
27. Hall T, David A, Geere J, Salvenson K. Relative Recruitment of the Abdominal Muscles During Three Levels of Exertion During Abdominal Hollowing. Gold Coast, Queensland: Manipulative Physiotherapists Association of Australia, 1995.
28. Miller MI, Medeiros JM. Recruitment of the internal oblique and transverse abdominis muscles on the eccentric phase of the curl-up. Phys Ther 1987;67(8):1213–1217.
29. O'Sullivan PE, Twomey L, Allison G. Evaluation of Specific Stabilizing Exercises in the Treatment of Chronic Low Back Pain With Radiological Diagnosis of Spondylolisthesis. Gold Coast, Queensland: Manipulative Physiotherapists Association of Australia, 1995.
30. Richardson CA, Jull G, Toppenberg R, Comerford M. Techniques for active lumbar stabilization for spinal protection. Aus J Physiother 1992;38:105–112.
31. Lewit K. Muscular and articular factors in movement restriction. Man Med 1985;1:83–85.
32. Lewit K. Manipulative therapy in the rehabilitation of the locomotor system. London: Butterworth, 1985.
33. Bullock-Saxton JE. Muscles and joint: inter-relationships with pain and movement dysfunction. Course Manual. Nov 1997.

Balance-Training Concepts

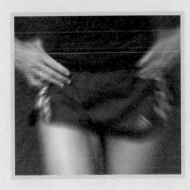

OBJECTIVES

After completing this chapter, you will be able to:

- Describe balance and its purpose.
- Rationalize the importance of balance training.
- Design a balance-training program for clients in any level of training.
- Perform, describe, and instruct various balance-training exercises.

KEY TERMS

Controlled instability	Dynamic joint stabilization	Multisensory condition

Concepts in Balance Training

THE IMPORTANCE OF BALANCE

Whether on a basketball court or a stability ball, or walking down stairs, maintaining balance is key to all functional movements. In functional activities, balance does not work in isolation. Therefore, it should not be thought of as an isolated component of function. Balance is a component of all movements, regardless of whether strength, speed, flexibility, or endurance dominates the movement.

Balance is often thought of as a static process. However, functional balance is a dynamic process involving multiple neurologic pathways. Maintenance of postural equilibrium (or balance) is an integrated process requiring optimal muscular balance (or length-tension relationships and force-couple relationships), joint dynamics (or arthrokinematics), and neuromuscular efficiency.

The integrated performance paradigm (Figure 9-1) shows that adequate force reduction and stabilization are required for optimum force production. The ability to reduce force at the right joint, at the right time, and in the right plane of motion requires optimum levels of functional dynamic balance and neuromuscular efficiency.

Importance of Properly Training the Balance Mechanism

Balance training should constantly stress an individual's limits of stability (or balance threshold). An individual's limit of stability is the distance outside of the base of support that he or she can go without losing control of his or her center of gravity. This threshold must be constantly stressed in a multiplanar, proprioceptively enriched environment, using functional movement patterns to improve dynamic balance and neuromuscular efficiency.

Training functional movements in a proprioceptively enriched environment (unstable, yet controllable) with appropriate progressions (floor, half foam roll, Airex pad, Dyna Disc), correct technique, and at varying speeds facilitates maximal sensory input to the central nervous system, resulting in the selection of the proper movement pattern.

Fitness professionals must implement progressive, systematic training programs to develop consistent, long-term changes in each client. Traditional program design often results in an incomplete training program, which does not challenge the proprioceptive mechanisms of the kinetic chain.

Balance training fills the gap left by traditional training. It focuses on functional movement patterns in a multisensory, unstable environment.[1,2] The design and implementation of balance into a program is critical for developing, improving, and restoring the synergy and synchronicity of muscle-firing patterns required for dynamic joint stabilization and optimal neural muscular control.[1-4]

SUMMARY

Balance is key to all functional movement. However, it does not work in isolation and is not static. Maintenance of postural equilibrium is an integrated, dynamic process requiring optimal muscular balance, joint dynamics, and neuromuscular

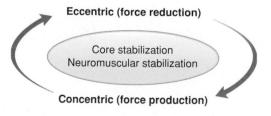

Figure 9.1 Integrated performance paradigm.

efficiency. Balance training should challenge an individual's ability to stabilize outside their normal base of support. By training in a multisensory environment, there will be more of a demand on the nervous system's ability to activate the right muscles at the right time in the right plane of motion.

Scientific Rationale for Balance Training

BENEFITS OF BALANCE TRAINING

Dynamic joint stabilization:
The ability of the kinetic chain to stabilize a joint during movement.

Balance training has been shown to be particularly beneficial to improve **dynamic joint stabilization**.[5-12] Dynamic joint stabilization refers to the ability of the kinetic chain to stabilize a joint during movement. Some examples of this include:

- The rotator cuff stabilizing the head of the humerus on the glenoid fossa while performing a push-up.
- The gluteus medius and adductor complex stabilizing the hip when performing a squat.
- The posterior tibialis and peroneus longus stabilizing the foot and ankle complex when performing a calf raise.

Multisensory condition:
Training environment that provides heightened stimulation to proprioceptors and mechanoreceptors.

Balance and neuromuscular efficiency are improved through repetitive exposure to a variety of **multisensory conditions**.[3,4] An example of this would be having a client balance on one foot on a half foam roll, while squatting down and reaching

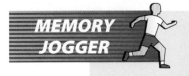

There are a number of training modalities on the market today that challenge one's balance and they all can be very useful tools. However, to ensure the safety and effectiveness of balance training, one must start in an environment they can control and go through the proper progression when using these modalities in a training program:

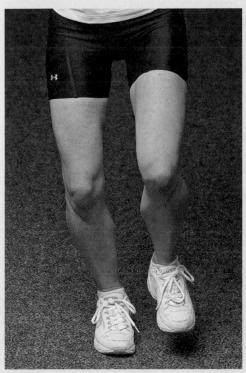

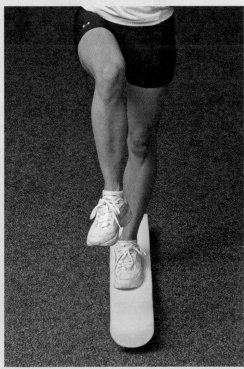

1. Floor

2. Half foam roll

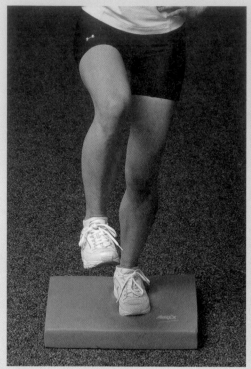

3. Airex pad

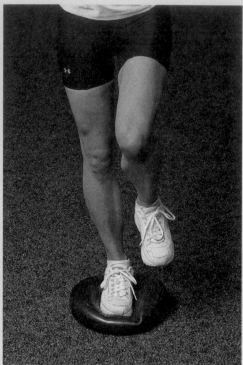

4. Dyna Disc

Not following the proper progression can cause movement compensations and improper execution of the exercise, decreasing the effectiveness of the exercise and increasing the risk for injury.

across the body, toward the floor. This helps facilitate the nervous system to achieve maximal sensorimotor integration, resulting in the selection of the proper movement pattern.

The main goal of balance training is to continually increase the client's awareness of his or her limit of stability (or kinesthetic awareness) by creating **controlled instability**. An example of this could range from having a 65-year-old client balance on one foot on the floor, to having a 25-year-old client balance on one foot on a half foam roll or Dyna Disc.

Controlled instability:
Training environment that is as unstable as can safely be controlled by an individual.

BALANCE AND JOINT DYSFUNCTIONS

Research has demonstrated that specific kinetic chain imbalances (such as altered length-tension relationships, force-couple relationships, and arthrokinematics) in individuals lead to altered balance and neuromuscular efficiency.[13-22]

Alterations in the kinetic chain before, during, or after exercises further affect the quality of movement and perpetuate faulty movement patterns. The faulty movement patterns alter the firing order of the muscles involved, disturbing specific functional movement patterns and decreasing neuromuscular efficiency.[13,23,24] Prime movers may be slow to activate, whereas synergists and stabilizers substitute and become overactive (synergistic dominance). This leads to abnormal joint stress, which affects the structural integrity of the kinetic chain. This may lead to pain and joint dysfunction, and further decrease neuromuscular efficiency.[15]

Research has demonstrated that joint dysfunction creates muscle inhibition.[15,25,26] Joint injury results in joint swelling, which results in the interruption of sensory input from articular, ligamentous, and muscular mechanoreceptors to the central nervous system (Figure 9-2).[27] This results in a clinically evident disturbance in proprioception. It has been demonstrated that sensory feedback to the

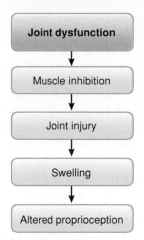

Figure 9.2 Effects of joint dysfunction.

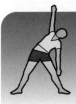

Evidence-Based Research

Injury Prevention, Performance Enhancement, and Balance Training

- Kovacs et al. (2004) in a prospective randomized controlled trial with 44 figure skaters found a significant effect on postural control when balance training versus traditional training (strength training alone) was incorporated into the off-ice training program.[1]

- Paterno et al. (2004) in a single-group pretest and posttest study with 41 healthy female high school athletes found statistically significant improvement in objective single-limb stability in female athletes who incorporated neuromuscular training into their preseason program.[2]

- Mandelbaum et al. (2002) in a prospective study with 1,041 female soccer players demonstrated an 88% decrease in ACL injuries by incorporating neuromuscular training (balance training).[3]

- Junge et al. (2002) in a prospective cohort study with 194 soccer players demonstrated a 20% decrease in injuries and 36% decrease in rate of injuries per player when neuromuscular training was incorporated into the training program.[4]

- Eils and Rosenbaum (2001) in a randomized clinical trial with 30 subjects demonstrated significant improvements in joint position sense, postural sway, and muscle reaction times during a 6-week multistation proprioceptive exercise program.[5]

- Hewett et al. (1999) in a prospective study with 41 female basketball, volleyball, and soccer players demonstrated increased strength (92% squat), increased single-leg hop (8–10 cm), improved 9.1-m sprint time (0.07 seconds), and three-dimensional motion analysis improvements when following a 6-week neuromuscular training program.[6]

1. Kovacs EJ, Birmingham TB, Forwell L, Litchfield RB. Effect of training on postural control in figure skaters: a randomized controlled trial of neuromuscular vs. basic off-ice training programs. Clin J Sport Med 2004;14(4):215–224.
2. Paterno MV, Myer GD, Ford KR, Hewett TE. Neuromuscular training improves single-leg stability in young female athletes. J Orthop Sports Phys Ther 2004;34:305–316.
3. Mandelbaum BR, Silvers HJ, Watanabe D, et al. Effectiveness of a neuromuscular and proprioceptive training program in preventing the incidence of ACL injuries in female athletes. American Orthopedic Society of Sports Medicine, 2002.
4. Junge A, Rosch D, Perterson L, Graf-Baumann T, Dvorak J. Prevention of soccer injuries: a prospective intervention study in youth amateur players. Am J Sports Med 2002;30(5):652–659.
5. Eils E, Rosenbaum D. A multi-station proprioceptive exercise program in patients with ankle instability. Med Sci Sports Exerc 2001;33(12):1991–1998.
6. Hewett TE, Lindenfeld TN, Riccobene JV, Noyes FR. The effect of neuromuscular training on the incidence of knee injury in female athletes: a prospective study. Am J Sports Med 1999;27(6):699–706.

central nervous system is altered after ankle sprains, ligamentous injuries to the knee, and low back pain.[15,17,18,28-32] This is critical for the fitness professional to understand because 85% of the adult U.S. population experiences low back pain and an estimated 80,000 to 100,000 anterior cruciate ligament (ACL) injuries and 2 million ankle sprains occur annually.

Thus, muscle imbalances, joint dysfunctions, pain, and swelling can lead to altered balance. Therefore, the majority of the clients that fitness professionals work with may have decreased neuromuscular efficiency. It is imperative to understand balance and how to design a balance routine that caters to the needs of today's client.

SUMMARY

Balance training benefits dynamic joint stabilization. Its main goal is to continually increase awareness of limits of stability. Repetitive exposure to varied multisensory conditions can improve balance and neuromuscular efficiency. Training should occur in an unstable environment in which an individual can still safely control movements.

Individuals with altered neuromuscular control likely have specific kinetic chain imbalances. These affect the quality of movement, create faulty movement patterns, and lead to lowered neuromuscular efficiency. This may contribute to synergistic dominance, which can cause joint dysfunction and pain elsewhere. Joint dysfunction creates muscle inhibition, which alters balance and leads to tissue overload and injury.

The majority of fitness clients have decreased neuromuscular efficiency and problems with balance.

Designing a Balance-Training Program

BALANCE-TRAINING DESIGN PARAMETERS

A balance-training program is a vital component of any integrated training program. It ensures optimum neuromuscular efficiency of the entire kinetic chain. The program must be systematic and progressive. Health and fitness professionals must follow specific program guidelines, proper exercise selection criteria, and detailed program variables (Figure 9-3).

Levels of Balance Training

There are three levels of training within the National Academy of Sports Medicine's OPT™ model—stabilization, strength, and power (Figure 9-4). A proper balance-training program follows the same systematic progression.

Stabilization Level

In balance stabilization training, exercises involve little joint motion. They are designed to improve reflexive joint stabilization contractions to increase joint stability. This means that when the body is placed in unstable environments, it must react by contracting the right muscles at the right time to maintain balance. Example exercises in this level include:

- Single-leg balance
- Single-leg balance reach
- Single-leg hip internal and external rotation
- Single-leg lift and chop

Exercise Selection:
- Safe
- Progressive
  - Easy to hard
  - Simple to complex
  - Known to unknown
  - Stable to unstable
  - Static to dynamic
  - Slow to fast
  - Two arms/legs to single arm/leg
  - Stable to unstable
  - Eyes open to eyes closed
- Systematic
- Proprioceptively challenging
  1. Floor
  2. Balance beam
  3. Half foam roll
  4. Airex pad
  5. Dyna Disc

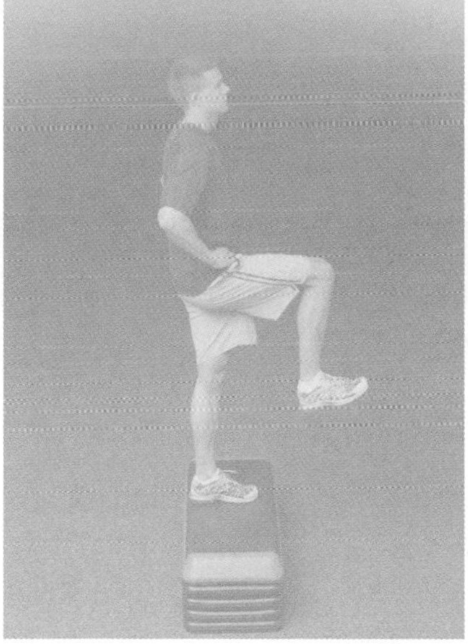

Variables
- Plane of motion
  - Sagittal
  - Frontal
  - Transverse
- Range of motion
  - Full
  - Partial
  - End-range
- Multisensory
  - Half foam roll
  - Airex pad
  - Dyna Disc
- Type of resistance
  - Body weight
  - Dumbbells
  - Tubing
  - Cable
- Body position
  - Two-leg/stable
  - Single-leg/stable
  - Two-legs/unstable
  - Single-leg/unstable
- Speed of motion
- Duration
- Frequency
- Amount of feedback

Figure 9.3 Program design parameters for balance training.

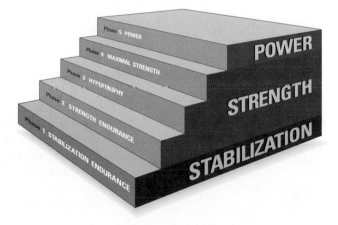

Figure 9.4 OPT™ model.

Single-Leg Balance

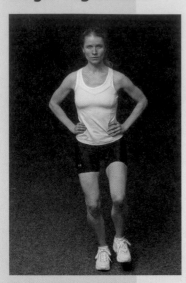

PREPARATION

1. Stand with feet shoulder-width apart and pointed straight ahead. Hips should be in a neutral position.
2. Lift chest, retract shoulders slightly, and tuck chin.

MOVEMENT

3. Draw navel in, activate glutes, and brace.
4. Lift one leg directly beside balance leg. Maintain optimal alignment, including level hips and shoulders.
5. Hold for 5 to 20 seconds.
6. Slowly return to original position.
7. Switch legs and repeat as instructed.

Technique   Make sure the gluteal musculature of the balance leg remains contracted while performing this and all balance exercises to help stabilize the lower extremity.

Single-Leg Balance Reach

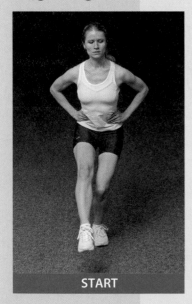

START

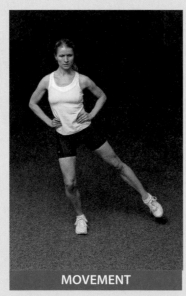

MOVEMENT

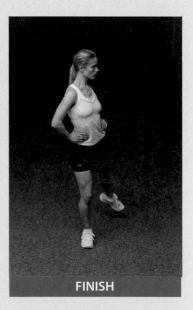

FINISH

PREPARATION

1. Stand with feet shoulder-width apart and pointed straight ahead. Hips should be in a neutral position.
2. Lift chest, retract shoulders slightly, and tuck chin.

MOVEMENT

3. Draw navel in and activate gluteals.
4. Lift one leg directly beside balance leg.
5. Move lifted leg to the front of the body. Hold for 2 seconds.
6. Slowly return to original position and repeat.
7. As a progression, reach the floating leg to the side of the body (frontal plane) and then reaching behind the body (transverse plane).

Keep the hips level when performing balance exercises. This will decrease stress to the lumbo-pelvic-hip complex.

Single-Leg Hip Internal and External Rotation

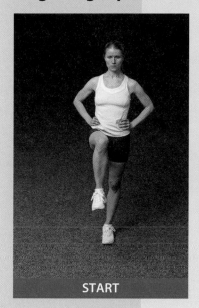
START

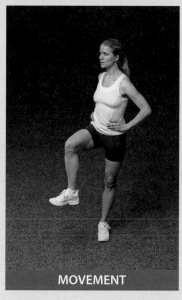
MOVEMENT

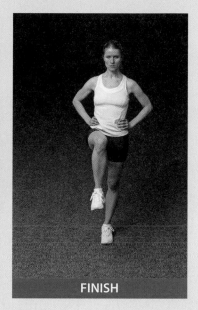
FINISH

PREPARATION

1. Stand with feet shoulder-width apart and pointed straight ahead. Hips should be in a neutral position.
2. Lift chest, retract shoulders slightly, and tuck chin.

MOVEMENT

3. Draw navel in and activate gluteals.
4. Lift one leg directly beside balance leg. Maintain optimal alignment, including level hips and shoulders.
5. Slowly internally and externally rotate hip of lifted leg, holding each end position for 2 seconds.
6. Slowly return to original position.
7. Switch legs and repeat as instructed.

Make sure when performing this exercise that one rotates through the hip of the balance leg versus the spine. This will decrease stress to the spine and enhance control of the lumbo-pelvic-hip complex.

Single-Leg Lift and Chop

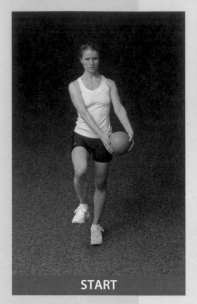
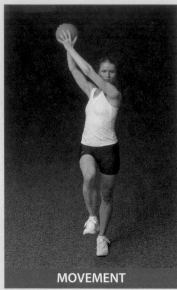
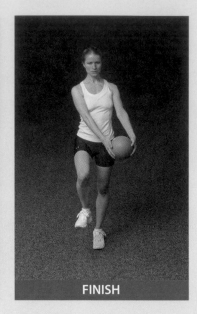

START

MOVEMENT

FINISH

PREPARATION

1. Stand with feet shoulder-width apart and pointed straight ahead. Hips should be in a neutral position.
2. Hold medicine ball in extended hands.
3. Lift chest, retract shoulders slightly, and tuck chin.

MOVEMENT

4. Draw navel in and activate gluteals.
5. Lift one leg directly beside balance leg.
6. Extend arms so that hands are at the outside of the balance leg.
7. Lift medicine ball in a diagonal pattern, rotating the body until medicine ball is overhead. Hold for 2 seconds.
8. Slowly return to original position and repeat.

Technique

When performing balance exercises, make sure the knee of the balance leg always stays in line with the toes.

Strength Level

In balance strength training, exercises involve more dynamic eccentric and concentric movement of the balance leg, through a full range of motion. Movements require dynamic control in mid-range of motion, with isometric stabilization at the end-range of motion. The specificity, speed, and neural demand are progressed in this level. These exercises are designed to improve the neuromuscular efficiency of the entire kinetic chain. Example exercises in this level include:

- Single-leg squat
- Single-leg squat touchdown
- Single-leg Romanian deadlift
- Step-up to balance
- Lunge to balance

Single-Leg Squat

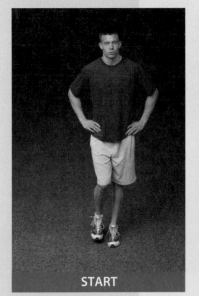

START

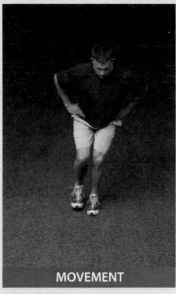

MOVEMENT

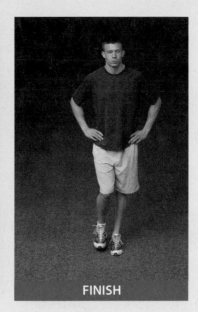

FINISH

PREPARATION

1. Stand with feet shoulder-width apart and pointed straight ahead. Hips should be in a neutral position.
2. Lift chest, retract shoulders slightly, tuck chin, and place hands on hips.

MOVEMENT

3. Draw navel in and activate gluteals.
4. Lift one leg directly beside balance leg and dorsiflex foot. Maintain optimal alignment, including level hips and shoulders.
5. Slowly squat as if sitting in a chair. Lower to first point of compensation. Hold for 2 seconds.
6. Slowly stand upright and contract gluteals.
7. Repeat as instructed.

Safety

As mentioned earlier, make sure the knee always stays in line with the toe and it does not move inside or outside the second and third toe. This will decrease stress to the knee.

Single-Leg Squat Touchdown

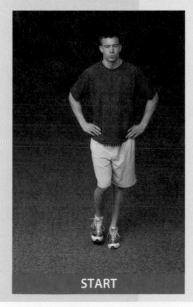

START

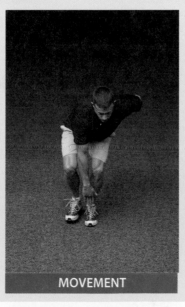

MOVEMENT

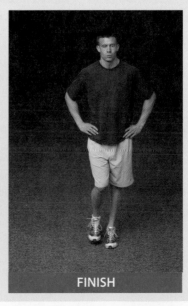

FINISH

PREPARATION

1. Stand with feet shoulder-width apart and pointed straight ahead. Hips should be in a neutral position.
2. Lift chest, retract shoulders slightly, tuck chin, and place hands on hips.

MOVEMENT

3. Draw navel in and activate gluteals.
4. Lift one leg directly beside balance leg.
5. Slowly squat as if sitting in a chair, reaching hand opposite of balance leg toward foot.
6. Slowly stand upright using abs and glutes.
7. Switch legs and repeat as instructed.

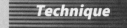

If individuals cannot touch their foot, have them first work on reaching to their knee, then to the shin, and then to the foot.

Single-Leg Romanian Deadlift

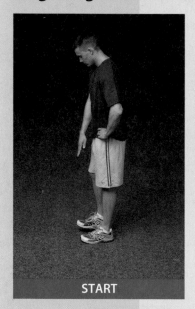

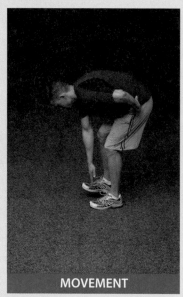

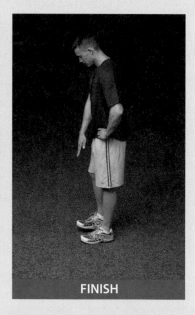

| START | MOVEMENT | FINISH |

PREPARATION

1. Stand with feet shoulder-width apart and pointed straight ahead. Hips should be in a neutral position.
2. Lift chest, retract shoulders slightly, tuck chin, and place hands on hips.

MOVEMENT

3. Draw navel in and activate gluteals.
4. Lift one leg directly beside balance leg.
5. Slowly reach hand down toward the toes of the balance leg.
6. Slowly stand upright using abs and gluteals.
7. Repeat as instructed.

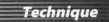

Technique

One can use the same progression with this exercise as that performed in the single-leg squat touchdown:

1. Reach to the knee
2. Reach to the shin
3. Reach to the foot

Step-Up to Balance

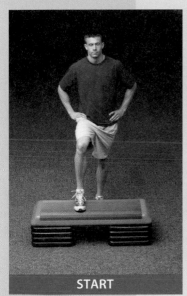

START

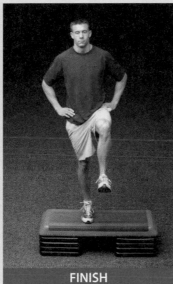

FINISH

PREPARATION

1. Stand in front of a box or platform with feet shoulder-width apart and pointed straight ahead. Hips should be in a neutral position.
2. Lift chest, retract shoulders slightly, and tuck chin.

MOVEMENT

3. Draw navel in and activate gluteals.
4. Step onto box with one leg, keeping toes pointed straight ahead and knee directly over the toes.
5. Push through front heel and stand upright, balancing on one leg.
6. Hold for 2 seconds.
7. Return lifted leg to the ground, keeping toes and knees aligned.
8. Repeat as instructed.
9. As a progression, use the same process and step up from the side (frontal plane) and turning (transverse plane).

Technique

Make sure at the end position that the balance leg is in full extension (knee extension and hip extension) for maximal recruitment of the gluteal musculature.

Lunge to Balance

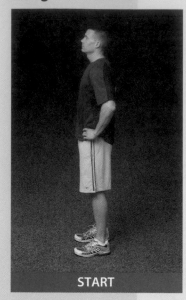

START

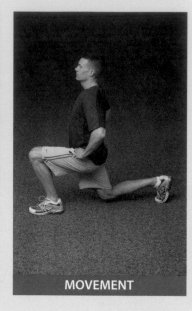

MOVEMENT

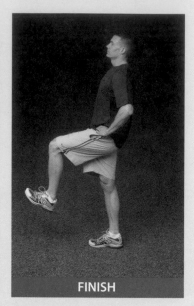

FINISH

PREPARATION

1. Stand with feet shoulder-width apart and pointed straight ahead. Hips should be in a neutral position.
2. Lift chest, retract shoulders slightly, tuck chin, and place hands on hips.

MOVEMENT

3. Draw navel in and activate gluteals.
4. Lunge forward with toes pointed straight ahead and knee directly over the toes.
5. Push off of front foot through heel onto back leg and maintain balance on the back leg.
6. Repeat as instructed.
7. As a progression, use the same process and lunge to the side (frontal plane) and turning (transverse plane).

Sefety When performing a lunge, make sure the stride length is not too large, particularly if one has tight hip flexors. This can force the spine into excessive extension, increasing stress to the low back.

Power Level

In balance power training, exercises are designed to develop high levels of eccentric strength, dynamic neuromuscular efficiency, and reactive joint stabilization. Exercises in this level include:

- Multiplanar hop with stabilization
- Box hop-up with stabilization
- Box hop-down with stabilization

Multiplanar Hop With Stabilization (Sagittal, Frontal, and Transverse)

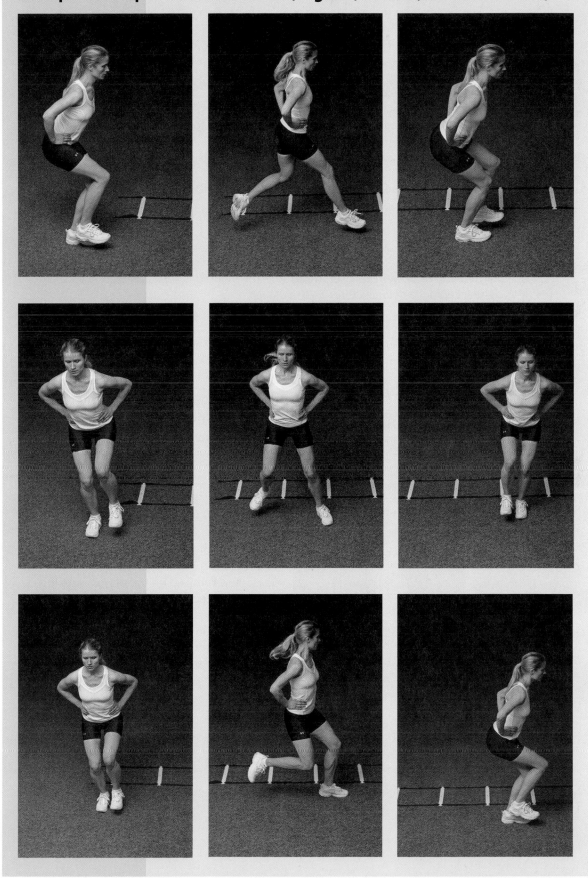

PREPARATION

1. Stand with feet shoulder-width apart and pointed straight ahead. Hips should be in a neutral position.
2. Lift chest, retract shoulders slightly, and tuck chin.

MOVEMENT

3. Draw navel in and activate gluteals.
4. Lift one leg directly beside balance leg.
5. Hop forward (sagittal plane), landing on opposite foot. Stabilize and hold for 3 to 5 seconds.
6. Hop backward (sagittal plane), landing on opposite foot in starting position. Stabilize and hold for 3 to 5 seconds.
7. As a progression, use the same process and hop side-to-side (frontal plane) and turning (transverse plane).

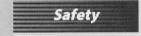

Safety   For all balance power exercises, make sure the landing is soft (quiet) to ensure efficient acceptance of forces through the tissues.

Single-Leg Box Hop-Up With Stabilization

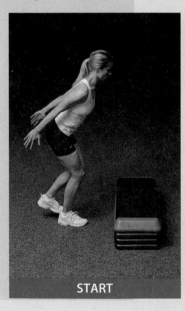

START

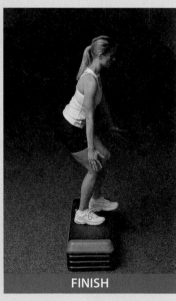

FINISH

PREPARATION

1. Stand in front of a box or platform with feet shoulder-width apart and pointed straight ahead. Hips should be in a neutral position.
2. Lift chest, retract shoulders slightly, and tuck chin.

MOVEMENT

3. Draw navel in and activate gluteals.
4. Lift one leg directly beside balance leg.
5. Hop up and land on top of box, keeping toes pointed straight ahead and knee directly over the toes.
6. Repeat as instructed.
7. As a progression, use the same format to hop in the frontal and transverse planes.

Single-Leg Box Hop-Down With Stabilization

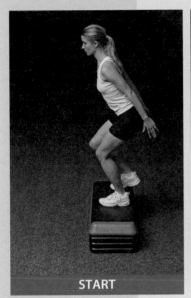

START

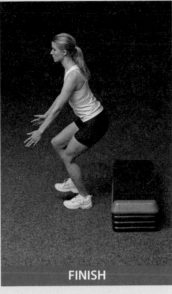

FINISH

PREPARATION

1. Stand on a box or platform with feet shoulder-width apart and pointed straight ahead. Hips should be in a neutral position.
2. Lift chest, retract shoulders slightly, and tuck chin.

MOVEMENT

3. Draw navel in and activate gluteals.
4. Lift one leg directly beside balance leg.
5. Hop off box and land on ground on one leg, keeping toes pointed straight ahead and knee directly over the toes.
6. Repeat as instructed.
7. As a progression, use the same format to hop in the frontal and transverse planes.

Technique   Once again, keep the knee in line with the toes when landing!

SUMMARY

A balance-training program is designed to ensure optimum neuromuscular efficiency of the entire kinetic chain. Balance-training programs must be systematic and progressive, following specific program guidelines, proper exercise selection criteria, and detailed program variables.

A proper balance-training program follows the same systematic progression as the OPT™ model—**stabilization, strength,** and **power** levels of training. Exercises in the **stabilization level** of balance training do not involve much joint motion. They improve joint stability. In the **strength level** of balance training, the balancing leg moves dynamically through a full range of motion, with exercises that require greater specificity, speed, and neural demand. These movements require isometric stabilization at the end-range of motion. They improve neuromuscular efficiency of the entire kinetic chain. Exercises in the **power level** of balance training improve high levels of eccentric strength, dynamic neuromuscular efficiency, and reactive joint stabilization.

Implementing a Balance-Training Program

BALANCE-TRAINING DESIGN PARAMETERS

Implementing a balance-training program requires that health and fitness professionals follow the progression of the OPT™ model. For example, if a client is in the **stabilization level** of training (phase 1), select **balance-stabilization exercises.** For a client in the **strength level** of training (phase 2, 3 or 4), the health and

Table 9.1

Balance Training Program Design

OPT™ Level	Phase(s)	Exercise	Number of Exercises	Sets	Reps	Tempo	Rest
Stabilization	1	Balance-stabilization exercises	1–4	1–3	12–20 (or single-leg, 6–10 each)	Slow (4/2/1)	0–90 s
Strength	2, 3, 4	Balance-strength exercises	0–4[a]	2–3	8–12	Medium (3/2/1–1/1/1)	0–60 s
Power	5	Balance-power exercises	0–2[b]	2–3	8–12	Controlled (hold the landing position for 3–5 s)	0–60 s

[a]For some goals in this level of training (hypertrophy and maximal strength), balance exercises may not be required. Although recommended, balance training is optional in these phases of training.

[b]Because balance exercises are performed in the dynamic flexibility portion of this program and the goal of the program is power, balance training may not be necessary in this phase of training. Although recommended, balance training is optional.

fitness professional should select **balance-strength exercises.** For an advanced client in the **power level** of training (phase 5), select **balance-power exercises** (Table 9-1).

FILLING IN THE TEMPLATE

To fill in the program template, go to the section labeled **Balance** in step 2 of the template (Figure 9-5). You will then refer to Table 9-1 for the appropriate type of balance exercise (**stabilization, strength,** or **power**), the appropriate number of balance exercises, and the appropriate acute variables specific to the phase of training your client will be working in (1–5).

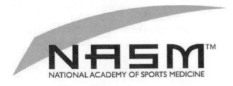

OPT For Fitness

Program Goal: Fat Loss

Name: John Smith	Month: 1
Date: 08/10/06	Week: 1
Professional Scott Lucett	Day: 1 of 12

STEP 1

A. Foam Roll

Foam Roll	Sets	Duration
Calves	1	30 sec.
IT Band	1	30 sec.
Adductors	1	30 sec.

B. Stretch

Static Stretching	Sets	Duration
Calves	1	30 sec.
Hip Flexors	1	30 sec.
Adductors	1	30 sec.

C. Cardiovascular

Treadmill	5-10 min.

STEP 2

A. Core

Exercise	Sets	Reps	Tempo	Rest
Floor Bridge	2	12	Slow	0
Floor Prone Cobra	2	12	Slow	0

B. Balance

Exercise	Sets	Reps	Tempo	Rest
Single-leg Balance	2	12	Slow	0

C. Reactive

Exercise	Sets	Reps	Tempo	Rest

Resistance Training Program

	Body Part Exercise		Sets	Reps	Intensity	Tempo	Rest
STEP 3	Total Body						
	Chest						
	Back						
	Shoulder						

Cool-Down

STEP 4	Repeat Steps 1A and 1B

Figure 9.5 OPT template.

Review Questions

1 *The integrated performance paradigm demonstrates that adequate force reduction and stabilization are required for optimum force production.*

    a. True

    b. False

2 *Joint dysfunction may lead to:*

    a. Synergistic dominance

    b. Muscle inhibition

    c. Decreased neuromuscular control

    d. All of the above

3 *What kind of exercises would you choose for a client in phase 3?*

    a. Balance-stabilization exercises

    b. Balance-strength exercises

    c. Balance-power exercises

4–7 *Match the exercises to either stabilization, strength, or power levels of training:*

    a. Stabilization

    b. Strength

    c. Power

4 *Single-leg balance*

5 *Multiplanar hop with stabilization*

6 *Single-leg squat*

7 *Lunge to balance*

REFERENCES

1. Tippet S, Voight M. Functional Progressions for Sports Rehabilitation. Champaign, IL: Human Kinetics, 1995.
2. Voight M, Cook G. Clinical application of closed kinetic chain exercise. J Sport Rehab 1996; 5(1):25–44.
3. Lephart SM. Re-establishing proprioception, kinesthesia, joint position sense, and neuromuscular control in rehabilitation. In: Prentice WE (ed). Rehabilitation Techniques in Sports, 2nd ed. St. Louis: Mosby, 1993.
4. Guskiewicz KM, Perrin DM. Research and clinical applications of assessing balance. J Sport Rehab 1996;5:45–63.
5. Balogun JA, Adesinasi CO, Marzouk DK. The effects of wobble board exercise training program on static balance performance and strength of the lower extremity muscles. Physiother Can 1992;44:23–30.
6. Barrack RL, Skinner HB. Proprioception in the ACL deficient knee. Am J Sports Med 1989;17:1–6.
7. Barret D. Proprioception and function after ACL reconstruction. J Bone Joint Surg 1991;73:833–837.
8. Blackburn TA. Rehabilitation of ACL injuries. Orthop Clin North Am 1985;16(2):241–269.

9. Freeman MAR, Wyke B. Articular reflexes at the ankle joint: an EMG study of normal and abnormal influences of ankle joint mechanoreceptors upon reflex activity in the leg muscles. Br J Surg 1967;54:990–1001.

10. Freeman MAR. Coordination exercises in the treatment of functional instability of the foot. Phys Ther 1964;44:393–395.

11. Hirokawa S, Solomonow M. Muscular co-contraction and control of knee stability. J Electromyogr Kinesiol 1991;1(3):199–208.

12. Ihara H, Nakayama A. Dynamic joint control training for knee ligament injuries. Am J Sports Med 1986;14:309–314.

13. Edgerton VR, Wolf S, Roy RR. Theoretical basis for patterning EMG amplitudes to assess muscle dysfunction. Med Sci Sports Exerc 1996;28(6):744–751.

14. Janda V. Muscle weakness and inhibition in back pain syndromes. In: Grieve GP (ed). Modern Manual Therapy of the Vertebral Column. New York: Churchill Livingstone, 1986.

15. Lewit K. Muscular and articular factors in movement restriction. Man Med 1985;1:83–85.

16. Janda V, Vavrova M. Sensory Motor Stimulation Video. Brisbane, Australia: Body Control Systems, 1990.

17. Hodges PW, Richardson CA. Neuromotor dysfunction of the trunk musculature in low back pain patients. In: Proceedings of the International Congress of the World Confederation of Physical Therapists. Washington, DC, 1995.

18. Hodges PW, Richardson CA. Inefficient muscular stabilization of the lumbar spine associated with low back pain. Spine 1996;21(22):2640–2650.

19. O'Sullivan PE, Twomey L, Allison G, Sinclair J, Miller K, Knox J. Altered patterns of abdominal muscle activation in patients with chronic low back pain. Aus J Physiother 1997;43(2):91–98.

20. Borsa PA, Lephart SM, Kocher MS, Lephart SP. Functional assessment and rehabilitation of shoulder proprioception for glenohumeral instability. J Sports Rehab 1994;3:84–104.

21. Janda V. Muscle Function Testing. London: Butterworth, 1983.

22. Janda V. Muscles, central nervous system regulation, and back problems. In: Korr IM (ed). Neurobiologic Mechanisms in Manipulative Therapy. New York: Plenum Press, 1978.

23. Liebenson C. Integrating rehabilitation into chiropractic practice (blending active and passive care). In: Liebenson C (ed). Rehabilitation of the Spine. Baltimore: Williams & Wilkins, 1996.

24. Sahrmann S. Diagnosis and treatment of muscle imbalances and musculoskeletal pain syndrome. Continuing Education Course. St. Louis, 1997.

25. Rowinski MJ. Afferent neurobiology of the joint. In: Gould JA (ed). Orthopedic and Sports Physical Therapy. St. Louis: Mosby, 1990.

26. Warmerdam ALA. Arthrokinetic therapy; manual therapy to improve muscle and joint function. Course manual. Marshfield, WI, 1996.

27. Fahrer H, Rentsch HU, Gerber NJ, Beyler C, Hess CW. Knee effusion and reflex inhibition of the quadriceps. A bar to effective retraining. J Bone Joint Surg 1988;70B:635–639.

28. Solomonow M, Barratta R, Zhou BH. The synergistic action of the ACL and thigh muscles in maintaining joint stability. Am J Sports Med 1987;15:207–213.

29. Bullock-Saxton JE, Janda V, Bullock M. Reflex activation of gluteal muscles in walking: an approach to restoration of muscle function for patients with low back pain. Spine 1993;18(6):704–708.

30. Janda V. Physical therapy of the cervical and thoracic spine. In: Grant R (ed). New York: Churchill Livingstone, 1988.

31. Jull G, Richardson CA, Comerford M. Strategies for the initial activation of dynamic lumbar stabilization. Proceedings of Manipulative Physiotherapists Association of Australia. New South Wales, 1991.

32. Jull G, Richardson CA, Hamilton C, Hodges PW, Ng J. Towards the validation of a clinical test for the deep abdominal muscles in back pain patients. Gold Coast, Queensland: Manipulative Physiotherapists Association of Australia, 1995.

Reactive (Power) Training Concepts

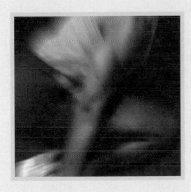

OBJECTIVES

After completing this chapter, you will be able to:

- Describe reactive training and its purpose.
- Rationalize the importance of reactive training.
- Design a reactive-training program for clients in any level of training.
- Perform, describe, and instruct various reactive-training exercises.

KEY TERMS

Rate of force production
Reactive training

Concepts in Reactive Training

The final component necessary in enhancing stability is reactive training. It is important to understand that an individual must possess proper core strength and have an ability to balance efficiently *before* performing reactive exercises. This chapter reviews the importance of reactive training and how to design and incorporate a reactive routine into your client's program regimen.

THE IMPORTANCE OF REACTIVE TRAINING

Enhanced performance during functional activities emphasizes the ability of muscles to exert maximal force output in a minimal amount of time (also known as *rate of force production*). Success in most functional activities depends on the speed at which muscular force is generated. Power and reactive neuromuscular control represents a component of function. It is perhaps the best measure of success in activities that require rapid force production.

Reactive training is defined as a quick, powerful movement involving an eccentric contraction, followed immediately by an explosive concentric contraction.[1] This is accomplished through the use of plyometric exercise and defines the stretch-shortening cycle of the integrated performance paradigm (Figure 10-1), which states that to move with precision, forces must be reduced (eccentrically), stabilized (isometrically), and then produced (concentrically). These exercises enhance the excitability, sensitivity, and reactivity of the neuromuscular system and increase the rate of force production (power), motor-unit recruitment, firing frequency (rate coding), and synchronization.

These training exercises are a progression that can be incorporated once a client has achieved proper core and balance stabilization capabilities. Ample isometric stabilization strength (developed through core and balance stabilization exercise) decreases the time between the eccentric contraction and concentric contraction, resulting in decreased tissue overload and potential injury when performing reactive training. Reactive exercises also use the stimulation of the body's proprioceptive mechanism and elastic properties to generate maximal force output in the minimal amount of time.

All movement patterns that occur during functional activities involve a series of repetitive stretch-shortening cycles (eccentric and concentric contractions). The neuromuscular system must react quickly and efficiently after an eccentric muscle action to produce a concentric contraction and impart the necessary force (or acceleration) in the appropriate direction. Muscles produce the necessary force to change the direction of an object's center of mass.[2] Therefore, specific functional exercises that emphasize a rapid change in direction must be used to prepare each client for the functional demands of a specific activity.

Reactive training provides the ability to train specific movement patterns in a biomechanically correct manner at a more functionally appropriate speed. This provides better functional strengthening of the muscle, tendon, and ligaments to meet the demands of everyday activities and sports. The ultimate goal of reactive training is to increase the reaction time of the muscle action spectrum (eccentric

Reactive training: Exercises that use quick, powerful movements involving an eccentric contraction immediately followed by an explosive concentric contraction.

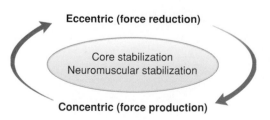

Figure 10.1 Integrated performance paradigm.

Eccentric (force reduction)

Core stabilization
Neuromuscular stabilization

Concentric (force production)

Integrated performance paradigm: To move with efficiency, forces must be reduced (eccentrically), stabilized (isometrically), and then produced (concentrically).

Rate of force production: Ability of muscles to exert maximal force output in a minimal amount of time.

deceleration, isometric stabilization, and concentric acceleration).[3] This is also known as **rate of force production**.

The speed of muscular exertion is limited by neuromuscular coordination. This means that the body will only move within a range of speed that the nervous system has been programmed to allow.[2] Reactive training improves neuromuscular efficiency and improves the range of speed set by the central nervous system. Optimum reactive performance of any activity depends on the speed at which muscular forces can be generated.

This is another component of program design that is often overlooked in traditional training programs. It is often perceived by many to be too dangerous, potentially increasing the risk of injury. However, reactive training has a systematic progression sequence that allows a client to begin with less demanding exercises and progress to more demanding exercises as he or she adapts. This is no different than any other form of training. If too-advanced exercises are assigned to a client, he or she will not have the ability to perform them correctly and will compensate. This leads to synergistic dominance and faulty movement patterns. When placed within the proper programming scheme with proper progression, reactive training can be a vital component to achieving optimal performance of any activity at any level of ability.

For example, a 60-year-old woman and a 25-year-old male professional athlete may not both need to train for maximal strength. However, they both need stabilization, strength, and endurance as well as the ability to produce force quickly to

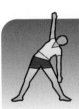

Stretch Your Knowledge

Evidence to Support the Use of Reactive Training for Injury Prevention and Performance Enhancement

- Chimera et al. (2004) in a pretest and posttest control group design with 20 healthy Division I female athletes found that a 6-week plyometric training program improved hip abductor and adductor coactivation ratios to help control varus and valgus moments at the knee during landing.[1]

- Wilkerson et al. (2004) in a quasi-experimental design with 19 female basketball players demonstrated that a 6-week plyometric training program improved hamstring to quadriceps ratio, which has been shown to enhance dynamic knee stability during the eccentric deceleration phase of landing.[2]

- Luebbers et al. (2003) in a randomized controlled trial with 19 subjects demonstrated that a 4-week and 7-week plyometric training program enhanced anaerobic power and vertical jump height.[3]

- Hewett et al. (1996) in a prospective study demonstrated decreased peak landing forces, enhanced muscle-balance ratio between the quadriceps and hamstrings, and decreased rate of anterior cruciate ligament injuries in female soccer, basketball, and volleyball players that incorporated reactive neuromuscular training into their program.[4]

1. Chimera NJ, Swanik KA, et al. Effects of plyometric training on muscle-activation strategies and performance in female athletes. J Athl Train 2004;39(1):24–31.
2. Wilkerson GB, Colston MA, et al. Neuromuscular changes in female collegiate athletes resulting from a plyometric jump training program. J Athl Train 2004;39(1):17–23.
3. Luebbers PE, Potteiger JA, Hulver MW, Thyfault JP, Carper MJ, Lockwood RH. Effects of plyometric training and recovery on vertical jump performance and anaerobic power. J Strength Cond Res 2003;17(4):704–709.
4. Hewett TE, Stroupe AL, Nance TA, Noyes FR. Plyometric training in female athletes. Decreased impact forces and increased hamstring torques. Am J Sports Med 1996;24(6):765–773.

perform daily activities efficiently. Therefore, the ability to react and produce sufficient force to avoid a fall or an opponent is paramount. The specificity of training concept dictates that both clients are trained in a more velocity-specific environment.[4] The speed of the repetition or movement is at a faster tempo, similar to movements seen in daily activities.

SUMMARY

The ability to react and generate force quickly is crucial to overall function and safety during movement. Reactive training is defined as a quick, powerful movement involving an eccentric contraction, followed immediately by an explosive concentric contraction. Reactive training can enhance one's ability to dynamically stabilize, reduce, and produce forces at speeds that are functionally applicable to the tasks at hand.

The nervous system only recruits muscles at speeds at which it has been trained. If it is not trained to recruit muscles quickly, when met with a demand for fast reaction, the nervous system will not be able to respond appropriately. The ultimate goal of reactive training is to increase the reaction time of muscle action spectrum (or rate of force production).

It is important to note, however, that reactive training should only be incorporated into an individual's exercise program once they have obtained proper flexibility, core strength, and balance capabilities. This reiterates the importance of using a progressive and systematic approach when designing the reactive component of your client's training regimen.

Designing a Reactive-Training Program

REACTIVE-TRAINING DESIGN PARAMETERS

A reactive-training program is a vital component of any integrated training program. The program must be systematic and progressive. A client must exhibit proper levels of core strength and balance before progressing into reactive training. Health and fitness professionals must follow specific program guidelines, proper exercise selection criteria, and detailed program variables (Figure 10-2).

LEVELS OF REACTIVE TRAINING

There are three levels of training within NASM's OPT™ model—stabilization, strength, and power (Figure 10-3).

Stabilization

In reactive-stabilization training, exercises involve little joint motion. They are designed to establish optimum landing mechanics, postural alignment, and reactive neuromuscular efficiency. When an individual lands during these exercises, he or she should hold the landing position (or stabilize) for 3 to 5 seconds before repeating. Exercises in this level include:

- Squat jump with stabilization
- Box jump-up with stabilization
- Box jump-down with stabilization
- Multiplanar jump with stabilization

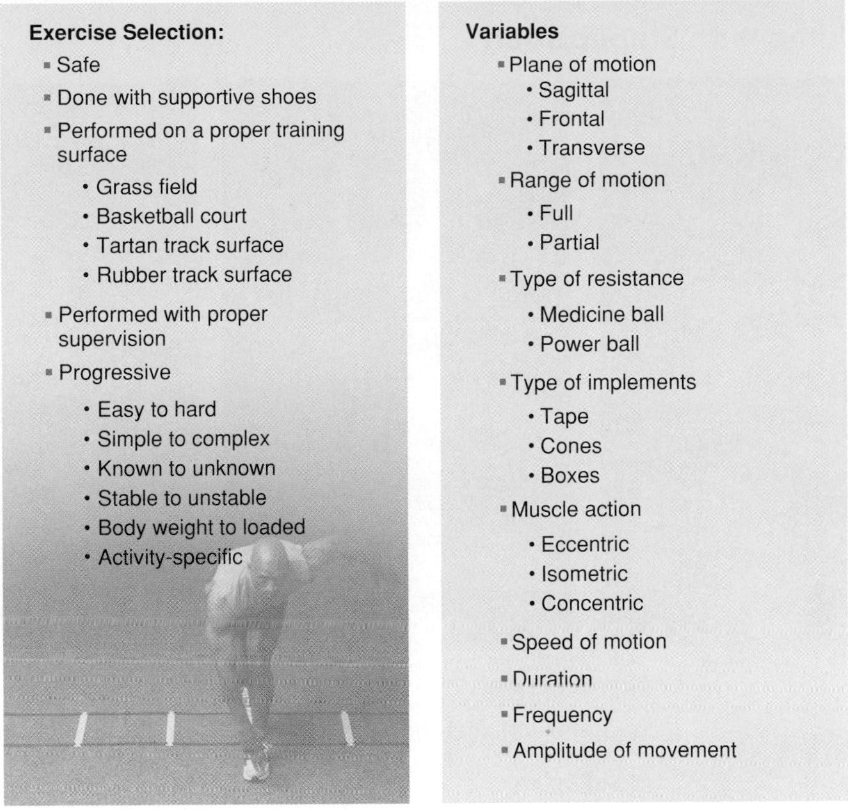

Exercise Selection:
Safe
Done with supportive shoes
Performed on a proper training surface
Grass field
Basketball court
Tartan track surface
Rubber track surface
Performed with proper supervision
Progressive
Easy to hard
Simple to complex
Known to unknown
Stable to unstable
Body weight to loaded
Activity-specific
Variables
Plane of motion
Sagittal
Frontal
Transverse
Range of motion
Full
Partial
Type of resistance
Medicine ball
Power ball
Type of implements
Tape
Cones
Boxes
Muscle action
Eccentric
Isometric
Concentric
Speed of motion
Duration
Frequency
Amplitude of movement

Figure 10.2 Program design parameters for reactive training.

Phase 5 POWER
Phase 4 MAXIMAL STRENGTH
Phase 3 HYPERTROPHY
Phase 2 STRENGTH ENDURANCE
Phase 1 STABILIZATION ENDURANCE
POWER
STRENGTH
STABILIZATION

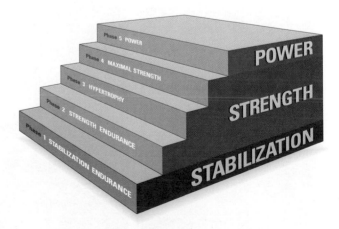

Figure 10.3 OPT™ model.

Squat Jump With Stabilization

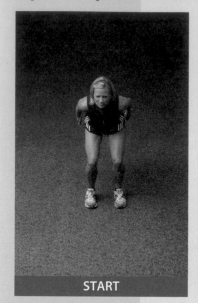

START

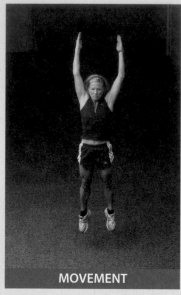

MOVEMENT

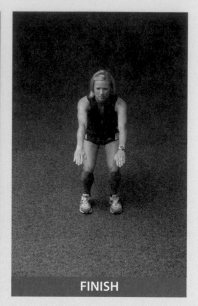

FINISH

PREPARATION

1. Stand with feet shoulder-width apart and pointed straight ahead.

MOVEMENT

2. Draw navel in and activate gluteals.
3. Jump up, extending arms overhead.
4. Land softly, maintaining optimal alignment and returning arms to sides. Stabilize and hold for 3 to 5 seconds.
5. Repeat as instructed.

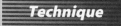 *Technique* Make sure the knees always stay in line with the toes, both before jumping and on the landing.

Box Jump-Up With Stabilization

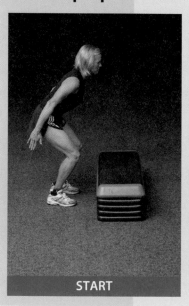

START

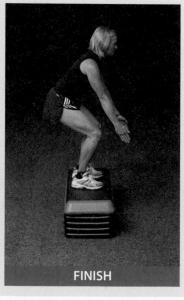

FINISH

PREPARATION

1. Stand in front of a box or platform with feet shoulder-width apart and pointed straight ahead.

MOVEMENT

2. Draw navel in and activate gluteals.
3. Using arms, jump up and land on top of box, keeping toes pointed straight ahead and knees directly over the toes. Hold for 3 to 5 seconds.
4. Step off box and repeat as instructed.
5. As a progression, perform in the frontal and transverse planes.

Adjust the height of the box to be consistent with the physical capabilities of the individual performing the exercise.

Box Jump-Down With Stabilization

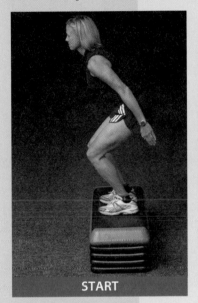

START

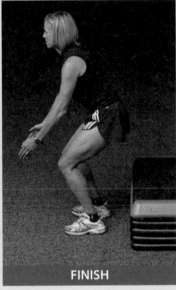

FINISH

PREPARATION

1. Stand on a box or platform with feet shoulder-width apart and pointed straight ahead.

MOVEMENT

2. Draw navel in and activate gluteals.
3. Using arms, jump off the box and land on floor, keeping toes pointed straight ahead and knees directly over the toes. Hold for 3 to 5 seconds.
4. Step onto box and repeat as instructed.
5. As a progression, perform in the frontal and transverse planes.

Make sure one lands softly and quietly on the ground to ensure proper force transmission through the tissues.

Horizontal Jump With Stabilization

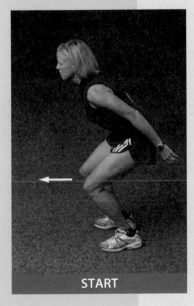

START

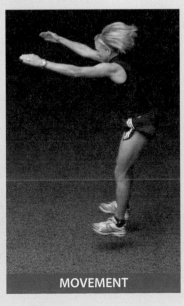

MOVEMENT

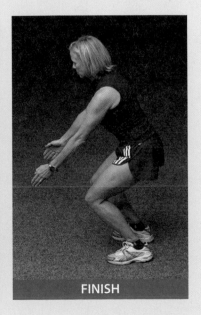

FINISH

PREPARATION

1. Stand with feet shoulder-width apart and pointed straight ahead.

MOVEMENT

2. Draw navel in and activate gluteals.
3. Jump forward (long jump) as far as can be controlled.
4. Land softly, maintaining optimal alignment and hold for 3 to 5 seconds.
5. Repeat as instructed.
6. As a progression, perform in the frontal (jump to the side) and the transverse (turning) planes.

Strength Level

In reactive-strength training, exercises involve more dynamic eccentric and concentric movement through a full range of motion. The specificity, speed, and neural demand are also progressed in this level. These exercises are designed to improve dynamic joint stabilization, eccentric strength, rate of force production, and neuromuscular efficiency of the entire kinetic chain. These exercises are performed in a more repetitive fashion (spending a short amount of time on the ground). Exercises in this level include:

- Squat jump
- Tuck jump
- Butt kick
- Power step-up

Squat Jump

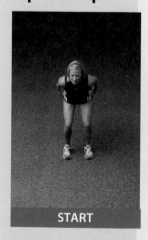
START

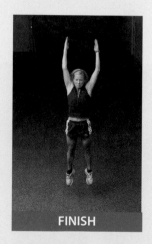
FINISH

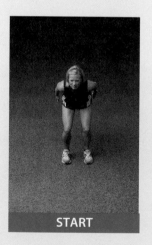
START

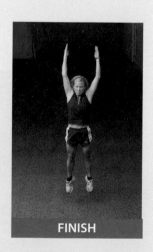
FINISH

PREPARATION

1. Stand with feet shoulder-width apart and pointed straight ahead.

MOVEMENT

2. Draw navel in and activate gluteals.
3. Jump up, extending arms overhead.
4. Land softly, maintaining optimal alignment and immediately repeat.

Technique Make sure to sit the hips back before jumping and upon landing. This will ensure optimal joint mechanics and muscle recruitment.

Tuck Jump

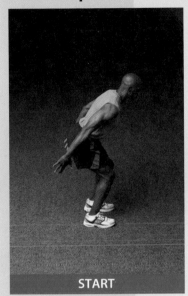

START

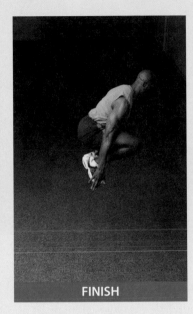

FINISH

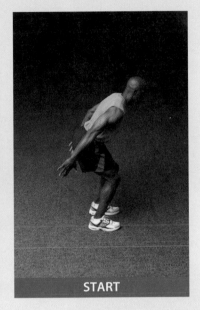

START

FINISH

PREPARATION

1. Stand with feet shoulder-width apart and pointed straight ahead.

MOVEMENT

2. Draw navel in and activate gluteals.
3. Jump up, bringing knees to chest.
4. Land softly, maintaining optimal alignment and immediately repeat.

Safety Now that the exercises are becoming more dynamic, proper alignment will be important to maximize force production.

Butt Kick

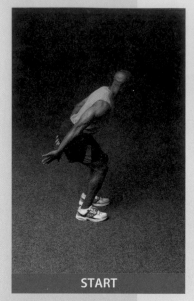

START

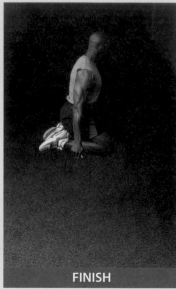

FINISH

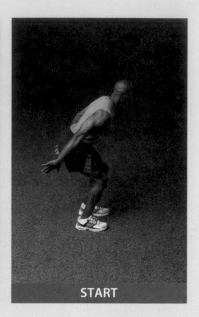

START

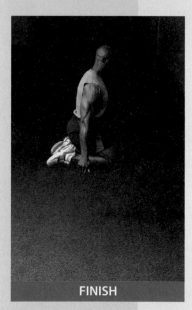

FINISH

PREPARATION

1. Stand with feet shoulder-width apart and pointed straight ahead.

MOVEMENT

2. Draw navel in and activate gluteals.
3. Jump up, bringing heels to glutes and avoiding arching of the lower back.
4. Land softly, maintaining optimal alignment and immediately repeat.

Safety   It is important that one has ample amounts of flexibility of the rectus femoris to ensure proper execution (avoid excessive lumbar extension).

Power Step-Up

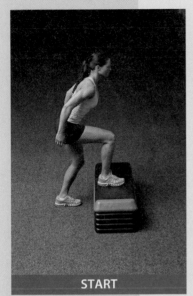

START

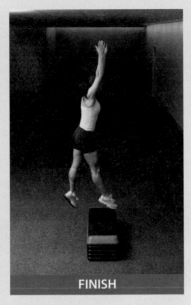

FINISH

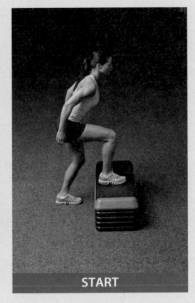

START

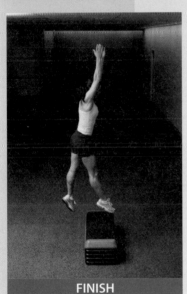

FINISH

PREPARATION

1. Stand in front of a box or platform with feet shoulder-width apart and pointed straight ahead.

MOVEMENT

2. Draw navel in and activate gluteals.
3. Place one foot on top of box.
4. Forcefully push off leg on top of box, putting leg into full extension.
5. Switch legs, keeping weight on the front leg and maintaining optimal alignment.
6. Repeat as instructed.

Technique   Make sure the knees always stay in line with the toes, both before jumping and on landing.

Power Level

In the power level of reactive training, exercises involve the entire muscle action spectrum and contraction-velocity spectrum used during integrated, functional movements. These exercises are designed to improve the rate of force production, eccentric strength, reactive strength, reactive joint stabilization, dynamic neuro-muscular efficiency, and optimum force production.[2,3] These exercises are performed as fast and as explosively as possible. Exercises in this level include:

- Ice skater
- Single-leg power step-up
- Proprioceptive plyometrics: cones and hurdles

Ice Skater

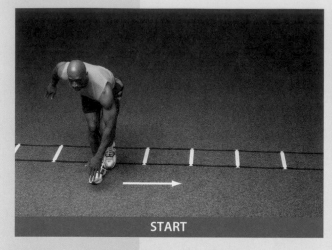

START

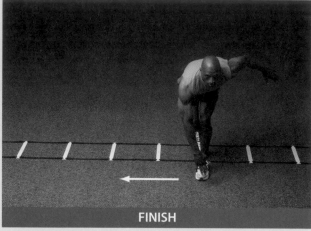

FINISH

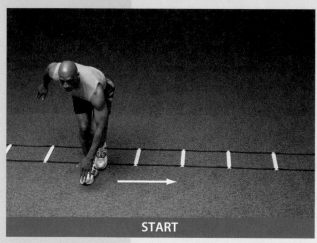

START

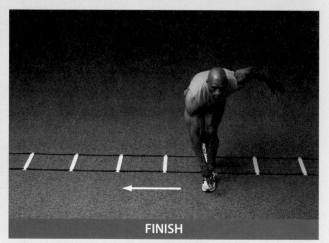

FINISH

PREPARATION

1. Stand with feet shoulder-width apart and pointed straight ahead.

MOVEMENT

2. Draw navel in and activate gluteals.
3. Quickly hop from side to side, switching legs and maintaining optimum alignment.
4. Repeat as instructed, as quickly as can be controlled.

Technique

One can start by hopping side-to-side from one foot to the other as fast as possible and then progress by adding a reach to make it more integrated.

Single-Leg Power Step-Up

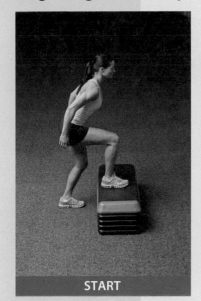

START

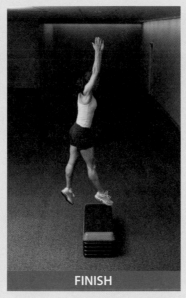

FINISH

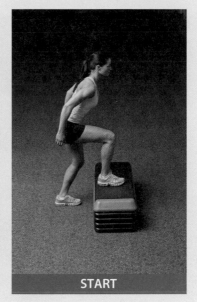

START

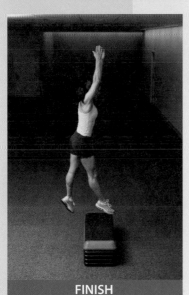

FINISH

PREPARATION

1. Stand in front of a box or platform with feet shoulder-width apart and pointed straight ahead.

MOVEMENT

2. Draw navel in and activate gluteals.
3. Place one foot on top of box.
4. Forcefully push off leg on top of box, putting leg into full extension.
5. Land on same leg, keeping weight on the upper leg and maintaining optimal alignment.
6. Repeat as instructed, as quickly as can be controlled.

Technique   One can progress this exercise by performing it in the frontal and transverse planes as well.

Proprioceptive Plyometrics

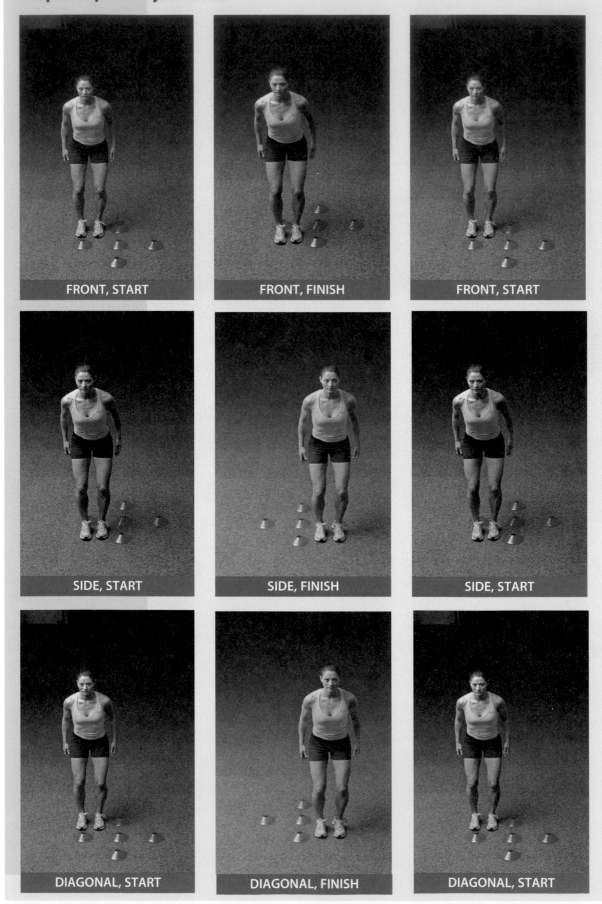

FRONT, START

FRONT, FINISH

FRONT, START

SIDE, START

SIDE, FINISH

SIDE, START

DIAGONAL, START

DIAGONAL, FINISH

DIAGONAL, START

PREPARATION

1. Stand with feet shoulder-width apart and pointed straight ahead.

MOVEMENT

2. Draw navel in and activate gluteals.
3. Jump (two legs) or hop (one leg) front-to-back, side-to-side, or in a diagonal pattern over cones, hurdles, or other implements.
4. Land softly, maintaining optimal alignment.
5. Repeat as instructed, as quickly as can be controlled.

Technique

If cones or hurdles are not available, you can also place tape on the floor in the form of an X and perform the exercises by jumping in different quadrants.

SUMMARY

A reactive-training program is designed to enhance neuromuscular efficiency, increase rate of force production, and improve functional eccentric strength. The program must:

- Be systematic.
- Be progressive.
- Follow specific program guidelines.
- Follow proper exercise selection criteria.
- Incorporate proper program variables.

A client must exhibit proper levels of core strength and balance before progressing into reactive training.

A proper reactive-training program follows the same systematic progression as the OPT™ model: stabilization, strength, and power levels of training. Exercises in the stabilization level of reactive training do not involve much joint motion. They improve landing mechanics, postural alignment, and reactive neuromuscular efficiency. In the strength level of reactive training, exercises involve more movement through a full range of motion, requiring greater specificity, speed, and neural demand. These movements improve dynamic joint stabilization, the rate of force production, and eccentric neuromuscular efficiency. Exercises in the power level of reactive training are performed as fast and explosively as possible. They improve rate of force production, reactive strength, dynamic neuromuscular efficiency, and optimum force production.

Designing a Reactive-Training Program

REACTIVE-TRAINING DESIGN PARAMETERS

Implementing a reactive training program requires that health and fitness professionals follow the progression of the OPT™ model. For example, if a client is in the stabilization level of training (phase 1), select reactive-stabilization exercises. For a client in the strength level of training (phases 2, 3, and 4), a health and fitness professional should select reactive-strength exercises. For an advanced client in the power level (phase 5), select reactive-power exercises. At this level, however, it may not be necessary to include reactive exercise into the routine as reactive-power exercises will be included in the resistance-training portion of the program.

FILLING IN THE TEMPLATE

To fill in the program template (Figure 10-4), go to the section labeled **Reactive** (step 2). You will then refer to Table 10-1 for the appropriate type of reactive exercise (stabilization, strength, or power), the appropriate number of reactive exercises, and the appropriate acute variables specific to the phase of training your client will be working in (phase 1–5).

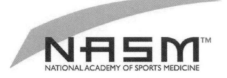

OPT For Fitness

NATIONAL ACADEMY OF SPORTS MEDICINE

Program Goal: Fat Loss

Name: John Smith	Month: 1
Date : 08/10/06	Week: 1
Professional Scott Lucett	Day: 1 of 12

STEP 1

A. Foam Roll

Foam Roll	Sets	Duration
Calves	1	30 sec.
IT Band	1	30 sec.
Adductors	1	30 sec.

B. Stretch

Static Stretching	Sets	Duration
Calves	1	30 sec.
Hip Flexors	1	30 sec.
Adductors	1	30 sec.

C. Cardiovascular

Treadmill	5-10 min.

STEP 2

A. Core

Exercise	Sets	Reps	Tempo	Rest
Floor Bridge	2	12	Slow	0
Floor Prone Cobra	2	12	Slow	0

B. Balance

Exercise	Sets	Reps	Tempo	Rest
Single-leg Balance	2	12	Slow	0

C. Reactive

Exercise	Sets	Reps	Tempo	Rest
Squat Jump w/ Stabilization	2	5	Controlled	90 sec.

STEP 3

Resistance Training Program

Body Part Exercise		Sets	Reps	Intensity	Tempo	Rest
Total Body						
Chest						
Back						
Shoulder						

STEP 4

Cool-Down

Repeat Steps 1A and 1B

Figure 10.4   OPT template.

REACTIVE (POWER) TRAINING CONCEPTS

Table 10.1

Reactive-Training Program Design

OPT™ Level	Phase(s)	Exercise	Number of Exercises	Sets	Reps	Tempo	Rest
Stabilization	1	Reactive-stabilization exercises	0–2[a]	1–3	5–8	Controlled (hold stabilization position for 3–5 seconds)	0–90 s
Strength	2 3 4	Reactive-strength exercises	0–4[b]	2–3	8–10	Medium (repeating)	0–60 s
Power	5	Reactive-power exercises	0–2[c]	2–3	8–12	As fast as possible	0–60 s

[a]Reactive exercises may not be appropriate for an individual in this phase of training if they do not possess the appropriate amount of core strength and balance capabilities.
[b]Because of the goal of certain phases in this level (hypertrophy and maximal strength), reactive training may not be necessary to do.
[c]Because one is performing reactive-power exercises in the resistance training portion of this phase of training, separate reactive exercises may not be necessary to perform.

Review Questions

1 *What kind of reactive exercise would you choose for a client in phase 2 of the OPT model?*

   a. Stabilization

   b. Strength

   c. Power

2 *Reactive training aims to generate <u>minimal/maximal</u> force output in a <u>minimal/maximal</u> amount of time.*

3–6 *Match the exercises to either stabilization, strength, or power levels of training:*

   a. Stabilization

   b. Strength

   c. Power

3 *Ice skater*

4 *Box jump-up with stabilization*

5 *Proprioceptive plyometrics*

6 *Power step-ups*

7 *Circle which safety guideline(s) must be taken into consideration when designing a reactive-training program?*

a. *Progressive*

b. *Performed alone*

c. *Performed on extremely hard surfaces*

d. *Performed with supportive shoes*

e. *Start in unstable environments*

REFERENCES

1. Wilk KE, Voight M. Plyometrics for the overhead athlete. In: Andrews JR, Wilk KE (eds). The Athletic Shoulder. New York: Churchill Livingstone, 1993.
2. Voight M, Draovitch P. Plyometrics. In: Albert M (ed). Eccentric Muscle Training in Sports and Orthopedics. New York: Churchill Livingstone, 1991.
3. Voight M, Brady D. Plyometrics. In: Devies GL (ed). A Compendium of Isokinetics in Clinical Usage, 4th ed. Onalaska: S&S Publishers, 1992.
4. Allman FL. Sports Medicine. New York: Academic Press, 1974.

Speed, Agility, and Quickness

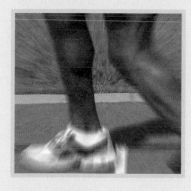

OBJECTIVES

After completing this chapter, you will be able to:

- Describe speed, agility, and quickness training and its purpose.
- Rationalize the importance of speed, agility, and quickness training.
- Design a speed, agility, and quickness training program for clients at any level of training.
- Perform, describe, and instruct various speed, agility, and quickness training exercises.

KEY TERMS

Agility	Quickness	Speed

Concepts in Speed, Agility, and Quickness (SAQ) Training

The programming component of speed, agility, and quickness (SAQ) training is similar to reactive training and follows the same concepts of the integrated performance paradigm. *Speed* in this text essentially refers to straight-ahead speed. *Agility* refers to short bursts of movement that involve change of direction. *Quickness* refers to the ability to react to a stimulus and change the motion of the body.

This form of training is often viewed as being beneficial only for the athlete. However, by using the proper progression as seen in the OPT™ model, the health and fitness professional can effectively use SAQ training to add intensity and complexity, increase the cardiorespiratory demand, and provide a simple and exciting variety to a routine workout.

SAQ training allows a client to enhance his or her ability to accelerate, decelerate, and dynamically stabilize the entire body during higher-velocity acceleration and deceleration movements in all planes of motion (such as running, cutting, and changing direction). It may further help the nervous system to respond or react more efficiently to demands placed on it and enhance muscular recruitment and coordination when performed with correct mechanics.[1]

SPEED

Speed: The ability to move the body in one intended direction as fast as possible.

Speed is the ability to move the body in one intended direction as fast as possible. It is the product of stride rate and stride length.[2,3] *Stride rate* is the number of strides taken in a given amount of time (or distance). It may be improved with proper core strength, reactive training, and technique. *Stride length* is the distance covered in one stride, during running. Research has found that optimum stride length at maximum velocity has a high correlation to leg length. It is approximately 2.1 to 2.5 times leg length.[1,3,4] Speed is an ability that can be learned and trained for by following an integrated training program seen in the OPT™ model.[5]

Proper Sprint Mechanics

Proper running mechanics allow the client to maximize forces generated by muscles, so that maximum velocity can be achieved in the shortest possible time.

This includes frontside and backside mechanics. *Frontside mechanics* is the emphasis on triple flexion of the front leg. Triple flexion includes the actions of:

- Ankle dorsiflexion
- Knee flexion
- Hip flexion
- Keeping the lumbar spine neutral

Backside mechanics is the emphasis on triple extension of the back leg. Triple extension includes the actions of:

- Ankle plantarflexion
- Knee extension
- Hip extension
- Keeping the lumbar spine neutral

AGILITY

Agility: The ability to accelerate, decelerate, stabilize, and change direction quickly, while maintaining proper posture.

Agility is the ability to start (or accelerate), stop (or decelerate and stabilize), and change direction quickly, while maintaining proper posture.[6] This requires high

Table 11.1

Kinetic Chain Checkpoints During Running Movements

Body Position	Comments
Foot/ankle complex	The foot and ankle should be pointing straight ahead in a dorsiflexed position when it hits the ground. Excessive flattening or external rotation of the foot will create abnormal stress throughout the rest of the kinetic chain and decrease overall performance.
Knee complex	The knees must remain straight ahead. If the athlete demonstrates excessive adduction and internal rotation of the femur during the stance phase, it decreases force production and leads to overuse injuries.
Lumbo-pelvic-hip complex (L-P-H-C)	The body should have a slight lean during acceleration. During maximum velocity, the L-P-H-C should be fairly neutral, without excessive extension or flexion, unless to reach for an object.
Head	The head should remain in line with the L-P-H-C, and the L-P-H-C should be in line with the legs. The head and neck should not compensate and move into extension, unless necessary to track an object (such as a ball), as this can affect the position of the L-P-H-C (pelvo-ocular reflex).

levels of neuromuscular efficiency because the client is constantly regaining a center of gravity over his or her base of support, while changing directions, at various speeds.

Agility training can enhance eccentric neuromuscular control, dynamic flexibility, dynamic postural control, functional core strength, and proprioception. Proper agility training can also help to prevent injury by enhancing the body's ability to effectively control eccentric forces in all planes of motion as well as by improving the structural integrity of the connective tissue. Proper technique for agility drills should follow the guidelines seen in Table 11-1.

QUICKNESS

Quickness: The ability to react and change body position with maximum rate of force production, in all planes of motion, from all body positions, during functional activities.

Quickness (or reaction time) is the ability to react and change body position with maximum rate of force production, in all planes of motion and from all body positions, during functional activities. Quickness involves the ability to react to visual, auditory, and kinesthetic feedback during functional activities with minimal hesitation. Proper technique for quickness drills should follow the guidelines seen in Table 11-1.

SUMMARY

Similar to reactive training, the programming component of speed, agility, and quickness training follows the same concepts of the integrated performance paradigm. It can add intensity, complexity, cardiorespiratory demand, and variety to a routine workout for regular clients as well as athletes. It enhances proprioceptive acceleration, deceleration, and dynamic stabilization of the entire body during higher-velocity movements.

Speed is the ability to move the body in one intended direction as fast as possible. It is the product of stride rate and stride length. It can be learned and trained for. Proper running mechanics (including frontside and backside mechanics) allow an athlete to maximize forces generated by muscles so that maximum velocity can be achieved in the shortest possible time.

Table 11.2

SAQ Program Design

OPT™ Level	Phase(s)	SAQ Exercise	Sets	Reps	Rest
Stabilization	1	4–6 speed ladder drills 1–2 cone drills	1–2 1–2	Half ladder[a]	0–60 s 0–90 s
Strength	2 3 4	6–9 speed ladder drills 1–2 cone drills	3–4 2–3	Half ladder[a]	0–60 s 0–90 s
Power	5	6–9 speed ladder drills 2–4 cone drills	3–6 3–6	Half ladder[a]	0–60 s 0–90 s

[a]Most speed ladders come in two sections that snap together. Half of a speed ladder consists of using only one section.

Agility refers to short bursts of movement that involve change of direction. It is the ability to start, stop, and change direction quickly, while maintaining proper posture. High levels of neuromuscular efficiency are required. It can help to prevent injury by enhancing control of eccentric forces in all planes of motion.

Quickness is the ability to react to a stimulus and change the motion of the body, with maximum rate of force production, in all planes of motion and from all body positions, during functional activities. Reactions are based on visual, auditory, and kinesthetic feedback and require minimal hesitation.

SAQ Drills and Programming Strategies

It must be stressed that the programming guidelines presented in Table 11-2 are only suggestions and should be gauged on the total volume of training for all components (core, balance, reactive, and resistance) in a workout. The success of a SAQ program is also dependent on the client's core, balance, and reactive capabilities. The higher these capabilities, the better and safer results a client will enjoy from his or her program. All exercises should be performed with precise technique and kinetic chain control to minimize risk of injury.

SAQ Speed Ladder Drills
One-Ins

Two-Ins

Side Shuffle

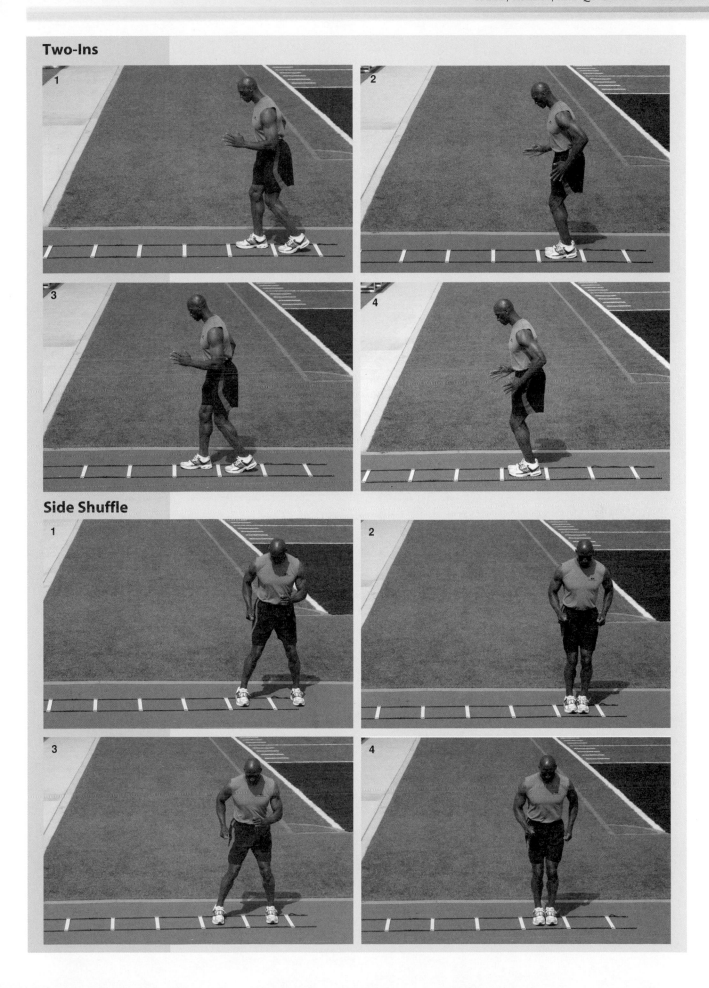

In-In-Out-Out

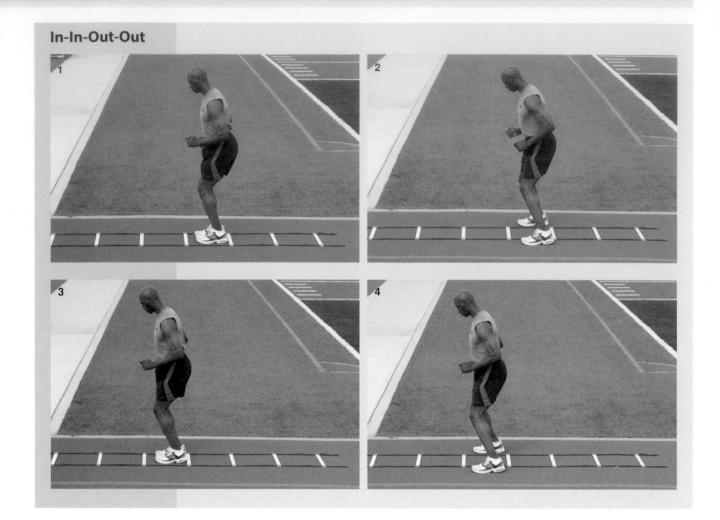

In-In-Out (Zigzag)

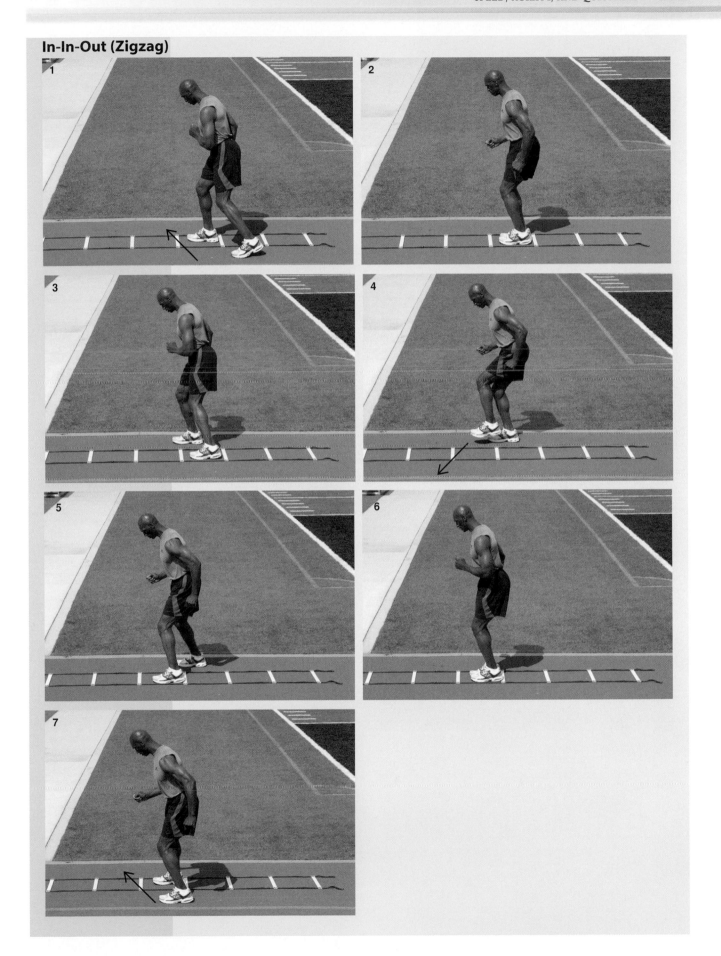

Ali Shuffle

SAQ Cone Drills

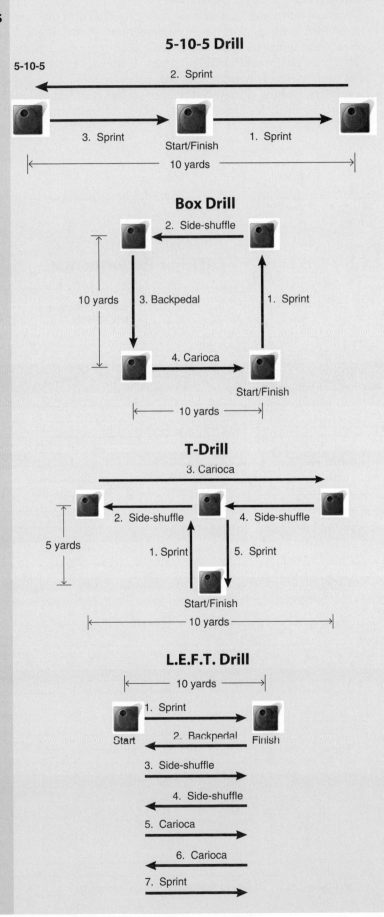

5-10-5 Drill

5-10-5

2. Sprint

3. Sprint

Start/Finish

1. Sprint

10 yards

Box Drill

2. Side-shuffle

10 yards

3. Backpedal

1. Sprint

4. Carioca

Start/Finish

10 yards

T-Drill

3. Carioca

2. Side-shuffle

4. Side-shuffle

5 yards

1. Sprint

5. Sprint

Start/Finish

10 yards

L.E.F.T. Drill

10 yards

1. Sprint

2. Backpedal

Start

Finish

3. Side-shuffle

4. Side-shuffle

5. Carioca

6. Carioca

7. Sprint

FILLING IN THE TEMPLATE

Program templates that include speed, agility, and quickness are typically reserved for those with performance enhancement goals. Figure 11-1 shows how a performance template would look and where speed, agility, and quickness training would be performed in the program. If speed, agility, and quickness training are to be used in the program, you will refer to Table 11-2 for the appropriate type of exercises (ladder or cones), the appropriate number of exercises, and the appropriate acute variables specific to the phase of training your client will be working in (phases 1–5).

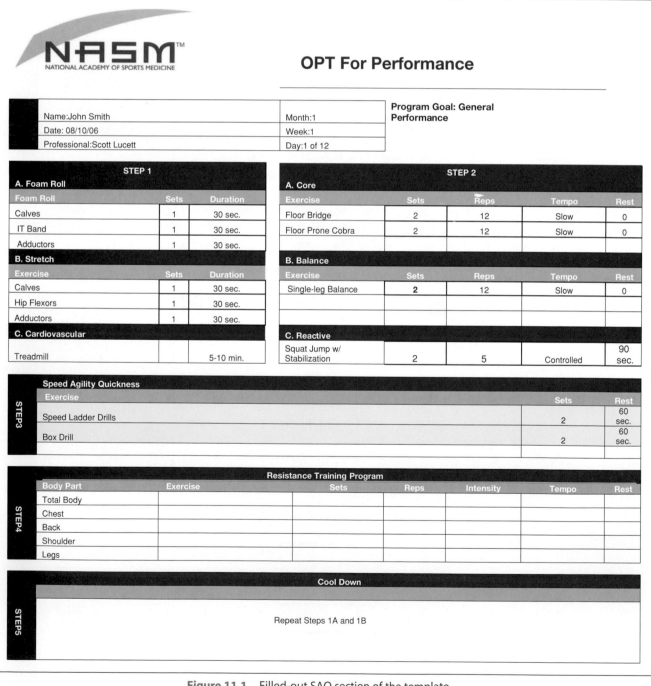

Figure 11.1 Filled-out SAQ section of the template.

SUMMARY

Programming guidelines must be gauged on the total volume of training for all components in a workout. A client's core, balance, and reactive capabilities will determine the success and safety of the program. Precise technique and kinetic chain control are required to minimize risk of injury. Various speed ladder and cone drills may be used in programming.

Review Questions

1 *Research has found that optimum stride length at maximum velocity is approximately how many times leg length?*

   a. 1.1–1.5

   b. 2.1–2.5

   c. 3.1–3.5

   d. 4.1–4.5

2 *Proper agility training can help to prevent injury by improving the structural integrity of connective tissue.*

   a. True

   b. False

3 *Select one: <u>Frontside mechanics/backside mechanics</u> includes the actions of ankle plantarflexion, knee extension, hip extension, and keeping the lumbar spine neutral.*

REFERENCES

1. Brown LE, Ferrigno VA, Santana JC. Training for Speed, Agility, and Quickness. Champaign, IL: Human Kinetics, 2000.
2. Luhtanen P, Komi PV. Mechanical factors influencing running speed. In: Asmussen E, Jorgensen K (eds). Biomechanics: VI-B. Baltimore: University Park Press, 1978:23–29.
3. Mero A, Komi PV, Gregor RJ. Biomechanics of sprint running. Sports Med 1992;13(6):376–392.
4. Leierer S. A guide for sprint training. Athlet J 1979;59(6):105–106.
5. McFarlane B. Developing maximal running speed. *Track Field Q Rev 1*985;83(2):4–9.
6. Parsons LS, Jones MT. Development of speed, quickness and agility for tennis athletes. Strength Cond J 1998;20:14–19.

Resistance-Training Concepts

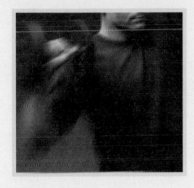

OBJECTIVES

After completing this chapter, you will be able to:

- Describe the stages of the general adaptation syndrome.
- Define and describe the principle of specificity.
- List and define the various stages of strength and training systems.

KEY TERMS

Alarm reaction

Exhaustion

General adaptation syndrome

Horizontal loading

Hypertrophy

Maximal strength

Mechanical specificity

Metabolic specificity

Muscular endurance

Neuromuscular specificity

Periodization

Power

Principle of specificity

Resistance development

Specific adaptation to imposed demands (SAID principle)

Stability

Strength

Strength endurance

Vertical loading

INTRODUCTION TO RESISTANCE TRAINING

The final component of the template that must be addressed is the resistance-training portion. This section of the OPT™ template is traditionally considered the "work-out" portion of a session. It consists of filling in the exercise for each body part (chest, back, shoulders, and so forth), the sets, repetitions, intensity (or weight), tempo (or speed of repetition), and the rest interval (or amount of rest given between each exercise). The resistance-training portion of the program is generally seen as the most important. However, it should be very evident by now that without a proper assessment and flexibility protocol and attention to the client's goals, resistance training can become more of a hindrance than help.

There is quite a bit of information that a health and fitness professional needs to review to create and understand an effective resistance-training program. The following modules will explore many concepts in resistance training, as well as address many misconceptions. They will focus on adaptations, progressive strength adaptations derived from resistance training, training systems used to acquire strength, and specific resistance-training exercise progressions.

Adaptation

PRINCIPLE OF ADAPTATION

There are many important training principles that a health and fitness professional must understand. The most important, perhaps, is that of adaptation (Figure 12-1).[1-7]

Adaptation

One of the many unique qualities that the human body displays is its ability to adapt or adjust its functional capacity to meet the desired needs. This is perhaps the root of all training and conditioning. The desire to seek an adaptation is the driving force behind most clients and training programs. Whether the goal is cosmetic in nature or health- or performance-related, resistance training has been shown to produce many desirable effects (Figure 12-2). A good understanding of this phenomenon is important for the health and fitness professional.

General Adaptation Syndrome

The kinetic chain seeks to maintain a state of physiologic balance (or homeostasis).[5] To do this, it must be able to adapt to stresses placed on it. This ability to adapt to stress is known as the **general adaptation syndrome**. This general pattern of adaptation was brought forth by Hans Selye, who showed that the kinetic chain responds and adapts to the stresses placed on it. To respond, however, the

> **General adaptation syndrome:** The kinetic chain's ability to adapt to stresses placed on it.

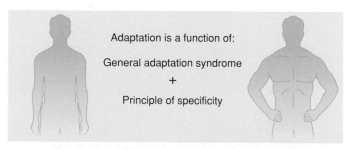

Figure 12.1 Resistance training principle of adaptation.

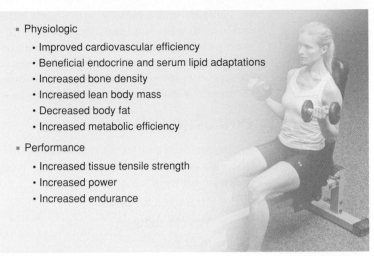

- Physiologic
  - Improved cardiovascular efficiency
  - Beneficial endocrine and serum lipid adaptations
  - Increased bone density
  - Increased lean body mass
  - Decreased body fat
  - Increased metabolic efficiency
- Performance
  - Increased tissue tensile strength
  - Increased power
  - Increased endurance

Figure 12.2   Adaptive benefits from resistance training.

body must be confronted with a stressor or some form of stress that creates the need for a response (Table 12-1).[6] Selye outlined three stages of response to stress:[6]

- Alarm reaction
- Resistance development
- Exhaustion

ALARM REACTION STAGE

Alarm reaction: The alarm reaction is the initial reaction to a stressor.

The **alarm reaction** is the initial reaction to a stressor. It allows for the activation of protective processes within the body. For example, a person who decides to begin resistance training places his or her body under the stress of increased amounts of force on his or her bones, joints, muscles, connective tissues, and nervous system. This creates a need for increased oxygen and blood supply to the right areas in his or her body, as well as an increased neural recruitment to the muscles. Initially, the individual's body is very inefficient at responding to the demands placed on it. Thus, the body must increase its ability to meet these new demands.[5,6]

RESISTANCE DEVELOPMENT STAGE

Resistance development: The body increases its functional capacity to adapt to the stressor.

During the **resistance development** stage, the body increases its functional capacity to adapt to the stressor. After repeated training sessions, the kinetic chain will increase its capability to efficiently recruit muscle fibers and distribute oxygen and blood to the proper areas in the body. However, once adapted, the body will require increased stress to produce a new response.[5,6]

Table 12.1

The General Adaptation Syndrome

Stage	Reaction
Alarm reaction	Initial reaction to stressor such as increased oxygen and blood supply to the necessary areas of the body
Resistance development	Increased functional capacity to adapt to stressor such as increasing motor unit recruitment
Exhaustion	A prolonged intolerable stressor produces fatigue and leads to a breakdown in the system or injury

Health and fitness professionals often understand this adaptation response, but use it with improper application. In this scenario, many professionals only manipulate or adjust the amount of weight the client uses when, in fact, this is only one of many ways that increased stress can be placed on the body. The Program Design chapter will discuss the importance of manipulating many acute variables to properly enhance the kinetic chain to avoid breakdown or exhaustion.

EXHAUSTION STAGE

Exhaustion: Prolonged stress or stress that is intolerable and will produce exhaustion or distress to the system.

Prolonged stress or stress that is intolerable to a client will produce **exhaustion** or distress. When the stressor is too much for the system to handle it causes a breakdown or injury such as:[5,6]

- Stress fractures
- Muscle strains
- Joint pain
- Emotional fatigue

In turn, many of these will lead to the initiation of the cumulative injury cycle.

This is the prime rationale for using the OPT™ model (a systematic, progressive training program) that is based on science and proven through application. Resistance training (and any other form of training) must be cycled through different stages that increase stress placed on the kinetic chain and also allow for sufficient rest and recuperation. More information about the **periodization** of training (OPT™ model) will be detailed in the Program Design chapter.

Periodization: Division of a training program into smaller, progressive stages.

In the above example, if the resistance is continually increased with the intention of stressing the muscles of the body to produce a size or strength change, it can lead to injury of the muscle, joint, or connective tissue. This is a result of the fact that connective tissues (such as ligaments and tendons) do not adapt as quickly as muscles as a result of their lack of blood supply.[8-11] It is important to have a complete understanding of how the kinetic chain functions to properly manipulate it for optimum adaptation with minimal risk of injury.

There are many different tissues in the body (muscle fibers, connective tissue, and so forth), and each have a different adaptive potential to stresses. This means that training programs should provide a variety of intensities and stresses to optimize the adaptation of each tissue to ensure the best possible results. Adaptation can be more specifically applied to certain aspects of the kinetic chain depending on the training technique(s) used. This is evident by the principle of specificity.

The Principle of Specificity: The SAID Principle

Principle of specificity *or* **specific adaptation to imposed demands (SAID principle):** Principle that states the body will adapt to the specific demands that are placed on it.

The **principle of specificity** is often referred to as the SAID principle, which stands for **specific adaptation to imposed demands**. Essentially, this means that the body will specifically adapt to the type of demand placed on it. For example, if someone repeatedly lifts heavy weights, that person will produce higher levels of maximal strength. If a person repeatedly lifts lighter weights for many repetitions, that person will develop higher levels of endurance.

This is a fairly simple concept to understand and implies that, in essence, you get what you train for. However, the principle of specificity is often used out of context and can become misleading to the health and fitness professional who does not remember the basic sciences previously discussed. That is, there are different tissues in the body that each respond to a different stimulus. To make the principle of specificity a safe and effective tool, it must be used appropriately.

The body must progress through different stages of adaptation to ensure that all of the necessary tissues are developed to properly meet the desired goal. Connective tissue recovers slower to training than muscle, but also must be strong for muscles to generate high levels of force. If emphasis is placed on training muscles to get big

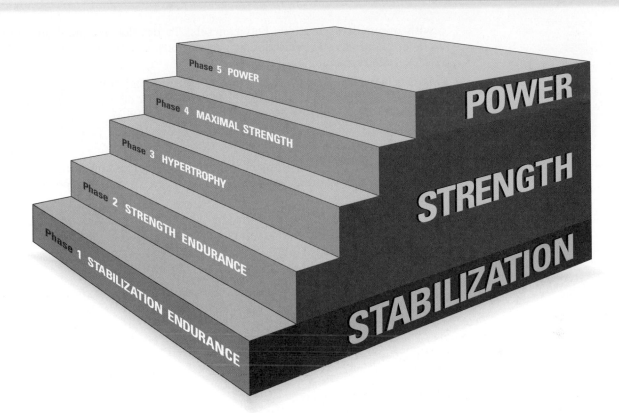

Figure 12.3   The OPT™ model.

or strong, before training for connective tissue strength and endurance, there is risk of increased injury.

Remember that type I muscle fibers function differently than type II muscle fibers and are vitally important for postural stabilization. To train with higher intensities, proper postural stabilization is required. Therefore, tissues need to be trained differently to prepare them for higher levels of training, which are necessary to achieve many of the goals in a planned, organized manner. This is the specific purpose behind the three main adaptations of training within the OPT™ model that will be discussed later in the chapter (Figure 12-3).

The degree of adaptation that occurs during training is directly related to the mechanical, neuromuscular, and metabolic specificity of the training program.[4,12–57] In other words, the more specifically a health and fitness professional manipulates the exercise routine to meet the actual goal, the greater the carryover the training program will have on that goal. It is important to remember that if a specific adaptation is required or desired, it must be trained for. The body can only adapt if it has a reason to adapt.

Mechanical specificity:
Refers to the weight and movements placed on the body.

Neuromuscular specificity:
Refers to the speed of contraction and exercise selection.

Metabolic specificity: Refers to the energy demand placed on the body.

- **Mechanical specificity** refers to the weight and movements placed on the body.[52,58] To develop endurance in the legs, light weights must be used over many repetitions with leg exercises. To develop maximal strength in the chest, heavy weights must be used during chest-related exercises.

- **Neuromuscular specificity** refers to the speed of contraction and exercise selection.[20,59–63] To develop higher levels of power in the legs, low-weight, high-velocity contractions must be performed in a plyometric manner (such as those seen in reactive-power level exercises). To develop higher levels of stability while pushing, chest exercises will need to be performed, with controlled, unstable exercises, at slower speeds. (An example would be a dumbbell chest press performed on a stability ball.)

- **Metabolic specificity** refers to the energy demand placed on the body.[64–69] To develop endurance, training will require prolonged bouts of exercise, with minimal rest periods between sets. To develop maximal strength or power, training will require longer rest periods, so the intensity of each bout of exercise remains high.

This is a very important concept for the health and fitness professional to understand and implement in their training program. A client must be trained to meet the specific demands of his or her daily life and goal(s).

As an example, imagine this concept were being applied to a client with the goal of body fat reduction. It is understood that: [70-72]

1. Mechanically, the body burns more calories when movements are performed in the standing position (versus a seated or lying position) with moderate weights.

2. Neuromuscularly, the body burns more calories when more muscles are being used for longer periods in controlled, unstable environments.

3. Metabolically, the body burns more calories when rest periods are controlled to minimize full recuperation.

Following these specificity guidelines, this client should perform more of the exercises in a standing position with moderate weight. The client should also recruit and use more muscles on each exercise, while metabolically monitoring rest periods. This method will get the client to effectively burn more calories and achieve the goal of body fat reduction.

SUMMARY

A well-designed, integrated training program produces optimum levels of:

- Strength
- Neuromuscular control
- Power
- Flexibility
- Endurance
- Alterations in body composition

To achieve this, the body is required to adapt to specifically imposed demands and stresses. The ability to adapt to stress is known as the general adaptation syndrome. There are three stages of response to stress: (1) alarm reaction (or initial activation of protective processes within the body), (2) resistance development (or an increase in the functional capacity to adapt to a stressor), and (3) exhaustion (or stress that is too much for the system and causes an injury). To avoid injury, adaptive programs must use a planned training methodology (periodization) that cycles through different stages and allows for sufficient rest and recuperation. Adaptive programs have several benefits, including:

- Physiologic
  - Improved cardiovascular efficiency
  - Decreased body fat
  - Increased lean body mass
  - Metabolic efficiency
  - Bone density
- Performance
  - Increased tissue tensile strength
  - Increased endurance
  - Increased power

Adaptation must relate to a client's goals and the design of the program. There are different types of strength and different systems of strength training that may be used to create a more individualized and systematic program for the client. There are also many different tissues in the body, and each responds to different stresses as seen in the principle of specificity or specific adaptation to imposed demands (or SAID principle). Training programs should provide a variety of intensities and stresses to optimize the adaptation of each tissue to ensure the best possible results. The degree of adaptation that occurs during training is directly related to the mechanical, neuromuscular, and metabolic specificity of the training program.

Progressive Strength Adaptations From Resistance Training

The concept of adaptation makes it clear that some type of change will occur based on the stresses placed on the body. Resistance-training programs are designed to produce changes that result in various strength adaptations. Whether the goal is to increase muscle mass, develop better athletic performance, or reduce body fat, the use of resistance training is an important component of any program. This will help ensure optimal health and longevity for the client. The healthier a client remains, the longer they can train. The longer they can train without entering the exhaustion stage (general adaptation syndrome) and developing tissue breakdown or injury, the greater amount of change or adaptation they will realize.

Following the concepts of the general adaptation syndrome and the principle of specificity, a health and fitness professional can plan the appropriate fitness, wellness, or performance program for their client.

DEFINITION OF STRENGTH

Strength: The ability of the neuromuscular system to produce internal tension to overcome an external force.

Strength is the ability of the neuromuscular system to produce internal tension (in the muscles and connective tissue that pull on the bones) to overcome an external force. Whether the external force demands the neuromuscular system to produce stability, endurance, maximal strength, or power, it still requires a form of internal tension. This internal tension produced is *strength adaptation*. The specific form of strength or internal tension that is produced from training is based on the style of training used by the client (principle of specificity).

Traditionally, resistance-training programs have focused on developing maximal strength in individual muscles, emphasizing one plane of motion. Because all muscles function eccentrically, isometrically, and concentrically in all three planes of motion at different speeds, a training program should use a progressive approach that emphasizes the appropriate exercise selection, all muscle actions, and repetition tempos (see Chapter 13).[1,4,13,51,73]

Strength adaptations obtained from resistance training can be divided into three main categories of stabilization, strength, and power as seen in the OPT™ model. Each adaptation can be defined by the emphasis that is placed on the neuromuscular system (principle of specificity), and all occur in a progressive sequence: stabilization before strength; strength before power. Each adaptation category can be further divided into more specific adaptations, summarized in Table 12-2, which are a result of resistance training.[1,60]

STABILIZATION LEVEL RESISTANCE TRAINING (PHASE 1)

Stabilization adaptations build the foundation for optimum human movement and should be the beginning point for all first-time clients. Stabilization adaptation should also be revisited periodically by advanced clients. Stabilization must be established before training for other adaptations because it specifically focuses on the recruitment

Table 12.2	
Specific Adaptations in the OPT™ Model	
Category	**Specific Adaptations**
Stabilization	Muscular endurance Stability
Strength	Strength-endurance Hypertrophy Maximal strength
Power	Power

of tissues in the body responsible for postural stability. This includes tissue such as type I muscle fibers and connective tissue. The general adaptation syndrome and principle of specificity both dictate that to maximize training for these tissues, a program must use high-repetition schemes with low to moderate volume and intensity in a postural position that challenges the stability of the body. This means, more simply, training for muscular endurance in unstable positions that can be safely controlled. This challenges the body's ability to structurally stabilize itself.

The emphasis is placed on the nervous system in this adaptation category. Initial gains that are noted in strength originate from within the nervous system.[40,55,74-76] For muscles to function properly they must be appropriately linked to the nervous system by motor units.

Recruitment of motor units is generally determined by their size (size principle).[77] Smaller motor units (type I) are recruited before larger motor units (type II). It has been noted that many clients who are new to resistance training have not established the ability to recruit a high percentage of motor units.[55,74] By focusing on high repetitions with low intensities at slow velocities, a beginning client can be taught precise exercise technique and establish the right connection between the brain and muscles, without placing improper stresses on the body.

The two primary adaptations that are achieved in this period of training are muscular endurance and stability. Both of these adaptations increase the ability of the body to produce internal tension and, as a result, increase specific forms of strength for each client.

Muscular Endurance

Muscular endurance: The ability of the body to produce low levels of force and maintain them for extended periods.

Muscular endurance is the ability to produce and maintain relatively low levels of force for prolonged periods. The ability to overcome gravity, ground reaction forces, and momentum on a continual basis is vital in the prevention of injury and allows proper kinetic chain alignment and performance.[1,13,57] This is most important for maintaining proper length-tension relationships in the muscles to minimize unwanted stress on the joints and reduce the risk of entering the exhaustion phase of the general adaptation syndrome and eventual injury. It promotes proper stabilization during training, as well as maintenance of better posture throughout the day, increasing a client's sense of well-being.

Stability

Stability: The ability of the body to maintain postural equilibrium and support joints during movement.

Stability is the ability of the kinetic chain's stabilizing muscles to provide optimal dynamic joint stabilization and maintain correct posture during all movements. This requires high levels of muscular endurance to allow for optimal recruitment of prime movers, increasing force production and force reduction.

Research has repeatedly demonstrated that training with controlled, unstable exercises increases the body's ability to stabilize or balance itself.[78-80] Conversely, if training is not performed with controlled unstable exercises, clients will not gain the same level of stability and may even worsen.[80,81]

Stability is arguably the most important adaptation because it increases the ability of the kinetic chain to stabilize the lumbo-pelvic-hip complex and joints during movement, to allow the arms and legs to work more efficiently.

STRENGTH LEVEL RESISTANCE TRAINING (PHASES 2–4)

Strength adaptations provide the necessary progression from the stabilization adaptations of training to increase the stress placed on the body, allowing for new adaptations to be achieved. Type II muscle fibers are more predominantly recruited to increase the body's capacity to produce internal tension. The general adaptation syndrome and principle of specificity both dictate that to maximize training for these tissues, a program must use low to moderate repetition schemes with moderate to high volume and intensity.

The emphasis in this adaptation category is on both the nervous and muscular systems. Heavier weights and higher volumes of training are used to increase the recruitment, synchronization, and firing rate of motor units, while placing necessary mechanical stress on the muscles to increase their size or strength.[40,55,74–76] Strength endurance, hypertrophy, and maximal strength are the primary adaptations seen in this period of training.

Strength Endurance (Phase 2)

Strength endurance: The ability of the body to repeatedly produce high levels of force for prolonged periods.

Strength endurance is the ability to repeatedly produce higher levels of force for relatively prolonged periods. Whereas muscular endurance involves lower intensities of force being used with higher repetitions (12 to 25) and minimal rest between sets, strength endurance allows the body to use higher levels of force with lower repetitions (6 to 12) and more sets, repeatedly, with minimal rest. This adaptation is often trained with the use of supersets (Program Design, Chapter 13).[57,73]

Hypertrophy (Phase 3)

Hypertrophy: Enlargement of skeletal muscle fibers in response to overcoming force from high volumes of tension.

Hypertrophy is the enlargement of skeletal muscle fibers in response to increased volumes of tension, as seen in resistance training.[82,83] Muscle hypertrophy is characterized by the increase in the cross-sectional area of individual muscle fibers and is believed to result from an increase in the myofibril proteins (myofilaments).[84–87] Although hypertrophy is not externally visible for many weeks (4 to 8 weeks) in a beginning client, the process begins in the early stages of training, regardless of the intensity.[21,58,88–98] However, muscle fibers must be recruited to induce hypertrophy.[7,99] The nervous system must establish the proper connection to effectively communicate with each muscle fiber. This provides the necessary rationale as to why clients should start and revisit the stabilization level of training before entering into the strength level.

Maximal Strength (Phase 4)

Maximal strength: The maximum force that a muscle can produce in a single, voluntary effort, regardless of velocity.

Maximal strength is the maximum force that a muscle can produce in a single, voluntary effort, regardless of how fast the load moves. For a muscle to produce maximal force, all of the muscle's motor units must be recruited.[40,55,74–76] This is necessary to ensure that as many possible muscle fibers are involved in the contraction. One means of increasing strength lies in the ability to recruit a maximal amount of motor units.

Maximum strength can be improved through stabilization training. This type of training improves the ability of the neuromuscular system to better recruit motor units within a muscle (intramuscular coordination) and in synergy with many other muscles (intermuscular coordination). This allows the nervous system to appropriately use muscles to stabilize a joint while other muscles are lifting maximal loads.[1,4,13,51,57,73]

POWER LEVEL RESISTANCE TRAINING (PHASE 5)

Power: Ability of the neuromuscular system to produce the greatest force in the shortest time.

Power is the ability of the neuromuscular system to produce the greatest possible force in the shortest possible time. This is represented by the simple equation of force multiplied by velocity.[100]

The adaptation of power uses the stabilization and strength adaptations and applies them at more realistic speeds and forces, seen in everyday and sporting activities. The focus is now on getting the neuromuscular system to generate force as quickly as possible (rate of force production).

An increase in either force or velocity will produce an increase in power. This can be achieved by increasing the weight (force), as seen in the strength adaptations, or increasing the speed with which weight is moved (velocity). Power training allows for increased rate of force production by increasing the number of motor units activated, the synchronization between them, and the speed at which they are activated.[74,75,101] The general adaptation syndrome and principle of specificity both dictate that to maximize training for this adaptation both heavy and light loads must be moved as fast and as controlled as possible.

SUMMARY

Resistance-training programs produce changes that result in various strength adaptations. Strength is the ability of the neuromuscular system to produce internal tension to overcome an external force. Traditionally, resistance-training programs have focused on developing maximal strength in individual muscles. However, today's training program should emphasize appropriate exercise selection, all muscle actions, and repetition tempos. Training adaptations can be divided into three main categories that are consistent with the OPT model: stabilization, strength, and power.

Stabilization adaptations should be the beginning point for all first-time clients. Use high repetitions with low to moderate volume and low to moderate intensity in a postural position that challenges the stability of the body. The two primary adaptations that are achieved are muscular endurance and stability.

Strength adaptations should use low to moderate repetition schemes with moderate to high volume and moderate to high intensity. Heavier weights and higher volumes of training are used to improve the function of motor units, while placing stress on the muscles to increase size or strength. Strength-endurance, hypertrophy, and maximal strength are the primary adaptations seen in this period of training.

Power is the ability of the neuromuscular system to produce the greatest possible force in the shortest possible time. An increase in either force (weight) or velocity (speed with which weight is moved) will produce an increase in power. To maximize training for this adaptation, both heavy and light loads must be moved as fast and as controlled as possible.

Resistance-Training Systems

Originally, power lifters, Olympic lifters, and bodybuilders were the ones who designed most resistance-training programs. Many of these styles of resistance-training programs remain popular today because of marketing or gym science, not because they scientifically demonstrate superiority over other programs in bringing about increases in stabilization, strength, and power.

Table 12.3	
Resistance-Training Systems	
Type	**Definition**
Single-set	Performing one set of each exercise
Multiple-set	Performing a multiple number of sets for each exercise
Pyramid	Increasing (or decreasing) weight with each set
Superset	Performing two exercises in rapid succession with minimal rest
Circuit training	Performing a series of exercises, one after the other, with minimal rest
Peripheral heart action	A variation of circuit training that uses different exercises (upper and lower body) for each set through the circuit
Split-routine	A routine that trains different body parts on separate days
Vertical loading	Performing exercises on the OPT™ template one after the other, in a vertical manner down the template
Horizontal loading	Performing all sets of an exercise (or body part) before moving on to the next exercise (or body part)

Following a systematic, integrated training program and manipulating key training variables are necessary to achieve optimal gains in specific forms of strength.[1,13,35,52,57,102] The OPT™ model follows a progressive, systematic approach that enables the health and fitness professional to make consistent gains with all clients. It can be manipulated in many ways to achieve various goals. There are many training systems that can be used to structure a resistance-training program for different effects. We will review several of the most common training systems that are currently used in the fitness industry (Table 12-3).

RESISTANCE-TRAINING SYSTEMS EXPLAINED

The Single-Set System

The single-set system is one of the oldest training methods.[25] The single-set system entails performance of one set of each exercise. Each set usually consists of 8 to 12 repetitions of each exercise at a controlled tempo. It is usually recommended that this system be performed two times per week to promote sufficient development and maintenance of muscle mass.[102] Although multiple-set training is promoted as being more beneficial for strength and hypertrophy gains in advanced clients, the single-set system has been shown to be as beneficial for a beginning-level client.[25,103–107]

This system of training should be explored by the health and fitness professional to help customize program design. Often in the training industry, single-set training is negatively perceived as not providing enough stimuli for adaptation. However, when reviewing the physiology of how the kinetic chain operates and current research, this may not be true.[25,104] In fact, most first-time clients *should* follow a single-set program to allow for proper adaptive responses of the connective tissue and nervous system before engaging in more-rigorous training systems. By not giving a client more than they can handle, synergistic dominance and injury can be avoided. Applying variation to rest periods, repetitions, and intensity, single-set training can make a program very demanding for even the advanced client.

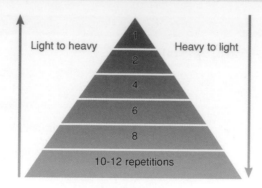

Figure 12.4 The pyramid system.

The Multiple-Set System

This resistance-training system has been popular since the 1940s.[73] The multiple-set system of training consists of performing a multiple number of sets for each exercise. The resistance, sets, and repetitions that are performed can be selected according to the goals and needs of the client.[73,108,109] Multiple-set training can be appropriate for both novice and advanced clients, but has specifically been shown to be superior to single-set training for the advanced client.[102,110–114] It appears that the increased volume (sets, reps, and intensity) is necessary for further improvement, but must be administered appropriately to avoid overtraining.[7,115,116]

The Pyramid System

The pyramid system involves a progressive or regressive step approach that either increases weight with each set or decreases weight with each set (Figure 12-4).[102]

In the *light-to-heavy system*, the individual performs 10 to 12 repetitions with a light load and increases the resistance for each following set, until the individual can perform one to two repetitions, usually in four to six sets. This system can easily be used for workouts that involve only two to four sets or higher repetition schemes (12 to 20 repetitions).

The *heavy-to-light system* works in the opposite direction. The individual begins with a heavy load (after a sufficient warm-up) for one to two repetitions, then decreases the load and increases the repetitions for four to six sets.[102]

The Superset System

The superset system uses a couple of exercises performed in rapid succession of one another. This system features the use of independent subsystems with similar principles (namely, compound-set and tri-set systems).[102]

Compound-sets involve the performance of two exercises for antagonistic muscles. For example, an individual may perform a set of bench presses followed by cable rows (chest and back). Working opposing musculature allows for better recovery before the start of another set. In addition, it is more time efficient.[102]

Tri-sets use three exercises in rapid succession for the same muscle group or body part. For example, an individual may perform incline dumbbell presses, cable chest presses, and ball push-ups, all in succession (chest superset).[102] This may also be performed with two exercises.

Typically, supersetting involves sets of 8 to 12 repetitions with no rest between sets or exercises. However, any number of repetitions can be used. The superset system is popular among bodybuilders and may be beneficial for muscular hypertrophy and muscular endurance.[102,112]

The Circuit-Training System

The circuit-training system consists of a series of exercises that an individual performs one after the other, with minimal rest (Figure 12-5). The typical acute variables

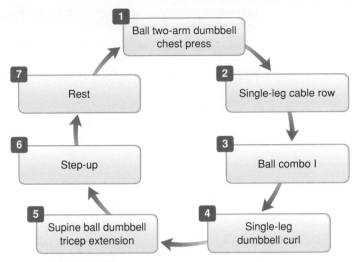

Figure 12.5 Example circuit.

for a circuit-training program include one to three sets of 8 to 15 repetitions with 15 to 60 seconds of rest between exercises.[102,117,118] However, these variables can be manipulated to enhance the desired effect.

Circuit training is a great training system for those individuals with limited time and for those who want to alter body composition.[13,102,117–119]

The Peripheral Heart Action System

The peripheral heart action system is another variation of circuit training that alternates upper body and lower body exercises throughout the circuit. The number of exercises per sequence varies with the program's goal. The individual performs 8 to 20 repetitions per exercise, depending on the desired adaptation and phase of training they are using in the OPT™ model. This system is very beneficial for incorporating an integrated, multidimensional program and for altering body composition.[102,119] An example for each of the three main adaptations is shown in Table 12-4.

The Split-Routine System

A split-routine system involves breaking the body up into parts to be trained on separate days. Many bodybuilders and mass-dominant and strength athletes (football, shot put, and so forth) use the split-routine system. Bodybuilders typically perform many exercises for the same body part to bring about optimal muscular hypertrophy. By breaking up the body into parts that can be trained on different

Table 12.4

Peripheral Heart Action System: Sample Workout

Set 1: Stabilization	Set 2: Strength	Set 3: Power
1. Ball dumbbell chest press	1. Bench press	1. Medicine ball chest pass
2. Ball squat	2. Barbell squat	2. Squat jump
3. Single-leg cable row	3. Seated row	3. Woodchop throw
4. Step-up to balance	4. Leg press	4. Power step-up
5. Single-leg dumbbell shoulder press	5. Seated dumbbell shoulder press	5. Side oblique throw

Table 12.5		
Split-Routine System: Sample Workouts		
Routine	**Day(s) Performed**	**Body Parts Trained**
2-Day	Monday Thursday	Chest/shoulders/triceps Back/biceps/legs
3-Day	Monday Wednesday Friday	Chest/shoulders/triceps Legs Back/biceps
4-Day	Monday and Thursday Tuesday and Friday	Chest/shoulders/triceps Back/biceps/legs
5-Day	Monday Tuesday Wednesday Thursday Friday	Chest Legs Back Shoulders Arms
6-Day	Monday and Friday Tuesday and Saturday Wednesday and Sunday	Chest/shoulders/triceps Legs Back/biceps

days, more work can be performed for the allotted time per workout. Split-routines come in all sizes and shapes. A few typical split-routines are shown in Table 12-5.

Any derivative of these outlined routines can be used. The important issue with some of these routines is recovery time. When training each body part more than once a week, volume and intensity should be accounted for.

Vertical Loading and Horizontal Loading

Vertical loading:

Alternating body parts trained from set to set, starting from the upper extremity and moving to the lower extremity.

Vertical loading is a resistance training system used by NASM and follows the OPT™ model. It progresses a workout vertically down the template by alternating body parts trained from set to set. Looking at the OPT™ template, it is seen that the resistance-training section involves the following exercises:

1. Total body exercise
2. Chest
3. Back
4. Shoulders
5. Biceps
6. Triceps
7. Legs

In a vertically loaded workout, the client would perform the first exercise (total body) for the required repetitions and then move to the chest exercise for the next set of repetitions. After the chest exercise, the client would move on to the back exercise and so forth, until all exercises have been completed. Once completed, the client would then start back at the first exercise (total body) and run through the exercises again for the desired amount of sets. This can also be done in a circuit style, by minimizing the rest periods in between exercises.

This system of training can be very beneficial for allowing maximal recovery to each body part while minimizing the amount of time wasted on rest. For example, if it takes 1 minute to perform each exercise, by the time the client returns to the chest exercise, 7 to 10 minutes could have passed, which is far more than necessary for full adenosine triphosphate–creatine phosphate (ATP/CP) recovery. Even though 7 to 10 minutes have passed, the client has been constantly moving and has performed one set of every exercise in his or her workout.

Horizontal loading refers to performing all sets of an exercise or body part before moving on to the next exercise or body part. For example, if performing three sets of a chest exercise and three sets of a back exercise, the client would perform all three sets of the chest exercise before moving on to the back exercise. The progression of exercises is therefore said to be horizontal across the template. This is the method most commonly used in the fitness environment.

The drawback to the horizontal loading system is the amount of time typically spent resting, which can often add up to more time then the actual workout itself. Horizontal loading can be a metabolic progression if rest periods are monitored and limited to 30 to 90 seconds between sets. It forces the same muscle group to work with minimal recovery. This can cause metabolic and hypertrophy-related adaptations to occur in the muscle.[65,69,102]

Horizontal loading:
Performing all sets of an exercise or body part before moving on to the next exercise or body part.

SUMMARY

The OPT™ method follows a progressive, systematic approach that enables the health and fitness professional to make consistent gains with all clients through training manipulations to achieve various goals. There are many training systems that can be used to structure a resistance-training program for different effects.

The single-set system entails performance of one set of each exercise, usually of 8 to 12 repetitions. This system has been shown to be beneficial for strength and hypertrophy gains in the beginning-level client.

The multiple-set system of training consists of performing a multiple number of sets for each exercise, with resistance, sets, and repetitions adjusted according to the goals or needs of the client. This system is superior to single-set training for the advanced client.

The pyramid system involves a progressive or regressive step approach that either increases weight with each set or decreases weight with each set.

The superset system uses a couple of exercises performed in rapid succession of one another, usually 8 to 12 repetitions with no rest between sets or exercises. This system can be performed as compound-sets or tri-sets. It is popular among bodybuilders for muscular hypertrophy and muscular endurance.

The circuit-training system programs consist of a series of exercises that an individual performs one immediately after the other, with minimal rest. It is a good system for clients with limited time and those who want to alter body composition.

The peripheral heart action system is another variation of circuit training that alternates upper body and lower body exercises (of varied numbers) throughout the circuit.

A split-routine system involves breaking the body up into parts to be trained on separate days so that more work can be performed for the allotted time per workout. When training each body part more than once a week, recovery period, volume, and intensity should be accounted for.

Vertical loading and horizontal loading progress a workout vertically or horizontally down the template by alternating body parts trained from set to set. In a vertically loaded workout, the client would perform each exercise until all exercises have been completed and then run through the exercises again for the desired amount of sets. This can also be done in a circuit style, by minimizing the rest periods in between exercises to allow maximal recovery to each body part and minimize the amount of time wasted on rest. In a horizontally loaded workout, the client would perform all sets of an exercise or body part before moving on to the next exercise or body part.

Exercises

TOTAL BODY EXERCISE DESCRIPTIONS

Example Total Body-Stabilization Exercises

Ball Squat, Curl to Press

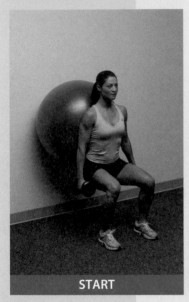 START

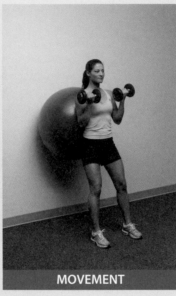 MOVEMENT

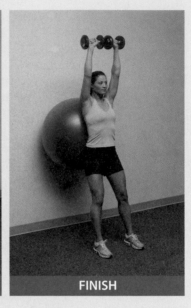 FINISH

PREPARATION

1. Begin with both feet shoulder-width apart, with feet pointing straight ahead and knees over the second and third toes. Position the ball on the low back region.
2. Hold two dumbbells in hands to the side of the body.

MOVEMENT

3. Perform a three-quarter squat, keeping lower extremity in proper alignment.
4. Before any compensation occurs, activate glutes and stand to a fully upright position.
5. Once stabilized, curl and press the dumbbells overhead until both arms are fully extended, with palms facing away. Keep navel drawn in at all times.
6. Slowly return the dumbbells to chest and repeat.
7. Regression
   a. Decrease range of motion
8. Progression
   a. Alternating-arm
   b. One-arm
   c. Single-leg

Technique

When performing any form of a ball squat, try to use the ball to *guide* one through the squatting motion (sitting into a chair) versus relying on the ball for support (leaning back on the ball).

Multiplanar Step-Up Balance to Overhead Press

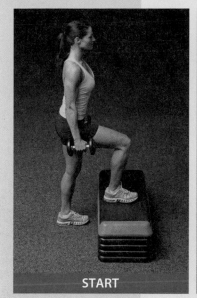
START

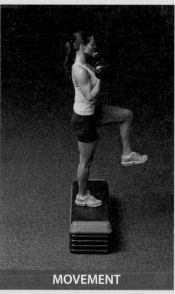
MOVEMENT

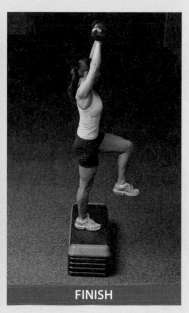
FINISH

PREPARATION

1. Stand in front of a box (6 to 18 inches high) with feet shoulder-width apart.

MOVEMENT

2. Step onto box with one leg, keeping foot pointed straight ahead and knee lined up over mid-foot.
3. Push through heel and stand up straight, balancing on one leg.
4. Flex the other leg at the hip and knee.
5. Once balance has been established, press the dumbbells overhead until both arms are fully extended. Keep navel drawn in at all times.
6. Slowly return the dumbbells to the starting position.
7. Return opposite leg to the ground and step off the box.
8. Repeat on other leg.
9. Regression
   a. Omit balance
10. Progression
    a. Frontal plane
    b. Transverse plane

Technique

When pressing overhead, make sure the low back does not arch. This may indicate tightness of the latissimus dorsi and weakness of the intrinsic core stabilizers.

Example Total Body-Strength Exercises

Lunge to Two-Arm Dumbbell Press

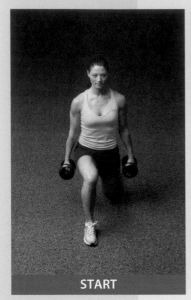

START

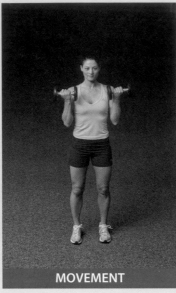

MOVEMENT

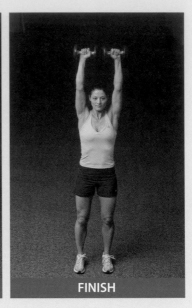

FINISH

PREPARATION

1. Begin with both feet shoulder-width apart.
2. Hold two dumbbells in hands at side of body.

MOVEMENT

3. Lunge forward, landing on the heel of lunge foot.
4. Then, come to a stabilized position with front foot pointing straight ahead and knee directly over second and third toes.
5. Both knees should now be bent at a 90-degree angle, front foot should be flat on the ground, and back foot should have the heel lifted off the ground.
6. From this position, drive off of front foot (heel first) and back into a standing position.
7. In this stable position, press the dumbbells overhead until arms are fully extended. Keep navel drawn in at all times.
8. Lower weight and repeat.

Technique   When performing any squatting or lunging motion, make sure the foot stays straight and the knees stay in line with the toes. This ensures proper joint mechanics (arthrokinematics) and optimal force generation (via proper length-tension relationships and force-couple relationships), increasing the benefit of the exercise and decreasing its risk.

Squat to Two-Arm Press

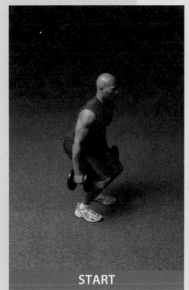
START

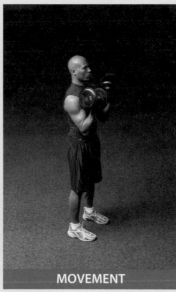
MOVEMENT

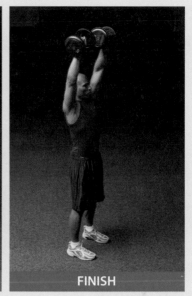
FINISH

PREPARATION

1. Begin with both feet shoulder-width apart and pointing straight ahead, and knees over second and third toes.

MOVEMENT

2. Perform a three-quarter squat, keeping lower extremity in proper alignment.
3. Before any compensation occurs, activate glutes and stand to a fully upright position.
4. Once stabilized, press the dumbbells overhead until both arms are fully extended, with palms facing away. Keep navel drawn in at all times.
5. Slowly return the dumbbells and repeat.

Example Total Body-Power Exercises

Two-Arm Push Press

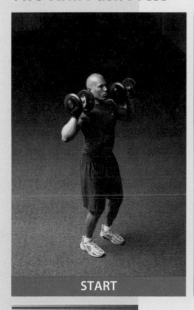
START

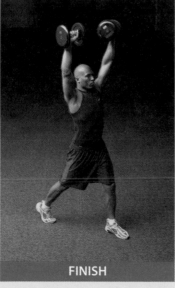
FINISH

PREPARATION

1. Stand with feet shoulder-width apart.
2. Hold two dumbbells in hands at shoulder level.

MOVEMENT

3. Quickly drive dumbbells up, as if doing a shoulder press. Keep navel drawn in at all times.
4. At the same time, drive the legs into a stagger stance position. Back leg should be in triple extension (plantarflexion, knee extension, hip extension) with the front leg bent slightly.
5. Maintain optimal alignment on the return to the starting position and repeat.

Safety

One must establish proper stability (stabilization level training) and prime mover strength (strength level training) before progressing to the power exercises.

Barbell Clean

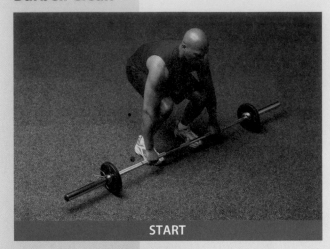

START

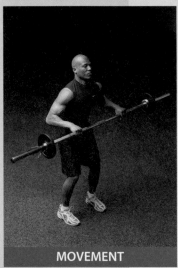

MOVEMENT

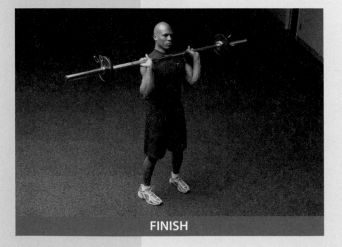

FINISH

PREPARATION

1. Stand with feet shoulder-width apart, toes pointing forward.
2. Bend the knees slightly.
3. Bend over at the waist, grasping the barbell with both hands slightly farther than shoulder-width apart (palms facing body).

MOVEMENT

4. Keeping the navel drawn-in, rapidly lift the barbell up to shoulder level.
5. Bend knees to a semi-squat position.
6. Contract glutes to stand upright and pull to bar from the ground.
7. Scoop the bar up towards the chest.
8. Catch the bar at chest level by dropping the elbows under the bar and stand upright.
9. Carefully lower the barbell back to the ground and repeat.

CHEST EXERCISE DESCRIPTIONS

Example Chest-Stabilization Exercises

Ball Dumbbell Chest Press

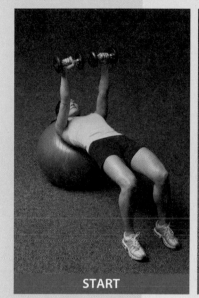
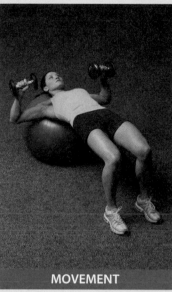
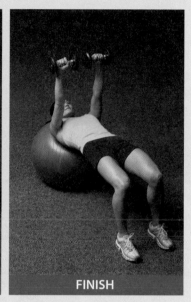

| START | MOVEMENT | FINISH |

PREPARATION

1. Lie on stability ball, with ball placed between shoulder blades.
2. Maintain a bridge position by contracting glutes and keeping shoulders, hips, and knees at the same level.
3. Feet should be shoulder-width apart with toes pointing straight ahead.
4. Hold one dumbbell in each hand, at chest level, slightly outside of body line, with elbows flexed.

MOVEMENT

5. Press both dumbbells straight up and then together, by extending elbows and contracting chest.
6. Hold.
7. Slowly return dumbbells toward body by flexing elbows.
8. Regression
   a. Dumbbell chest press progression on bench
9. Progressions
   a. Alternating-arm
   b. Single-arm

Technique   To ensure proper alignment, the ears, shoulders, hips, and knees should all be in line with one another.

Push-Up

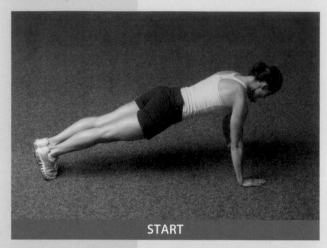

START

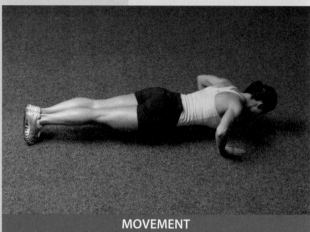

MOVEMENT

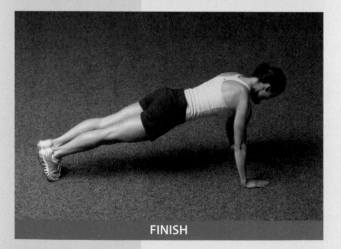

FINISH

PREPARATION

1. Begin in a push-up position with feet and hands on the floor slightly wider than shoulder-width apart.
2. Draw in navel and contract glutes.

MOVEMENT

3. Keeping back flat, slowly lower body toward ground, by flexing elbows and retracting and depressing shoulder blades.
4. Stop at first point of compensation.
5. Push back up to starting position, by extending elbows and contracting chest. Do not allow head to jut forward.
6. Regressions
   a. On knees
   b. Hands on bench, feet on floor
   c. Wall push-up
7. Progressions
   a. Lower extremity on ball
   b. Hands on medicine balls
   c. Hands on stability ball

Safety A common compensation that occurs when performing a push-up is the low back arching (stomach falls toward the ground). This is an indicator that the individual possesses weak intrinsic core stabilizers and the exercise must be regressed.

Example Chest-Strength Exercises

Flat Dumbbell Chest Press

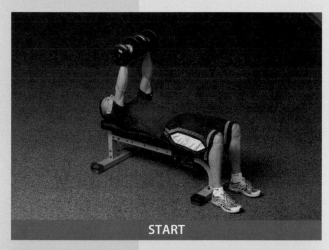

START

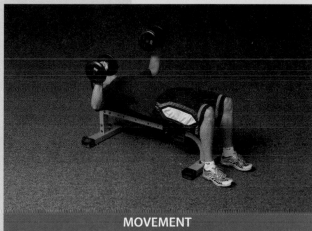

MOVEMENT

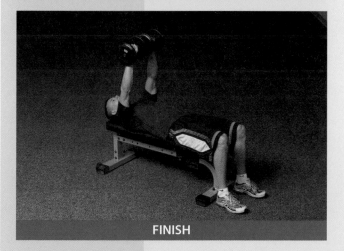

FINISH

PREPARATION

1. Lie on flat bench with knees bent.
2. Feet should be flat on the floor, shoulder-width apart with toes pointing straight ahead.
3. Hold one dumbbell in each hand, at chest level, slightly outside of body line, with elbows flexed.

MOVEMENT

4. Press both dumbbells straight up and then together, by extending elbows and contracting chest. Keep navel drawn in.
5. Hold.
6. Slowly return dumbbells toward body by flexing elbows and allowing shoulders to retract and depress.

Technique When performing chest presses, the range of motion at the shoulder joint (how far the elbows go down) will be determined by the load one is lifting (control) and tissue extensibility. The key is to only go as far as one can control without compensating.

Barbell Bench Press

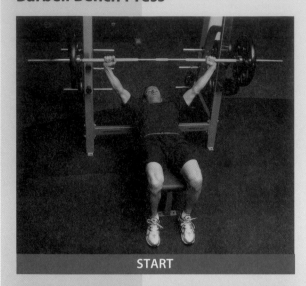

START

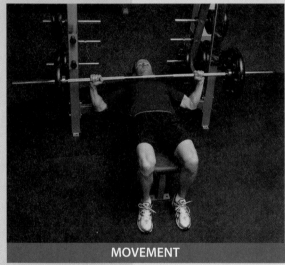

MOVEMENT

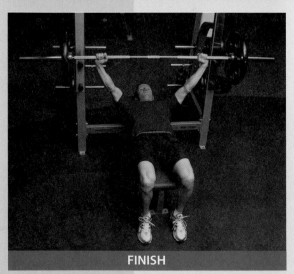

FINISH

PREPARATION

1. Lie on flat bench, feet flat on floor and toes pointing straight ahead.
2. Navel should be drawn in.
3. Hold a barbell and grasp the bar with hands slightly wider than shoulder-width apart.

MOVEMENT

4. Slowly lower the bar toward the chest by flexing elbows. Avoid letting the back arch or the head jut off the bench.
5. Press the bar back up, extending arms and contracting chest, until elbows are fully extended.

Example Chest-Power Exercises

Two-Arm Medicine Ball Chest Pass

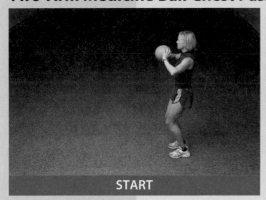
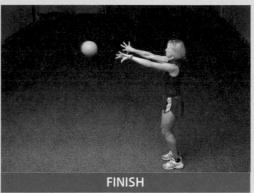

START | FINISH

PREPARATION

1. Stand, facing wall, and establish a squared stance position.
2. Hold a medicine ball (5 to 10% of body weight) with both hands, elbows flexed, at chest level.
3. Without moving the core or lower extremities, draw in navel.

MOVEMENT

4. Push and release the ball toward the wall as hard as possible, by extending the elbows and contracting the chest. Do not allow the shoulders to elevate.
5. Repeat as quickly as possible, under control.

Technique   If it is not an option to be able to perform power exercises with a medicine ball (facility-dependent, equipment), this exercise can also be done using tubing or cable. Just make sure to adjust the weight or resistance accordingly so one can still perform the movement quickly and under control without compensation.

Rotation Chest Pass

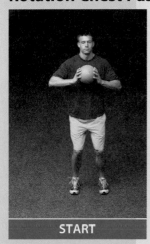
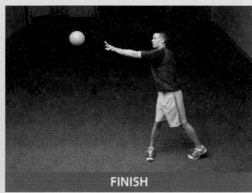

START | FINISH

PREPARATION

1. Stand, with body turned at a 90-degree angle from a wall.
2. Feet should be shoulder-width apart, toes pointing straight ahead.
3. Hold a medicine ball (5 to 10% of body weight) with both hands, elbows flexed, at chest level.

MOVEMENT

4. Use abs, hips, and glutes to rotate body quickly and explosively toward the wall.
5. As body turns, pivot back leg and allow it to go into triple extension.
6. With the upper body, push the medicine ball (as if doing a chest pass). Use the arm farthest from the wall to extend and apply force.
7. Repeat as quickly as possible, under control.

BACK EXERCISE DESCRIPTIONS

Example Back Stabilization Exercises

Standing Cable Row

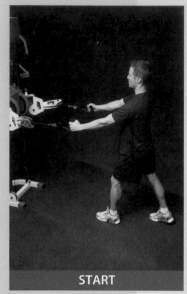

START

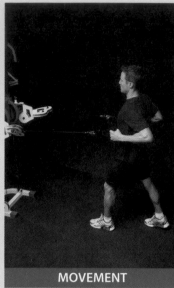

MOVEMENT

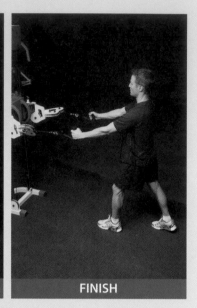

FINISH

PREPARATION

1. Stand facing a cable machine, with feet staggered and pointing straight ahead, and knees over second and third toes.
2. Hold cables, with arms extended at chest level.

MOVEMENT

3. With knees slightly flexed, row cable by flexing elbows, retracting and depressing the shoulder blades.
4. Bring thumbs toward the armpits, keeping the shoulder blades retracted and depressed.
5. Keep navel drawn in. Do not allow the head to jut forward or shoulders to elevate.
6. Hold.
7. Slowly return arms to original position, by extending the elbows.
8. Regression
   a. Seated
9. Progressions
   a. Two-legs, alternating-arm
   b. Two-legs, one-arm
   c. Single-leg, two-arms
   d. Single-leg, alternating-arm
   e. Single-leg, one-arm

Technique

When performing rows, initiate the movement by retracting and depressing the shoulder blades (scapulae). Do not allow the shoulders to elevate.

Ball Dumbbell Row

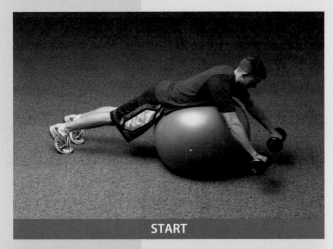

START

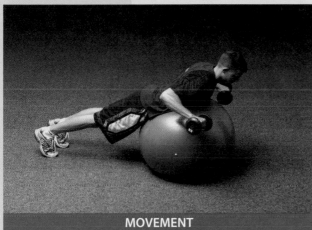

MOVEMENT

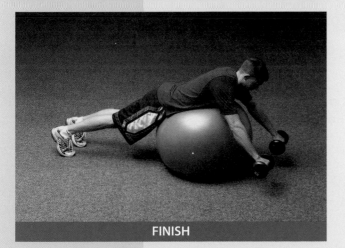

FINISH

PREPARATION

1. Begin in a prone position, with stability ball under abdomen.
2. Keep feet pointed down, legs completely straight, and navel drawn in.
3. Hold dumbbells in each hand and extend arms in front of body.

MOVEMENT

4. Contract glutes and quadriceps.
5. Row the dumbbells by retracting and depressing shoulder blades.
6. Flex elbows, bringing thumbs toward armpits.
7. Hold.
8. Return dumbbells slowly to ground, by extending elbows and allowing shoulders to protract at end range.
9. Regression
   a. Kneeling over ball
10. Progression
    a. Alternating-arm
    b. One-arm

Technique Performing exercises in a prone position can be uncomfortable. When working with overweight individuals, it may be more appropriate to perform these exercises in a seated or standing position.

Example Back Strength Exercises

Seated Cable Row

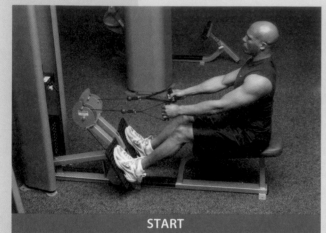
START

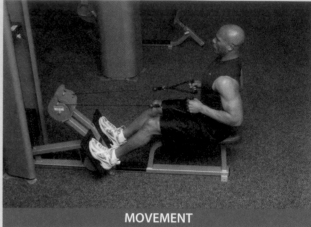
MOVEMENT

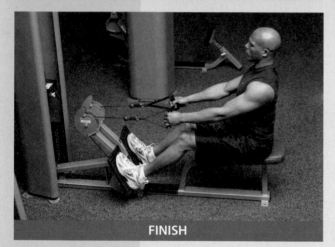
FINISH

PREPARATION

1. Sit facing a cable machine, with feet shoulder-width apart and pointing straight ahead and knees over second and third toes.
2. Hold cables, with arms extended at chest level.

MOVEMENT

3. Row cable by flexing elbows and pulling the handles toward the trunk.
4. Bring thumbs toward the armpits, keeping the shoulder blades retracted and depressed.
5. Keep navel drawn in. Do not allow the head to jut forward.
6. Hold.
7. Slowly return arms to original position, by extending the elbows.

Technique To increase the effectiveness of the exercise and decrease the risk of injury, keep the torso stationary throughout the execution of the exercise; flexing and extending the torso while performing the row creates momentum, which decreases the effectiveness of the exercise and places stress on the low back.

Seated Lat Pull-Down

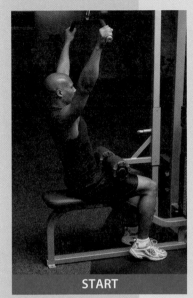

START

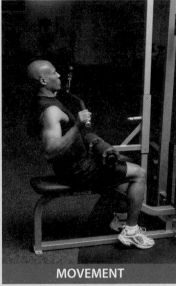

MOVEMENT

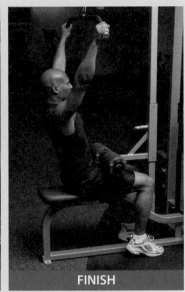

FINISH

PREPARATION

1. Sit upright with navel drawn in.

MOVEMENT

2. Pull handles toward the body, by flexing elbows and depressing the shoulder blades. Do not arch back, allow head to jut forward, or elevate the shoulders.
3. Hold at end range.
4. Slowly return weight to original position, by extending elbows and elevating the shoulder blades.

Safety

Performing lat pull-downs behind the neck are not advised as this places stress to the shoulder joint and cervical spine.

Example Back Power Exercises

Ball Medicine Ball Pullover Throw

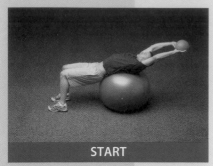

START

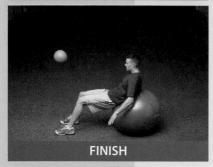

MOVEMENT

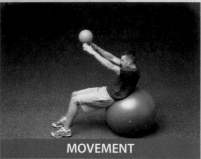

FINISH

PREPARATION

1. Place stability ball under low back, bend knees at a 90-degree angle, and keep feet flat and toes pointing straight ahead.
2. Hold a medicine ball (5 to 10% of body weight) overhead with both hands, with arms extended.

MOVEMENT

3. Using abdominals, quickly crunch forward. Keep navel drawn in.
4. Throw the medicine ball off the wall.
5. As the ball releases, continue pulling the arms through all the way to the sides of the body.
6. Keep chin tucked throughout the exercise.
7. Repeat as quickly as possible, under control.

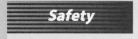

Safety   To decrease stress to the shoulder and low back, it will be important that one has optimal extensibility through the latissimus dorsi musculature before performing these back-power exercises.

Woodchop Throw

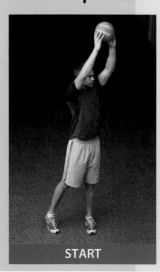

START

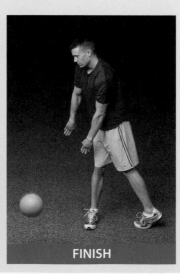

FINISH

PREPARATION

1. Stand perpendicular a wall or partner with feet shoulder-width apart.
2. Hold a medicine ball (5 to 10% of body weight) overhead.

MOVEMENT

3. Quickly rotate and throw the medicine ball toward the floor, throwing the ball toward the opposite foot (in a woodchop motion). Keep navel drawn in.
4. Repeat.

SHOULDER EXERCISE DESCRIPTIONS

Example Shoulder Stabilization Exercises

Single-Leg Dumbbell Scaption

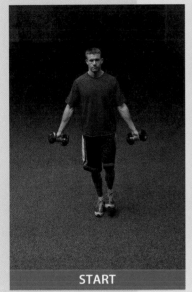

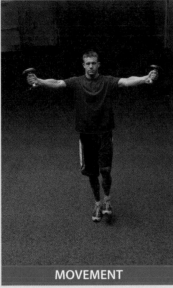

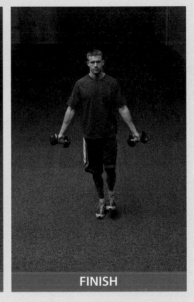

| START | MOVEMENT | FINISH |

PREPARATION

1. Stand with feet shoulder-width apart, pointing straight ahead, and knees over second and third toes.
2. Hold dumbbells at side, with palms facing side of body.
3. Keep navel drawn in.
4. Raise one foot off the floor.

MOVEMENT

5. Raise both arms, thumbs up, at a 45-degree angle in front of the body, until hands reach eye level.
6. Keep shoulder blades retracted and depressed throughout the exercise. Do not allow the back to arch.
7. Hold.
8. Slowly return arms back to sides of body and repeat.
9. Regression
   a. Two-legs
   b. Seated
10. Progression
    a. Single-leg, alternating-arm
    b. Single-leg, single-arm
    c. Proprioceptive modalities

Technique   Performing shoulder exercises in the scapular plane decreases the risk of supraspinatus muscle becoming impinged between the head of the humerus and the coracoacromial arch of the scapula.

Seated Stability Ball Military Press

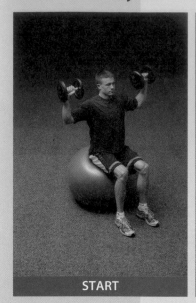
START

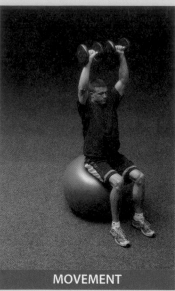
MOVEMENT

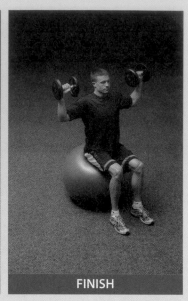
FINISH

PREPARATION

1. Sit on a stability ball, keeping the toes pointed straight ahead, feet hip width apart.
2. Hold dumbbells at shoulder level, with palms away.

MOVEMENT

3. Press the dumbbells overhead until both arms are fully extended, with palms facing away. Keep navel drawn in at all times.
4. Hold.
5. Slowly return dumbbells back to chest and repeat.
6. Regression
   a. Seated on a bench
7. Progression
   a. Alternating-am
   b. One-arm
   c. Standing

Safety Performing exercises on a stability ball can be uncomfortable for some people. It may be required for the health and fitness professional to hold the ball while the individual performs the exercise to provide some additional support (both mentally and physically).

Example Shoulder Strength Exercises

Seated Dumbbell Shoulder Press

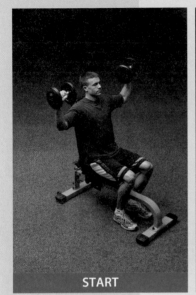
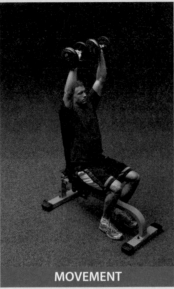
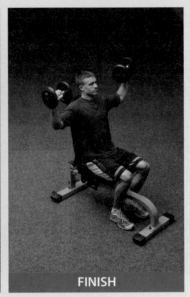

| START | MOVEMENT | FINISH |

PREPARATION

1. Sit on a bench, feet flat on floor, shoulder-width apart, and toes pointing straight ahead.
2. Hold one dumbbell in each hand, with palms facing away from body.
3. Keep navel drawn in.
4. Begin with elbows near sides of body and hands at chest level. Shoulders should be externally rotated as far as possible with scapula in a retracted and depressed position.

MOVEMENT

5. Press arms directly overhead by extending elbow. Do not allow head to jut forward or back to arch.
6. Slowly return to starting position and repeat.

Safety   When performing overhead presses, make sure the cervical spine stays neutral (head drawn back). Do not allow the head to migrate forward as this places excessive stress on the posterior neck muscles and cervical spine.

Seated Shoulder Press Machine

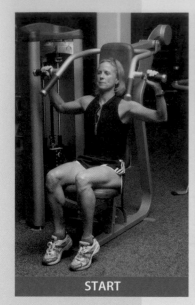
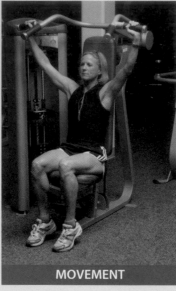
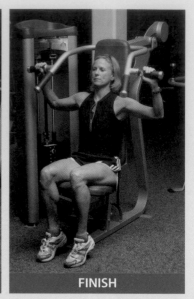

START MOVEMENT FINISH

PREPARATION

1. Sit at machine.
2. Make any adjustments necessary to fit body.
3. Select desired weight.
4. Keep navel drawn in.
5. Keep the chin tucked.

MOVEMENT

6. Press weight overhead until arms are fully extended.
7. Hold.
8. Slowly return weight to original position by flexing elbows and allowing shoulder blades to retract and depress.

Example Shoulder Power Exercises

Medicine Ball Scoop Toss

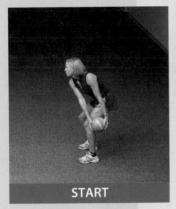
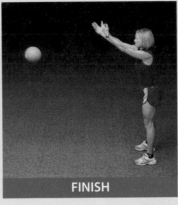

START

FINISH

PREPARATION

1. Stand with feet straight ahead, hip-width apart, knees slightly bent and lined up over second and third toes, hip neutral with abdomen drawn in, shoulders slightly retracted, and chin tucked.
2. Have a partner stand in front of you to receive and toss back the medicine ball.
3. Hold a medicine ball at the side of the hip.

MOVEMENT

4. Maintaining body alignment, rotate the body using the glutes and abs.
5. Toss the medicine ball to a partner as body rotates.
6. Use a scooping motion to catch ball as the partner tosses it back and repeat in a quick yet controlled fashion.
7. Repeat on both sides.

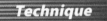

Technique   If a partner is unavailable, you can perform the exercise by tossing the medicine ball against a wall.

Medicine Ball Side Oblique Throw

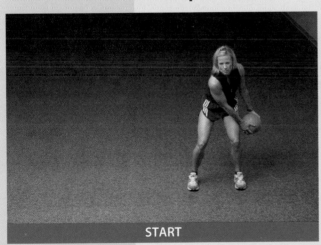
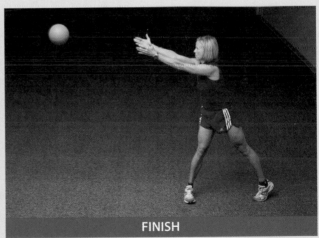

START

FINISH

PREPARATION

1. Stand with a partner positioned to the side.
2. Feet should be shoulder-width apart, toes pointing straight ahead, and knees flexed slightly over second and third toes.
3. Hold a medicine ball at the hip on the opposite side to the partner.

MOVEMENT

4. Maintaining body alignment, rotate the body using the glutes and abs, allowing the trailing leg to pivot. Keep navel drawn in.
5. Toss the medicine ball to a partner as body rotates.
6. Use a scooping motion to catch ball as the partner tosses it back and repeat in a quick yet controlled fashion.
7. Repeat on both sides.

BICEPS EXERCISE DESCRIPTIONS

Example Biceps Stabilization Exercises

Single-Leg Dumbbell Curl

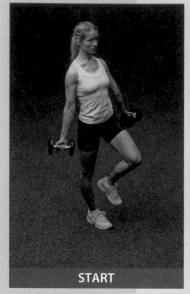
START

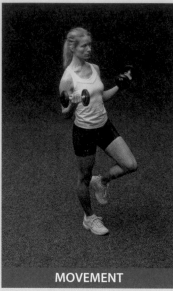
MOVEMENT

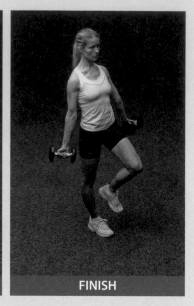
FINISH

PREPARATION

1. Stand on one foot with foot pointed straight ahead, and knee slightly flexed over second and third toes.
2. Allow arms to extend and hang to the sides of the body with a dumbbell in each hand.
3. Keep navel drawn in and keep hips level.

MOVEMENT

4. Perform a biceps curl by flexing the elbow.
5. Slowly return dumbbells to their original position by extending at the elbow.
6. Regression
   a. Two-leg
7. Progression
   a. Alternating-arm
   b. Single-arm
   c. Proprioceptive modalities

Technique

Keeping the scapula retracted during the exercise ensures proper scapular stability, placing more of an emphasis on the biceps musculature.

Single-Leg Barbell Curl

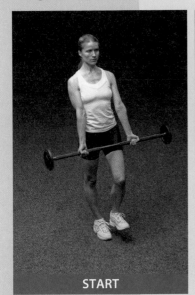
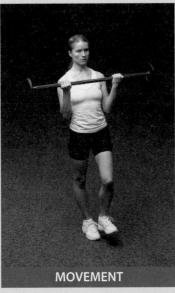
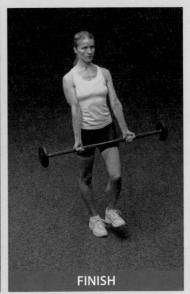

START   MOVEMENT   FINISH

PREPARATION

1. Stand on one foot with foot pointed straight ahead, and knee slightly flexed over second and third toes.
2. Hold a barbell in both hands (palms facing up) with arms extended in front of body.
3. Keep navel drawn in and keep hips level.

MOVEMENT

4. Perform a barbell curl by flexing both elbows, keeping the shoulder blades retracted.
5. Curl bar up to chest level.
6. Slowly lower the bar back to original position by extending the elbows.
7. Regression
   a. Two-leg
8. Progression
   a. Proprioceptive modalities

Safety   To decrease stress on the elbow, do not grip too close or too wide on the bar. To determine grip width, extend your elbows so your hands fall naturally to your sides, palms facing forward. Where your hands fall at your sides is the position where they should be when they grip the bar.

Example Biceps Strength Exercises

Seated Two-Arm Dumbbell Biceps Curl

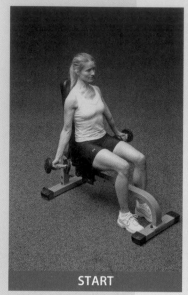

START

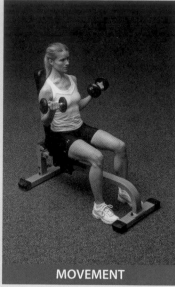

MOVEMENT

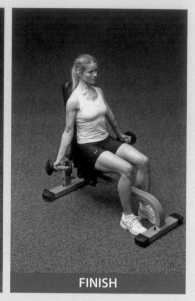

FINISH

PREPARATION

1. Sit on a bench with feet shoulder-width apart, pointing straight ahead.
2. Hold dumbbell in each hand with arms at sides.
3. Keep navel drawn in and keep hips level.

MOVEMENT

4. Perform a biceps curl by flexing the elbow.
5. Keep shoulder blades retracted throughout the exercise.
6. Slowly return dumbbells to their original position by extending at the elbow.

Biceps Curl Machine

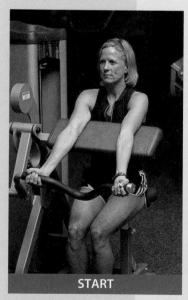

START

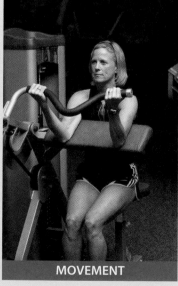

MOVEMENT

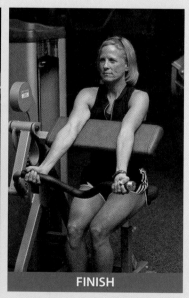

FINISH

PREPARATION

1. Sit at machine.
2. Make any adjustments necessary to fit body.

3. Select desired weight.
4. Keep navel drawn in.

MOVEMENT

5. Perform a curl by flexing elbows, while keeping shoulder blades retracted. Do not allow head to jut forward.
6. Curl until end range.
7. Slowly return weight to original position by extending elbows.

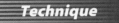

Technique   Make sure the seat is adjusted appropriately so the elbow is lined up with the axis of the machine and it is not too low, forcing elevation of the shoulders.

TRICEPS EXERCISE DESCRIPTIONS
Example Triceps Stabilization Exercises

Supine Ball Dumbbell Triceps Extensions

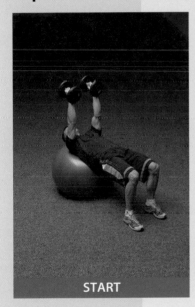
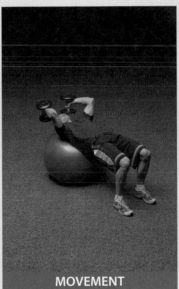
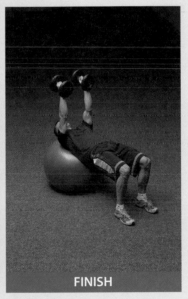

| START | MOVEMENT | FINISH |

PREPARATION

1. Lie on a stability ball, with ball between shoulder blades.
2. Maintain a bridge position by contracting glutes and keeping shoulders, hips, and knees level.
3. Feet should be shoulder-width apart with toes pointing straight ahead.
4. Hold dumbbells in each hand with the elbows in line with the shoulders.

MOVEMENT

5. Extend elbows until arms are straight.
6. Return dumbbells slowly toward chest by flexing elbows.
7. Regression
   a. On bench
8. Progressions
   a. Alternating-arms
   b. One-arm

Safety   When performing stability ball exercises in a supine position, make sure position is such that head comfortably rests on the ball. This will decrease stress to the cervical spine.

Prone Ball Dumbbell Triceps Extensions

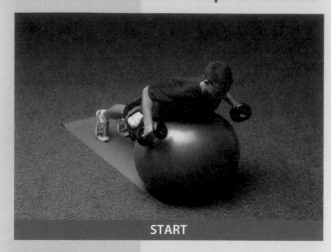

START

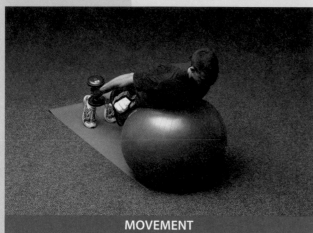

MOVEMENT

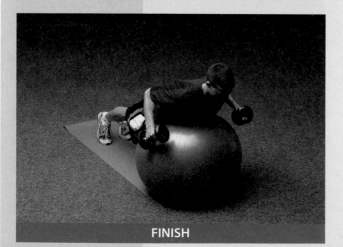

FINISH

PREPARATION

1. Lie in a prone position, with stability ball under abdomen.
2. Keep feet pointed down, legs completely straight, and navel drawn in.
3. Hold dumbbells in each hand with elbows bent and shoulder blades retracted and depressed.

MOVEMENT

4. Maintaining a retracted position, extend elbows so that they are parallel to the side of body.
5. Hold.
6. Slowly return dumbbells to original position by flexing elbows.
7. Regression
   a. Standing with cable
8. Progression
   a. Alternating-arms
   b. Single-arm

Technique

To ensure optimal alignment, make sure the ankle, knee, hips, elbow, shoulders, and ears are all in alignment and maintained throughout the exercise.

Example Triceps Strength Exercises

Cable Pushdown

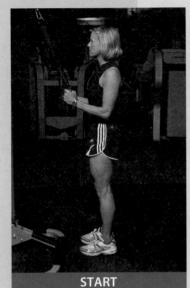 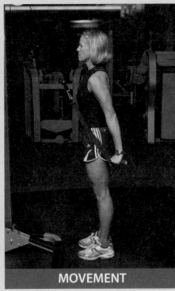 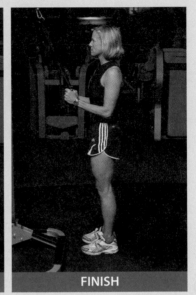

START   MOVEMENT   FINISH

PREPARATION

1. Stand with feet shoulder-width apart, pointed straight ahead, and knees slightly flexed over second and third toes.
2. Grasp a cable, with elbows flexed.
3. Keep shoulder blades retracted and depressed.
4. Keep navel drawn in.

MOVEMENT

5. Extend triceps by pushing hands toward the ground until arms are fully extended.
6. Hold.
7. Slowly return to the starting position.
8. Repeat.

Technique Using a rope when performing cable pushdowns will allow the elbows to track through their natural path of motion versus having the hands closely fixed on a bar. This may help decrease the risk of compensation when performing the exercise.

Supine Bench Barbell Triceps Extension

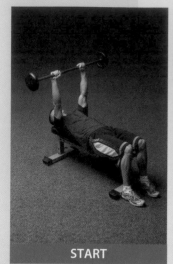

START

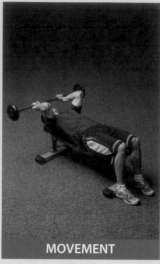

MOVEMENT

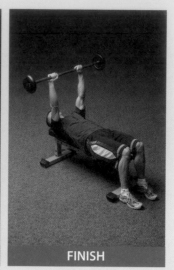

FINISH

PREPARATION

1. Lie on flat bench.
2. Feet should be flat and shoulder-width apart, with toes pointing straight ahead.
3. Hold barbell with elbows in line with the shoulders.
4. Maintain a drawn-in position.

MOVEMENT

5. Extend elbows until arms are straight.
6. Hold.
7. Slowly lower barbell toward forehead by flexing the elbows.
8. Repeat.

Safety

As with barbell curls, keeping the hands too close on the bar can increase stress on the elbow. Having your hands closer to shoulder width apart can help to decrease stress to the elbow and compensation.

LEG EXERCISE DESCRIPTIONS

Example Leg Stabilization Exercises

Ball Squat

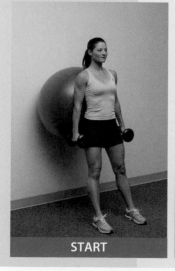

START

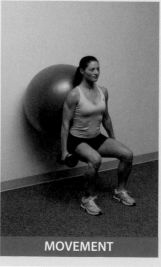

MOVEMENT

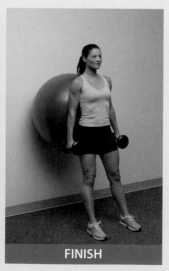

FINISH

PREPARATION

1. Stand with feet shoulder-width apart, toes pointing forward, and knees over second and third toes. Hold dumbbells to the side of the body.
2. Rest back against a stability ball, which is placed on a wall.
3. Ideally, keep feet under the knees. For individuals who lack ankle dorsiflexion (tight calves), place the feet slightly in front of the knees.

MOVEMENT

4. Slowly begin to squat down, bending knees and flexing hips, keeping feet straight (as if sitting into a chair). Keep the knees in line with the toes and the navel drawn in.
5. Allow the pelvis to sit back under the ball while maintaining a neutral spine.
6. Keep the chest up and put pressure through the heels. Do not rely solely on the ball for support.
7. To rise back up, contract glutes and place pressure through the heels as knees are extended.
8. Stand up straight until hips and legs are fully extended. Avoid compensation in the low back or lower extremities.
9. Regression
   a. Decrease range of motion
   b. Holding on to a stable support
10. Progression
    c. Squat without stability ball

Safety

Ball squats are a great way to teach individuals how to squat properly with the goal to have them to eventually progress to squats without the stability ball.

Multiplanar Step-Up to Balance

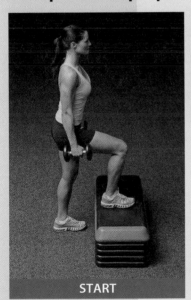 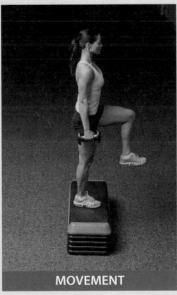 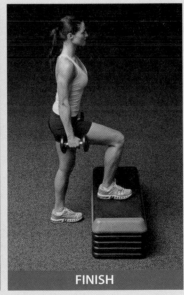

| START | MOVEMENT | FINISH |

PREPARATION

1. Stand in front of box, with feet shoulder-width apart and pointed straight ahead. Hold dumbbells to the side.

MOVEMENT

2. Step onto box with one leg, keeping foot pointed straight ahead and knee lined up over mid-foot.
3. Push through heel and stand up straight, balancing on one leg. Keep navel drawn in.
4. Flex the other leg at the hip and knee.

5. Dorsiflex the foot.
6. Return "floating" leg to the ground and step off the box, maintaining optimal alignment.
7. Repeat on other leg.
8. Regression
   a. Omit balance
   b. Decrease step height
9. Progression
   a. Frontal plane step-up
   b. Transverse plane step-up

Technique Lunges are excellent lower extremity strengthening exercises; however, many individuals lack the flexibility and stabilization requirements to execute the exercise properly. Step-ups are a great way to regress the lunge until one develops proper flexibility and stabilization capabilities to perform the lunge.

Example Leg Strength Exercises

Leg Press

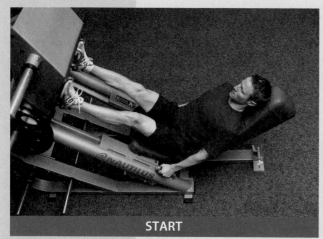
START

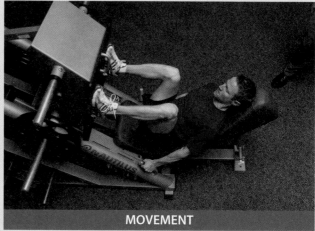
MOVEMENT

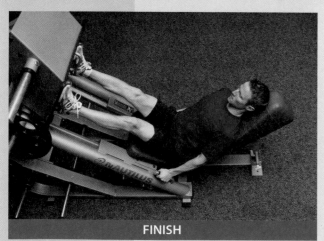
FINISH

PREPARATION

1. Sit in machine.
2. Make any adjustments necessary to fit body.
3. Place feet shoulder-width apart, with toes pointing forward and knees directly over second and third toes.
4. Keep the navel drawn in.

MOVEMENT

5. Slowly lower weight toward body by flexing at the knees and hips. Keep optimal alignment of the lower extremity throughout the movement.
6. Before any compensation occurs, activate glutes and apply pressure through heels to push the load up and extend legs.

Technique Make sure the feet are positioned on the platform hip-to-shoulder-width apart, toes are pointed straight, and the knees track in line with the toes. This will decrease stress to the knees, hips, and low back.

Barbell Squat

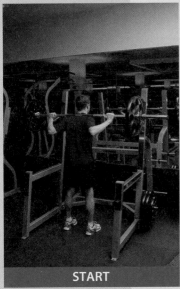

START

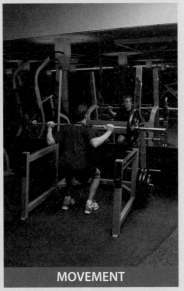

MOVEMENT

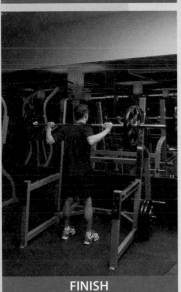

FINISH

PREPARATION

1. Stand with feet shoulder-width apart, toes pointing straight ahead, and knees over second and third toes.
2. Rest barbell on shoulders, behind neck, with hands grasping the bar wider than shoulder-width apart.

MOVEMENT

3. Slowly begin to squat down, bending knees and flexing hips, keeping feet straight. Do not allow the knees to move inward, and keep the navel drawn in.
4. Keep the chest up and put pressure through the heels.
5. Squat to a three-quarter position.
6. To rise back up, contract glutes and place pressure through the heels as knees are extended.
7. Stand up straight until hips and legs are fully extended. Avoid compensation in the low back or lower extremities.

Safety How far down should you squat? Only as far as can be controlled without compensating. As one develops more flexibility and stabilization strength, the range of motion can be increased assuming no compensation occurs.

Example Leg Power Exercises

Squat Jump

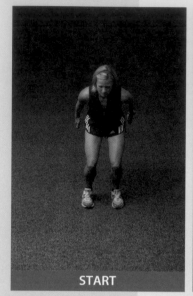

START

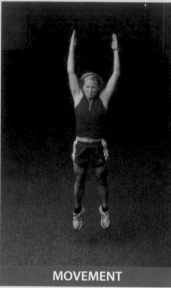

MOVEMENT

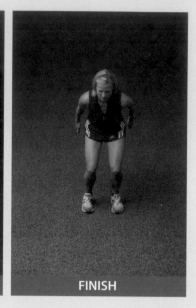

FINISH

PREPARATION

1. Stand with feet shoulder-width apart and pointed straight ahead and knee slightly flexed over second and third toes.
2. Place arms by sides.

MOVEMENT

3. Squat down slightly, keeping your navel drawn in.
4. Jump up into the air, using arms and extending them overhead.
5. Bring arms back to sides during landing.
6. Land softly on the mid-foot in a controlled manner with feet straight, knees over mid-foot. Repeat as quickly as can be controlled.

Tuck Jump

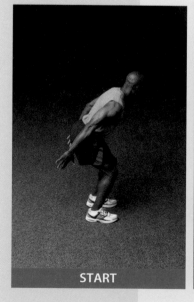

START

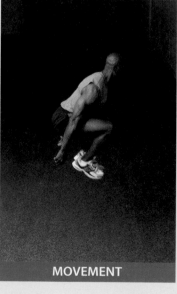

MOVEMENT

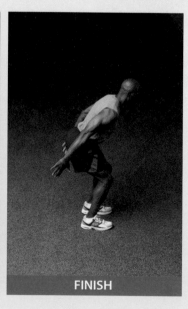

FINISH

PREPARATION

1. Draw navel in.
2. Stand with feet shoulder-width apart and pointed straight ahead, and knees aligned over mid-foot with arms by sides.

MOVEMENT

3. Jump up off the ground and, while in the air, bring knees up to chest.
4. Land softly on the midpoint of the feet, in a controlled manner, with feet straight and knees over mid-foot. Maintain control of entire body.
5. Repeat immediately, as quickly as can be controlled.

Technique When performing power exercises, make sure you land behind the ball of the foot (not on the ball of the foot or on the heel). This will ensure proper force distribution through the foot and lower extremity, improving force production capabilities.

FILLING IN THE TEMPLATE

The information contained in this chapter provides the health and fitness professional with the essentials to more effectively manipulate clients' programs. Having an understanding of how the body works, the different types of strengths, and different ways to train allows the health and fitness professional to gain insight into the construction of a properly designed integrated training program. This information combined with that of the following chapter allows the fitness professional to properly fill in the resistance-training portion of the OPT™ program template. Fill in the template according to the example in Figure 12-6.

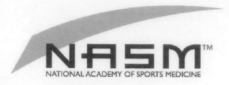

OPT For Fitness

Name: John Smith	Month: 1
Date : 08/10/06	Week: 1
Professional Scott Lucett	Day: 1 of 12

Program Goal: Fat Loss

STEP 1

A. Foam Roll

Foam Roll	Sets	Duration
Calves	1	30 sec.
IT Band	1	30 sec.
Adductors	1	30 sec.

B. Stretch

Static Stretching	Sets	Duration
Calves	1	30 sec.
Hip Flexors	1	30 sec.
Adductors	1	30 sec.

C. Cardiovascular

Treadmill	5-10 min.

STEP 2

A. Core

Exercise	Sets	Reps	Tempo	Rest
Floor Bridge	2	12	Slow	0
Floor Prone Cobra	2	12	Slow	0

B. Balance

Exercise	Sets	Reps	Tempo	Rest
Single-leg Balance	2	12	Slow	0

C. Reactive

Exercise	Sets	Reps	Tempo	Rest
Squat Jump w/ Stabilization	2	5	Controlled	90 sec.

STEP 3

Resistance Training Program

Body Part	Exercise	Sets	Reps	Intensity	Tempo	Rest
Total Body	Ball Squat, Curl to Press	2	12	60%	4-2-1	0
Chest	Push Up	2	12	60%	4-2-1	0
Back	Standing Cable Row	2	12	60%	4-2-1	0
Shoulder	Single-leg Dumbbell Scaption	2	12	60%	4-2-1	0
Biceps	*Optional*					
Triceps	*Optional*					
Legs	Front Step Up to Balance	2	12	60%	4-2-1	90 sec.

STEP 4

Cool-Down

Repeat Steps 1A and 1B

Figure 12.6 Filled-out resistance-training section of the template.

Review Questions

1 In which category does the specific adaptation of muscular endurance fall?

a. Power

b. Strength

c. Stability

2 Connective tissues (such as ligaments and tendons) adapt just as quickly as muscles.

a. True

b. False

3 _____ training is promoted as being more beneficial for strength and hypertrophy gains in advanced clients.

a. Single-set

b. Multiple-set

4 _____ loading refers to performing all sets of an exercise or body part before moving on to the next exercise or body part.

a. Vertical

b. Horizontal

5 Strength endurance allows the body to use lower levels of force with lower repetitions and fewer sets.

a. True

b. False

REFERENCES

1. Fleck SJ, Schutt RC. Types of strength training. Clin Sports Med 1985;4:159–167.
2. Pearson D, Faigenbaum A, Conley M, Kraemer WJ. The NSCA Basic Guidelines for the Resistance Training of Athletes. Strength Cond J 2000;22(4):14–27.
3. Stone MH, Collins D, Plisk S, Haff G, Stone ME. Training principles: evaluation of modes and methods of resistance training. Strength Cond J 2000;22(3):65–76.
4. Tan B. Manipulating resistance training program variables to optimize maximum strength in men: a review. J Strength Cond Res 1999;13(3):289–304.
5. Brooks GA, Fahey TD, White TP. Exercise Physiology: Human Bioenergetics and Its Application, 2nd ed. Mountain View, CA: Mayfield Publishing Company, 1996.
6. Selye H. The Stress of Life. New York: McGraw-Hill, 1976.
7. Kraemer WJ, Ratamess NA. Physiology of resistance training. Ortho Phys Ther Clin North Am 2000;9(4):467–513.
8. Alter MJ. Science of Flexibility, 2nd ed. Human Kinetics, 1996.
9. Gross J, Fetto J, Rosen E. Musculoskeletal Examination. Malden, MA: Blackwell Sciences, 1996.
10. Nordin M, Lorenz T, Campello M. Biomechanics of tendons and ligaments. In: Nordin M, Frankel VH (eds). Basic Biomechanics of the Musculoskeletal System,3rd ed. Philadelphia: Lippincott Williams & Wilkins, 2001.
11. Kannus P. Structure of the tendon connective tissue. Scand J Med Sci Sports 2000;10(6):312–320.
12. Adams K, O'Shea JP, O'Shea KL, Climstein M. The effect of six weeks of squat, plyometric and squat-plyometric training power production. J Appl Sports Sci Res 1992;6:36–41.
13. Bompa TO. Theory and Methodology of Training. Dubuque, IA: Kendall/Hunt, 1983.

14. Bompa TO. Variations of periodization of strength. Strength Cond J 1996;18:58–61.
15. Canavan PK, Garret GE, Armstrong LE. Kinematic and kinetic relationships between an Olympic style lift and the vertical jump. J Strength Cond Res 1996;10:127–130.
16. Ebben WP, Watts PB. A review of combined weight training and plyometric training modes: complex training. Strength Cond J 1998;20(5):18–27.
17. Fees MA. Complex training. Athl Ther Today 1997;2(1):18.
18. Fleck S, Kontor K. Complex training. Strength Cond J 1986;8(5):66–68.
19. Graves JE, Pollock ML, Jones AE, Colvin AB, Leggett SH. Specificity of limited range of motion variable resistance training. Med Sci Sports Exerc 1989;21:84–89.
20. Haff GG, Stone MH, O'Bryant HS, et al. Force-time dependent characteristics of dynamic and isometric muscle contractions. J Strength Cond Res 1997;11:269–272.
21. Hakkinen K, Allen M, Komi PV. Changes in isometric force—and relaxation—time, electromyographic and muscle fiber characteristics of human skeletal muscle during strength training and detraining. Acta Physiol Scand 1985;125:573–585.
22. Hennessey LC, Watson AW. The interference effects of training for strength and endurance simultaneously. J Strength Cond Res 1994;8:12–19.
23. Hickson RC. Interference of strength development by simultaneously training for strength and endurance. Eur J Appl Physiol 1980;45:255–263.
24. Hickson RC, Rosenkoetter MA, Brown MM. Strength training effects on aerobic power and short term endurance. Med Sci Sports Exerc 1980;12:336–339.
25. Hurley BF, Seals DR, Ehsani AA, Cartier LJ, Dalsky GP, Hagberg JM, Hollososzy JO. Effects of high-intensity strength training on cardiovascular function. Med Sci Sports Exerc 1984;16:483–488.
26. Kaneko M, Fuchimoto T, Toji H, Suei K. Training effect of different loads on the force-velocity relationship and mechanical power output in human muscle. Scand J Sports Sci 1983;5(2):50–55.
27. Lyttle AD, Wilson GJ, Ostrowski KJ. Enhancing performance: maximal power versus combined weights and plyometric training. J Strength Cond Res 1996;10:173–179.
28. Mateeva L. The speed strength correlation with the explosive strength development (abstract). Teniorska Missal 1988;6:23–24.
29. McBride J, Triplett-McBride T, Davie A, Newton RU. A comparison of strength and power characteristics between power lifters, Olympic lifters, and sprinters. J Strength Cond Res 1999;13:58–66.
30. Morrissey MC, Harman EA, Johnson MJ. Resistance training modes: specificity and effectiveness. Med Sci Sports Exerc 1986;18:612–624.
31. Moss BM, Refsnes PE, Abildgaard A, Nicolayysen K, Jensen J. The effects of maximal effort strength training with different loads on dynamic strength, cross-sectional area, load-power and load-velocity relationships. Eur J Appl Physiol 1997;75:193–199.
32. Newton RU, Kraemer WJ. Developing explosive muscular power: implications for a mixed methods training strategy. Strength Cond J 1994;16(5):20–31.
33. Newton RU, Kraemer WJ, Hakkinene K, Humphries BJ, Murphy AJ. Kinematics, kinetics and muscle activation during explosive upper body movements. J Appl Biomech 1996;12:31–43.
34. Newton RU, Murphy AJ, Humphries BJ, Wilson GJ, Kraemer WJ, Hakkinen K. Influence of load and stretch shortening cycle on the kinematics, kinetics and muscle activation that occurs during explosive upper-body movements. Eur J Appl Physiol 1997;75:333–342.
35. O'Shea P. Effects of selected weight training programs on the development of strength and muscle hypertrophy. Res Q 1966;37:95–102.
36. Paavolainen L, Hakkinen K, Hamalainen I, et al. Explosive strength training improves 5-km running time by improving running economy and muscle power. J Appl Physiol 1999;86:1527–1533.
37. Polhemus R, Burkherdt E, Osina M, Patterson M. The effect of plyometric training with ankle and vest weights on conventional weight training programs for men. Track Field Q Rev 1980;80(4):59–61.
38. Robinson JM, Stone MH, Johnson RL, Penland CM, Warren BJ, Lewis RD. Effects of different weight training exercise/rest intervals on strength, power, and high intensity exercise endurance. J Strength Cond Res 1995;9:216–221.
39. Rutherford OM, Greig CA, Sargent AJ, Jones DA. Strength training and power output: transference effects in the human quadriceps muscle. J Sport Sci 1986;4:101–107.
40. Sale DG. Influence of exercise and training on motor unit activation. Exer Sport Sci Rev 1987;15:95–151.
41. Schmidtbleicher D. Training for power events. In: Komi PV (ed). Strength and Power in Sports. Boston: Blackwell Scientific, 1992.
42. Schmidtbleicher D, Haralambie G. Changes in contractile properties of muscle after strength training in a man. Eur J Appl Physiol 1981;46:221–228.
43. Sforzo GA, Touey PR. Manipulating exercise order affects muscular performance during a resistance exercise training session. J Strength Cond Res 1996;10:20–24.
44. Verkhoshansky Y. Perspectives in the improvement of speed—strength preparation of jumpers. Track Field 1966;9:11–12.
45. Verkhoshansky Y. Speed-strength preparation and development of strength endurance of athletes in various specializations. Sov Sports Rev 1986;21:120–124.
46. Verkhoshansky Y, Tatyan V. Speed-strength preparation of future champions. Legkaya Atletika 1973;2:12–13.

47. Wenzel RR, Perfetto EM. The effect of speed versus non-speed training in power development. J Appl Sport Sci Res 1992;6:82–87.
48. Wilson GJ, Newton RU, Murphy AJ, Humphries BJ. The optimal training load for the development of dynamic athletic performance. Med Sci Sports Exerc 1993;25:1279–1286.
49. Yessis M. Integrating plyometrics with strength training. Fitness Sports Rev Int 1995; 28(4):113–116.
50. Young WB. Training for speed-strength: heavy versus light loads. Strength Cond J 1993;15 (5):34–42.
51. Zatsiorsky VM. Science and Practice of Strength Training. Champaign, IL: Human Kinetics, 1995.
52. Behm DG. Neuromuscular implications and applications of resistance training. J Strength Cond Res 1995;9:264–274.
53. Kovaleski JE, Heitman RH, Trundle TL, Gilley WF. Isotonic preload versus isokinetic knee extension resistance training. Med Sci Sports Exerc 1995;27:895–899.
54. Noose LJ, Hunter GR. Free weights: a review supporting their use in rehabilitation. Athl Train 1985;Fall:206–209.
55. Sale DG. Neural adaptation in strength and power training. In: Jones NL, McCartney N, McComas AJ (eds). Human Muscle Power. Champaign, IL: Human Kinetics, 1986.
56. Wilson GJ, Murphy AJ, Walshe A. The specificity of strength training: the effect of posture. Eur J Appl Physiol 1996;73:346–352.
57. Siff MC, Verkhoshansky Y. Supertraining. Escondido, CA: Sports Training, 1994.
58. Rutherford OM, Jones DA. The role of learning and coordination in strength training. Eur J Appl Physiol 1986;55:100–105.
59. Hakkinen K. Neuromuscular adaptation during strength training, aging, detraining and immobilization. Crit Rev Phys Rehab Med 1994;6:161–198.
60. Siff MC, Verkhoshansky Y. Supertraining. Escondido, CA: Sports Training, 1994.
61. McEvoy KP, Newton RU. Baseball throwing speed and base running speed: the effects of ballistic resistance training. J Strength Cond Res 1998;12(4):216–221.
62. Moritani T, Muro M, Ishida K, Taguchi S. Electrophysiological analyses of the effects of muscle power training. Res J Phys Educ Jap 1987;1:23–32.
63. Miller J. Medicine ball training for throwers. Strength Cond J 1987;9(1):32–33.
64. Hamilton MT, Booth FW. Skeletal muscle adaptation to exercise: a century of progress. J Appl Physiol 2000;88(1):327–331.
65. Franklin BA, Roitman JL. Cardiorespiratory adaptations to exercise. In: American College of Sports Medicine (ed). ACSM's Resource Manual for Guidelines for Exercise Testing and Prescription, 3rd ed. Baltimore: Williams & Wilkins, 1998.
66. Viru A, Viru M. Nature of training effects. In: Garrett WE, Kirkendall DT (eds). Exercise and Sport Science. Philadelphia: Lippincott Williams & Wilkins, 2000.
67. MacDougall JD, Hicks AL, MacDonald JR, McKelvie RS, Green HJ, Smith KM. Muscle performance and enzymatic adaptations to sprint interval training. J Appl Physiol 1998;84(6):2138–2142.
68. Harmer AR, McKenna MJ, Sutton JR, Snow RJ, Ruell PA, Booth J, Thompson MW, Mackay NA, Stathis CG, Crameri RM, Carey MF, Eager DM. Skeletal muscle metabolic and ionic adaptations during intense exercise following sprint training in humans. J Appl Physiol 2000;89(5): 1793–1803.
69. Parra J, Cadefau JA, Rodas G, Amigo N, Cusso R. The distribution of rest periods affects performance and adaptations of energy metabolism induced by high-intensity training in human muscle. Acta Physiol Scand 2000;169(2):157–165.
70. Ogita F, Stam RP, Tazawa HO, Toussaint HM, Hollander AP. Oxygen uptake in one-legged and two-legged exercise. Med Sci Sports Exerc 2000;32(10):1737–1742.
71. Williford HN, Olson MS, Gauger S, Duey WJ, Blesing DL. Cardiovascular and metabolic costs of forward, backward, and lateral motion. Med Sci Sports Med 1998;30(9):1419–1423.
72. Heus R, Wertheim AH, Havenith G. Human energy expenditure when walking on a moving platform. Eur J Appl Physiol Occup Physiol 1998;100(2):133–148.
73. Fleck SJ, Kraemer WJ. Designing Resistance Training Programs, 2nd ed. Champaign, IL: Human Kinetics, 1997.
74. Sale DG. Neural adaptation to resistance training. Med Sci Sports Exerc 1988;20(5 Suppl): S135–S145.
75. Sale DG, MacDougall JD, Upton AR, McComas AJ. Effect of strength training upon motorneuron excitability in man. Med Sci Sports Exerc 1983;15(1):57–62.
76. Enoka RM. Muscle strength and its development: new perspectives. Sports Med 1988;6:146–168.
77. Henneman E. Relation between size of motor neurons and their susceptibility to discharge. Science 1957,126.1345–1347.
78. Cosio-Lima LM, Reynolds KL, Winter C, Paolone V, Jones MT. Effects of Physioball and conventional floor exercises on early adaptations in back and abdominal core stability and balance in women. J Strength Cond Res 2003;17(4):721–725.
79. Behm DG, Anderson K, Curnew RS. Muscle force and activation under stable and unstable conditions. J Strength Cond Res 2002;16(3):416–422.
80. Heitkamp HC, Horstmann T, Mayer F, Weller J, Dickhuth HH. Gain in strength and muscular balance after balance training. Int J Sports Med 2001;22:285–290.

81. Bellew JW, Yates JW, Gater DR. The initial effects of low-volume strength training on balance in untrained older men and women. J Strength Cond Res 2003;17(1):121–128.

82. MacDougall JD, Sale DG, Always SE, Sutton JR. Muscle ultrastructural characteristics of elite powerlifters and bodybuilders. Eur J Appl Physiol 1982;48:117–126.

83. Always SE, Grumby WH, Stray-Gunderson J, Gonyea WJ. Effects of resistance training on elbow flexors of highly competitive bodybuilders. J Appl Physiol 1992;72:1512–1521.

84. Thorstenson A, Hultren B., von Dobeln W, Karlsson J. Effect of strength training on enzyme activities and fibre characteristics in human skeletal muscle. Acta Physiol Scand 1976;96:392–398.

85. MacDougal JD, Elder GCB, Sale DG, Moroz JR, Sutton JR. Effects of strength training and immobilization on human muscle fibers. Eur J Appl Physiol 1980;43:25–34.

86. Abernathy PJ, Jurimae J, Logan PA, Taylor AW, Thayer RE. Acute and chronic response of skeletal muscle to resistance exercise. Sports Med 1994;17(1):22–38.

87. McDonagh MJM, Davies CTM. Adaptive response to mammalian muscle to exercise with high loads. Eur J Appl Physiol 1984;52:139–159.

88. Hakkinen K, Komi PV. Electromyographic changes during strength training and detraining. Med Sci Sports Exerc 1983;15(6):455–460.

89. Narici MV, Roi GS, Landoni L, Minetti AE, Cerretelli P. Changes in force, cross-sectional area and neural activation during strength training and detraining of the human quadriceps. Eur J Appl Physiol 1989;59:310–319.

90. Moritani T, deVries HA. Neural factors versus hypertrophy in the time course of muscle strength gain. Am J Phys Med 1979;58(3):115–129.

91. Komi PV, Viitasalo JT, Rauramaa R, Vihko V. Effect of isometric strength training on mechanical, electrical, and metabolic aspects of muscle function. Eur J Appl Physiol 1978;40:45–55.

92. Mayhew TP, Rothstein JM, Finucane SD, Lamb RL. Muscular adaptation to concentric and eccentric exercise at equal power levels. Med Sci Sports Exerc 1995;27:868–873.

93. Staron RS, Karapondo DL, Kraemer WJ, et al. Skeletal muscle adaptations during early phase of heavy resistance training in men and women. J Appl Physiol 1994;76:1247–1255.

94. Chelsey A, Macdougal JD, Tarnopolsky MA, Atkinson SA, Smith K. Changes in human muscle protein synthesis after resistance exercise. J Appl Physiol 1992;73:1383–1388.

95. Booth FW, Thomason DB. Molecular and cellular adaptation of muscle in response to exercise: perspectives of various models. Physiol Rev 71:541–585.

96. Fry AC, Allemeier CA, Staron CS. Correlation between percentage fiber type area and myosin heavy chain content in human skeletal muscle. Eur J Appl Physiol 1994;68:246–251.

97. Kraemer WJ, Fleck SJ, Evans WJ. Strength and power training: physiological mechanisms of adaptation. In: Holloszy JO (ed). Exercise and Sport Science Reviews, vol 24. Baltimore: Williams & Wilkins, 1998:363–397.

98. Staron RS, Leonardi MJ, Karapondo DL, et al. Strength and skeletal muscle adaptations in heavy-resistance-trained women after detraining and retraining. J Appl Physiol 1991;70:631–640.

99. Enoka RM. Neuromechanical Basis of Kinesiology, 2nd ed. Champaign, IL: Human Kinetics, 1994.

100. Enoka RM. Neuromechanics of Human Movement, 3rd ed. Champaign, IL: Human Kinetics, 2002.

101. Brown HS, Stein RB, Yemm R. Changes in firing rate of human motor units during linearly changing voluntary contractions. J Physiol (Lond) 1973;230:371–390.

102. Marx JO, Kraemer WJ, Nindl BC, Gotshalk LA, Duncan ND, Volek JS, Hakkinen K, Newton RU. The effect of periodization and volume of resistance training in women (abstract). Med Sci Sports Exerc 1998;30(5):S164.

103. Kraemer WJ, Ratamess N, Fry AC, Triplett-McBride T, Koziris LP, Bauer JA, Lynch JM, Fleck SJ. Influence of resistance training volume and periodization on physiological and performance adaptations in college women tennis players. Am J Sports Med 2000;28(5):626–633.

104. Starkey DB, Pollock ML, Ishida Y, et al. Effect of resistance training volume on strength and muscle thickness. Med Sci Sports Exerc 1996;28:1311–1320.

105. Jacobson BH. A comparison of two progressive weight training techniques on knee extensor strength. Athl Train 1986;21:315–319.

106. Reid CM, Yeater RA, Ullrich IH. Weight training and strength, cardiorespiratory functioning and body composition of men. Br J Sports Med 1987;21:40–44.

107. American College of Sports Medicine. Position stand: the recommended quantity and quality of exercise for developing and maintaining cardiorespiratory and muscular fitness in healthy adults. Med Sci Sports Exerc 1990;22:265–274.

108. Stone MH, Plisk SS, Stone ME, Schilling BK, O'Bryant HS, Pierce KC. Athletic performance development: volume load-1 set vs. multiple sets, training velocity and training variation. Strength Cond J 1998;20(6):22–31.

109. Logan GA. Differential applications of resistance and resultant strength measured at varying degrees of knee flexion. Doctoral dissertation, University of Southern California, Los Angeles, CA, 1960.

110. Harris GR, Stone MH, O'Bryant H, Proulx CM, Johnson R. Short-term performance effects of high speed, high force and combined weight training. J Strength Cond Res 2000;14:14–20.

111. Kraemer WJ. A series of studies: the physiological basis for strength training in American football: fact over philosophy. J Strength Cond Res 1997;11:131–142.

112. Kraemer WJ, Newton RU, Bush J, Volek J, Triplett NT, Koziris LP. Varied multiple set resistance training produces greater gains than single set program (abstract). Med Sci Sports Exerc 1995;27(5 Suppl):S195.
113. O'Bryant H, Byrd R, Stone MH. Cycle ergometer and maximum leg and hip strength adaptations to two different methods of weight training. J Appl Sports Sci Res 1988;2(2):27–30.
114. Schoitz MK, Potteiger JA, Huntsinger PG, Denmark DC. The short-term effects of periodized and constant-intensity training on body composition, strength and performance. J Strength Cond Res 1998;12(3):173–178.
115. Hakkinen K, Pakarinen A, Alen M, et al. Relationships between training volume, physical performance capacity, and serum hormone concentrations during prolonged training in elite weight lifters. Int J Sports Med 1987;8(Suppl):61–65.
116. Hakkinen K, Pakarinen A, Alen M, et al. Neuromuscular and hormonal responses in elite athletes to two successive strength training sessions in one day. Eur J Appl Physiol 1988;57:133–139.
117. Haltom RW, Kraemer R, Sloan R, Hebert EP, Frank K, Tryniecki JL. Circuit weight training and its effects on postexercise oxygen consumption. Med Sci Sports Exerc 1999;31(11):1613–1618.
118. Burleson MA, O'Bryant HS, Stone MH, Collins MA, Triplett-McBride T. Effect of weight training exercise and treadmill exercise on post-exercise oxygen consumption. Med Sci Sports Exerc 1998;30(4):518–522.
119. Gambetta V. The Gambetta Method: Common Sense Training for Athletic Performance. Sarasota, FL: Gambetta Sports Training Systems, 1998.

Program Design Concepts

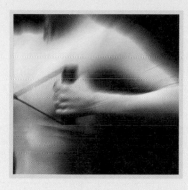

OBJECTIVES

After completing this chapter, you will be able to:

- Define and describe the acute training variables within the Optimum Performance Training (OPT™) model.
- Describe the phases within the OPT™ model.
- Design programs for each phase of training.

KEY TERMS

Acute variables
Annual plan
Exercise selection
Monthly plan
Program design

Repetition
Repetition tempo
Rest interval
Set
Training duration

Training frequency
Training intensity
Training plan
Weekly plan

Program Design

INTRODUCTION TO PROGRAM DESIGN

Traditionally, most training programs are based on the experiences of the health and fitness professional (whether he or she is a bodybuilder, group exercise instructor, power lifter, Olympic lifter, or an athlete). This has led to many scientifically unsupported training programs that have created confusion for health and fitness professionals. Indeed, science has been slow to validate anecdotal evidence that still continues to be used in the fitness world.[1,2]

To be safe, effective, and productive, all health and fitness professionals must be competent at designing resistance-training programs for a variety of clients. This entails the proper utilization of acute variables (repetitions, sets, and so forth) and exercises in a structured, progressive manner. For many health and fitness professionals, this can become a daunting task, causing them to ask, "How many exercises should I use? How many sets and repetitions should I use? How many days per week should my client train?" When using a structured, scientifically based program design model, answers to these questions become very simple.

WHAT IS PROGRAM DESIGN?

Program design: A purposeful system or plan put together to help an individual achieve a specific goal.

Program design simply means creating a purposeful system or plan to achieve a specific goal. The key words here are "purposeful system." The purpose of a training program is to provide a path for the client to achieve his or her goal. Providing a path requires the health and fitness professional to have a comprehensive understanding of a few key concepts:

Acute Variables

- What are they?
- How do they affect the desired adaptation?
- How do they affect the overall training program?

The OPT™ Model (Planned Fitness Training—Periodization)

- How and why must the physiologic, physical, and performance adaptations of stabilization, strength, and power take place in a planned, progressive manner to establish the proper foundation for each subsequent adaptation?

The Five Phases of Training in the OPT™ Model

- How do these phases promote specific adaptations?
- What are the acute variables for each of the phases?

Application

- Selecting the right exercises.
- Selecting the right acute variables.
- Applying both in a systematic manner to different populations with different goals.

IS THERE AN EASIER WAY?

Taking the Guesswork Out

If a health and fitness professional has a proven system that he or she can follow, the needed information can simply be plugged in, without the worry of using the correct formula for success. This is exactly what the OPT™ model provides (Figure 13-1).

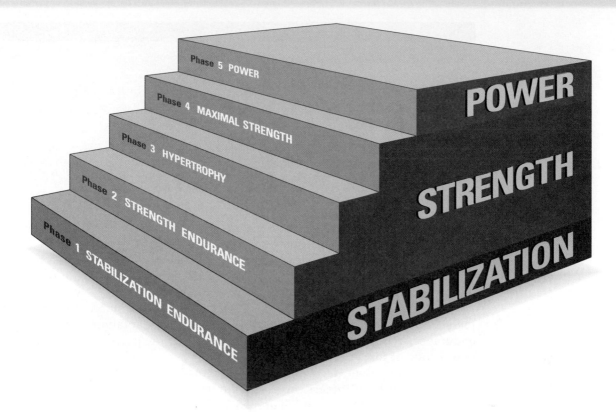

Figure 13.1 The OPT™ model.

NASM designed the OPT™ model as a planned, systematic, periodized training program. It was established to concurrently improve all functional abilities, such as flexibility, core stabilization, balance, power, strength, and cardiorespiratory endurance. The OPT™ program has been extremely successful in helping all populations to reduce body fat, increase lean muscle mass and strength, and improve performance and overall health.

The remaining modules of this chapter will detail acute variables of planned fitness training (or periodization) as it relates to the OPT™ model, the five phases of the OPT™ model, and how to apply the OPT™ program design model to various goals.

SUMMARY

Health and fitness professionals must be competent at designing training programs for a variety of clients, using acute variables and exercises in a structured, progressive manner. A structured, scientifically based program design model makes this easy. The Optimum Performance Training (OPT™) model provides the health and fitness professional with a proven system in which a client's information can simply be plugged in. Program design is creating a purposeful system or plan to achieve a specific goal. To do so, the health and fitness professional must understand acute variables, the OPT™ model, and its phases, as well as how to apply it all.

Acute Variables of Training

Acute variables: Important components that specify how each exercise is to be performed.

Acute variables are the most fundamental components of designing a training program. They determine the amount of stress placed on the body and, ultimately, what adaptations the body will incur.

The body will specifically adapt to the demands placed on it (known also as the principle of specificity). The acute variables dictate these demands.

Table 13.1

Program Design Continuum

Adaptation	Reps	Sets	Intensity	Rest Period
Power	1–10	3–6	30–45% of one rep max or ≤10% of body weight	3–5 min
Strength	1–12	2–6	70–100%	45 s–5 min
Stabilization	12–25	1–3	50–70%	0 s–1.5 min

The OPT™ model takes the guesswork out of program design and allows for a planned, systematic progression by preassigning specific acute variables for each of the five phases of training to elicit the desired adaptation.[3-11] Collectively, the acute variables are the foundation of program design and fall within the program design continuum seen in Table 13-1.

As discussed in Chapter 12—Resistance Training, the stabilization adaptation includes both endurance and stability, the strength adaptation includes strength endurance, hypertrophy, and maximal strength, and the power adaptation includes power (rate of force production).

To ensure proper development and progression of an integrated training program, the health and fitness professional must understand the acute training variables, which are shown in Figure 13-2. Each of the acute variables will be explained in this module as they relate to the OPT™ model.

REPETITIONS

Repetition (or "rep"): One complete movement of a single exercise.

A **repetition** is one complete movement of a particular exercise. Most repetitions will involve the three muscle actions, concentric, isometric, and eccentric (not necessarily in that order).

These muscle actions can be seen in the example of a biceps curl. A single repetition includes raising the dumbbell up against the direction of resistance (a concentric contraction), pausing for any specified amount of time (an isometric contraction), and then lowering the dumbbell with the direction of resistance back to its starting position (an eccentric contraction).

Another example of this can be seen when performing a squat. Starting from a standing position, one repetition includes lowering the body (with the direction of resistance) toward the ground (eccentric), pausing for any specified amount of time (isometric), and then raising back up (against the direction of resistance) to the starting position (concentric).

Repetitions are simply a means to count the number of movements performed in a given amount of time. They can therefore be a means to count the time the muscles are under tension (*time under tension*).

Each phase of training in the OPT™ model has specific goals and therefore requires a specific number of repetitions to achieve these goals. The number of repetitions performed in a given set is dependent on the client's work capacity, intensity of the exercise, and the specific phase of training.

- Repetitions
- Sets
- Training intensity
- Repetition tempo
- Training volume
- Rest interval
- Training frequency
- Training duration
- Exercise selection

Figure 13.2 Acute variables of training.

Table 13.2	
Repetition Continuum	
Training Adaptation	**Repetition Range**
Power	1–10
Strength	1–12
Stabilization	12–25

The health and fitness professional must keep in mind that all acute variables are interdependent. This means that the specific use of one will affect the others. For example, the more intense the exercise or heavier the load, the fewer the number of repetitions that the individual can perform.[11-17]

Research demonstrates that training in a specific repetition range yields specific adaptations.[11-15,17,18] Therefore, depending on the goal of the individual and the phase of training, it is possible to define a specific repetition range (Table 13-2).

- Power adaptations require 1 to 10 repetitions at 30 to 45% of the one-repetition maximum (1RM), or approximately 10% of body weight.
- If maximal strength adaptations are desired, the repetition range is one to five at 85 to 100% of the 1RM.
- Hypertrophy is best achieved using 8 to 12 repetitions at 70 to 85% of the 1RM.
- Endurance is best achieved by performing 12 to 25 repetitions at 50 to 70% of the 1RM.[11-17]

The OPT™ model uses the specified repetition continuum to provide the desired adaptations in a systematic manner. The beginning phases consist of higher repetition schemes necessary to build proper connective tissue strength, stability, and endurance. This is especially important for the beginning client. However, a common mistake of many advanced clients is to not use a planned training program that provides periods of low-repetition training alternated with periods of high-repetition training. Higher intensities of training (lower repetitions) can only be sustained for a short period without running the risk of overtraining.[19,20] Using the OPT™ model enables the health and fitness professional to use a systematic training approach to prevent overtraining and yield specific results by using planned intervals of training.[21]

SETS

Set: A group of consecutive repetitions.

A **set** is a group of consecutive repetitions.[14,16,17,22] The quantities of the other acute variables (i.e., repetitions, training intensity, number of exercises, training level, and recoverability) determine the number of sets an individual performs.[14,16,17,23]

There is an inverse relationship between sets, repetitions, and intensity. The individual usually performs fewer sets when performing higher repetitions at a lower intensity (endurance and hypertrophy adaptations) and more sets when performing lower repetitions at a higher intensity (strength and power adaptations), as seen in Table 13-3.[11,13,22]

- For power adaptations, three to six sets of between 1 and 10 repetitions at an intensity of 30 to 45% of 1RM or approximately 10% of body weight are recommended.
- For maximal strength adaptation, four to six sets of between one and five repetitions at an intensity of 85 to 100% of 1RM are recommended.

Table 13.3

Set Continuum

Training Adaptation	Set Range
Power	3–6
Strength	2–6
Stabilization	1–3

- Hypertrophy adaptations require three to four sets of 8 to 12 repetitions at 70 to 85% of 1RM intensity level.
- Endurance is best developed with one to three sets of 12 to 25 repetitions at 50 to 70% of 1RM intensity.[11,13,16,17,22]

It has been suggested that, to prevent overtraining, 24 to 36 total sets should be performed in a given workout (24 total sets for low volume or up to 36 total sets for high volume).[15] For the beginning client, this number may be as low as 5 to 12 total sets (one set of 5 to 12 exercises).

As a training program advances and the desired adaptations change from stabilization and endurance to hypertrophy or maximal strength, the number of sets capable of being performed will also change.

When training for strength adaptations, the number of sets performed needs to increase to place enough stress on the tissues to provoke the desired changes.[11,12,15] As shown in Table 13-4, a beginning client may perform one to two exercises per body part for two to three sets per exercise, whereas an advanced client may perform three to four exercises per body part for three to five sets per exercise. This manipulation will have a large impact on the total training volume and must be planned (periodized) with phases that include a higher and lower number of sets over the course of the training program. Also, using the numbers in Table 13-4 in conjunction with the total number of sets per workout discussed above (24 to 36 sets), it is clear that the intermediate and advanced client may only train two to three body parts per workout, owing to the total volume of training in a given workout and time constraints.

TRAINING INTENSITY

Training intensity: An individual's level of effort, compared with their maximal effort, which is usually expressed as a percentage.

Training intensity is one of the most important acute variables to consider when designing an integrated training program.[11,13,16,17,22] **Training intensity** is defined as an individual's level of effort compared with their maximum effort.[11,13]

The specific training phase and an individual's training goal will determine the number of sets and repetitions for an exercise. Intensity is then determined by the number of sets and repetitions to be performed, which is based on the individual's specific training goals (Table 13-5).

Table 13.4

Set Manipulations per Body Part

Client Level	Exercises per Body Part	Sets Each Exercise	Total Sets per Body Part
Beginning	1–2	2–3	2–6
Intermediate	2–3	3–4	6–12
Advanced	3–4	3–5	9–20

Table 13.5

Intensity Continuum

Training Adaptation	Intensity Range
Power	30–45% of 1RM or approximately 10% of body weight
Strength	70–100% of 1RM
Stabilization	50–70% of 1RM

1RM, one repetition maximum.

- Power (high velocity) adaptations are best attained with 30 to 45% of 1RM when using conventional weight training, or approximately 10% of body weight when using medicine balls.
- Maximum strength adaptations require training with 85 to 100% of 1RM.
- Hypertrophy is best achieved by training with 70 to 85% of 1RM.
- Endurance is best developed with a training intensity of 40 to 70% of 1RM.[8,14,22–33]

Training intensity can also be derived from the percent of maximal oxygen consumption, as in the case of cardiorespiratory training programs.[34,35]

Training in an unstable environment, as seen in the stabilization phases of the OPT™ model, can also increase the training intensity because it requires more motor unit recruitment. This leads to more energy expenditure per exercise,[36–39] which allows for optimum development of neuromuscular efficiency. Changing other acute training variables such as rest periods and tempo also changes the training intensity. In short, intensity is a function of more than just external resistance. An integrated training program must focus on a holistic approach to force continued adaptations.[32,40]

REPETITION TEMPO

Repetition tempo: The speed with which each repetition is performed.

Repetition tempo refers to the speed with which each repetition is performed. This is an important variable that can be manipulated to achieve specific training objectives such as power, hypertrophy, stability, and endurance.[11,13,16,17,41–47]

Movements also occur at different velocities. Therefore, to get the appropriate results from training, the health and fitness professional must select the appropriate speed of movement for the exercise, based on the repetition tempo spectrum (Table 13-6).[47]

Table 13.6

Repetition Tempo Spectrum

Training Adaptation	Repetition Tempo (Eccentric/Isometric/Concentric)
Power	Explosive (x/x/x)
Strength	Moderate (2/0/2)
Stabilization	Slow (4/2/1)

x/x/x, As fast as possible.

The amount of time that a muscle is under tension yields a specific result (*time under tension*). For example, the optimum tempo for hypertrophy is approximately 20 to 70 seconds per set (8 to 10 repetitions in a range between 4/2/1 and 2/0/2 tempos).[48] The optimum tempo for power is as fast as the individual can move.[41-44,47] Therefore, based on the client's specific goals, the health and fitness professional must use the entire repetition tempo spectrum to achieve the desired results.[11,15-17,42,43]

The OPT™ model places a major emphasis on the repetition tempo spectrum as it has a significant impact on the functional outcome of the stressed tissues. By emphasizing eccentric and isometric muscle actions at slower velocities during the initial stabilization phases of training, more demand is placed on the connective tissue (as well as the stabilizing muscles) and better prepares the nervous system for functional movements. This is important for building the appropriate structural and functional foundation for more specific forms of strength and power training that will follow.

REST INTERVAL

Rest interval: The time taken to recuperate between sets.

The **rest interval** is the time taken to recuperate between sets or exercises and has a dramatic effect on the outcome of the training program.[11,16,17,22,33,47] Each exercise that is performed requires energy. The primary type of energy used during training depends on the training phase, intensity, and goal (Table 13-7).[13,14]

Power and maximal strength adaptations may require up to 5 minutes of rest between sets and exercises, depending on the client's level of fitness. Hypertrophy adaptations are maximized by decreasing the rest interval to 45 to 90 seconds between sets and exercises, but are dependent on the load being used. Stability and endurance adaptations should involve 30 to 90 seconds of rest.

Dynamic resistance training, as well as isometric training, can significantly reduce adenosine triphosphate (ATP) and creatine phosphate (CP) supplies.[49,50] The ability to replenish these supplies is crucial for optimal performance and the desired adaptation. By adjusting the rest interval, energy supplies can be regained according to the goal of the training program. Rest intervals of:[51]

- 20 to 30 seconds will allow approximately 50% recovery of ATP and CP.
- 40 seconds will allow approximately 75% recovery of ATP and CP.
- 60 seconds will allow approximately 85 to 90% recovery of ATP and CP.
- 3 minutes will allow approximately 100% recovery of ATP and CP.

The rest interval between sets determines to what extent the energy resources are replenished before the next set.[13,14,47] The shorter the rest interval, the less ATP and CP will be replenished and consequently less energy will be available for the next set.[11] In the beginner client, this can result in fatigue, which can lead to decreased neuromuscular control, force production, and stabilization by decreasing motor unit recruitment.[52,53] Therefore, inadequate rest intervals can decrease performance and could lead to excessive compensation and even injury. As the

Table 13.7		
Rest Interval Continuum		
Training Adaptation	**Rest Interval**	**Energy Source**
Power	3–5 min	ATP-CP
Strength	45 s–5 min	ATP-CP and glycolysis
Stabilization	0 s–1.5 min	Oxidative and glycolysis

ATP, adenosine triphosphate; *CP*, creatine phosphate.

- Training experience
- Training intensity
- Tolerance of short rest periods
- Muscle mass
- General fitness level
- Training goals
- Nutritional status
- Recoverability

Figure 13.3   Factors for appropriate rest intervals.

client advances, this can be used as a means to increase the intensity of the workout and promote better adaptations especially for stability, endurance, and hypertrophy.

Conversely, if rest periods are too long between sets or exercises, the potential effects include decreased neuromuscular activity and decreased body temperature. If the beginner client is then asked to perform an intense bout of exercise, this could entail a potential increased risk of injury. For the advanced client, this may be necessary if heavy weight is being used repetitively. The goal of the training program should establish the appropriate rest periods.[11,14,15] There are several factors to consider when prescribing appropriate rest intervals (Figure 13-3). [11,13,15]

Individuals who are beginning an integrated training program may respond better to longer rest periods (60 to 90 seconds) until they adjust to the demands of their program. This also helps to ensure proper neuromuscular efficiency. By decreasing the amount of fatigue experienced by the client, that individual will be able to recruit the appropriate motor units and perform each exercise with greater precision. Individuals who are at advanced levels of training and have larger muscle mass or higher fitness levels may respond better to shorter rest periods, but it is still dependent on the phase of training and the goal.

TRAINING VOLUME

Training volume: Amount of physical training performed within a specified period.

Training volume is the total amount of work performed within a specified time.[13,16,17,23,34] It is extremely important to plan and control training volume to prevent overtraining, as all training is cumulative.[19-21] Training volume varies among individuals and is based on:

- Training phase
- Goals
- Age
- Work capacity
- Recoverability
- Nutritional status
- Injury history

For an individual to achieve optimum results from an integrated training program, the program must provide them with the appropriate planned training volume for extended periods (Table 13-8).[21]

One of the most important training concepts to remember is that volume is always inversely related to intensity. In other words, you cannot safely perform high volumes of high-intensity exercises for any extended length of time.[13,14,23,24] For example, when working with loads exceeding 90% of an individual's maximum, one rarely exceeds a workout volume of 20 repetitions (four sets of three to five repetitions) per exercise. However, when working with loads of 60% of maximum, the trainee can easily perform a workout volume of 36 to 60 repetitions per exercise

Table 13.8

Volume Continuum

Training Adaptation	Total Volume of Reps per Exercise (Sets × Repetitions)
Power	6–30
Strength	8–36
Stabilization	36–75

(three sets of 12 to 20 repetitions). The exception here is the beginning client who may only perform 12 to 20 total repetitions per exercise (one set of each exercise).

The training phase and the training goal dictate the repetitions, sets, intensity, rest, and tempo, and these combined dictate the volume.[11,13–17,21,22,23] Research demonstrates that higher volume training (three to four sets of 9 to 20 repetitions) produces cellular adaptations shown (Table 13-9).[54–59] Conversely, high-intensity training with low training volumes (four to six sets of one to five repetitions) produces greater neurologic adaptations (Table 13-9).[11,13,15–17,32]

TRAINING FREQUENCY

Training frequency refers to the number of training sessions that are performed during a given period (usually 1 week). There is considerable debate concerning the adequate number of training sessions per body part per week necessary for optimum results.[13,14,17,22] The number of training sessions per week per body part is determined by many factors, including training goals, age, general health, work capacity, nutritional status, recoverability, lifestyle, and other stressors.[16,17]

For example, a first-time client may begin by training his or her entire body two times a week.[11,13,14,60] However, an experienced bodybuilder with the specific goal of hypertrophy may have a training cycle in which he or she trains with a split routine of six sessions per week, training each body part two times per week with a larger volume per session.

The specific training goal dictates the program design. Research on training frequency indicates that the optimum training frequency for improvements in strength is three to five times per week. There is no significant difference noted between three days and five days.[11,13,16,17,60] Other research indicates that training at least one to two times per week is sufficient to maintain the physical, physiologic, and performance improvements that were achieved during other phases of training.[11,13,16,17,60]

Table 13.9

Training Volume Adaptations

High Volume (Low Intensity)	Low Volume (High Intensity)
Increased muscle cross-sectional area	Increased neuromuscular efficiency
Improved blood lipid serum profile	Increased rate of force production
Improved lean body mass	Increased motor unit recruitment
Decreased body fat	Increased rate coding
Increased metabolic rate	Increased motor unit synchronization

Table 13.10

Durations for a General Fitness Program

Sets	3
Reps	12
Tempo	4/2/1
Rest interval	30 s between sets
Number of exercises	7
Total duration	25–40 min of workout (excluding warm-up and cool-down)

TRAINING DURATION

Training duration has two prominent meanings:

1. The timeframe from the start of the workout to the finish of the workout, including the warm-up or cool-down.
2. The length of time (number of weeks) spent in one phase (or period) of training.

The training duration for a workout is a function of the number of repetitions, number of sets, number of exercises, and the length of the rest intervals (Table 13-10).

Training programs that exceed 60 to 90 minutes are associated with rapidly declining energy levels.[11,18,22,61,62] This causes alterations in hormonal and immune system responses that can have a negative effect on a training program.[18,47,61,62]

The training duration for a phase of training is dictated by the client's level of physical ability, goal, and compliance to the program. Typically, a phase of training will last between 4 and 8 weeks as this is the amount of time it generally takes for the body to adapt to a given stimulus.[63-73]

EXERCISE SELECTION

Exercise selection is the process of choosing exercises for program design that allow for the optimal achievement of the desired adaptation. It has a tremendous impact on the outcome of the training program.[13,16,17,22,33,47]

The kinetic chain is a highly adaptable organism and readily adjusts to the imposed demands of training (principle of specificity). Therefore, exercises should be specific to the training goals and based on the principles of the exercise selection continuum (Table 13-11).[13,16,17,22,33,47]

In the OPT™ model, exercises from all components (core, balance, reactive, and resistance training) are categorized by the adaptation for which they are primarily

Table 13.11

The Exercise Selection Continuum

Training Adaptation	Training Level	Exercise Selection
Power	Power level	Total body; multijoint (explosive)
Strength	Strength level	Total body; multijoint or single joint
Stabilization	Stabilization level	Total body; multijoint or single joint; controlled unstable

Table 13.12

Exercise Selection—Examples

Level	Total Body	Multijoint	Single Joint
Power	Squat jump	Two-arm medicine ball chest pass Medicine ball pullover Medicine ball oblique throw	N/A
Strength	Squat to two-arm dumbbell press	Bench press Seated row machine Shoulder press machine Squat	Standing two-arm dumbbell curl
Stabilization	Step-up, balance to overhead press	Ball dumbbell chest press Ball dumbbell row Standing overhead press	Single-leg dumbbell curl

used. For example, exercises that are used in phase 1 of the OPT™ model (stabilization) are termed *stabilization level* exercises because they are used and progressed for the stabilization adaptation. Similarly, the exercises used in phases 2 to 4 are termed *strength level* exercises, and exercises used in phase 5 are termed *power level* exercises (Table 13-11).

Exercises can be broken down simplistically into three different types on the basis of the number of joints used, movements performed, and adaptation desired (Table 13-12):[47]

1. Total body: These exercises include multiple joint movements such as a squat, biceps curl, to a shoulder press (squat, curl, and press).
2. Multijoint: These exercises use the involvement of two or three joints.
3. Single joint: These exercises focus on isolating one major muscle group or joint.

The OPT™ model enables the health and fitness professional to effectively select the appropriate exercise for each client. Completing a fitness assessment and reviewing the specific training goals will allow the health and fitness professional to implement these exercises into a properly planned, integrated training program.

For example, to develop optimum stability, traditional exercises can be *progressed* to a more-unstable environment, such as standing up (two-leg, staggered-stance, single-leg) or from a stable environment to an unstable environment (stability ball). Research has shown that exercises performed in unstable environments produce superior results for the goal of stabilization and training the core stabilizing muscles.[65,66,67] Stabilization exercise examples include:

- Crunch on a stability ball
- Cobra on a stability ball
- Chest press on a stability ball
- Cable rows on one leg
- Shoulder press or lateral raise on a stability ball
- Step-up to balance

To develop optimum strength, the use of total body and multijoint exercises has been shown most beneficial.[10,17] Strength exercise examples include:

- Bench press (barbell or dumbbell)
- Row (machine or free weight; seated or bent over)
- Shoulder press (barbell, dumbbell, machine, seated or standing)
- Squat

Table 13.13		
The Progression Continuum		
Stabilization Continuum	**Lower Body**	**Upper Body**
Floor	Two-leg Staggered-stance	Two-arm Alternating arms
Sport beam	Single-leg	Single-arm
Half foam roll Airex pad Dyna Disc 3D-board		

To develop optimum power, explosive medicine ball and body weight exercises can be performed during functional movement patterns.[13,16,17,22,33,47] Power exercise examples include:

- Overhead medicine ball throw
- Medicine ball chest pass
- Medicine ball soccer throw
- Squat jump
- Tuck jump
- Box jump

All exercises, once selected, can be progressed or regressed in a systematic fashion by following the progression continuum (Table 13-13).

SUMMARY

Designing the appropriate program for a client is the primary function of the health and fitness professional. Programs should be individualized to meet the needs and goals of each client. Therefore, it is important that a scientifically based, systematic, and progressive model is used. The OPT™ model provides the health and fitness professional with all the necessary tools to properly use acute variables (repetitions, sets, and so forth), scientific concepts, and exercises to design programs.

Acute variables determine the amount of stress placed on the body and, ultimately, what adaptation the body will incur. The acute variables to consider when designing a program are as follows:

- Repetitions: The more intense the exercise, the fewer the number of repetitions that the individual should perform.
- Sets: The individual usually performs fewer sets when performing higher repetitions at a lower intensity (endurance and hypertrophy adaptations) and more sets when performing lower repetitions at a higher intensity (strength and power adaptations). Twenty-four to 36 total sets should be performed in a given workout.
- Training intensity: This should be determined after sets and reps. Altering other variables (such as environment stability, rest periods, and tempo) changes the training intensity.
- Repetition tempo: Different times under tension yield specific results. By emphasizing eccentric and isometric muscle actions at slower velocities, more demand is placed on the connective tissue.
- Rest interval: This has a dramatic effect on the outcome of the training program. By adjusting the rest interval, energy supplies can be regained

according to the goal of the training program. The shorter the rest interval, the less ATP and CP will be replenished, and consequently less energy will be available for the next set. To avoid making rests too long or short, consider the following factors: training experience, training intensity, tolerance to short rest periods, muscle mass, general fitness level, training goals, nutritional status, and recoverability.

- Training volume: Plan and control training volume to prevent overtraining. Volume is always inversely related to intensity.
- Training frequency: Optimum training frequency for improvements in strength is three to five times per week. Training at least one to two times per week is sufficient to maintain improvements achieved during other phases of training.
- Training duration: Programs should not exceed 90 minutes. Typically, a phase of training will last between 4 and 8 weeks.
- Exercise selection: Exercises should be specific to the training goals and based on the principles of the exercise selection continuum.

Periodization and the OPT™ Model (Planned Fitness Training)

Understanding the need for program design and the purpose of acute variable manipulation is important fundamental information for all health and fitness professionals. Applying this knowledge will determine the success of a health and fitness professional. A system is required to properly organize this base level of information.

The science behind the OPT™ model of program design lies in the concept of periodization. As discussed in Chapter 12 (resistance training), periodization is a systematic approach to program design that uses the general adaptation syndrome and principle of specificity to vary the amount and type of stress placed on the body to produce adaptation and prevent injury. Periodization (or planned fitness training) varies the focus of a training program at regularly planned periods of time (weeks, months, and so forth) to produce optimal adaptation. It involves two primary objectives:

1. Dividing the training program into distinct periods (or phases) of training.
2. Training different forms of strength in each period (or phase) to control the volume of training and to prevent injury.[11-14,74,75]

TRAINING PLANS

Training plan: The specific outline, created by a fitness professional to meet a client's goals, that details the form of training, length of time, future changes, and specific exercises to be performed.

Annual plan: Generalized training plan that spans 1 year to show when the client will progress between phases.

To accomplish these objectives, a client's training program should be organized into a training plan that involves long-term and short-term planning. A **training plan** is a specific plan that a health and fitness professional uses to meet the client's goal. It will determine the forms of training to be used, how long it will take, how often it will change, and what specific exercises will be performed. The long-term plan of a training plan in the OPT™ model is known as an *annual plan* whereas the short-term plans are termed *monthly and weekly plans*. By providing a training plan, the client will be able to see the future achievement of his or her goal in a timely, organized fashion.

An **annual plan** organizes the training program for a 1-year period (Figure 13-4). The annual plan allows the health and fitness professional to provide the client with a blueprint (or map) that specifically shows how the OPT™ training program will progress for the long term, from month-to-month, to meet the desired goal.

	PHASE	JAN	FEB	MAR	APR	MAY	JUN	JUL	AUG	SEP	OCT	NOV	DEC
Stabilization	1												
Strength	2												
	3												
	4												
Power	5												
Cardio													

Figure 13.4 Annual plan.

This gives the client a clear representation of how the health and fitness professional plans to get the client to his or her goal and how long it will take to get there.

In Figure 13-4, the column on the far left represents the period or main strength adaptation. The second column shows the specific phases of the OPT™ model that make up each specific adaptation of training.

Each month within the annual plan is further broken down into periods of training called **monthly plans** (Figure 13-5). The monthly plan details the specific days of each workout, showing the client exactly what phase of the OPT™ model (type of training) will be required each day of the week as well as when the reassessment will occur. The monthly plan also shows the client the necessary cardio and flexibility requirements.

Each monthly plan will also illustrate one's **weekly plans**, which are the specific workouts that the client will do for that week (Figure 13-5). The weekly plan gives the client a picture of exactly what phases will be used in his or her workout for that period.

Much of the literature regarding periodization refers to dividing the training program into specific cycles termed macro-, meso-, and microcycles (Figure 13-6). For ease of understanding, a *macrocycle* is the largest cycle and, typically, covers a year-long period of training (or annual plan). The macrocycle is divided into *mesocycles,* which are typically 1 to 3 months in length (or monthly plans). Each mesocycle in turn is divided into *microcycles,* which are usually a week in length (or weekly plans).[48,76]

Periodization has been shown to be an effective form of program design for many fitness-related goals, and yet, to date, it is not a common practice among fitness professionals.[48,77-79] It provides for the repeated use of different forms of training at specific times in an annual training program to elicit different adaptations in the body (stabilization, strength, and power). By intentionally cycling through different periods (or phases) of training, the acute variables are manipulated to adjust the volume of training. By controlling the volume of training as a function of time in any given program, periodization allows for maximal levels of adaptation, while minimizing overtraining. This is a primary benefit of periodization, because overtraining will lead to fatigue and eventual injury.[48,74,77,78,80]

Monthly plan: Generalized training plan that spans 1 month and shows which phases will be required each day of each week.

Weekly plan: Training plan of specific workouts that spans 1 week, to show which exercises are required each day of the week.

Week				1							2							3							4				
Day	M	T	W	T	F	S	S	M	T	W	T	F	S	S	M	T	W	T	F	S	S	M	T	W	T	F	S	S
Phase 1																												
Phase 2																												
Phase 3																												
Phase 4																												
Phase 5																												
Cardio																												
Flexibility																												
Re-assess																												

Figure 13.5 The monthly or weekly plan.

Annual Plan = Macrocycle
Monthly Plan = Mesocycle
Weekly Plan = Microcycle

Figure 13.6 Periodization cycles.

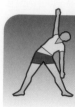

Stretch Your Knowledge

What is the Evidence to Support the use of Planned, Periodized, Integrated Training Programs?

- Making gradual increases in volume and decreases in intensity was the most effective program for increasing muscular endurance (Rhea et al., 2003).[1]

- A 9-month periodized resistance-training program was superior for enhancing strength and motor performance in collegiate women tennis players (Kraemer et al., 2003).[2]

- Making program alterations on a daily basis was more effective in eliciting strength gains than doing so every 4 weeks (Rhea et al., 2002).[3]

- Planned, integrated strength-training programs led to superior physical, physiologic, and performance improvements compared with nonperiodized training programs (Kraemer and Ratamess, 2000).[4]

- Planned variations in an integrated training program are essential because they enable continuous adaptations to occur during a training period and prevent injury (Tan, 1999).[5]

1. Rhea MR, Phillips WT, Burkett LN, Stone WJ, Ball SD, Avlar BA, Thomas AB. A comparison of linear and daily undulating periodized programs with equated volume and intensity for local muscular endurance. J Strength Cond Res 2003;17(1):82–87.
2. Kraemer, WJ, Hakkinen K, Triplett-McBride NT, Fry AC, Koziris LP, Ratamess NA, Bauer E, Volek JS, McConnell T, Newton RU, Girdon SE, Cummings D, Hauth J, Pullo F, Lynch JM, Mazetti SA, Knuttgen HG. Physiological changes with periodized resistance training in women tennis players. Med Sci Sports Exerc 2003;35 (1):157–168.
3. Rhea MR, Phillips WT, Burkett LN, Stone WJ, Ball SD. A comparison of daily and undulating periodized programs with equated volume and intensity for strength. J Strength Cond Res 2002;16(2):250–255.
4. Kraemer WJ, Ratamess NA. Physiology of resistance training. Ortho Phys Ther Clin North Am 2000;9 (4):467–513.
5. Tan B. Manipulating resistance training program variables to optimize maximum strength in men: a review. J Strength Cond Res 1999;13(3):289–304.

SUMMARY

Planned fitness training (or periodization) shifts the focus of a training program at regularly planned intervals of time to vary stress placed on the body to produce adaptation and prevent injury.

A training plan clarifies what forms of training will be used, how long it will take, how often it will change, and what specific exercises will be performed. An annual plan organizes the training program for a 1-year period to show when the client is in which phase. The annual plan is further broken down into periods of training called monthly plans, which detail the specific days of each workout, showing the client exactly what type of training will be required each day of the month. Weekly plans are the specific workouts and exercises that the client will do for that week.

The OPT™ Model

The different periods (or phases) of training seen in a traditional periodization model include a preparatory period (termed *anatomic adaptation*), a hypertrophy period, a maximum strength period, and a power period.

In the OPT™ model, these are simplified into stabilization (anatomic adaptation), strength (strength endurance, hypertrophy, and maximum strength), and power. The OPT™ model seen in a phase-specific model of training includes five different phases of training. These phases systematically progress all clients through the three main adaptations of stabilization, strength, and power (Figures 13-1 and 13-7).

Think of the OPT™ model as a staircase, guiding a client to different adaptations. This journey will involve going up and down the stairs, stopping at different steps, and moving to various heights, depending on the client's goals, needs, and abilities. This module will detail the various phases of training in the OPT™ model.

STABILIZATION

The first level of training in the OPT™ model focuses on the main adaptation of stabilization (or anatomic adaptation) and is designed to prepare the body for the demands of higher levels of training that may follow. This period is crucial for all beginners. It is also necessary to cycle back through after periods of strength and power training to maintain a high degree of core and joint stability. In addition, it allows the body to rest from more intense bouts of training. The focus of stabilization training includes:[74,76]

- Correcting muscle imbalances
- Improving stabilization of the core musculature
- Preventing tissue overload by preparing muscles, tendons, ligaments, and joints for the upcoming imposed demands of training
- Improving overall cardiorespiratory and neuromuscular condition
- Establishing proper movement patterns or exercise technique

The above goals are accomplished through low-intensity, high-repetition training programs, emphasizing core and joint stabilization (as opposed to increasing the strength of the arms and legs). This will incorporate exercises that progressively challenge the body's stability requirements (or proprioception), as opposed to how much weight is being used.[74,76]

Therefore, the primary means of progressing (or increasing the intensity of training) in this period is by increasing the proprioceptive demands of the exercises. This form of training has been shown to be extremely effective for increasing neuromuscular efficiency in the healthy,[80] elderly,[81] and unhealthy populations.[82–85] Another important component of stabilization training is that it may help to ensure

Period of training (main adaptation)	Specific adaptation	Phases used	Method of progression
Stabilization	• Endurance • Stability	1	Proprioception (controlled instability)
Strength	• Strength endurance • Hypertrophy • Maximal strength	2, 3, and 4	Volume Load
Power	• Power	5	Speed Load

Figure 13.7 Summary chart for the OPT™ system.

activity-specific strength adaptations (such as standing on one leg to kick a ball, climbing up stairs, or simply walking).[86]

The stabilization period of training in the OPT™ model consists of one phase of training: stabilization endurance (Figures 13-1 and 13-7).

Stabilization Endurance Training (Phase 1)

Stabilization endurance should be used for beginning clients who may possess muscle imbalances, lack postural control, and stability (Table 13-14). Although this phase is the first phase of training in the OPT™ model, it will also be important to cycle back through this phase of training between periods of higher-intensity training seen in phases 2 through 5. This will allow for proper recovery and maintenance of high levels of stability that will ensure optimal strength and power adaptations. This phase of training focuses on:

- Increasing stability
- Increasing muscular endurance
- Increasing neuromuscular efficiency of the core musculature
- Improving intermuscular and intramuscular coordination

The primary focus when progressing in this phase is on increasing the proprioception (controlled instability) of the exercises, rather than just the load.

Acute variables can be progressed if the client is starting in the stabilization endurance phase, with minimal to no training background, and is also fairly conditioned, with no major muscle imbalances (Table 13-15). The health and fitness professional will want to increase repetitions and challenge proprioception to establish the necessary levels of endurance in core muscles. The intensity of the weight will remain low, to allow the client to focus on proprioception.

A client in this category will generally stay in this phase of training for a 4-week duration. This will prepare the client for the demands of the strength endurance phase (phase 2). This progression is beneficial for any client, but especially for those with the goal of body fat reduction or general fitness.

Table 13.14

Phase 1: Stabilization Endurance Acute Variables

Stabilization Endurance

	Reps	Sets	Tempo	% Intensity	Rest Interval	Frequency	Duration	Exercise Selection
Flexibility	1	1–3	30-s hold	n/a	n/a			SMR and static
Core	12–20	1–4	slow 4/2/1	n/a	0–90 s	2–4 times/ week	4–6 weeks	1–4 stabilization level
Balance	12–20 6–10 (SL)	1–3	slow 4/2/1	n/a	0–90 s	2–4 times/ week	4–6 weeks	1–4 stabilization level
Reactive	5–8	1–3	3–5 s hold	n/a	0–90 s	2–4 times/ week	4–6 weeks	0–2 stabilization level
Resistance	12–20	1–3	4–2–1	50–70%	0–90 s	2–4 times/ week	4–6 weeks	1–2 stabilization progression
Comments:								

SL, single leg; *SMR*, self myofascial release; *n/a*, not applicable.

Table 13.15

Phase 1: Stabilization Endurance Progressions for Beginning Clients

Weekly Progression

		Week 1	Week 2	Week 3	Week 4
Core	Sets	1	2	2	3
	Reps	12	15	20	20
Balance	Sets	1	2	2	3
	Reps	12	15	20	20
Reactive	Sets	1	2	2	2
	Reps	5	5	6	8
Resistance	Sets	1	2	2	3
	Reps	12	15	20	20
	Intensity	60%	60%	60%	60%

Acute variables can be progressed if the client is fairly conditioned and has a good level of training background (Table 13-16). The health and fitness professional should slowly progress by increasing intensity and decreasing the repetitions to establish the necessary levels of endurance and strength in stabilizing muscles.

This progression is beneficial for the client who has the goal of increasing lean body mass and general performance. A client in this category will generally stay in this phase of training for a 4-week duration.

Table 13.16

Phase 1: Stabilization Endurance Progressions for Clients Who Are Fairly Conditioned With Good Training Background

Weekly Progression

		Week 1	Week 2	Week 3	Week 4
Core	Sets	1	2	3	3
	Reps	20	20	15	15
Balance	Sets	1	2	3	3
	Reps	20	20	15	15
Reactive	Sets	1	2	3	3
	Reps	6	6	6	8
Resistance	Sets	1-2	2	3	3
	Reps	20	15	15	12
	Intensity	60%	65%	65%	70%

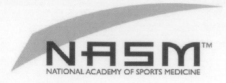

OPT For Fitness

Name: John Smith	Month: 1
Date: 8/10/06	Week: 1
Professional: Scott Lucett	Day: 1 of 12

Program Goal
PHASE 1: STAB. ENDURANCE
Total Body

STEP 1

A. Foam Roll

Foam Roll	Sets	Duration
Calves	1	30 sec
IT Band	1	30 sec
Latissimus Dorsi	1	30 sec

B. Stretch

Static Stretching	Sets	Duration
Gastrocnemius	1	30 sec
Kneeling Hip Flexor Stretch	1	30 sec
Latissimus Dorsi Ball Stretch	1	30 sec

C. Cardiovascular

Treadmill	1	5 min

STEP 2

A. Core

Exercise	Sets	Reps	Tempo	Rest
Supine Marching	2	15	Slow	0
Floor Bridge	2	15	Slow	0

B. Balance

Exercise	Sets	Reps	Tempo	Rest
Single-leg Balance	2	x	Slow	0

C. Reactive

Exercise	Sets	Reps	Tempo	Rest
Squat Jump w/Stabilization	2	5	Slow	60 sec

STEP 3

Resistance Training Program

Body Part	Exercise	Sets	Reps	Intensity	Tempo	Rest
Total Body	Ball Squat Curl to Press	2	15	60%	Slow	0
Chest	Push Up	2	15	60%	Slow	0
Back	Standing Cable Row	2	15	60%	Slow	0
Shoulder	Single-leg Scaption	2	15	60%	Slow	0
Biceps	*Optional*					
Triceps	*Optional*					
Legs	Step Up to Balance	2	15	60%	Slow	60 sec

STEP 4

Cool-Down

Repeat Steps 1A and/or 1B

Example Phase 1 Program

STRENGTH

The second level of training in the OPT™ model focuses on the main adaptation of strength, which includes strength endurance, hypertrophy, and maximal strength. It is designed to maintain stability while increasing the amount of stress placed on the body for increased muscle size and strength. This period of training is a necessary progression from stabilization for anyone who desires to increase caloric expenditure, muscle size, muscle strength, and bone mineral density. The focus of the strength period of training is to:

- Increase the ability of the core musculature to stabilize the pelvis and spine under heavier loads, through more-complete ranges of motion
- Increase the load-bearing capabilities of muscles, tendons, ligaments, and joints
- Increase the volume of training with more reps, sets, and intensity
- Increase metabolic demand by taxing the ATP and CP and glycolysis energy systems to induce cellular changes in muscle (weight loss or hypertrophy)
- Increase motor unit recruitment, frequency of motor unit recruitment, and motor unit synchronization (maximal strength)

The strength period of training in the OPT™ model consists of three phases: phase 2, strength endurance; phase 3, hypertrophy; and phase 4, maximal strength (Figures 13-1 and 13-7).

Strength Endurance Training (Phase 2)

Strength endurance is a hybrid form of training that promotes increased stabilization endurance, hypertrophy, and strength. This form of training entails the use of superset techniques in which a more-stable exercise (such as a bench press) is immediately followed with a stabilization exercise with similar biomechanical motions (such as a standing cable chest press). Thus, for every set of an exercise or body part performed according to the acute variables, there are actually two exercises or two sets being performed. High amounts of volume can be generated in this phase of training (Table 13-17).

Acute variables can be progressed if a client with the goal of general fitness or body fat reduction has properly progressed through phase 1 of the OPT™ model (Table 13-18). Because the goal does not require hypertrophy, sets, repetition, and intensity ranges will remain moderate.

Table 13.17

Phase 2: Strength Endurance Acute Variables

Strength Endurance

	Reps	Sets	Tempo	% Intensity	Rest Interval	Frequency	Duration	Exercise Selection
Flexibility	5–10	1–2	1–2 s hold	n/a	n/a	3–7 times/ week	4–6 weeks	SMR and active
Core	8–12	2–3	3-2-1–1/1/1 medium	n/a	0–60	2–4 times/ week	4–6 weeks	1–3 strength
Balance	8–12	2–3	3-2-1–1/1/1 medium	n/a	0–60	2–4 times/ week	4-6 weeks	1–3 strength
Reactive	8–10	2–3	Repeating medium	n/a	0–60	2–4 times times/ week	4–6 weeks	1–3 strength
Resistance	8–12	2–4	(Str) 2-0-2 (Stab) 4-2-1	70–80%	0–60	2–4 times times/ week	4–6 weeks	1 strength superset 1 stabilization
Comments:	Each resistance-training exercise is a superset of a strength level exercise immediately followed by a stabilization level exercise.							

SMR, self myofascial release; *n/a*, not applicable.

Table 13.18

Phase 2: Strength Endurance
Progressions for Clients With Goals of Body Fat Reduction or General Fitness

Weekly Progression

		Week 1	Week 2	Week 3	Week 4
Core	Sets	2	2	2	2
	Reps	12	12	12	12
Balance	Sets	2	2	2	2
	Reps	12	12	12	12
Reactive	Sets	2	2	2	2
	Reps	8	8	8	8
Resistance	Sets	2	2	2	2
	Reps	12 strength 12 stabilization	12 strength 12 stabilization	10 strength 10 stabilization	10 strength 10 stabilization
	Intensity	70%	70%	75%	75%

Acute variables can be progressed if a client with the goal of increasing lean body mass and general performance has properly progressed through phase 1 of the OPT™ model (Table 13-19). Because the goal of this phase of training is strength and hypertrophy, the health and fitness professional will want to increase intensity and decrease the repetitions to establish the necessary levels of strength. A client in this category will generally stay in this phase of training for a 4-week duration.

Table 13.19

Phase 2: Strength Endurance
Progressions for Clients With Goals of Increased Lean Body Mass or General Performance

Weekly Progression

		Week 1	Week 2	Week 3	Week 4
Core	Sets	2	2	3	3
	Reps	12	12	10	8
Balance	Sets	2	2	3	3
	Reps	12	12	10	8
Reactive	Sets	2	3	3	3
	Reps	8	8	10	10
Resistance	Sets	2	3	3	4
	Reps	12 strength 12 stabilization	10 strength 10 stabilization	8 strength 8 stabilization	8 strength 8 stabilization
	Intensity	70%	75%	80%	80%

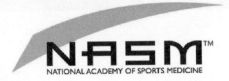

OPT For Fitness

Name: John Smith	Month: 2
Date:	Week: 1
Professional: Scott Lucett	Day: 1 of 12

Program Goal
PHASE 2: STRENGTH ENDURANCE
Total Body

STEP 1

A. Foam Roll

Foam Roll	Sets	Duration
Calves	1	30 sec
IT Band	1	30 sec
Latissimus Dorsi	1	30 sec

B. Stretch

Active Stretching	Sets	Duration
Active Gastrocnemius Stretch	1	5 reps
Active Kneeling Hip Flexor Stretch	1	5 reps
Active Latissimus Dorsi Ball Stretch	1	5 reps

C. Cardiovascular

	Sets	Duration
Treadmill	1	5 min

STEP 2

A. Core

Exercise	Sets	Reps	Tempo	Rest
Ball Crunch	2	10	Medium	0
Reverse Crunch	2	10	Medium	0

B. Balance

Exercise	Sets	Reps	Tempo	Rest
Single-leg Squat	2	10	Medium	60 sec

C. Reactive

Exercise	Sets	Reps	Tempo	Rest
Squat Jump	2	10	Medium	60 sec

STEP 3

Resistance Training Program

Body Part Exercise		Sets	Reps	Intensity	Tempo	Rest
Total Body	*Optional*					
Chest	1. Bench Press 2. Push Up	2	12	75%	Medium Slow	0 60 sec
Back	1. Seated Cable Row 2. Ball Dumbbell Row	2	12	75%	Medium Slow	0 60 sec
Shoulder	1. Shoulder Press Machine 2. Single-leg Scaption	2	12	75%	Medium Slow	0 60 sec
Biceps	*Optional*					
Triceps	*Optional*					
Legs	1. Barbell Squat 2. Step Up to Balance	2	12	75%	Medium Slow	0 60 sec

STEP 4

Cool-Down

Repeat Steps 1A/or 1B, but use static stretches

NOTE: Resistance training portion can be split into a 2-, 3-, or 4-day workout routine - Ex. 3-day routine: day 1 (chest/back), day 2 (shoulders and legs), day 3 (biceps and triceps)

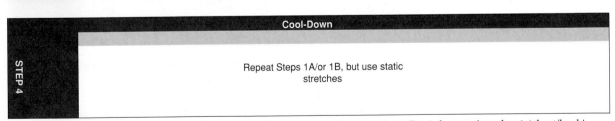

Example Phase 2 Program

Hypertrophy Training (Phase 3)

Hypertrophy training is specific for the adaptation of maximal muscle growth, focusing on high levels of volume with minimal rest periods to force cellular changes that result in an overall increase in muscle size (Table 13-20).

Acute variables can be progressed if a client with the goal of increasing lean body mass and general performance has properly progressed through phases 1 and

Table 13.20

Phase 3: Hypertrophy
Acute Variables

Hypertrophy

	Reps	Sets	Tempo	% Intensity	Rest Interval	Frequency	Duration	Exercise Selection
Flexibility	5–10	1–2	1–2 s hold	n/a	n/a	3–7 times/ week	4 weeks	SMR and active
Core	8–12	2–3	3-2-1–1/1/1 medium	n/a	0–60 s	3–6 times/ week	4 weeks	0–4 strength
Balance	8–12	2–3	3-2-1–1/1/1 medium	n/a	0–60 s	3–6 times/ week	4 weeks	0–4 strength
Reactive	8–10	2–3	Repeating	n/a	0–60 s	3–6 times/ week	4 weeks	0–4 strength
Resistance	6–12	3–5	2-0-2	75–85%	0–60 s	3–6 times/ week	4 weeks	2–4 strength level exercises/body part
Comments:	Total of 24–36 sets per workout Light day = 20–24 total sets Moderate day = 24–30 total sets Heavy day = 30–36 total sets							

2 of the OPT™ model (Table 13-21). Because the goal of this phase of training is primarily hypertrophy, the health and fitness professional will want to increase intensity and volume.

A client in this category will generally stay in this phase of training for a 4-week duration, before cycling back through phase 1 or 2 or progressing on to phase 4 or 5.

Table 13.21

Phase 3: Hypertrophy
Progressions for Clients With Goals of Increased Lean Body Mass or General Performance

Weekly Progression

		Week 1	Week 2	Week 3	Week 4
Core	Sets	2	2	3	3
	Reps	12	12	10	8
Balance	Sets	2	2	3	3
	Reps	12	12	10	8
Reactive	Sets	2	3	3	3
	Reps	8	8	10	10
Resistance	Sets	3	3	4	5
	Reps	12	10	8	6
	Intensity	75%	80%	80%	85%

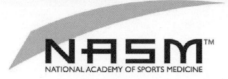

OPT For Fitness

Name: John Smith	Month: 3
Date:	Week: 1
Professional: Scott Lucett	Day: 1

Program Goal
PHASE 3: HYPERTROPHY
Total Body

STEP 1

A. Foam Roll

Foam Roll	Sets	Duration
Calves	1	30 sec
IT Band	1	30 sec
Latissimus Dorsi	1	30 sec

B. Stretch

Active Stretching	Sets	Duration
Active Gastrocnemius Stretch	1	5 reps
Active Kneeling Hip Flexor Stretch	1	5 reps
Active Latissimus Dorsi Ball Stretch	1	5 reps

C. Cardiovascular

Treadmill	1	5 min

STEP 2

A. Core

Exercise	Sets	Reps	Tempo	Rest
Ball Crunch	2	12	Medium	0
Back Extension	2	12	Medium	0

B. Balance

Exercise	Sets	Reps	Tempo	Rest
Single-leg Squat Touchdown	2	12	Medium	60 sec

C. Reactive

Exercise	Sets	Reps	Tempo	Rest
Optional				

STEP 3

Resistance Training Program						
Body Part	Exercise	Sets	Reps	Intensity	Tempo	Rest
Total Body	*Optional*					
Chest	Flat Dumbbell Chest Press	3	10	80%	Medium	60 sec
Back	Lat Pulldown	3	10	80%	Medium	60 sec
Shoulder	Shoulder Press Machine	3	10	80%	Medium	60 sec
Biceps	Standing Two-arm Dumbbell Curl	3	10	80%	Medium	60 sec
Triceps	Cable Pressdown	3	10	80%	Medium	60 sec
Legs	Leg Press	3	10	80%	Medium	60 sec

STEP 4

Cool-Down
Repeat Steps 1A/or 1B, but use static stretches

NOTE: Resistance training portion can be split into a 2-, 3-, or 4-day workout routine - Ex. 3-day routine: day 1 (chest/back), day 2 (shoulders and legs), day 3 (biceps and triceps)

Example Phase 3 Program

Maximal Strength Training (Phase 4)

The maximal strength training phase focuses on increasing the load placed upon the tissues of the body (Table 13-22). Maximal intensity improves:

- Recruitment of more motor units
- Rate of force production
- Motor unit synchronization

Table 13.22

Phase 4: Maximal Strength Training
Acute Variables

Maximal Strength Training

	Reps	Sets	Tempo	% Intensity	Rest Interval	Frequency	Duration	Exercise Selection
Flexibility	5–10	1–2	2–4 s hold	n/a	n/a	3–7 times/week	4 weeks	SMR and active
Core	8–12	2–3	1-1-1 medium	n/a	0–60 s	2–4 times/week	4 weeks	0–3 strength
Balance	8–12	2–3	1-1-1 medium	n/a	0–60 s	2–4 times/week	4 weeks	0–3 strength
Reactive	8–10	2–3	Repeating medium	n/a	0–60 s	2–4 times/week	4 weeks	0–3 strength
Resistance	1–5	4–6	X-X-X	85–100%	3–5 min	2–4 times/week	4 weeks	1–3 strength
Comments:								

SMR, self myofascial release; *n/a,* not applicable. X-X-X, as fast as can be controlled.

Maximal strength training has also been shown to help increase the benefits of forms of power training used in phase 5.[60]

Acute variables can be progressed if the client with the goal of increasing lean body mass and general performance has properly progressed through phases 1 and 2 (and possibly phase 3; Table 13-23). Because the goal of this phase of training is primarily maximal strength, the health and fitness professional will want to increase intensity.

A client in this category will generally stay in this phase of training for a 4-week duration before cycling back through phase 1 or 2 or progressing on to phase 5.

Table 13.23

Phase 4: Maximal Strength Training (MST)
Progressions for Clients With Goals of Increased Lean Body Mass
or General Performance

Weekly Progression

		Week 1	Week 2	Week 3	Week 4
Core	*Sets*	2	2	3	3
	Reps	12	12	10	8
Balance	*Sets*	2	2	3	3
	Reps	12	12	10	8
Reactive	*Sets*	2	3	3	3
	Reps	8	8	10	10
Resistance	*Sets*	4	5	5	6
	Reps	5	5	4	3
	Intensity	85%	85%	89%	93%

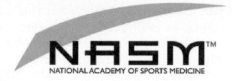

OPT For Fitness

Name: John Smith	Month: 1
Date:	Week: 1
Professional: Scott Lucett	Day: 1 of 12

Program Goal
PHASE 4: MAX STRENGTH
Total Body

STEP 1

A. Foam Roll

Foam Roll	Sets	Duration
Calves	1	30 sec
IT-Band	1	30 sec
Latissimus Dorsi	1	30 sec

B. Stretch

Active Stretching	Sets	Duration
Active Gastrocnemius Stretch	1	5 reps
Active Kneeling Hip Flexor Stretch	1	5 reps
Active Latissimus Dorsi Ball Stretch	1	5 reps

C. Cardiovascular

	Sets	Duration
Treadmill	1	5 min

STEP 2

A. Core

Exercise	Sets	Reps	Tempo	Rest
Cable Rotations	3	8	Medium	0
Back Extension	3	8	Medium	60 sec

B. Balance

Exercise	Sets	Reps	Tempo	Rest
Optional				

C. Reactive

Exercise	Sets	Reps	Tempo	Rest
Optional				

STEP 3

Resistance Training Program

Body Part	Exercise	Sets	Reps	Intensity	Tempo	Rest
Total Body	Barbell Clean	3	5	85%	Medium	3 min
Chest	Bench Press	3	5	85%	Medium	3 min
Back	Lat Pulldown	3	5	85%	Medium	3 min
Shoulder	Seated Dumbbell Shoulder Press	3	5	85%	Medium	3 min
Biceps	*Optional*					
Triceps	*Optional*					
Legs	Barbell Squat	3	5	85%	Medium	3 min

STEP 4

Cool-Down

Repeat Steps 1A and/or 1B, but use static stretches

NOTE: Resistance training portion can be split into a 2-, 3-, or 4-day workout routine - Ex. 3-day routine: day 1 (chest/back), day 2 (shoulders and legs), day 3 (biceps and triceps)

Example Phase 4 Program

POWER

The third level of training is power and is designed to increase the rate of force production (or speed of muscle contraction). This form of training uses the adaptations of stabilization and strength acquired in the previous phases of training and applies them with more realistic speeds and forces that the body will encounter in everyday life and in sports.

Power training is usually not common practice in the fitness environment, but has a very viable and purposeful place in a properly planned training program.

Power is simply defined as force multiplied by velocity $(P = F \times V)$.[60] Therefore, any increase in either force or velocity will produce an increase in power. This is accomplished by either increasing the load (or force) as in progressive strength training or increasing the speed with which you move a load (or velocity). The combined effect is a better rate of force production in daily activities and sporting events.[60]

To develop optimum levels of power, it has been shown that individuals must train both with heavy loads (85 to 100%) and light loads (30 to 45%) at high speeds.[8,25,26,29,31,63] The focus of power training is to increase the rate of force production by increasing the number of motor units activated, the synchrony between them, and the speed at which they are excited.[63,87,88]

The power level of training in the OPT™ model consists of one phase of training: phase 5: power (Figures 13-1 and 13-7).

Power Training (Phase 5)

The power training phase focuses on both high force and velocity to increase power (Table 13-24). This is accomplished by combining a strength exercise with a power exercise for each body part (such as performing a barbell bench press superset with a medicine ball chest pass).

Don't let the intensities confuse you. The 85 to 100% refers to the intensity for traditional strength training exercises. It increases power by increasing the *force* side of the power equation (force multiplied by velocity).

The 30 to 45% intensity, on the other hand, is used for "speed" exercises such as speed squats in which the squats are performed as fast as possible with a low load.[93] The approximately 10% intensity is used for medicine ball training that will require the throwing or release of a medicine ball. These last two forms of training affect the *velocity* side of the power equation (force multiplied by velocity).

By using heavy weight with explosive movement and low resistance with a high velocity, you can produce high power outputs.[12,89–92]

Table 13.24								
Phase 5: Power **Acute Variables**								
Power								
	Reps	**Sets**	**Tempo**	**% Intensity**	**Rest Int.**	**Frequency**	**Duration**	**Exercise Selection**
Flexibility	10–15	1–2	Controlled	n/a	n/a	3–7 times/ week	4 weeks	SMR and dynamic 3–5 exercises
Core	8–12	2–3	fast as can be controlled	n/a	0–60 s	2–4 times/ week	4 weeks	0–2 power level
Balance	8–12	2–3	controlled	n/a	0–60 s	2–4 times/ week	4 weeks	0–2 power level
Reactive	8–12	2–3	X-X-X as fast as possible	n/a	0–60 s	2–4 times/ week	4 weeks	0–2 power level
Resistance	1–5 (S) 8–10 (P)	3–5	X-X-X (S) X-X-X (P)	85–100% (S) up to 10% BW or 30–45% 1RM (P)	1–2 min b/w pairs 3–5 min b/w circuits	2–4 times/ week	4 weeks	1 strength superset 1 power
Comments:								

BW, body weight; *1RM*, 1 repetition maximum; *X-X-X*, as fast as can be controlled; *SMR*, self myofascial release; *n/a*, not applicable.

Table 13.25					
Phase 5: Power **Progressions for Clients With Goals of Increased Lean Body Mass or General Performance**					
Weekly Progression					
		Week 1	**Week 2**	**Week 3**	**Week 4**
Core	*Sets*	2	2	3	3
	Reps	12	12	10	8
Balance	*Sets*	2	2	3	3
	Reps	12	12	10	8
Reactive	*Sets*	2	3	3	3
	Reps	8	8	10	10
Resistance	*Sets*	3	4	4	5
	Reps	5 strength 10 power	4 strength 10 power	4 strength 8 power	3 strength 8 power
	Intensity	Strength 85% Power 2% BW	Strength 89% Power 3% BW	Strength 89% Power 4% BW	Strength 93% Power 4% BW
Comments:					

BW, body weight; *1RM*, 1 repetition maximum.

Acute variables can be progressed if the client with the goal of increasing general performance has properly progressed through the rest of the OPT™ model (Table 13-25). Because the goal of this phase of training is primarily power, the health and fitness professional will want to progress by increasing intensity and velocity.

A client in this category will generally stay in this phase of training for a 4-week duration before cycling back through phase 1 or 2.

SUMMARY

The different levels of training seen in a traditional periodization model include anatomic adaptation, hypertrophy, maximum strength, and power. In the OPT™ model, these are simplified into stabilization, strength, and power. These are further broken down into five different phases of training.

The first level, stabilization, is crucial for all beginners as it is designed to prepare the body for the demands of higher levels of training. For advanced clients, this level allows for rest from more-intense bouts of training. It involves low-intensity, high-repetition training, emphasizing core and joint stabilization (as opposed to increasing the strength of the arms and legs). Exercises progressively challenge proprioception.

The stabilization level of consists of one phase of training: phase 1, stabilization endurance. This phase focuses on increasing core stability and endurance of all major muscles. It also optimizes the amount of continuous blood flow in the muscles during exercise to reduce tissue adhesions. The phase usually lasts 4 weeks.

The second level, strength, is designed to increase strength endurance, muscle size, and strength. The strength period of training in the OPT™ model consists of three phases: phase 2, strength endurance; phase 3, hypertrophy; and phase 4, maximal strength. Phase 2 uses superset techniques with high volume, for about 4 weeks. Phase 3 stresses maximal hypertrophy, focusing on high levels of volume

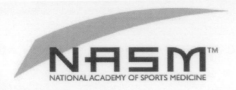

OPT For Fitness

Name: John Smith	Month: 2
Date:	Week: 1
Professional: Scott Lucett	Day: 1 of 12

Program Goal
PHASE 5: POWER
Total Body

STEP 1

A. Foam Roll

Foam Roll	Sets	Duration
Calves	1	30 sec
Adductors	1	30 sec
Latissimus Dorsi	1	30 sec

B. Stretch

Dynamic Stretching	Sets	Duration
Tube Walking	1	10 reps
Multiplanar Lunges	1	10 reps

C. Cardiovascular

Treadmill	1	5 min

STEP 2

A. Core

Exercise	Sets	Reps	Tempo	Rest
Rotation Chest Pass	3	8	Fast	0 sec
Ball MB Pullover Throw	3	8	Fast	0 sec

B. Balance

Exercise	Sets	Reps	Tempo	Rest
Single-leg Hop w/Stabilization	3	8	Fast	60 sec

C. Reactive

Exercise	Sets	Reps	Tempo	Rest
Optional				

STEP 3

Resistance Training Program

Body Part	Exercise	Sets	Reps	Intensity	Tempo	Rest
Total Body	*Optional*					
Chest	1. Bench Press 2. Medicine Ball Chest Pass	3	5 10	85% 5% of BW	Fast	0 2 min
Back	1. Seated Row 2. Woodchop Throw	3	5 10	85% 5% of BW	Fast	0 2 min
Shoulder	2. Shoulder Press Machine 2. Medicine Ball Scoop Toss	3	5 10	85% 5% of BW	Fast	0 2 min
Biceps	*Optional*					
Triceps	*Optional*					
Legs	2. Barbell Squat 2. Ice Skater	3	5 10	85% 5% of BW	Fast	0 2 min

STEP 4

Cool-Down

Repeat Steps 1A/ and/or 1B, but
use static stretches

Example Phase 5 Program

with minimal rest periods, for about 4 weeks. Phase 4 focuses on increasing the load placed on the tissues of the body, for about 4 weeks.

The third level of training, power, is designed to increase the rate of force production. To develop optimum levels of power, it has been shown that individuals must train both with heavy and light loads at high speeds. The power level consists of one phase of training: phase 5, power. This phase focuses on both high force and velocity to increase power and lasts about 4 weeks.

Applying the OPT™ Model

The concepts of program design, periodization, and the OPT™ model have all been described. Program design was defined as creating a purposeful system or plan to achieve a goal. Periodization is the scientific basis that allows health and fitness professionals to strategically plan, design programs, and achieve goals, without the risk of placing improper stresses on the body.

The OPT™ model is a proven, easy-to-use system of periodization that can be used to create programs for clients with various goals. Although the understanding of these concepts is paramount, what matters most is the ability to apply the information in multiple situations to a variety of clients. This module will demonstrate how to specifically apply the OPT™ model to goals. These include body fat reduction, increase in lean body mass, and enhanced general performance.

APPLYING THE MODEL FOR THE GOAL OF BODY FAT REDUCTION

The goal of reducing body fat requires clients to follow the simple principle of burning more calories than they consume (see Chapter 15, Nutrition). The best way to increase the calories burned is to move more. Weight training provides an extremely potent means to burn calories when it is combined with cardiorespiratory training. It also provides the added benefit of increased muscle strength.[93-96]

The following program is a general representation of how the OPT™ model is used for clients with the goal of body fat reduction. Figure 13-8 shows the annual plan. Because the goal is not for hypertrophy or to gain maximal strength and power, the client only needs to be cycled through the first two phases of the OPT™ model. The client will start in January in phase 1, to ensure proper muscle balance and endurance of the stabilization muscles. He or she will remain there for approximately 4 weeks before moving on to phase 2.

The remainder of the annual plan shows the client cycling back and forth between phases 1 and 2 (Figure 13-8). Phase 2 will promote times of greater metabolic demand and more volume for increased caloric expenditure. Phase 1 will allow the client proper recovery time before entering back into phase 2. Cardiorespiratory training can be performed each month. During phase 1, the client may be inclined to do more cardiorespiratory work (in conjunction with weight training) to sustain good caloric expenditure without the higher intensity of weight training seen in phase 2. This will also provide proper periodization of the client's cardiorespiratory training.

Figure 13-9 illustrates the monthly plan for January. This plan demonstrates a 3-day-per-week workout plan, with scheduled workouts on Mondays, Wednesdays, and Fridays. This monthly plan can easily be performed twice a week. The client

	PHASE	JAN	FEB	MAR	APR	MAY	JUN	JUL	AUG	SEP	OCT	NOV	DEC
Stabilization	1	X		X		X		X		X		X	
Strength	2		X		X		X		X		X		X
	3												
	4												
Power	5												
Cardio		X	X	X	X	X	X	X	X	X	X	X	X

Figure 13.8 Annual plan for the goal of body fat reduction.

Week	1							2							3							4						
Day	M	T	W	T	F	S	S	M	T	W	T	F	S	S	M	T	W	T	F	S	S	M	T	W	T	F	S	S
Phase 1	X		X		X			X		X		X			X		X		X			X		X		X		
Phase 2																												
Phase 3																												
Phase 4																												
Phase 5																												
Cardio	X		X		X			X		X		X			X		X		X			X		X		X		
Flexibility	X	X	X	X	X	X	X	X	X	X	X	X	X	X	X	X	X	X	X	X	X	X	X	X	X	X	X	X

Figure 13.9 Monthly plan for the goal of body fat reduction, January—phase 1: stabilization endurance.

can perform flexibility exercises every day of the week, if desired. Cardio can be done on the workout days (or any other day during the week, depending on the client's schedule).

Figure 13-10 illustrates the monthly plan for February. As with the previous month, this plan demonstrates a 3-day-per-week workout plan with scheduled workouts on Mondays, Wednesdays, and Fridays. Again, this monthly plan could easily be performed twice a week. The client can perform flexibility exercises every day of the week, if desired. Cardio can be done on the workout days (or any other day during the week depending on the client's schedule).

Week	1							2							3							4						
Day	M	T	W	T	F	S	S	M	T	W	T	F	S	S	M	T	W	T	F	S	S	M	T	W	T	F	S	S
Phase 1																												
Phase 2	X		X		X			X		X		X			X		X		X			X		X		X		
Phase 3																												
Phase 4																												
Phase 5																												
Cardio	X		X		X			X		X		X			X		X		X			X		X		X		
Flexibility	X	X	X	X	X	X	X	X	X	X	X	X	X	X	X	X	X	X	X	X	X	X	X	X	X	X	X	X

Figure 13.10 Monthly plan for the goal of body fat reduction, February —phase 2: strength endurance.

APPLYING THE MODEL FOR THE GOAL OF INCREASING LEAN BODY MASS

The goal of increasing lean body mass (or hypertrophy) requires the client to increase caloric intake to exceed the amount that is burned to put weight on. The training will need to be progressed to higher volumes (more sets, reps, and intensity) to force muscles to increase their cellular makeup and produce increased size.

The following program is a general representation of how the OPT™ model is used for clients with the goal of increased lean body mass. With the goal of hypertrophy the client can be cycled through the first four phases of the OPT™ model, depending on the needs and wants of the client.

Figure 13-11 shows the annual plan. The client will start January in phase 1 to ensure proper muscle balance and endurance of the stabilization muscles. He or she will remain there for approximately 4 weeks before moving into phase 2. Phase 1 is vital for this client, as it will prepare the connective tissues and muscles for the high demands of training required for this goal. Without proper preparation, injury will be imminent.

	PHASE	JAN	FEB	MAR	APR	MAY	JUN	JUL	AUG	SEP	OCT	NOV	DEC
Stabilization	1	X						X					
Strength	2		X		X				X				X
	3			X		X				X		X	
	4						X				X		
Power	5												
Cardio													

Figure 13.11 Annual plan for the goal of muscle gain.

The remainder of the annual plan shows the client cycling through phases 2 through 4. Phase 2 will promote greater strength endurance and more volume to prepare the client for the greater demands of phases 3 and 4.

Phase 3 is specific for maximal hypertrophy and will place larger volumes of stress through the body to force cellular changes that result in muscle hypertrophy. Phase 4 is used to increase the strength capacity to allow the client to train with heavier weights in the future. This will equate to higher volumes of training and greater hypertrophy.

Returning to phase 1 will allow the client proper recovery time before entering back into phases 2 through 4. Cardiorespiratory training can be performed each month to ensure the cardiorespiratory system is efficient and promoting optimal tissue recovery.

Figure 13-12 illustrates the monthly plan for January. This plan demonstrates a 3-day-per-week workout plan, with scheduled workouts on Mondays, Wednesdays, and Fridays. The client can perform flexibility exercises every day of the week, if desired. Cardio can be done on the workout days (or any other day during the week, depending on the client's schedule).

Figure 13-13 illustrates the monthly plan for February. As with the previous month, this plan demonstrates a 3-day-per-week workout plan, with scheduled

Day	M	T	W	T	F	S	S	M	T	W	T	F	S	S	M	T	W	T	F	S	S	M	T	W	T	F	S	S
Phase 1	X		X		X			X		X		X			X		X		X			X		X		X		
Phase 2																												
Phase 3																												
Phase 4																												
Phase 5																												
Cardio	X		X		X			X		X		X			X		X		X			X		X		X		
Flexibility	X	X	X	X	X	X	X	X	X	X	X	X	X	X		X	X	X	X	X	X	X	X	X		X	X	X

Figure 13.12 Monthly plan for the goal of muscle gain, January—phase 1: stabilization endurance.

Week	1							2							3							4						
Day	M	T	W	T	F	S	S	M	T	W	T	F	S	S	M	T	W	T	F	S	S	M	T	W	T	F	S	S
Phase 1																												
Phase 2	X		X		X			X		X		X			X		X		X			X		X		X		
Phase 3																												
Phase 4																												
Phase 5																												
Cardio	X		X		X			X		X		X			X		X		X			X		X		X		
Flexibility	X	X	X	X	X	X	X	X	X	X	X	X	X	X	X	X	X	X	X	X	X	X	X	X	X	X	X	X

Figure 13.13 Monthly plan for the goal of muscle gain, February—phase 2: strength endurance.

Week	1							2							3							4						
Day	M	T	W	T	F	S	S	M	T	W	T	F	S	S	M	T	W	T	F	S	S	M	T	W	T	F	S	S
Phase 1																												
Phase 2																												
Phase 3	X	X		X	X			X	X		X	X			X	X		X	X			X	X		X	X		
Phase 4																												
Phase 5																												
Cardio																												
Flexibility	X	X	X	X	X	X	X	X	X	X	X	X	X	X	X	X	X	X	X	X	X	X	X	X	X	X	X	X

Figure 13.14 Monthly plan for the goal of muscle gain, March—phase 3: hypertrophy.

workouts on Mondays, Wednesdays, and Fridays. This monthly plan could easily be performed four times per week, with a split routine for the body parts. The client can perform flexibility exercises every day of the week, if desired. In this phase of training, the workouts require more time and energy, so cardio can be done on the days opposite the workout days. This does not mean, however, that the client should not also do cardio on workout days.

Figure 13-14 illustrates the monthly plan for March. This plan demonstrates a 4-day-per-week workout plan (split routine) with scheduled workouts on Mondays, Tuesdays, Thursdays, and Fridays. The client can perform flexibility exercises every day of the week, if desired.

Figure 13-15 illustrates the monthly plan for June when the individual will introduce phase 4 into his routine. This plan demonstrates a 4-day-per-week workout plan (split routine) with scheduled workouts on Mondays, Tuesdays, Thursdays, and Fridays. The client can perform flexibility exercises every day of the week, if desired.

Week	1							2							3							4						
Day	M	T	W	T	F	S	S	M	T	W	T	F	S	S	M	T	W	T	F	S	S	M	T	W	T	F	S	S
Phase 1																												
Phase 2																												
Phase 3																												
Phase 4	X	X		X	X			X	X		X	X			X	X		X	X			X	X		X	X		
Phase 5																												
Cardio																												
Flexibility	X	X	X	X	X	X	X	X	X	X	X	X	X	X	X	X	X	X	X	X	X	X	X	X	X	X	X	X

Figure 13.15 Monthly plan for the goal of muscle gain, June—phase 4: maximal strength

APPLYING THE MODEL FOR THE GOAL OF IMPROVING GENERAL PERFORMANCE

The goal of improving general performance requires the client to increase overall proprioception, strength, and power output (or rate of force production). The training will need to be progressed from stabilization through power phases of training and use the entire OPT™ model.

The following program is a general representation of how the OPT™ model is used for clients with the goal of improving general performance. The client can be cycled through the entire OPT™ model, depending on the needs and wants of the client. However, for the typical client, phases 1, 2, and 5 will be the most important.

	PHASE	JAN	FEB	MAR	APR	MAY	JUN	JUL	AUG	SEP	OCT	NOV	DEC
Stabilization	1	X		X		X		X		X		X	
Strength	2		X	X	X	X	X	X	X	X	X	X	X
	3												
	4												
Power	5			X	X	X	X	X	X	X	X	X	X
Cardio		X	X	X	X	X	X	X	X	X	X	X	X

Figure 13.16 Annual plan for the goal of general performance.

Because phase 3 is dedicated to maximal hypertrophy, it will not be necessary for the goal of general performance. Phase 4 can be used in moderation to help increase the initial strength levels required to optimize the adaptation in phase 5, if necessary.

Figure 13-16 shows the annual plan. The client will start January in phase 1 to ensure proper muscle balance and endurance of the stabilization muscles. He or she will remain there for approximately 4 weeks before moving on to phase 2. Phase 1 is vital for this client, as it will prepare the connective tissues and muscles for the high demands of training required for this goal. Without proper preparation, injury will be eminent for the athletic client.

The remainder of the annual plan shows the client cycling through phases 1, 2, and 5. Phase 2 will promote greater overall strength and more volume to prepare the client for the greater demands of phase 5. As previously mentioned, phase 4 can be used to increase the strength capacity of the client, but is not vitally necessary for general performance.

From March on, phases 1 or 2 and 5 are used in the same month or week. This is a hybrid form of periodization known as *undulating periodization*. Undulating periodization allows the client to train at various intensities during the course of a week, eliciting multiple adaptations once a certain level of fitness is achieved.[65,77] In this program, stabilization (phase 1), strength (phase 2), and power (phase 5) are all being trained together. Cardiorespiratory training can be performed each month to ensure the cardiorespiratory system is efficient and promoting optimal tissue recoverability.

Figure 13-17 illustrates the monthly plan for January. This plan demonstrates a 3-day-per-week workout plan with scheduled workouts on Mondays, Wednesdays, and Fridays. The client can perform flexibility exercises every day of the week, if desired. Cardio can be done on the workout days (or any other day during the week, depending on the client's schedule).

Week	1							2							3							4						
Day	M	T	W	T	F	S	S	M	T	W	T	F	S	S	M	T	W	T	F	S	S	M	T	W	T	F	S	S
Phase 1	X		X		X			X		X		X			X		X		X			X		X		X		
Phase 2																												
Phase 3																												
Phase 4																												
Phase 5																												
Cardio	X		X		X			X		X		X			X		X		X			X		X		X		
Flexibility	X	X	X	X	X	X	X	X	X	X	X	X	X	X	X	X	X	X	X	X	X	X	X	X	X	X	X	X

Figure 13.17 Monthly plan for the goal of general performance, January—phase 1: stabilization endurance.

Week	1							2							3							4						
Day	M	T	W	T	F	S	S	M	T	W	T	F	S	S	M	T	W	T	F	S	S	M	T	W	T	F	S	S
Phase 1																												
Phase 2	X		X		X			X		X		X			X		X		X			X		X		X		
Phase 3																												
Phase 4																												
Phase 5																												
Cardio	X		X		X			X		X		X			X		X		X			X		X		X		
Flexibility	X	X	X	X	X	X	X	X	X	X	X	X	X	X	X	X	X	X	X	X	X	X	X	X	X	X	X	X

Figure 13.18 Monthly plan for the goal of general performance, February —phase 2: strength endurance.

Figure 13-18 illustrates the monthly plan for February. As with the previous month, this plan demonstrates a 3-day-per-week workout plan with scheduled workouts on Mondays, Wednesdays, and Fridays. This monthly plan could easily be four times a week, with a split routine for the body parts. The client can perform flexibility exercises every day of the week, if desired. Cardio can be done on the workout days (or any other day during the week, depending on the client's schedule).

Figure 13-19 illustrates the monthly plan for March. As with the previous month, this plan demonstrates a 3-day-per-week workout plan with scheduled workouts on Mondays, Wednesdays, and Fridays. In this month, however, phases 1, 2, and 5 are all used in the same week. This helps to introduce power training at a slower, more moderate pace, with low weekly volumes, while ensuring optimal levels of stabilization and strength necessary to increase power. The client can perform flexibility exercises every day of the week, if desired.

Week	1							2							3							4						
Day	M	T	W	T	F	S	S	M	T	W	T	F	S	S	M	T	W	T	F	S	S	M	T	W	T	F	S	S
Phase 1			X							X							X							X				
Phase 2	X							X							X							X						
Phase 3																												
Phase 4																												
Phase 5					X							X							X							X		
Cardio	X		X		X			X		X		X			X		X		X			X		X		X		
Flexibility	X	X	X	X	X	X	X	X	X	X	X	X	X	X	X	X	X	X	X	X	X	X	X	X	X	X	X	X

Figure 13.19 Monthly plan for the goal of general performance, March—hybrid phases 1, 2, and 5.

FILLING IN THE TEMPLATE

Now that all the necessary components of the OPT™ template have been discussed, the resistance-training section of the template can be completed. The beauty of the OPT™ system is that it eliminates the guesswork. When filling in the resistance-training portion of the OPT™ template, just simply choose which phase of training the client will work on. In this manner, all of the major acute variables are already predetermined. Therefore, *sets, reps, intensity, tempo,* and *rest interval* are already given.

In the *exercises* box, simply choose an exercise that fits the desired body part as well as the guidelines of the specific phase of training. For example, phase 2, strength endurance, consists of a strength exercise, followed by a stabilization exercise. Thus, in the *chest* section, a bench press followed by a stability ball push-up would be appropriate exercise selections.

Using information from Chapter 12 (resistance training), the health and fitness professional can choose a particular system of training (such as using a circuit-training or vertical-loading method) to increase the intensity of the workout. If the client works out 2 to 6 days a week, a split routine may be used with varying body parts. Essentially, the possibilities are endless and only limited by creativity. The most important thing, however, is to follow the physiologic guidelines of the OPT™ model. After becoming more familiar with the system and the information, begin to experiment and try new approaches.

Figure 13-20 shows example program templates for the goals of body fat reduction, lean body mass gain and general performance.

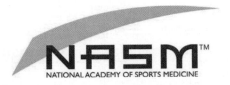

OPT For Fitness

Name: John Smith	Month: 1
Date: 08/10/06	Week: 1
Professional: Scott Lucett	Day: 1of 12

Program Goal:
PHASE 1: FAT LOSS

STEP 1

A. Foam Roll

Foam Roll	Sets	Duration
Calves	1	30 sec
IT Band	1	30 sec
Adductors	1	30 sec

B. Stretch

Static Stretching	Sets	Duration
Calves	1	30 sec
Hip Flexors	1	30 sec
Adductors	1	30 sec

C. Cardiovascular

	Sets	Duration
Treadmill	1	5 min

STEP 2

A. Core

Exercise	Sets	Reps	Tempo	Rest
Floor Bridge	2	15	Slow	0
Floor Prone Cobra	2	15	Slow	0

B. Balance

Exercise	Sets	Reps	Tempo	Rest
Single-leg Balance Reach	2	15	Slow	0

C. Reactive

Exercise	Sets	Reps	Tempo	Rest
Squat Jump w/ Stabilization	2	8	Controlled	60 sec

STEP 3

Resistance Training Program

Body Part	Exercise	Sets	Reps	Intensity	Tempo	Rest
Total Body	Ball Squat, Curl to Press	2	15	60%	Slow	0
Chest	Ball Dumbbell Chest Press	2	15	60%	Slow	0
Back	Standing Cable Row	2	15	60%	Slow	0
Shoulder	Single-leg Dumbbell Scaption	2	15	60%	Slow	0
Biceps	*Optional*					
Triceps	*Optional*					
Legs	Step Up to Balance	2	15	60%	Slow	60 sec

STEP 4

Cool Down

Repeat Steps 1A and/or 1B

Figure 13.20   Filled out strength-training section of the template. (*continued*)

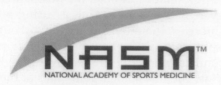

OPT For Fitness

Name: John Smith	Month: 2
Date: 08/10/06	Week: 1
Professional: Scott Lucett	Day: 1 of 12

Program Goal:
PHASE 2: FAT LOSS

STEP 1		
A. Foam Roll		
Foam Roll	Sets	Duration
Calves	1	30 sec
IT Band	1	30 sec
Latissimus Dorsi	1	30 sec
B. Stretch		
Active Stretching	Sets	Duration
Active Gastrocnemius Stretch	1	5 reps
Active Kneeling Hip Flexors Stretch	1	5 reps
Active Latissimus Dorsi Stretch	1	5 reps
C. Cardiovascular		
Treadmill	1	5 min

STEP 2				
A. Core				
Exercise	Sets	Reps	Tempo	Rest
Ball Crunch	2	12	Medium	0
Back Extension	2	12	Medium	0
B. Balance				
Exercise	Sets	Reps	Tempo	Rest
Single-leg Squat	2	12	Medium	0
C. Reactive				
Exercise	Sets	Reps	Tempo	Rest
Squat Jump	2	8	Medium	60 sec

Resistance Training Program						
Body Part Exercise		Sets	Reps	Intensity	Tempo	Rest
Total Body	*Optional*					
Chest	1. Bench Press	2	12	75%	Medium	0
	2. Push Up				Slow	0
Back	1. Lat Pulldown	2	12	75%	Medium	0
	2. Ball Dumbbell Row				Slow	0
Shoulder	1. Shoulder Press Machine	2	12	75%	Medium	0
	2. Single-leg Scaption				Slow	0
Biceps	*Optional*					
Triceps	*Optional*					
Legs	1. Leg Press	2	12	75%	Medium	0
	2. Step up to Balance				Slow	60 sec

STEP 3

Cool Down
Repeat Steps 1A and/or 1B, but use static stretches

STEP 4

Figure 13.20 (*continued*).

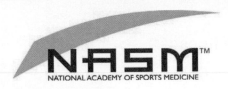

OPT For Fitness

Name: John Smith	Month: 1
Date: 08/10/06	Week: 1
Professional: Scott Lucett	Day: 1 of 12

Program Goal:
PHASE 1: LEAN BODY MASS GAIN

STEP 1

A. Foam Roll

Foam Roll	Sets	Duration
Calves	1	30 sec
IT-Band	1	30 sec
Latissimus Dorsi	1	30 sec

B. Stretch

Static Stretching	Sets	Duration
Gastrocnemius Stretch	1	30 sec
Kneeling Hip Flexor Stretch	1	30 sec
Latissimus Dorsi Ball Stretch	1	30 sec

C. Cardiovascular

	Sets	Duration
Treadmill	1	5 min

STEP 2

A. Core

Exercise	Sets	Reps	Tempo	Rest
Prone Iso Abs	2	15	Slow	0
Floor Bridges	2	15	Slow	0

B. Balance

Exercise	Sets	Reps	Tempo	Rest
Single-leg Balance Reach	2	15	Slow	60 sec

C. Reactive

Exercise	Sets	Reps	Tempo	Rest
optional				

STEP 3

Resistance Training Program

Body Part	Exercise	Sets	Reps	Intensity	Tempo	Rest
Total Body	Optional					
Chest	Ball Dumbbell Chest Press	2	15	65%	Slow	0
Back	Standing Cable Row	2	15	65%	Slow	0
Shoulder	Single-leg Scaption	2	15	65%	Slow	0
Biceps	Single-leg Barbell Curl	2	15	65%	Slow	0
Triceps	Supine Ball Dumbbell Extensions	2	15	65%	Slow	0
Legs	Ball Squat	2	15	65%	Slow	90 sec

STEP 4

Cool Down

Repeat Steps 1A and/or 1B

Figure 13.20 (*continued*).

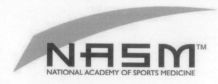

OPT For Fitness

Name: John Smith	Month: 2
Date: 08/10/06	Week: 1
Professional: Scott Lucett	Day: 1 of 12

Program Goal:
PHASE 2: LEAN BODY MASS GAIN

STEP 1

A. Foam Roll

Foam Roll	Sets	Duration
Calves	1	30 sec
IT Band	1	30 sec
Latissimus Dorsi	1	30 sec

B. Stretch

Active Stretching	Sets	Duration
Active Gastrocnemius Stretch	1	5 reps
Active Kneeling Hip Flexors Stretch	1	5 reps
Active Latissimus Dorsi Ball Stretch	1	5 reps

C. Cardiovascular

	Sets	Duration
Treadmill	**1**	**5 min**

STEP 2

A. Core

Exercise	Sets	Reps	Tempo	Rest
Ball Crunch	2	12	Medium	0
Back Extension	2	12	Medium	0

B. Balance

Exercise	Sets	Reps	Tempo	Rest
Single-leg Squat	2	12	Medium	0

C. Reactive

Exercise	Sets	Reps	Tempo	Rest
Squat Jump	2	8	Medium	60 sec

STEP 3

Resistance Training Program

Body Part Exercise		Sets	Reps	Intensity	Tempo	Rest
Total Body	*Optional*					
Chest	1. Flat Dumbbell Chest Press				Medium	0
	2. Ball Dumbbell Chest Press	2	10	80%	Slow	60 sec
Back	1. Seated Cable Row				Medium	0
	2. Ball Dumbbell Row	2	10	80%	Slow	60 sec
Shoulder	1. Seated Dumbbell Shoulder Press				Medium	0
	2. Single-leg Dumbbell Scaption	2	10	80%	Slow	60 sec
Biceps	1. Bicep Curl Machine				Medium	0
	2. Single-leg Dumbbell Curl	2	10	80%	Slow	60 sec
Triceps	1. Cable Pushdown				Medium	0
	2. Prone Ball Dumbbell Tricep Extensions	2	10	80%	Slow	60 sec
Legs	1. Leg Press				Medium	0
	2. Ball Squat	2	10	80%	Slow	60 sec

STEP 4

Cool Down

Repeat Steps 1A and/or 1B, but use
static stretches

NOTE: Resistance training portion can be split into a 2-, 3-, or 4-day workout routine - Ex. 3-day routine: day 1 (chest/back), day 2 (shoulders and legs), day 3 (biceps and triceps)

Figure 13.20 (*continued*).

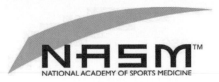

OPT For Fitness

Name: John Smith	Month: 3
Date: 08/10/06	Week: 1
Professional: Scott Lucett	Day: 1 of 12

Program Goal:
PHASE 3: LEAN BODY MASS GAIN
Chest, Shoulders, and Triceps

STEP 1

A. Foam Roll

Foam Roll	Sets	Duration
Calves	1	30 sec
IT Band	1	30 sec
Latissimus Dorsi	1	30 sec

B. Stretch

Active Stretching	Sets	Duration
Active Gastrocnemius Stretch	1	5 reps
Active Kneeling Hip Flexors Stretch	1	5 reps
Active Latissimus Dorsi Ball Stretch	1	5 reps

C. Cardiovascular

Treadmill		5 min

STEP 2

A. Core

Exercise	Sets	Reps	Tempo	Rest
Ball Crunch	2	12	Medium	0
Back Extension	2	12	Medium	60 sec

B. Balance

Exercise	Sets	Reps	Tempo	Rest
Optional				

C. Reactive

Exercise	Sets	Reps	Tempo	Rest
Optional				

STEP 3

Resistance Training Program

Body Part	Exercise	Sets	Reps	Intensity	Tempo	Rest
Total Body	*Optional*					
Chest	1. Barbell Bench Press	3	8	85%	Medium	60 sec
	2. Flat Dumbbell Chest Press	3	8	85%	Medium	60 sec
Back						
Shoulder	1. Seated Dumbbell Shoulder Press	3	8	85%	Medium	60 sec
	2. Shoulder Press Machine	3	8	85%	Medium	60 sec
Biceps						
Triceps	1. Cable Pushdown	3	8	85%	Medium	60 sec
	2. Supine Bench Barbell Tricep Extension	3	8	85%	Medium	60 sec
Legs						

STEP 4

Cool Down

Repeat Steps 1A and/or 1B, but use
static stretches

Figure 13.20 (*continued*).

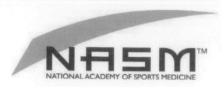

OPT For Fitness

Name: John Smith	Month: 3
Date: 08/10/06	Week: 1
Professional: Scott Lucett	Day: 2 of 12

Program Goal:
PHASE 3: LEAN BODY MASS GAIN
Back, Biceps, and Legs

STEP 1		
A. Foam Roll		
Foam Roll	**Sets**	**Duration**
Calves	1	30 sec
IT Band	1	30 sec
Latissimus Dorsi	1	30 sec
B. Stretch		
Active Stretching	**Sets**	**Duration**
Active Gastrocnemius Stretch	1	5 reps
Active Kneeling Hip Flexors Stretch	1	5 reps
Active Latissimus Dorsi Ball Stretch	1	5 reps
C. Cardiovascular		
Treadmill		**5 min**

STEP 2				
A. Core				
Exercise	**Sets**	**Reps**	**Tempo**	**Rest**
Reverse Crunch	2	12	Medium	0
Back Extension	2	12	Medium	60 sec
B. Balance				
Exercise	**Sets**	**Reps**	**Tempo**	**Rest**
Optional				
C. Reactive				
Exercise	**Sets**	**Reps**	**Tempo**	**Rest**
Optional				

Resistance Training Program						
Body Part Exercise		**Sets**	**Reps**	**Intensity**	**Tempo**	**Rest**
Total Body	*Optional*					
Chest						
Back	1. Lat Pulldown	3	8	85%	Medium	60 sec
	2. Seated Cable Row	3	8	85%	Medium	60 sec
Shoulder						
Biceps	1. Seated Dumbbell Curls	3	8	85%	Medium	60 sec
	2. Bicep Curl Machine	3	8	85%	Medium	60 sec
Triceps						
Legs	1. Barbell Squat	3	8	85%	Medium	60 sec
	2. Leg Press	3	8	85%	Medium	60 sec

STEP 3

Cool Down
Repeat Steps 1A and/or 1B, but use static stretches

STEP 4

Figure 13.20 *(continued)*.

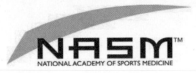

OPT For Performance

Name: John Smith	Month: 1
Date: 08/10/06	Week: 1
Professional: Scott Lucett	Day: 1 of 12

Program Goal:
PHASE 1: GENERAL PERFORMANCE

STEP 1

A. Foam Roll

Foam Roll	Sets	Duration
Calves	1	30 sec
IT Band	1	30 sec
Latissimus Dorsi	1	30 sec

B. Stretch

Static Stretching	Sets	Duration
Gastrocnemius Stretch	1	30 sec
Kneeling Hip Flexors Stretch	1	30 sec
Latissimus Dorsi Ball Stretch	1	30 sec

C. Dynamic Warm Up

	Sets	Duration
Tube Walking	1	10 reps
Prisoner Squat	1	10 reps

STEP 2

A. Core

Exercise	Sets	Reps	Tempo	Rest
Floor Bridge	2	15	Slow	0
Prone Iso Abs	2	15	Slow	0

B. Balance

Exercise	Sets	Reps	Tempo	Rest
Single-leg Balance Reach	2	15	Slow	0

C. Reactive

Exercise	Sets	Reps	Tempo	Rest
Box Jump w/ Stabilization	2	8	Controlled	60 sec

STEP 3

Speed/Agility/Quickness

Exercise	Sets	Rest
Speed Ladder (1 in's, 2 in's, side shuffle, ali shuffle)	2	60 sec
Box Drill	2	60 sec

STEP 4

Resistance Training Program

Body Part	Exercise	Sets	Reps	Intensity	Tempo	Rest
Total Body	*Optional*					
Chest	Ball Dumbbell Chest Press	2	15	60%	Slow	0
Back	Standing Cable Row	2	15	60%	Slow	0
Shoulders	Single-leg Scaption	2	15	60%	Slow	0
Biceps	*Optional*					
Triceps	*Optional*					
Legs	Step-up to balance	2	15	60%	Slow	90 sec

STEP 5

Cool Down

Repeat Steps 1A and/or 1B

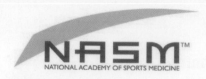

OPT For Performance

Name: John Smith	Month: 2
Date: 08/10/06	Week: 1
Professional: Scott Lucett	Day: 1 of 12

Program Goal:
PHASE 2: GENERAL PERFORMANCE

STEP 1

A. Foam Roll

Foam Roll	Sets	Duration
Calves	1	30 sec
IT Band	1	30 sec
Latissimus Dorsi	1	30 sec

B. Stretch

Active Stretching	Sets	Duration
Active Gastrocnemius Stretch	1	5 reps
Active Kneeling Hip Flexors Stretch	1	5 reps
Active Latissimus Dorsi Ball Stretch	1	5 reps

C. Dynamic Warm Up

	Sets	Duration
Tube Walking	1	10 reps
Prisoner Squat	1	10 reps

STEP 2

A. Core

Exercise	Sets	Reps	Tempo	Rest
Ball Crunch	2	10	Medium	0
Back Extension	2	10	Medium	0

B. Balance

Exercise	Sets	Reps	Tempo	Rest
Step-up to Balance	2	10	Medium	0

C. Reactive

Exercise	Sets	Reps	Tempo	Rest
Squat Jump	2	10	Medium	60 sec

STEP 3

Speed/Agility/Quickness

Exercise	Sets	Rest
Speed Ladder (1 in's, 2 in's, side shuffle, ali shuffle, zig zag, in-in-out-out)	2	60 sec
T- Drill	2	60 sec

STEP 4

Resistance Training Program

Body Part	Exercise	Sets	Reps	Intensity	Tempo	Rest
Total Body	*Optional*					
Chest	1. Flat Dumbbell Chest Press 2. Push up	2	10	75%	Medium Slow	0 60 sec
Back	1. Lat Pulldown 2. Ball Dumbbell Row	2	10	75%	Medium Slow	0 60 sec
Shoulders	1. Seated Dumbbell Shoulder Press 2. Single-leg Scaption	2	10	75%	Medium Slow	0 60 sec
Biceps	*Optional*					
Triceps	*Optional*					
Legs	1. Leg Press 2. Step up to Balance	2	10	75%	Medium Slow	0 60 sec

STEP 5

Cool Down

Repeat Steps 1A and/or 1B, but using static stretches

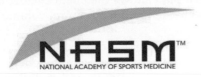

OPT For Performance

Name: John Smith	Month: 3
Date: 08/10/06	Week: 1
Professional: Scott Lucett	Day: 1 of 12

Program Goal:
PHASE 5: GENERAL PERFORMANCE

STEP 1

A. Foam Roll

Foam Roll	Sets	Duration
Calves	1	30 sec
IT Band	1	30 sec
Latissimus Dorsi	1	30 sec

B. Stretch

Dynamic Stretching	Sets	Duration
See Dynamic Warm Up		

C. Dynamic Warm Up

	Sets	Duration
Tube Walking	1	10 reps
Prisoner Squat	1	10 reps
Multiplanar Lunges	1	10 reps

STEP 2

A. Core

Exercise	Sets	Reps	Tempo	Rest
Ball MB Pullover Throw	2	12	Fast	0
Rotation Chest Pass	2	12	Fast	0

B. Balance

Exercise	Sets	Reps	Tempo	Rest
Multiplanar Hop w/Stabilization	2	10	Controlled	60 sec

C. Reactive

Optional				

STEP 3

Speed/Agility/Quickness

Exercise	Sets	Rest
Speed Ladder (1 in's, 2 in's, side shuffle, ali shuffle, zig zag, in-in-out-out)	2	60 sec
5-10-5 Drill	2	60 sec

STEP 4

Resistance Training Program

Body Part	Exercise	Sets	Reps	Intensity	Tempo	Rest
Total Body	*Optional*					
Chest	1. Bench Press		5	85%		0
	2. Medicine Ball Chest Pass	3	10	5% of BW	Fast	2 min
Back	1. Lat Pulldown		5	85%		0
	2. Woodchop Throw	3	10	5% of BW	Fast	2 min
Shoulders	1. Shoulder Press Machine		5	85%		0
	2. Single-leg Scaption	3	10	5% of BW	Fast	2 min
Biceps	*Optional*					
Triceps	*Optional*					
	1. Squat		5	85%		0
	2. Single Leg Power Step Ups	3	10	5% of BW	Fast	2 min

STEP 5

Cool Down

Repeat Steps 1A and/or 1B, but using static stretches

SUMMARY

The OPT™ model is a planned fitness-training system that can be used to create programs for clients with various goals. Health and fitness professionals must be able to apply the information in multiple situations to a variety of clients. The OPT™ model can be used to reduce body fat, increase lean body mass, and improve general performance.

To reduce body fat, clients must burn more calories than they consume by moving more with resistance and cardiorespiratory training. The client will work in phase 1 for 4 weeks, to ensure proper muscle balance and endurance of the stabilization muscles. The remainder of the annual plan shows the client cycling back and forth between phases 1 and 2 (metabolic demand and more volume for increased caloric expenditure).

To increase lean body mass, clients must consume more calories than are burned by working with higher volumes to increase muscle size. The client will work in phase 1 for 4 weeks, to ensure proper muscle balance and endurance of the stabilization muscles. The remainder of the annual plan shows the client cycling through phase 1 (recovery time), phase 2 (greater strength endurance and more volume), phase 3 (larger volumes of stress for hypertrophy), and phase 4 (increased strength capacity with even higher volumes of training and more hypertrophy). Cardiorespiratory training can be performed each month to ensure the cardiorespiratory system is efficient and promoting optimal tissue recoverability.

To improve general performance, clients must increase overall proprioception, strength, and rate of force production. The training will use the entire OPT™ model, although for the typical client, phases 1, 2, and 5 will be the most important. The client will work in phase 1 for 4 weeks, to ensure proper muscle balance and endurance of the stabilization muscles. The remainder of the annual plan shows the client cycling through phases 1, 2 (greater overall strength and more volume), and 5. After the first 4 months, undulating periodization is used, and stabilization (phase 1), strength (phase 2), and power (phase 5) are used in the same month and week. Cardiorespiratory training can be performed each month as well.

Review Questions

1 *The OPT™ model has been extremely successful in helping all populations to reduce body fat, increase lean muscle mass and strength, improve performance, and improve overall health.*

   a. True

   b. False

2 *A typical client with the goal of improving general performance should specifically be cycled through which phases?*

3 *Beginning clients should perform lower repetition schemes.*

   a. True

   b. False

4 *How long does it take for the body to replenish 100% of its ATP and creatine phosphate (CP) supplies?*

   a. 20 seconds

   b. 40 seconds

   c. 60 seconds

   d. 3 minutes

5 *Training volume is always inversely related to intensity.*

   a. True

   b. False

6 *Which phase(s) of training uses superset techniques?*

a. Phase 1: stabilization endurance

b. Phase 2: strength endurance

c. Phase 3: hypertrophy

d. Phase 4: maximal strength

e. Phase 5: power

REFERENCES

1. Rose DL, Radzyminski SF, Beaty RR. Effect of brief maximal exercise on the strength of the quadriceps femoris. Arch Phys Med Rehabil 1957;Mar:157–164.
2. Rutherford OM, Jones DA. The role of learning and coordination in strength training. Eur J Appl Physiol 1986;55:100–105.
3. Hickson RC. Interference of strength development by simultaneously training for strength and endurance. Eur J Appl Physiol 1980;45:255–263.
4. Hickson RC, Rosenkoetter MA, Brown MM. Strength training effects on aerobic power and short term endurance. Med Sci Sports Exerc 1980;12:336–339.
5. Issurin VB, Liebermann DG, Tenenbaum G. Effect of vibratory stimulation training on maximal force and flexibility. J Sports Sci 1994;12:561–566.
6. O'Shea P. Throwing speed. Sports Fitness 1985;August:66–67, 89–90.
7. Ostrowski KJ, Wilson GJ, Weatherby R, Murphy PW, Lyttle AD. The effect of weight training volume on hormonal output and muscular size and function. J Strength Cond Res 1997;11:148–154.
8. Ploutz LL, Tesch PA, Biro RL, Dudley GA. Effect of resistance training on muscle use during exercise. J Appl Physiol 1994;76:1675–1681.
9. Stone MH, O'Bryant HS, Schilling BK, Johnson RL, Pierce KC, Haff GG, Koch AJ, Stone M. Periodization: effects of manipulating volume and intensity. Part 2. NSCA J 1999;21(3):54–60.
10. Stone MH, Plisk SS, Stone ME, Schilling BK, O'Bryant HS, Pierce KC. Athletic performance development: volume load-1 set vs. multiple sets, training velocity and training variation. NSCA J 1998;20(6):22–31.
11. Tan B. Manipulating resistance training program variables to optimize maximum strength in men: A review. J Strength Cond Res 1999;13(3):289–304.
12. Baker D, Wilson G, Carlyon R. Periodization: the effect on strength of manipulating volume and intensity. J Strength Cond Res 1994;8(4):235–242.
13. Bompa TO. Theory and Methodology of Training. Dubuque, IA: Kendall/Hunt, 1983.
14. Bompa TO. Variations of periodization of strength. Strength Cond 1996;18:58–61.
15. Poliquin C. Five steps to increasing the effectiveness of your strength training program. Natl Strength Cond Assoc J 1998;10:34–39.
16. Siff MC, Verkhoshansky Y. Supertraining. Escondido, CA: Sports Training, 1994.
17. Fleck SJ, Kraemer WJ. Designing Resistance Training Programs, 2nd ed. Champaign, IL: Human Kinetics, 1997.
18. Kraemer WJ, Patton JF, Gordon SE, Harman EA, Deschenes KR, Reynolds K, Newton RU, Triplett NT, Dziados JE. Compatibility of high-intensity strength and endurance training on hormonal and skeletal muscle adaptations. J Appl Physiol 1995;78:976–989.
19. Hakkinen K, Pakarinen A, Alen M, et al. Relationships between training volume, physical performance capacity, and serum hormone concentrations during prolonged training in elite weight lifters. Int J Sports Med 1987;8(Suppl):61–65.
20. Hakkinen K, Pakarinen A, Alen M, et al. Neuromuscular and hormonal responses in elite athletes to two successive strength training sessions in one day. Eur J Appl Physiol 1988;57:133–139.
21. Stone MH, Fry AC. Responses to increased resistance training volume. In: Kreider R, Fry AL, O'Toole M (eds). Overtraining and Overreaching in Sport. Champaign, IL: Human Kinetics, 1997.
22. Zatsiorsky VM. Science and Practice of Strength Training. Champaign, IL: Human Kinetics, 1995.
23. Berger RA. Effect of varied weight training programs on strength. Res Q 1962;33:169–181.
24. Hakkinen K. Neuromuscular adaptation during strength training, aging, detraining and immobilization. Crit Rev Phys Rehab Med 1994;6:161–198.
25. Kaneko M, Fuchimoto T, Toji H, Suei K. Training effect of different loads on the force-velocity relationship and mechanical power output in human muscle. Scand J Sports Sci 1983;5(2):50–55.
26. Sale DG. Neural adaptation in strength and power training. In: Jones NL, McCartney N, McComas AJ (eds). Human Muscle Power. Champaign, IL: Human Kinetics, 1986:289–307.

27. Sale DG. Influence of exercise and training on motor unit activation. Exer Sport Sci Rev 1987;15:95–151.
28. Sale DG. Neural adaptation to strength training. In: Komi PV (ed). Strength and Power in Sport. London: Blackwell Scientific, 1992:249–265.
29. Schmidtbleicher D. Training for power events. In: Chem PV (ed). Strength and Power in Sports. Boston: Blackwell Scientific, 1992:381–396.
30. Schmidtbleicher D, Haralambie G. Changes in contractile properties of muscle after strength training in a man. Eur J Appl Physiol 1981;46:221–228.
31. Stone MH. Considerations in gaining a strength power training effect. NSCA J 1982;4(1):22–24, 54.
32. Stone MH, Borden RA. Modes and methods of resistance training. Strength Cond 1997;19(4):18–24.
33. Stone MH, O'Bryant HS. Weight Training: A Scientific Approach. Minneapolis: Burgess, 1987.
34. Holly RG, Shaffrath JD. Cardiorespiratory endurance. In: American College of Sports Medicine (ed). ACSM's Resource Manual for Guidelines for Exercise Testing and Prescription, 3rd ed. Baltimore: Williams & Wilkins, 1998.
35. American College of Sports Medicine. ACSM's Guidelines for Exercise Testing and Prescription, 5th ed. Philadelphia: Williams & Wilkins, 1995.
36. Heus R, Wertheim AH, Havenith G. Human energy expenditure when walking on a moving platform. Eur J Appl Physiol Occup Physiol 1998;100(2):133–148.
37. Williford HN, Olson MS, Gauger S, Duey WJ, Blessing DL. Cardiovascular and metabolic costs of forward, backward, and lateral motion. Med Sci Sports Exerc 1998;30(9)1419–1423.
38. Ogita F, Stam RP, Tazawa HO, Toussaint HM, Hollander AP. Oxygen uptake in one-legged and two-legged exercise. Med Sci Sports Exerc 2000;32(10):1737–1742.
39. Willoughby DS. Training volume equated: a comparison of periodized and progressive resistance weight training programs. J Hum Move Studies 1991;21:233–248.
40. Gambetta V. The Gambetta Method: Common Sense Training for Athletic Performance. Sarasota, FL: Gambetta Sports Training Systems, 1998.
41. Hakkinen K, Komi PV, Allen M. Effect of explosive type strength training on isometric force- and relaxation-time, electromyographic and muscle fiber characteristics of leg extensor muscles. Acta Physiol Scand 1985;125:587–600.
42. Bauer T, Thayer TE, Boras G. Comparison of training modalities for power development in the lower extremity. J Appl Sports Sci Res 1990;4:115–121.
43. Burkhardt E, Barton B, Garhammer J. Maximal impact and propulsion forces during jumping and explosive lifting exercise. J Appl Sports Sci Res 1990;4(3):107.
44. Chu DA. Plyometrics: the link between strength and speed. NSCA J 1983;5(2):20–21.
45. Housh DJ, Housh TJ, Johnson GO, et al. Hypertrophic response to unilateral concentric isokinetic resistance training. J Appl Physiol 1992;73:65–70.
46. Ballor DL, Becque MD, Katch VL, et al. Metabolic responses during hydraulic resistance exercise. Med Sci Sports Exerc 1987;19:363–367.
47. Kraemer WJ, Ratamess NA. Physiology of resistance training. Orthop Phys Ther Clin North Am 2000;9(4):467–513.
48. Stone MH, O'Bryant H, Garhammer J. A hypothetical model for strength training. J Sports Med Phys Fitness 1981;21:341–352.
49. Tesch PA, Colliander EB, Kaiser P. Muscle metabolism during intense, heavy resistance exercise. Eur J Appl Physiol 1986;55:362–366.
50. Tesch PA, Karlsson J. Lactate and fast and slow twitch skeletal muscle fibers of man during isometric contraction. Acta Physiol Scand 1977;99:230–236.
51. Fleck SJ. Bridging the gap: interval training physiological basis. NSCA J 1983;5:57–62.
52. Brooks GA, Fahey TD, White TP. Exercise Physiology: Human Bioenergetics and Its Application, 2nd ed. Mountain View, CA: Mayfield Publishing, 1996.
53. Fitts RH. Cellular mechanisms of muscle fatigue. Physiol Rev 1994;74:49–94.
54. Thorstenson A, Hultren B, von Dobeln W, Karlsson J. Effect of strength training on enzyme activities and fibre characteristics in human skeletal muscle. Acta Physiol Scand 1976;96:392–398.
55. MacDougal JD, Elder GCB, Sale DG, Moroz JR, Sutton JR. Effects of strength training and immobilization on human muscle fibers. Eur J Appl Physiol 1980;43:25–34.
56. Abernathy PJ, Jurimae J, Logan PA, Taylor AW, Thayer RE. Acute and chronic response of skeletal muscle to resistance exercise. Sports Med 1994;17(1):22–38.
57. Kim JR, Oberman A, Fletcher GF, Lee JY. Effect of exercise intensity and frequency on lipid levels in men with coronary heart disease: Training Level Comparison Trial. Am J Cardiol 2001;87(8):942–946.
58. Tsukui S, Kanda T, Nara M, Nishino M, Kondo T, Kobayashi I. Moderate-intensity regular exercise decreases serum tumor necrosis factor-alpha and HbA1c levels in healthy women. Int J Obes Relat Metab Disord 2000;24(9):1207–1211.
59. Van Etten LMLA, Westerterp KR, Verstappen FTJ, et al. Effect of an 18-week training program on energy expenditure and physical activity. J Appl Physiol 1997;82:298–304.
60. Gillam GM. Effects of frequency of weight training on muscle strength enhancement. J Sports Med Phys Fitness 1981;21:432–436.

61. Kraemer WJ, Marchitelli L, Gordon SE, Harman E, Dziados JE, Mello R, Frykman P, McCrury D, Fleck SJ. Hormonal growth factor responses to heavy resistance protocols. J Appl Physiol 1990;69:1442–1450.
62. Kraemer WJ, Fleck SJ, Callister R, Shealy M, Dudley GA, Maresh CM, Marchitelli L, Cruthirds C, Murray T, Falkel JE. Training responses of plasma beta-endorphin, adrenocorticotropin, and cortisol. Med Sci Sports Exerc 1989;21:146–153.
63. Cosio-Lima LM, Reynolds KL, Winter C, Paolone V, Jones MT. Effects of Physioball and conventional floor exercises on early adaptations in back and abdominal core stability and balance in women. J Strength Cond Res 2003;17(4):721–725.
64. Behm DG, Anderson K, Curnew RS. Muscle force and activation under stable and unstable conditions. J Strength Cond Res 2002;16(3):416–422.
65. Heitkamp HC, Horstmann T, Mayer F, Weller J, Dickhuth HH. Gain in strength and muscular balance after balance training. Int J Sports Med 2001;22:285–290.
66. Haff GG, Stone MH, O'Bryant HS, et al. Force-time dependent characteristics of dynamic and isometric muscle contractions. J Strength Cond Res 1997;11:269–272.
67. Schmidt RA. Motor Learning Performance. Champaign, IL: Human Kinetics, 1991.
68. Sale DG. Neural adaptation to resistance training. Med Sci Sports Exerc 1988;20(5 Suppl):S135–S145.
69. Enoka RM. Muscle strength and its development: new perspectives. Sports Med 1988;6:146–168.
70. Henneman E. Relation between size of motor neurons and their susceptibility to discharge. Science 1957;126:1345–1347.
71. Sale DG. Neural adaptation to resistance training. Med Sci Sports Exerc 1988;20(5 Suppl):S135–S145.
72. Enoka RM. Muscle strength and its development. New perspectives. Sports Med 1988;6: 146–168.
73. Westerterp KR, Meijer GAL, Janssen GME, Saris WHM, Hoor F. Long-term effect of physical activity on energy balance and body composition. Br J Nutr 1992;68(1):21–30.
74. Bompa TO. Periodization of Strength: The New Wave in Strength Training. Toronto: Verita Publishing, 1993.
75. Plisk SS, Stone MH. Periodization strategies. Strength Cond J 2003;25(6):19–37.
76. Graham J. Periodization research and an example application. Strength Cond J 2002;24(6): 62–70.
77. Herrick AB, Stone WJ. The effects of periodization versus progressive resistance exercise on upper and lower body strength in women. J Strength Cond Res 1996;10:72–76.
78. Dolezal BA, Potteiger JA. Concurrent resistance and endurance training influence basal metabolic rate (BMR) in non-dieting individuals. J Appl Physiol 1998;85:695–700.
79. Rhea MR, Phillips WT, Burkett LN, Stone WJ, Ball SD, Alvar BA, Thomas AB. A comparison of linear and daily undulating periodized programs with equated volume and intensity for local muscular endurance. J Strength Cond Res 2003;17(1):82–87.
80. Heitkamp HC, Horstmann T, Mayer F, Weller J, Dickhuth HH. Gain in strength and muscular balance after balance training. Int J Sports Med 2001;285–290.
81. Wolf B, Feys H, Weerdt D, Van der Meer J, Noom M, Aufdemkampe G, Noom M. Effect of a physical therapeutic intervention for balance problems in the elderly: a single-blind, randomized, controlled multicentre trial. Clin Rehab 2001:15(6):624–636.
82. Fitzgerald GK, Childs JD, Ridge TM, Irrgang JJ. Agility and perturbation training for a physically active individual with knee osteoarthritis. Phys Ther 2002;82(4):372–382.
83. Luoto S, Aalto H, Taimela S, Hurri H, Pyykko I, Alaranta H. One footed and externally disturbed two footed postural control in patients with chronic low back pain and health control subjects. A controlled study with follow-up. Spine 1998;23(19):2081–2089.
84. Borsa PA, Lephart SM, Kocher MS, Lephart SP. Functional assessment and rehabilitation of shoulder proprioception for glenohumeral instability. J Sports Rehab 1994;3:84–104.
85. Hirsch M, Toole T, Maitland CG, Rider RA. The effects of balance training and high-intensity resistance training on persons with idiopathic Parkinson's disease. Arch Phys Med Rehab 2003;84:1109–1117.
86. Behm DG, Anderson K, Curnew RS. Muscle force and activation under stable and unstable conditions. J Strength Cond Res 2002;16(3):416–422.
87. DeRenne C, Hetzler RK, Buxton BP, Ho KW. Effects of training frequency on strength maintenance in pubescent baseball players. J Strength Cond Res 1996;10:8–14.
88. Hoffman JR, Fry AC, Howard R, Maresh CM, Armstrong LE, Kraemer WJ. Effects of off-season and in-season resistance training programs on a collegiate male basketball team. J Hum Muscle Perform 1991;1:48–55.
89. Baker D. Selecting the appropriate exercises and loads for speed-strength development. Strength Cond Coach 1995;3(2):8–16.
90. Ebben WP, Watts PB. A review of combined weight training and plyometric training modes: complex training. Strength Cond 1998;20(5):18–27.
91. Fleck S, Kontor K. Complex training. NSCA J 1986;8(5):66–68.
92. Ebben WP, Blackard DO. Complex training with combined explosive weight and plyometric exercises. Olympic Coach 1997;7(4):11–12.

93. Kaikkonen H, Yrlama M, Siljander E, Byman P, Laukkanen R. The effect of heart rate controlled low resistance circuit weight training and endurance training on maximal aerobic power in sedentary adults. Scand J Med Sci Sports 2000;10(4):211–215.

94. Jurimae T, Jurimae J, Pihl E. Circulatory response to single circuit weight and walking training sessions of similar energy cost in middle-aged overweight females. Clin Physiol 2000;20(2):143–149.

95. Burleson MA, O'Bryant HS, Stone MH, Collins MA, Triplett-McBride T. Effect of weight training exercise and treadmill exercise on post-exercise oxygen consumption. Med Sci Sports Exerc 1998;30(4):518–522.

96. Gillette CA, Bullough RC, Melby CL. Postexercise energy expenditure in response to acute aerobic or resistive exercise. Int J Sport Nutr 1994;4(4):347–360.

Special Populations

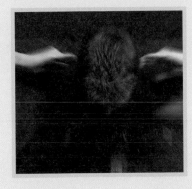

OBJECTIVES

After completing this chapter, you will be able to:

- Define and describe conditions, dysfunctions, or diseases common in the special populations of clients.
- Understand how these conditions affect the acute training variables within the OPT™ model.
- Alter program design for clients with various conditions.

KEY TERMS

Arthritis	Obesity	Osteoporosis
Cancer	Obstructive lung disease	Pregnancy
Diabetes	Osteoarthritis	Restrictive lung disease
Hypertension	Osteopenia	Rheumatoid arthritis

INTRODUCTION TO SPECIAL POPULATIONS

Up to this point, the information studied has been based on the assumption that the clients being worked with are apparently healthy adults. These individuals do not seem to have conditions, dysfunctions, or diseases that would necessitate an alteration in their assessment or program design.

However, in some cases, application of exercise principles for the apparently healthy adult could be potentially dangerous. This could easily be the case for an individual with underlying coronary heart disease, or osteoporosis. In other instances, such as obesity, application of these principles might not harm the participant, but may not be the optimal course of exercise treatment. Thus, the consideration of individuals with special needs is twofold: to provide a margin of safety and to optimize training.

In this chapter, a variety of common conditions and diseases encountered in exercise training programs will be reviewed. The list is by no means inclusive. There are considerably more diseases that may require different assessment techniques or altered program design (those with neuromuscular disease, for example). Additional excellent resources are available for other special populations.[1–3]

Age Considerations

YOUTH TRAINING

Health and fitness professionals are confronted with an increasing variance in clientele seeking assistance in fitness venues. One such growing population is youth clients. Realistically, this population can range between the ages of 6 and 20 years of age. However, owing to biomechanical and physiologic variations in growth, it is difficult to precisely determine maturity and the exact age of "youth" training. A 1994 consensus paper by Sallis and colleagues[4] defines adolescence as ages 11 to 21 years. As such, the guidelines for youth training are largely based on that age range, although physical development and maturation can vary.

Most established guidelines for exercise in the youth population have previously been focused on sport training. Given the alarming increase in childhood obesity and diabetes, increased attention has recently been directed to the development of guidelines to promote a healthy threshold for physical activity (including federal guidelines for school and community programs).[5] Consistent with the recommendations made for adults, adolescents should engage in moderate to vigorous physical activity for a minimum of 20 minutes, three or more days of the week, to promote health and chronic disease prevention as adults.[2] Emphasizing the need to initiate high levels of physical activity in even younger children, the National Association for Sport and Physical Education promotes physical activity of at least 30 to 60 minutes on most, or all, days of the week for elementary school children, focusing on developmentally appropriate activities.[6] The American College of Sports Medicine has published a summary of appropriate field fitness tests for children, as well as specific exercise testing protocols.[7]

Physiologic Differences Between Children and Adults

It is important to appreciate that there are fundamental physiologic differences between children and adults. Children are not miniature adults. Although they may experience similar effects as a result of training, they do not demonstrate the same capabilities or progressions. Therefore, the youth population will still use the OPT™ model for training purposes, but will progress in a fashion more specific to their physiologic capabilities.

Table 14.1

Physiologic and Training Considerations for Youth

Physiologic Considerations	Implication of Exercise Compared With Adult	Considerations for Health and Fitness	Considerations in Sport and Athletic Training
"$\dot{V}O_2$ peak" is similar to adult when adjusted for body weight	Able to perform endurance tasks relatively well	Physical activity of 30–60+ minutes on most or all days of the week for elementary school children, emphasizing developmentally appropriate activities[5]	Progression of aerobic training volume should not exceed 10% per period of adaptation (if weekly training volume was 200 minutes per week, increase to 220 minutes before further increases in intensity)
Submaximal oxygen demand is higher compared with adults for walking and running	Greater chance of fatigue and heat production in sustained higher-intensity tasks	Moderate to vigorous physical activity for adolescents, for a minimum of 20 minutes three or more days of the week[3]	Intensive anaerobic exercise exceeding 10 seconds is not well tolerated (if using stage II or III training, provide sufficient rest and recovery intervals between intense bouts of training)
Glycolytic enzymes are lower than adult	Decreased ability to perform longer-duration (10–90 s), high-intensity tasks	Resistance exercise for muscular fitness: 1–2 sets of 8–10 exercises 8–12 reps per exercise[7]	Resistance exercise should emphasize proprioception, skill, and controlled movements. Repetitions should not exceed: 6–8 per set for strength development 20 for enhanced muscular endurance
Sweating rate	Decreased tolerance to environmental extremes, particularly heat and humidity	2–3 days per week Duration = 30 minutes, with added time for warm-up and cool-down	2–3 days per week, with increases in overload occurring through increases in reps first, then resistance

$\dot{V}O_2$, oxygen consumption.

The fitness professional should be aware of some simple physiologic differences between children and adults that impact physical performance and include (Table 14-1):[8]

- Peak oxygen uptake—The term "maximum oxygen uptake" should not be used to describe peak assessed values in children because they do not exhibit a plateau in oxygen uptake at maximum exercise. Thus, "peak" is a more appropriate term. When adjusted for body weight, peak oxygen consumption is similar for young and mature males, and slightly higher for young females (compared to mature females). A similar interpretation can be made for force production, or strength.
- Submaximal oxygen demand —Economy of movement
- Glycolytic enzymes—Enzymes used in the glycolysis energy pathway
- Sweating rate

The similarity in peak oxygen uptake values between children and adults allows for children to perform endurance-related tasks fairly well. This enables youths to train in the stabilization level of the OPT™ model (phase 1).

A higher submaximal oxygen demand, combined with a lower absolute sweating rate (and other factors beyond the scope of this text), contributes to children having less of a tolerance for temperature extremes. Vigorous exercise in the presence of high temperature and humidity should be restricted to less than 30 minutes. As in adults, adequate hydration is important.

The lower glycolytic enzymes seen in children decrease their ability (or efficiency) to perform higher intensity (or anaerobic) tasks for prolonged periods of time (10 to 90 seconds). This requires that children have adequate rest intervals when training at high intensities.

Resistance Training in the Youth Population

Overcoming the perception that resistance training is inappropriate for children has resulted in research that has demonstrated that resistance training is both safe and effective in children.[9-11] It has been shown that resistance training for health and fitness conditioning in the youth population results in a lower risk of injury when compared with many popular sports (including soccer, football, and basketball).[12] Furthermore, resistance training in the 5- to 14-year-old age group has been associated with a decrease in the number of common injuries.[13] The most common injuries related to resistance training in the youth population have been sprains and strains.[14] These injuries have been attributed to lack of qualified supervision, poor technique, and improper progression.[15]

This information reiterates the importance of following a systematic approach to exercise training. To promote a safe and effective training environment, health and fitness professionals must first use a simple movement assessment to observe a youth's movement ability.

This movement assessment can easily be done by having the youth perform 10 body-weight squats and 10 push-ups. Follow the kinetic chain checkpoints from Chapter 5 (Fitness Assessment) to gather information regarding movement imbalances. This information will allow for the selection of exercises that are appropriate for each individual youth client. Adherence to these kinetic chain checkpoints during regular exercise will also ensure safe and effective training technique and proper progression.

Results in youth physiologic adaptation are similar to those in adults.[16] A review of literature by Faigenbaum and colleagues[9] suggests that, on average, untrained children have increased strength by 30 to 40%. It has also been suggested that resistance training has positive effects on motor skills (sprinting and jumping), body composition, and bone mineral density.[9,16,17] The source of strength gains and improvements in performance for this population appear to be attributed to neural adaptations in contrast to hypertrophy.[11,18] Relating to flexibility in youth populations, it has been shown that there is a decline as they get older.[19,20]

Collectively, this information is extremely important for a health and fitness professional to understand in regard to program design. It suggests the importance of assessing each youth for movement deficiencies, incorporating the flexibility continuum, and training in the stabilization phase of the OPT™ model. Progression into phases 2 through 5 should be predicated on maturity level, dynamic postural control (flexibility and stability), and advice from a licensed physician. Perhaps the most important aspect of training, especially for the youth population, is to make it fun.

Recommendations for youth training parameters are outlined in Tables 14-1 and 14-2.

SENIORS

By the middle of this century, it is estimated that the number of Americans older than the age of 65 will reach approximately 70 million (nearly one in five residents will be considered elderly). As America's population ages, it is increasingly faced with the issue of mortality, longevity, and quality of life.[21] This upward drift in average age has significant implications for health and fitness professionals. As the importance of exercise for functional independence becomes more widely known and accepted, opportunities to evaluate and provide meaningful physical training for older adults will increase.

Table 14.2	
Basic Exercise Guidelines for Youth Training	
Mode	Walking, jogging, running, games, activities, sports, water activity, resistance training
Frequency	2–5 days per week
Intensity	50–90% of maximum heart rate for cardiorespiratory training
Duration	30–120 minutes per day (for sports).
Movement Assessment	Overhead squats 10 push-ups (if 10 cannot be performed, do as many as can be tolerated Single-leg stance (if can tolerate perform 3–5 single-leg squats per leg)
Flexibility	Follow the flexibility continuum specific for each phase of training
Resistance Training	1–2 sets of 6–20 repetitions at 40–70% on 2–3 days per week. Phase 1 of OPT™ model should be mastered before moving on. Phases 2–5 should be reserved for mature adolescents on the basis of dynamic postural control and a licensed physician's recommendation.
Special Considerations	Progression for the youth population should be based on postural control and not on the amount of weight that can be used. Make exercising fun!

Unfortunately, aging has come to be associated with degeneration and the limited functional ability of the older adult.[22] Typical forms of degeneration in the older adult include osteoporosis, arthritis (osteoarthritis),[23,24] low back pain (LBP),[25,26] and obesity.[27] Although special considerations for those specific diseases will be addressed in subsequent modules, considerations for apparently healthy older adults help provide the fitness professional with the fundamental knowledge to effectively evaluate and design programs for this population.

With this being said, it is important to draw a distinction between what is observed in older adults and what is abnormal. For example, it is not unusual to find increased blood pressure at rest and during exercise, owing to a combination of physiologic aging and behavioral factors. However, blood pressure reaching prehypertensive (135 mm Hg systolic, 85 mm Hg diastolic) or higher levels should be referred to a physician for further evaluation and treatment, regardless of the client's age.

Likewise, an important observation about older adults lies in the adaptive capability for physiologic improvement in fitness. It is known that as adults age all of the following functions decrease:[28,29]

- Maximum attainable heart rate
- Cardiac output
- Muscle mass
- Balance
- Coordination (neuromuscular efficiency)
- Connective tissue elasticity
- Bone mineral density

This obviously affects the central component to fitness. These degenerative processes can lead to a decrease in the functional capacity of the older adult, as defined by overall strength (cardiorespiratory and muscular) and proprioceptive responses.[30,31] Perhaps the most important functional capacity affected is walking. The decreased ability to move freely in one's own environment not only reduces the physical and emotional independence of an individual, it also can lead to an increase in the degenerative cycle.[16]

Many people who exhibit one or more of these degenerative conditions may tend to shy away from known remedies (such as resistance training) out of fear of injury or feelings of inadequacy.[32] However, research shows that musculoskeletal degeneration may not be entirely age-related and that certain measures can be taken to prevent functional immobility.[33-36] It has also been demonstrated that many of the structural deficits responsible for decreased functional capacity in the older adult (loss of muscle strength and proprioception) can be slowed and even reversed.

By adhering to the OPT™ model, health and fitness professionals can make a dramatic impact on the overall health and well-being of the older adult. Training must begin with a Physical Activity Readiness Questionnaire (PAR-Q) and movement assessment such as a squat, sitting and standing from a seated position, or a single-leg stance. This assessment will provide information about quality of movement as well as a person's functional capacity for activities of daily living. Flexibility will be paramount, as older adults lose the elasticity of their connective tissue. Self-myofascial release and static stretching are advised for this population, provided there is sufficient ability to perform the necessary movements. Otherwise, simple forms of active or dynamic stretching may be required to simply get the client to move their joints and "warm-up."

Stages I and II will be appropriate levels of cardiorespiratory training for this population and should progress slowly; however, medications and other comorbidities must be taken into consideration. Phases 1 and 2 of the OPT™ model will be applicable for this population and should be progressed slowly, with an emphasis

Table 14.3

Physiologic and Training Considerations for Seniors

Physiologic Considerations	Implications of Health and Fitness Training
Maximum oxygen uptake, maximum exercise heart rate, and measures of pulmonary function will all decrease with increasing age	Initial exercise workloads should be low and progressed more gradually 3–5 days per week Duration = 20–45 minutes Intensity = 45–80% of peak
Percentage of body fat will increase, and both bone mass and lean body mass will decrease with increasing age	Resistance exercise is recommended, with lower initial weights and slower progression (For example: 1–3 sets of 8–10 exercises, 8–20 reps Session length = 20–30 minutes)
Balance, gait, and neuromuscular coordination may be impaired	Exercise modalities should be chosen and progressed to safeguard against falls and foot problems Cardio options include stationary or recumbent cycling, aquatic exercise, or treadmill with handrail support Resistance options include seated machines progressing to standing exercises
There is a higher rate of both diagnosed and undetected heart disease in the elderly	Knowledge of pulse assessment during exercise is critical, as is monitoring for chronic disease signs and symptoms
Pulse irregularity is more frequent	Careful analysis of medication use and possible exercise effects

Table 14.4

Basic Exercise Guidelines for Seniors

Mode	Stationary or recumbent cycling, aquatic exercise, or treadmill with handrail support
Frequency	2–5 days per week
Intensity	40–85% of $\dot{V}O_2$ peak
Duration	30–60 minutes per day or 8- to 10-min bouts
Movement Assessment	Push, pull, OH squat, *or* Sitting and standing into a chair Single-leg balance
Flexibility	Self-myofascial release and static stretching (see Special Considerations)
Resistance Training	1–3 sets of 8–20 repetitions at 40–80% on 3–5 days per week Phases 1 and 2 of OPT™ model should be mastered before moving on Phases 2–5 should be based on dynamic postural control and a licensed physician's recommendation
Special Considerations	Progression should be slow, well monitored, and based on postural control Exercises should be progressed if possible toward free sitting (no support) or standing Make sure client is breathing in normal manner and avoid holding breath as in a Valsalva maneuver If client cannot tolerate SMR or static stretches because of other conditions, perform slow rhythmic active or dynamic stretches

SMR, self-myofascial release; *OH*, overhead squats.

on stabilization training (core, balance, and progression to standing resistance exercises). As always, consult with a licensed physician for specific information regarding the older adult client.

The physiologic considerations and their implications for training apparently healthy older adults are listed in Tables 14-3 and 14-4. Resources that further detail the physiologic changes that occur in the older adult are available.[37]

SUMMARY

The guidelines for youth training are largely based on an 11- to 21-year-old age range, although physical development and maturation can vary. Adolescents should engage in moderate to vigorous physical activity for a minimum of 20 minutes, three or more days of the week. Elementary school children should engage in 30 to 60 minutes of physical activity on most days of the week.

Children have lower body weight and peak oxygen uptake than adults. Special considerations must be given to musculoskeletal growth issues as well as children's lower tolerance for temperature extremes. High-volume aerobic training is not advisable in children. Instead, physiologic adaptations should be developed through resistance training that emphasizes skill and controlled movements.

In older adults, it is important to draw a distinction between what is observed and what is abnormal. These individuals may have increased blood pressure as a result of a combination of physiologic aging and behavioral factors. In addition, maximum attainable heart rate decreases and cardiac output declines, although peripheral adaptation remains intact. Resistance training is recommended 3 to 5 days per week, using lighter weights and slower progressions.

Obesity

Obesity: The condition of subcutaneous fat exceeding the amount of lean body mass.

Obesity is the fastest growing health problem in America and most other industrialized cultures. The trends in the United States are especially alarming. Currently, it is estimated that approximately 33% of the adult population and 15% of children older than the age of 6 are obese.[38,39] However, it has been demonstrated that perhaps two thirds of the adult population may be considered overweight.[40] Not only is obesity associated with many chronic diseases discussed in this chapter, it is emotionally difficult as well.

Body Mass Index

The most reliable measure of overweight and obesity in adults is body mass index (BMI). BMI is defined as total body weight in kilograms divided by the height in meters squared. For example, a client with a body weight of 200 pounds (91 kg) and height of 70 inches (178 cm, or 3.16 m^2) would have a BMI of 28.79 (91/3.16). This is not to suggest that body composition measurements (such as skin-fold calipers or circumference measurements) cannot be used to assist in developing goals and providing realistic feedback to clients. However, in the obese population, the actual computation of body fat is less clinically accurate or relevant. Although BMI is not a perfect measure, it does provide reliable values for comparison and for reasonable goal setting. For example, once the BMI is established, setting a goal of a weight associated with a BMI that is two units less is easy to derive and monitor.

When BMI is considered, a value of 18.5 to 24.9 is considered within normal limits, 25 to 29.9 is overweight, and more than 30 is obese. It is estimated that more than two thirds of adults in the United States have a BMI of more than 25. The risk of chronic disease increases in proportion to BMI in the obese population. Yet, radical treatment for obesity (such as medically supervised fasting, or pharmacologic or surgical intervention) is generally reserved for individuals with a BMI of more than 40.

Causes of Obesity

The causes of obesity are the subject of considerable debate, but virtually all experts agree that the fundamental problem (with respect to both prevention and treatment) is energy balance. As such, it is critically important for health and fitness professionals to refer clients to a registered dietitian or nutritionist who can provide reasonable and achievable dietary recommendations to coincide with their exercise regimen. Evans and Rosenburg[41] suggest that adults who are not involved in exercising regimens will lose approximately 5 pounds of muscle per decade, while simultaneously adding 15 pounds of fat per decade. This is exacerbated by the fact that the average person will have an approximate 15% decrease in fat-free mass (FFM) between the ages of 30 and 80. When the concept of age-related fat gain was investigated, it was determined that body fat was not an age-related issue, but rather was attributed to the number of hours individuals spent exercising per week.[42] It has also been shown in sedentary individuals that the daily-activity level accounts for more than 75% of the variability of body-fat storage in men.[43]

Obesity and Training

With respect to functional movement, research has also shown a correlation between the weight of an individual and the functional capacity of their gait. In a study involving more than 200 75-year-old women, the relationship between balance, muscular strength, and gait was investigated. It was shown that the heavier individuals exhibited poorer balance, slower gait velocity, and shorter steps, regardless of their higher level of muscular strength.[44] It can be inferred that because of the higher level of strength in the heavier individuals, strength training alone is not the prime issue. Rather, emphasis on balance or proprioceptive training may better facilitate the obese individual, as demonstrated by lack of balance and stepping parameters.

For effective weight loss, caloric expenditure should approximate 200 to 300 kcal per day, with a minimum weekly output of more than 1,250 kcal associated with exercise.[2] This should be progressively increased to 2,000 kcal per week of exercise expenditure. Resistance training should be part of any exercise regimen to promote weight loss. In Chapter 7 (Cardiorespiratory Training), it was shown that circuit-style resistance training (when compared with walking at a fast pace) produced nearly identical caloric expenditure for the same given time span.[45] Other researchers have noted much higher values in similar studies.[46,47] Furthermore, resistance training helps to produce lean body mass. Lean body mass helps to maintain basic metabolic rate, which improves the effectiveness of an energy-balance weight-loss program. The same guidelines that are used for adults with normal weight should be used for resistance training in the obese population, with emphasis on correct form and breathing.

This points to the importance of following the OPT™ model for the obese client. When working with this population, it may be advisable to use exercises in a standing or seated position. Health and movement assessments should always be performed to establish pertinent program design parameters. However, assessing the obese client can be challenging. After the fitness assessment seen in Chapter 5, using a pushing, pulling, and squatting exercise is suggested. These may be best performed with cables, exercise tubing, or body weight from a standing or seated position. Also, using a single-leg balance assessment may be more appropriate versus a single-leg squat for this population. Flexibility exercises should also be performed from a standing or seated position. For example, using the standing hip flexor (rather than the kneeling hip flexor stretch), standing hamstring, calf stretch, and seated adductor stretch would be advised. Self-myofascial release should be used with caution and may need to be done from a standing position or at home (see Psychosocial Aspects of Working With Obese Clients). This population can progress through the flexibility continuum as needed.

Core and balance training will be very important for this population because of their lack of balance and walking speed. Health and fitness professionals must be cautious when placing a client in a prone or supine position to perform many of these exercises because of the high probability that these clients will also exhibit hypertension or high blood pressure. These positions may be contraindicated. Performing many of these exercises in the standing position may be more appropriate. For example, performing prone iso-abs on an incline or cobras in a standing position would be suggested. Other examples include performing crunches or back extensions from a standing position, using a cable resistance. Resistance training may need to be started in a seated position and progress to a standing position.

Phases 1 and 2 of the OPT™ model will be appropriate for the obese population. The health and fitness professional should always ensure that the client is breathing normally and not straining to exercise or overgripping (squeezing too tightly) the exercise equipment, as this can increase blood pressure.

Psychosocial Aspects of Working With Obese Clients

Obesity is a unique chronic disease because it brings with it many issues that affect a person's sense of emotional well-being.[48] It can alter the emotional and social aspects of a person's life just as much as the physical. Health and fitness professionals must be very aware of this when training an obese client to ensure that the client feels socially and emotionally safe. This will help to create trust between the client and professional and assist the client in adhering to a program.

Proper exercise selections and positions will be very important to the client's sense of well-being. For example, machines are often not the best choice for exercises

Table 14.5	
Physiologic and Training Considerations for Individuals Who Are Overweight or Obese	
Physiologic Considerations	**Considerations for Health and Fitness**
May have other comorbidities (diagnosed or undiagnosed), including hypertension, cardiovascular disease, or diabetes	Initial screening should clarify the presence of potential undiagnosed comorbidities
Maximum oxygen uptake and ventilatory (anaerobic) threshold is typically reduced	Consider testing and training modalities that are weight-supported (such as cycle ergometer, swimming). If a client does not have these limitations, consider a walking program to improve compliance
Coexisting diets may hamper exercise ability and result in significant loss of lean body mass	Initial programming should emphasize low intensity, with a progression in exercise duration (up to 60 minutes as tolerable) and frequency (5–7 days per week), before increases are made in intensity of exercise. Exercise intensity should be no greater than 60–80% of work capacity, with weekly caloric volume a minimum of 1,250 kcal per week and a progression to 2,000, as tolerable.
Measures of body composition (hydrostatic weighing, skin-fold calipers) may not accurately reflect degree of overweight or obesity	Body mass index (BMI), scale weight, or circumference measurements are recommended measures of weight loss

because they may require a fair amount of mobility to get in and out of. Using dumbbell, cable, or exercise tubing exercises work quite well. The use of self-myofascial release should be done with caution as many clients will not feel comfortable rolling or lying on the floor. This may be done in the privacy of their own home if they agree. In addition, it is commonly recommended that obese clients engage in weight-supported exercise (such as cycling or swimming) to decrease orthopedic stress. However, walking is often both a preferred activity for many clients and one that is more easily engaged in. Thus, if the benefits of walking, particularly adherence, exceed the perceived risk of an orthopedic injury, walking might well be a primary exercise recommendation. When working with this population, the health and fitness professional must make sure to be aware of the situations, positions, and locations in the training facility they are placing the client. Exercise considerations are given in Tables 14-5 and 14-6.

SUMMARY

Obesity is the fastest growing health problem in the United States. Health and fitness professionals must be prepared to work with obese clients. First, body mass must be measured to chart progress. The most reliable measure of overweight and obesity in adults is body mass index (BMI). Once BMI is established, setting a goal weight associated with it is easy to derive and monitor.

When designing programs for overweight and obese clients, their adherence to the type of exercise should be considered. Walking is often a good recommendation if there is little risk of orthopedic injury. For effective weight loss, aerobic exercise

Table 14.6	
Basic Exercise Guidelines for Individuals Who Are Overweight or Obese	
Mode	Low-impact or step aerobics (such as treadmill walking, rowing, stationary cycling, and water activity)
Frequency	At least 5 days per week
Intensity	60–80% of maximum heart rate. Use the Talk Test[a] to determine exertion Stage I cardiorespiratory training progressing to stage II (intensities may be altered to 40–70% of maximum heart rate if needed)
Duration	40–60 minutes per day, or 20- to 30-minute sessions twice each day
Assessment	Push, pull, squat Single-leg balance (if tolerated)
Flexibility	SMR (only if comfortable to client) Flexibility continuum
Resistance Training	1–3 sets of 10–15 repetitions on 2–3 days per week Phases 1 and 2 will be appropriate performed in a circuit-training manner (higher repetitions such as 20 may be used)
Special Considerations	Make sure client is comfortable—be aware of positions and locations in the facility your client is in Exercises should be performed in a standing or seated position May have other chronic diseases; in such cases a medical release should be obtained from the individual's physician

[a]The "Talk Test" is a method of measuring intensity if the health and fitness professional is unable to assess intensity via heart rate. If the client can comfortably carry on a conversation while exercising, he or she is probably at the lower ranges of training heart rate. If he or she is having difficulty finishing a sentence, the client is probably at the high range. Depending on the individual's response and exercise status, adjust intensity accordingly.

SMR, self-myofascial release.

should approximate 200 to 300 kcal per day, with a minimum weekly output of more than 1,250 kcal associated with exercise. In addition, resistance training should be part of any exercise regimen to promote weight loss. Although it burns fewer calories than aerobic exercise, it preserves lean body mass, which is important for maintaining metabolism. The same resistance-training guidelines used for adults with normal weight should be used in the obese population, focusing on correct form and breathing.

Diabetes

Diabetes: Chronic metabolic disorder, caused by insulin deficiency, which impairs carbohydrate usage and enhances usage of fat and protein.

Diabetes is a metabolic disorder in which the body's ability to produce *insulin* (a hormone secreted by the pancreas to help deliver glucose to cells) or to utilize *glucose* (blood sugar) is altered. It is estimated that nearly 6% of the U.S. population has diabetes, with about one million new cases per year. This number is expected to double in the next 15 to 20 years. Diabetes is also the seventh leading cause of death in the United States.[49] It has been shown that people who develop diabetes before the age of 30 are 20 times more likely to die by age 40 than those who do not have diabetes.[50]

There are two primary forms of diabetes: type 1 (insulin-dependent diabetes) and type 2 (adult-onset diabetes). Type 2 is also referred to as "non–insulin-dependent diabetes," although that is technically incorrect. Some type 2 diabetics cannot manage their blood glucose levels and do require additional insulin. Coupled with an increase in obesity is the risk of type 2 diabetes.

Type 1 diabetes is typically found in normal (or even underweight) younger individuals and is rooted in a primary disease that impairs normal glucose management. As a result of this lack of insulin, blood sugar is not optimally delivered into the cells (particularly muscle and fat cells), resulting in *hyperglycemia* (high levels of blood sugar). To control this high level of blood sugar, the type 1 diabetic must inject insulin to compensate for what their pancreas cannot produce. This is important to note because exercise increases the rate in which cells utilize glucose. If the type 1 diabetic does not control his or her blood glucose levels (via insulin injections and dietary carbohydrates) before, during, and after exercise, blood sugar levels can drop rapidly and cause a condition called *hypoglycemia* (low blood sugar), leading to weakness, dizziness, and fainting. Although insulin, proper diet, and exercise are the primary components prescribed for type 1 diabetics, these individuals must still be monitored throughout exercise to ensure safety.

Type 2 diabetes is associated with obesity, particularly abdominal obesity. The incidence and prevalence of adult type 2 diabetes in the United States has increased sharply in recent years. There is significant public health concern about the rising incidence of type 2 diabetes in children, associated with both the increase in abdominal obesity and decrease in voluntary physical activity.

Type 2 diabetics usually produce adequate amounts of insulin; however, their cells are resistant to the insulin (that is, they do not allow insulin to bring adequate amounts of blood sugar into the cell). This condition can lead to *hyperglycemia* (high blood sugar). Chronic hyperglycemia is associated with a number of diseases associated with damage to the kidneys, heart, nerves, eyes, and circulatory system. Although type 2 diabetics do not experience the same fluctuations in blood sugar as type 1 diabetics, it is still important to be aware of the symptoms, particularly with type 2 diabetics using insulin medications.

Exercise and Diabetes

The overriding issue in diabetes is glucose control. Exercise training is effective in that regard, because it acts much like insulin by enhancing the uptake of circulating glucose by skeletal muscle. Studies show that exercise improves a variety of glucose measures, including tissue sensitivity, improved glucose tolerance, and even a decrease in insulin requirements.[51,52] Thus, exercise has been shown to have a substantial positive effect on the prevention of type 2 diabetes.

There are fairly specific recommendations to follow in this population to prevent hypoglycemic and hyperglycemic events during or after exercise, as well as when to defer exercise based on blood glucose levels or symptoms. In most cases, the exercise management and goals should be the same as would be developed to treat the underlying causes of inactivity and excess body weight. However, in contrast to the obesity recommendation to emphasize walking as the primary mode, care must be taken to prevent blisters and foot microtrauma that could result in foot infection. Special note should be taken with respect to advice about carbohydrate intake or insulin use, not only before exercise but afterward, to reduce the risk of a hypoglycemic event after exercise.

The parameters for exercise generally follow those advised for obese adults, as many type 2 diabetic patients are obese and because daily exercise is recommended for more stable glucose management (Tables 14-7 and 14-8). Lower impact exercise

Table 14.7

Physiologic and Training Considerations for Individuals With Diabetes

Physiologic Considerations	Considerations for Health and Fitness	Considerations in Sport and Athletic Training
Frequently associated with comorbidities (including cardiovascular disease, obesity, and hypertension)	Program should target weekly caloric goal of 1,000–2,000 kcal, progressing as tolerable, to maximize weight loss and cardio protection	Screening for comorbidities is important
Exercise exerts an effect similar to that of insulin	Increased risk of exercise-induced hypoglycemia	Be cognizant of signs and symptoms of hypoglycemia
Hypoglycemia may occur several hours after exercise, as well as during exercise	For those recently diagnosed, glucose should be measured before, during, and after exercise	Restoration of glucose after the event may be necessary to prevent nocturnal hypoglycemia
Clients taking β-blocking medications may be unable to recognize signs and symptoms of hypoglycemia	Some reduction in insulin and increase in carbohydrate intake may be necessary and proportionate to exercise intensity and duration	Substantial insulin dose reduction may be necessary before exercise Carbohydrate intake before and during exercise may be necessary
Exercise in excessive heat may mask signs of hypoglycemia	Post-exercise carbohydrate consumption is advisable	Initial exercise prescription should emphasize low intensity, with a progression in exercise duration (up 60 minutes as tolerable) and frequency (5–7 days per week), for consistent glucose control. Intensity should be no greater than 50–90% of work capacity to start with.
Increased risk for retinopathy	Be cognizant of signs and symptoms of hypoglycemia	Resistance training guidelines may follow those for normal weight healthy adults (e.g., 1–3 sets of 8–10 exercises, 10–15 reps per set, 2–3 days per week)
Peripheral neuropathy may increase risk for gait abnormalities and infection from foot blisters that may go unnoticed	Use weight-bearing exercise cautiously and wear appropriate footwear	Check daily for blisters or skin injury and appropriate footwear

modalities reduce the risk of injury, and resistance exercise is advised as part of an overall exercise plan for health and fitness. Assessment procedures should follow those outlined in Chapter 5 (Fitness Assessment). Flexibility exercises can be used as suggested; however, special care should be given to self-myofascial release, and this may be contraindicated for anyone with peripheral neuropathy (loss of protective sensation in feet and legs). Obtain the advice of a licensed physician concerning self-myofascial release (foam rolling) and specific clients. Phases 1 and 2 of the OPT™ model are appropriate for this population; however, the use of reactive training may be inappropriate.

SUMMARY

Diabetes impairs the body's ability to produce insulin. Type 1 diabetes (insulin-dependent diabetes) is typically found in younger individuals. If the type 1 diabetic does not control blood glucose levels (via insulin injections and dietary carbohydrates)

	Table 14.8
Basic Exercise Guidelines for Individuals With Diabetes	
Mode	Low-impact activities (such as cycling, treadmill walking, low-impact or step aerobics)
Frequency	4–7 days per week
Intensity	50–90% of maximum heart rate Stage I cardiorespiratory training progressing to stage II and III (may be adjusted to 40–70% of maximum heart rate if needed)
Duration	20–60 minutes
Assessment	Push, pull, OH squat Single-leg balance or single-leg squat
Flexibility	Flexibility continuum
Resistance Training	1–3 sets of 10–15 repetitions 2–3 days a week Phases 1 and 2 of the OPT™ model (higher repetitions such as 20 may be used)
Special Considerations	Make sure client has appropriate footwear and have client or physician check feet for blisters or abnormal wear patterns Advise client or class participant to keep a snack (quick source of carbohydrate) available during exercise, to avoid sudden hypoglycemia Use SMR with special care and licensed physician's advice Avoid excessive reactive training, and higher-intensity training is not recommended for typical client

SMR, self-myofascial release; *OH*, overhead squat.

before, during, and after exercise, blood sugar levels can drop rapidly and cause hypoglycemia leading to weakness, dizziness, and fainting. Type 2 diabetes (adult-onset diabetes) is associated with obesity, particularly abdominal obesity. Type 2 diabetics usually produce adequate amounts of insulin; however, their cells are resistant to the insulin, which can lead to hyperglycemia.

Exercise is effective for glucose control. Exercise recommendations generally follow those advised for obese adults, as many type 2 diabetic patients are obese and daily exercise is recommended for more stable glucose management. However, weight-bearing activities may need to be avoided to prevent blisters and foot microtrauma that could result in foot infection. Carbohydrate intake or insulin use should be stressed before exercise as well as afterward to reduce the risk of a postexercise hypoglycemic event.

Follow exercise guidelines for obese adults, using lower impact exercise modalities. Special care should be given to self-myofascial release and this may be contraindicated for anyone with a loss of protective sensation in feet and legs. Phases 1 and 2 of the OPT™ model are appropriate for this population, but reactive training may be inappropriate.

Hypertension

The definition of **hypertension** is blood pressure with the systolic (top number) reading greater than or equal to 140 mm Hg and the diastolic (bottom number) reading greater than or equal to 90 mm Hg. (Of course, if a client is taking medication

Hypertension: Raised systemic arterial blood pressure, which, if sustained at a high enough level, is likely to induce cardiovascular or end-organ damage.

to control blood pressure, that individual is considered hypertensive regardless of a normal blood pressure reading at rest.) More recent guidelines emphasize that a measurement of 135/85 mm Hg should be considered prehypertensive and should be lowered through appropriate lifestyle modifications. Average, healthy blood pressure is 120/80 mm Hg. Some of the most common contributors to hypertension include smoking, a diet high in fat (particularly saturated fat), and excess weight. The health risks of hypertension are well known and include increased risk for stroke, cardiovascular disease, chronic heart failure, and kidney failure.

One traditional method of controlling hypertension is through antihypertensive medications. Although medications have been proven effective, proper cardiorespiratory exercise and diet have also been shown to reduce blood pressure, potentially allowing for the elimination of medications. Fortunately, there is ample evidence to suggest that exercise can have a significant impact on the lowering of elevated blood pressure.[53-55] It may also cause the body to produce a more appropriate response to exercise or other physiologic stressors. The changes appear mild, on the order of 3 to 4 mm Hg (or more with higher resting blood pressure), but any lowering of pressure conveys a lowered overall health risk and is important. Interestingly, low to moderate cardiorespiratory exercise has been shown to be just as effective as high-intensity activity in reducing blood pressure. This is important for elderly or obese individuals with high blood pressure and who are not physically capable of performing high-intensity cardiorespiratory exercise.

It is important to emphasize the importance of an overall plan to reduce blood pressure that includes exercise, diet, weight loss (if appropriate), and, importantly, compliance with the medical regimen prescribed by a physician. Often, compliance with medication is a serious problem with hypertensive individuals because they do not "feel sick." The health and fitness professional must monitor and stress medication compliance.

It is also important for the health and fitness professional to evaluate the client's heart rate response to exercise, as measured during a submaximal exercise test or even a simple assessment of heart rate, during a comfortable exercise load. Hypertensive clients frequently take medications (most commonly β-blockers, but others may have similar effects) that blunt the heart rate response to exercise, thus invalidating prediction equations or estimates of exercise heart rate.

When training the hypertensive client, it is imperative that the health and fitness professional also monitor the body position. Similar to the obese and diabetic client, body position can dramatically increase the effects of hypertension. Often, supine or prone positions (especially when the head is lower in elevation than the heart) can increase blood pressure. These positions may be contraindicated.

For assessment of a hypertensive client, the health and fitness professional should follow the guidelines in Chapter 5 (Fitness Assessment). Use of a single-leg balance (or squat) exercise can also be beneficial, if tolerated by the client. If possible, all other exercises should be performed in a seated or standing position (Tables 14-9 and 14-10). Clients may use the full flexibility continuum; however, static and active stretching may be the easiest and safest. Self-myofascial release may be contraindicated as it requires lying down. Consult with specific clients' physicians for specific recommendations. Cardiorespiratory training should focus on stage I and progress only on physician's approval.

Core exercises in the standing position would include performing prone iso-abs on an incline, or cobras in a standing position (two-leg or single-leg). Other examples include performing crunches or back extensions from a standing position using a cable resistance. Use reactive training with care for this population.

Resistance training should be performed in a seated or standing position as well. Phases 1 and 2 of the OPT™ model will be appropriate for this population. The programs should be performed in a circuit-style or Peripheral Heart Action (PHA) training system (see Chapter 12, Resistance Training) to distribute blood flow between the upper and lower extremities. The health and fitness professional should always ensure that the client is breathing normally and not straining to

Table 14.9	
Physiologic and Training Considerations for Individuals With Hypertension	
Physiologic Considerations	**Considerations for Health and Fitness, Sport and Athletic Training**
Blood pressure response to exercise may be variable and exaggerated, depending on the mode and level of intensity	A program of continuous, lower-intensity (50–85% of work capacity) aerobic exercise is initially recommended. Frequency and duration parameters should be at minimum 3–5 days per week, 20–45 minutes per day, with additional increases in overall volume of exercise if weight loss is also desired
Despite medication, clients may arrive with pre-exercise hypertension	Resistance exercise should consist of a Peripheral Heart Action or circuit-training style Avoid Valsalva maneuvers, emphasize rhythmic breathing and a program design for muscular fitness (e.g., 1–3 sets of 8–10 exercises, 10–20 reps, 2–3 days per week)
Hypertension frequently is associated with other comorbidities, including obesity, cardiovascular disease, and diabetes	Screening for comorbidities is important. Exercise should target a weekly caloric goal of 1,500–2,000 kcal, progressing as tolerable, to maximize weight loss and cardio protection
Some medications, such as β-blockers, for hypertension will attenuate the heart rate at rest and its response to exercise	For clients taking medications that will influence heart rate, do not use predicted maximum heart rate or estimates for the exercise. Instead, use actual heart rate response or the Talk Test. Accepted blood pressure contraindications for exercise include an SBP of 200 mm Hg and a DBP of 115 mm Hg. Always check with any other lower guidelines the fitness facility may have in place.

SBP, systolic blood pressure; *DBP,* diastolic blood pressure.

exercise or overgripping (squeezing too tightly) the exercise equipment as this can increase blood pressure. In addition, the health and fitness professional should monitor the client when rising from a seated or lying position as he or she may experience dizziness.

SUMMARY

Normal blood pressure is 120/80 mm Hg. Hypertension is defined as a blood pressure greater than 140/90 mm Hg, although 135/85 mm Hg is considered prehypertensive. Hypertension can be controlled through cardiorespiratory exercise and diet. However, clients must also be sure to follow any prescribed medication or physician's recommendations.

Individuals with hypertension should engage in low-intensity aerobic exercise, but may want to avoid heavy resistance training. Health and fitness professionals should measure hypertensive clients' heart rate response to exercise, instead of relying on estimates or equations.

Monitoring body position is very important. Supine or prone positions (especially when the head is lower in elevation than the heart) may be contraindicated. Most exercises should be performed in a seated or standing position. The full

Table 14.10	
Basic Exercise Guidelines for Individuals With Hypertension	
Mode	Stationary cycling, treadmill walking, rowers
Frequency	3–7 days per week
Intensity	50–85% of maximum heart rate Stage I cardiorespiratory training
Duration	30–60 minutes
Assessment	Push, pull, OH squat Single-leg balance (squat if tolerated)
Flexibility	Static and active in a standing or seated position
Resistance Training	1–3 sets of 10–20 repetitions 2–3 days per week Phases 1 and 2 of the OPT™ model Tempo should not exceed 1 s for isometric and concentric portions (e.g., 4/1/1 instead of 4/2/1 or 3/2/1) Use circuit or PHA weight training as an option, with appropriate rest intervals
Special Considerations	Avoid heavy lifting and Valsalva maneuvers—make sure client breathes normally Do not let client overgrip weights or clench fists when training Modify tempo to avoid extended isometric and concentric muscle action Perform exercises in a standing or seated position Allow client to stand up slowly to avoid possible dizziness Progress client slowly

OH, overhead squats; *PHA*, Peripheral Heart Action.

flexibility continuum can be used, but static and active stretching may be easiest and safest. Self-myofascial release may be contraindicated depending on body position. Cardiorespiratory training should focus on stage I and progress only with physician's approval. Reactive training should be used with care for this population. Resistance training should be performed in a seated or standing position as well. Phases 1 and 2 of the OPT™ model are appropriate. Programs should be performed in a circuit style or using the Peripheral Heart Action (PHA) training system.

Coronary Heart Disease

Since reaching epidemic proportions in the mid-20th century, deaths from heart disease have steadily declined in the United States, but still account for approximately 40% of all deaths annually. Importantly, most recent statistics suggest nearly 18 million individuals in the United States have coronary artery disease or chronic heart failure, with another 50 million diagnosed with high blood pressure.[56]

For individuals with coronary artery disease, the underlying pathologic condition of concern has traditionally been plaque accumulation in the coronary arteries, and the eventual obstruction of the artery, resulting in a myocardial infarction (or heart attack). The procedures that have evolved over the years have all been designed with this in mind.

In recent years, there has been increased emphasis on improving the health of the internal lining of the coronary artery, resulting in plaque "stabilization." More recent research has suggested that it is unstable coronary lesions that rupture and precipitate most coronary events. Not surprisingly, factors such as stress and smoking are known to destabilize arterial endothelium. Exercise is a major factor that appears to improve the stability of the endothelium.

It is logical that in increasing numbers, individuals with diagnosed heart disease (as well as a small percentage of individuals with undiagnosed heart disease) engage in regular exercise in health and fitness facilities or seek the advice of the

Table 14.11

Physiologic and Training Considerations for Individuals With Coronary Heart Disease

Physiologic Considerations	Considerations for Health and Fitness, Sport and Athletic Training
The nature of heart disease may result in a specific level of exercise, above which it is dangerous to perform	The upper safe limit of exercise, preferably by heart rate, must be obtained. Heart rate should never be estimated from existing prediction formulas for clients with heart disease. Consult their physician.
Clients with heart disease may not have angina (chest pain equivalent) or other warning signs	Clients must be able to monitor pulse rate or use an accurate monitor to stay below the upper safe limit of exercise
Between the underlying disease and medication use, the heart rate response to exercise will nearly always vary considerably from age-predicted formulas, and will almost always be lower	Although symptoms should always supersede anything else as a sign to decrease or stop exercising, some clients may not have this warning system, so monitoring of heart rate becomes increasingly important
Clients may have other comorbidities (such as diabetes, hypertension, peripheral vascular disease, or obesity)	Screening for comorbidities is important and modifications to exercise made based on these diagnoses
Peak oxygen uptake (as well as ventilatory threshold) is often reduced because of the compromised cardiac pump and peripheral muscle deconditioning	The exercise prescription should be low intensity, to start, and based on recommendations provided by a certified exercise specialist or physical therapist with specialty training. Aerobic training guidelines should follow, at minimum, 20–30 minutes 3–5 days per week at 40–85% of maximum capacity, but below the upper safe limits prescribed by the physician.
	A weekly caloric goal of 1,500–2,000 kcal is usually recommended, progressing as tolerable, to maximize cardio protection
	Resistance training may be started after the patient has been exercising asymptomatically and comfortably for >3 months in the aerobic exercise program. A circuit-training format is recommended, 8–10 exercises, 1–3 sets of 10–20 reps per exercise, emphasizing breathing control and rest as needed between sets.

health and fitness professional. The cardiovascular complication rate is low in exercise programs, probably owing to the fact that the clients are well managed by their physicians and that healthier clients are more likely to engage in exercise. Nonetheless, health and fitness professionals must be aware of the presence of clients with heart disease and help design effective exercise programs with the knowledge that exercise *can* pose a risk for clients with heart disease (Table 14-11).

In some cases, clients will begin a fitness program after completing a cardiac rehabilitation program. However, research shows that less than 30% of heart patients (and a far lower percentage of women) are referred to and participate in cardiac rehabilitation programs.[57] In any case, the health and fitness professional must have a clear understanding about the client's disease, medication use, and most importantly, the upper safe limit of exercise—and any other restrictions—imposed by the client's physician. The health and fitness professional must not compromise on obtaining this information, and client participation must not proceed until the information is received. In many cases, the client can facilitate obtaining this information.

Clients must be able to find and monitor their own pulse rate or use an accurate monitor to stay below their safe upper limit of exercise. It is important to note that the heart rate response to exercise will almost always vary considerably from age-predicted formulas, and will often be lower. Although symptoms should always supersede anything else as a sign to decrease or stop exercising, some clients may not have this warning system, so monitoring of heart rate becomes increasingly important. Another option in this situation is using rate of perceived exertion to assess exercise intensity (Table 14-12), which allows the health and fitness professional to gage the intensity of the exercise without having to assess

Table 14.12			
Rating of Perceived Exertion			
Original Scale		**Category – Ratio Scale**	
6		0.0 Nothing at all	No intensity
7	Very, very light	0.3	
8		0.5 Extremely weak	Just noticeable
9	Very light	0.7	
10		1.0 Very weak	
11	Fairly light	1.5	
12		2.0 Weak	Light
13	Somewhat hard	2.5	
14		3.0 Moderate	
15	Hard	4.0	
16		5.0 Strong	Heavy
17	Very hard	6.0	
18		7.0 Very strong	
19	Very, very hard	8.0	
20		9.0	
		10.0 Extremely strong	Strongest intensity
		11.0	
		Absolute maximum	Highest possible

heart rate. The individual will rate the level of intensity based upon the values provided in the table, at which time the health and fitness professional can adjust the intensity accordingly.

Clients with stable coronary artery disease (and especially those who have participated in a cardiac rehabilitation program) understand the essential benefits of exercise, which include a lower risk of dying, increased exercise tolerance, muscle strength, reduction in angina and heart failure symptoms, and improved psychological status and social adjustment.[58] There is also evidence that heart disease may be slowed (or even reversed) when a multifactor intervention program of intensive education, exercise, counseling, and lipid lowering medications are used, as appropriate.[59-61]

Health and fitness professionals must be careful to not overstate the benefits of exercise as a singular intervention and must emphasize to clients the importance of a multidisciplinary approach to heart disease. That said, exercise is critically important and can be safely conducted in most health and fitness settings (Table 14-13).

The health and fitness professional should follow the guidelines in Chapter 5 (Fitness Assessment) for assessment of these clients. Use of a single-leg balance (or squat) exercise can also be beneficial, if tolerated by the client. If possible, all other

Table 14.13

Basic Exercise Guidelines for Individuals With Coronary Heart Disease

Mode	Large muscle group activities, such as stationary cycling, treadmill walking, or rowing
Frequency	3–5 days/week
Intensity	40–85% of maximal heart rate reserve The Talk Test may also be more appropriate as medications may effect heart rate Stage I cardiorespiratory training
Duration	5–10 minutes warm up, followed by 20–40 minutes of exercise, followed by a 5–10 minute cool-down
Assessment	Push, pull, OH squat Single-leg balance (squat if tolerated)
Flexibility	Static and active in a standing or seated position
Resistance Training	1–3 sets of 10–20 repetitions 2–3 days per week Phases 1 and 2 of the OPT™ model Tempo should not exceed 1 s for isometric and concentric portions (e.g., 4/1/1 instead of 4/2/2 or 4/2/1 or 3/2/1) Use circuit or PHA weight training as an option, with appropriate rest intervals
Specific Considerations	Be aware that clients may have other diseases to consider as well, such as diabetes, hypertension, peripheral vascular disease, or obesity Modify tempo to avoid extended isometric and concentric muscle action Avoid heavy lifting and Valsalva maneuvers —make sure client breathes normally Do not let client overgrip weights or clench fists when training Perform exercises in a standing or seated position Progress exercise slowly

OH, overhead squat; *PHA*, Peripheral Heart Action.

exercises should be performed in a seated or standing position. Clients should stay with static and active stretching in a standing or seated position because they may be the easiest and safest to perform. Consult with a licensed physician for specific recommendations concerning self-myofascial release. Cardiorespiratory training should focus on stage I and only progress with physician's advice.

Core exercises in the standing position would include performing prone iso-abs on an incline or cobras in a standing position (two-leg or single-leg). Other examples include performing crunches or back extensions from a standing position, using a cable resistance. Reactive training would not be recommended for this population in the initial months of training.

Resistance training should be performed in a seated or standing position, as well. Phases 1 and 2 of the OPT™ model will be appropriate for this population. The programs should be performed in a circuit-style or Peripheral Heart Action (PHA) training system (see Chapter 12, Resistance Training). The health and fitness professional should always ensure that the client is breathing normally and not straining to exercise or overgripping (squeezing too tightly) the exercise equipment, as this can increase blood pressure.

SUMMARY

Nearly 18 million individuals in the United States have coronary artery disease or chronic heart failure, with another 50 million diagnosed with high blood pressure. The cardiovascular complication rate is low in exercise programs; however, health and fitness professionals must be aware of the presence of clients with heart disease and help design effective exercise programs with the knowledge that exercise *can* pose a risk for clients with heart disease.

A health and fitness professional must have a clear understanding about a client's disease, medication use, and upper safe limit of exercise imposed by the client's physician. Participation must not proceed until the information is received.

Aerobic low-intensity exercise is recommended, with a weekly caloric expenditure goal of 1,500 to 2,000 kcal. Resistance training should not be started until the client has been exercising without any problems for at least 3 months.

Most exercises should be performed in a seated or standing position. Flexibility exercises should be limited to static and active stretching in a seated position. Self-myofascial release should be preapproved by a physician. Cardiorespiratory training should focus on stage I and progress only with the physician's approval. Reactive training would not be recommended for this population in the initial months of training. Resistance training should be performed in a seated or standing position as well. Phases 1 and 2 of the OPT™ model are appropriate. Programs should be performed in a circuit style or using the Peripheral Heart Action (PHA) training system.

Osteoporosis

Osteopenia: A decrease in the calcification or density of bone as well as reduced bone mass.

Osteoporosis: Condition in which there is a decrease in bone mass and density as well as an increase in the space between bones, resulting in porosity and fragility.

Osteopenia is the precursor to osteoporosis and is indicated on screening by a lowered bone mass. **Osteoporosis** is divided into two types (1 and 2), and in the vast majority of cases, fitness professionals are much more likely to see clients with type 1, as the onset of type 2 typically occurs in clients 70 years and older. Health and fitness professionals will encounter an increasing number of clients with osteopenia and osteoporosis. Although the vast majority of clients will be women, men can, in fact, have either of these diseases.[62]

Type 1 osteoporosis is most commonly associated with, and is most prevalent in, postmenopausal women. A principal observation in type 1 osteoporosis is a deficit in estrogen (usually secondary to menopause). The disease is characterized by an increase in bone reabsorption (removal of old bone) with a decrease in bone remodeling (formation of new bone). This leads to a decrease in bone mineral density.

Osteoporosis commonly affects the neck of the femur and the lumbar vertebrae. These structures are considered part of the core and are located in the region of the body where all forces come together. Thus, decreased bone mineral density places the core in a weakened state and thus, more susceptible to injury, such as a fracture.[62] Research has shown that the risk of hip fractures doubles every 5 years in postmenopausal women older than the age of 50.[62] Furthermore, osteoporosis affects more than 25 million people each year, resulting in approximately 1.5 million hip fractures. Of these 1.5 million hip fractures, only 20% of the patients return to a normal functional status.[63]

There are a variety of risk factors that influence osteoporosis. One of the most important is the amount of peak bone mass (or density). Peak bone mass is the highest amount of bone mass a person is able to achieve during his or her lifetime.[64] New bone formation (remodeling) occurs as the result of stress placed on the musculoskeletal system. To maintain consistent bone remodeling, people must remain active enough to ensure adequate stress is being placed on their bodies. This is imperative for adolescents and young adults to reach a high peak bone mass.

Other risk factors include a lack of physical activity, smoking, excess alcohol consumption, and low dietary calcium intake. The key for the health and fitness professional is to recognize that these factors can be influenced through a comprehensive health and fitness program (Table 14-14). In addition to exercise

Table 14.14

Physiologic and Training Considerations for Individuals With Osteoporosis

Physiologic Considerations	Considerations for Health and Fitness, Sport and Athletic Training
Maximum oxygen uptake and ventilatory threshold is frequently lower, as a result of chronic deconditioning	Typical exercise loads prescribed are consistent with fitness standards: 40–70% of maximum work capacity, 3–5 days per week, approximately 20–30 minutes per session
Gait and balance may be negatively affected	Physiologic and physical limitations point to low-intensity, weight-supported exercise programs that emphasize balance training
Chronic vertebral fractures may result in significant lower back pain	For clients with osteopenia (and no contraindications to exercise), resistance training is recommended to build bone mass. For clients who can engage in resistance exercise, recommended loads are relatively high intensity (>75% of 1RM). A circuit-training format is recommended, 8–10 exercises, 1 set of 8–12 reps per exercise, with rest as needed between sets.
Age, disease, physical stature, and deconditioning may place the client at risk for falls	For clients with severe osteoporosis, exercise modality should be shifted to water exercise to reduce risk of loading fracture. If aquatic exercise is not feasible, use other weight-supported exercise, such as cycling, and monitor signs and symptoms.
	Reinforce other lifestyle behaviors that will optimize bone health, including smoking cessation, reduced alcohol intake, and increased dietary calcium intake.

1RM, one repetition maximum.

programs, clients should be encouraged to increase dietary intake of calcium, decrease alcohol intake, and to cease smoking.

With respect to physical activity, it is important to know whether the diagnosis is osteopenia or osteoporosis and, if the latter, to what degree the client may engage in weight-bearing activities or resistive exercise training. That is, there is a balance between the benefit of providing exercises that are designed to increase bone through the provision of bone stress (weight-bearing exercise or heavier resistive exercises) and the risk of fracture that might be precipitated by advanced osteoporosis.

It has been demonstrated that individuals who partake in resistance training have a higher bone mineral density than those who do not.[65-67] Resistance training, however, has been shown to improve bone mineral density by no more than 5%, and some researchers believe that this does not represent a high enough increase to prevent fractures from occurring.[68] In fact, it has been estimated that a 20% increase in bone mineral density is necessary to offset fractures. Thus, it has been suggested that training that focuses on the prevention of falls, rather than strength alone, is more advantageous for the elderly. Therefore, exercise regimens that combine resistance training to increase bone mineral density with flexibility, core, and balance training to enhance proprioception (as seen in the OPT™ model) might better facilitate the needs of this population (Table 14-15).[69]

When using the OPT™ model with this population, the health and fitness professional must follow some precautionary measures. If the client demonstrates the ability to move fairly well without assistance, the movement assessments may be followed (overhead squat, single-leg squat or balance, push, pull). If the client is not able to get around very well, use more stable, machine-based equipment. Follow the kinetic chain checkpoints as closely as possible with this population, but realize that there may be degenerative deformations in their posture that cannot be corrected. Get clients to their own ideal position, not a general ideal position. Exercises should be performed in a seated or standing position.

Table 14.15	
Basic Exercise Guidelines for Individuals With Osteoporosis	
Mode	Treadmill with handrail support
Frequency	2–5 days per week
Intensity	50–90% of max HR Stage I cardiorespiratory training progressing to stage II
Duration	20–60 minutes per day or 8- to 10-min bouts
Assessment	Push, pull, overhead squat, *or* sitting and standing into a chair
Flexibility	Static and active stretching
Resistance Training	1–3 sets of 8–20 repetitions at up to 85% on 2–3 days per week Phases 1 and 2 of OPT™ model should be mastered before moving on
Special Considerations	Progression should be slow, well monitored, and based on postural control Exercises should be progressed if possible toward free sitting (no support) or standing Focus exercises on hips, thighs, back, and arms Avoid excessive spinal loading on squat and leg press exercises Make sure client is breathing in normal manner and avoid holding breath as in a Valsalva maneuver.

VO$_2$, oxygen consumption.

Flexibility should be limited to static and active stretching. The use of self-myofascial release may be contraindicated for this population. Cardiorespiratory training should begin in stage I (with a walking program, if tolerated). Weight-bearing activities may be more beneficial to increasing bone mineral density. Progression to stage II cardiorespiratory training should be based on physician's advice and client's ability.

Example core exercises in the standing position would include performing prone iso-abs on an incline, or cobras in a standing position (two-leg or single-leg). Other examples include performing back extensions from a standing position, using a cable resistance (being cautious of excessive extension). Care should be taken with crunches or movements with a lot of spinal flexion. Monitor range of motion and check with a licensed physician. Reactive training would not be recommended for this population.

Resistance training should be performed in a seated or standing position, as well. Phases 1 and 2 of the OPT™ model will be appropriate for this population. Research has indicated that higher intensities (75 to 85%) are needed to stimulate bone formation. Furthermore, it appears that the load (rather than the amount of repetitions) is the determining factor in bone formation.[70] However, to ensure proper kinetic chain preparation for these higher intensities, the health and fitness professional should progress clients through the OPT™ model. Stabilization training (especially balance exercises) will be just as important to counter a lack of balance that can lead to falls and hip fractures. For training to have an effect on bone mass it will require approximately 6 months of consistent exercise at high enough intensities. This means that the client will be making a long-term commitment to the exercise program. If the client is not progressed appropriately (following the OPT™ model), he or she may acquire injuries that will be a setback. The programs may be performed in a circuit-style or Peripheral Heart Action (PHA) training system (see Chapter 12, Resistance Training), focusing on hips, thighs, back, and arms. Progressing exercises to the standing position will help increase stress to the hips, thighs, and back as well as increase the demand for balance. Both components are necessary to overcome the effects of osteoporosis.

SUMMARY

Clients with osteopenia show a lowered bone mass. This is the precursor to osteoporosis. Osteoporosis is divided into two types. Fitness professionals are much more likely to see clients with type 1, the vast majority of these being female.

Physical inactivity, smoking, excess alcohol consumption, and low dietary calcium intake are factors that contribute to the risk of osteoporosis. In addition to exercise, clients should be encouraged to increase dietary intake of calcium, lower alcohol intake, and quit smoking.

If the diagnosis is osteoporosis, a physician must dictate to what degree the client may engage in weight-bearing activities or resistance training. The benefit of exercises designed to increase bone density may be outweighed by the risk of fracture. Exercise regimens that combine resistance training to increase bone mineral density with flexibility, core, and balance training to enhance proprioception might better facilitate the needs of this population.

Clients who can move fairly well, without assistance, can use the Integrated Fitness Profile assessment. Those not able to get around very well should use more stable, machine-based equipment. Kinetic chain checkpoints should be followed, taking into consideration that degenerative deformations in posture may not be able to be corrected. Exercises should be performed in a seated or standing position.

Flexibility exercises should be limited to static and active stretching in a seated position. Self-myofascial release may be contraindicated for this population. Cardiorespiratory training should focus on stage I (with a walking program, if tolerated). Progression to stage II cardiorespiratory training should be based on a physician's advice and client's ability. Care should be taken with crunches or movements with a lot of spinal flexion. Reactive training would not be recommended for this population. Resistance training should be performed in a seated or standing position. Phases 1 and 2 of the OPT™ model are appropriate. Six months of consistent exercise at high intensities, progressed appropriately, will be required for training to have an effect on bone mass. This means that the client will be making a long-term commitment to the exercise program. Programs should be performed in a circuit style or using the Peripheral Heart Action (PHA) training system, focusing on hips, thighs, back, and arms and progressing exercises to the standing position.

Arthritis

Arthritis: Chronic inflammation of the joints.

Osteoarthritis: Arthritis in which cartilage becomes soft, frayed, or thins out, as a result of trauma or other conditions.

Rheumatoid arthritis: Arthritis primarily affecting connective tissues, in which there is a thickening of articular soft tissue, and extension of synovial tissue over articular cartilages that have become eroded.

Arthritis is an inflammatory condition that mainly affects the joints of the body. It is estimated that arthritis is the most common chronic condition, affecting 50% of persons older than the age of 65 and more than 15% of the American population.[71] By the year 2020, arthritis is predicted to reach approximately 18% of the American population.[72] Two of the most common types of arthritis are *osteoarthritis* and *rheumatoid arthritis.*

Osteoarthritis is caused by degeneration of cartilage in joints. This lack of cartilage creates a wearing on the surfaces of articulating bones, causing inflammation and pain at the joint. Some of the most commonly affected joints are in the hands, knees, hips, and spine.

Rheumatoid arthritis is a degenerative joint disease in which the body's immune system mistakenly attacks its own tissue (in this case, tissue in the joint or organs). This can cause an inflammatory response in multiple joints, leading to pain and stiffness. The condition is systemic and may affect both a variety of joints and organ systems. Joints most commonly affected by this condition include the hands, feet, wrists, and knees. It is usually characterized by morning stiffness, lasting more than a half hour, which can be both acute and chronic, with eventual loss of joint integrity.

It is important for the health and fitness professional to understand the difference between rheumatoid arthritis and osteoarthritis, and be aware of the signs and symptoms of an acute rheumatoid arthritis exacerbation. In the presence of an arthritic flare-up, even flexibility exercises may be curtailed (Table 14-16).

In addition, health and fitness professionals should monitor the progress of clients with arthritis to assess the effects of the exercise program on joint pain. Pain persisting for more than 1 hour after exercise is an indication that the exercise should be modified or eliminated from the routine. Moreover, exercises of higher intensity or involving high repetitions are to be avoided to decrease joint aggravation. In that regard, a circuit program or multiple session format is suitable for clients with arthritis (Table 14-17).

Health and fitness professionals need to be aware of the medications being taken by clients with arthritis. Clients taking oral corticosteroids, particularly over time, may have osteoporosis, increased body mass, and, if there is a history of gastrointestinal bleeding, anemia. Steroids also increase fracture risk.

Research indicates that people exhibiting osteoarthritis have a decrease in strength and proprioception.[44,73] Wegner and colleagues have demonstrated that individuals with arthritis have a decreased ability to balance while standing.[58] In addition, Slemenda and colleagues noted that loss in knee-extensor strength was a strong predictor of osteoarthritis.[44,73] Furthermore, researchers have shown that patients with osteoarthritis exhibit increased muscle inhibition of knee extensors and were not able to effectively activate their knee-extensor musculature to optimal levels.[74,75]

Balance (or proprioception) and muscle strength are vital components of walking, and therefore any deficit in these areas could potentially have a negative effect

Table 14.16

Physiologic and Training Considerations for Individuals With Arthritis

Physiologic Considerations	Considerations for Health and Fitness, Sport and Athletic Training
Maximum oxygen uptake and ventilatory threshold is frequently lower as a result of decreased exercise associated with pain and joint inflammation	Multiple sessions or a circuit format, using treadmill, elliptical trainer, or arm and leg cycles, are a better alternative than higher-intensity, single-modality exercise formats. The usual principles for aerobic exercise training apply (60–80% peak work capacity, 3–5 days per week). Duration of exercise should be an accumulated 30 minutes, following an intermittent or circuit format, 3–5 days per week.
Medications may significantly influence bone and muscle health	Incorporate functional activities in the exercise program wherever possible
Tolerance to exercise may be influenced by acute arthritic flare-ups	Awareness of the signs and symptoms that may be associated with acute arthritic flare-ups should dictate a cessation or alteration of training, and joint pain persisting for more than 1 hour should result in an altered exercise format
Rheumatoid arthritis results, in particular, in early morning stiffness	Avoid early morning exercise for clients with rheumatoid arthritis
Evaluate for presence of comorbidities, particularly osteoporosis	Resistive exercise training is recommended, as tolerable, using pain as a guide. Start with very low number of repetitions and gradually increase to the number usually associated with improved muscular fitness (e.g., 10–12 reps, before increasing weight, 1 set of 8–10 exercises, 2–3 days per week).

on one's ability to exercise and perform activities of daily living. This claim was supported by a study that showed a significant decrease in dynamic balance for elderly people who had a history of falling.[76]

It used to be common practice for arthritic patients to avoid strenuous exercise. However, research on the effects of training on the symptoms of arthritis have led to a paradigm shift.[77,78] Tufts University showed that a 12-week strength-training program provided relief from arthritic symptoms.[78] Hurley and colleagues[74] demonstrated that a 4-week training regimen (including proprioceptive training) decreased muscle inhibition and increased muscle strength in patients with moderate muscle inhibition.

Therefore, individuals with arthritis are advised to participate in a regular exercise program that follows the OPT™ methodology for increasing stabilization and strength, while also increasing activities of daily living. In spite of the risks associated with exercise in the arthritic client, it is very important in restoring functional mobility and endurance in a deconditioned client who has joint limitations secondary to arthritis. Symptoms of arthritis (such as joint pain and stiffness) are heightened through inactivity as a result of muscle atrophy and lack of tissue flexibility. Progressing exercises so that they are performed in the seated position (without support) and standing position will increase functional capacity and balance of clients.

Table 14.17	
Basic Exercise Guidelines for Individuals With Arthritis	
Mode	Treadmill walking, stationary cycling, rowers, and low-impact or step aerobics
Frequency	3–5 days per week
Intensity	60–80% of maximum heart rate Stage I cardiorespiratory training progressing to stage II (may be reduced to 40–70% of maximum heart rate if needed)
Duration	30 minutes
Assessment	Push, pull, overhead squat Single-leg balance or single-leg squat (if tolerated)
Flexibility	SMR and static and active stretching
Resistance Training	1–3 sets of 10–12 repetitions 2–3 days per week Phase 1 of OPT™ model with reduced repetitions (10–12) May use a circuit or PHA training system
Special Considerations	Avoid heavy lifting and high repetitions Stay in pain-free ranges of motion *Only use SMR if tolerated by the client There may be a need to start out with only 5 minutes of exercise and progressively increase, depending on the severity of conditions

SMR, self-myofascial release; *PHA*, Peripheral Heart Action.

A methodical approach is important in the assessment and activity recommendations to reduce symptoms of flare-ups. Follow the guidelines for assessment in Chapter 5 (Fitness Assessment) and note the pain-free range of motion that clients exhibit during these exercises. Improving muscle strength and enhancing flexibility through exercise can assist in decreasing symptoms associated with arthritis. Static and active forms of stretching can be used and may be better tolerated from a seated or standing position. The use of self-myofascial release can be used if tolerated. Cardiorespiratory training should begin in stage I and may progress to stage II or stage III, depending on the client's capabilities and a physician's advice. Core and balance exercises will be very important for this population to increase levels of stability. Reactive training is not recommended for arthritic clients. Phase 1 of the OPT™ model will be used for this population with modified repetitions (10 to 12) to avoid heavy, repetitive joint loading that increases stress to the affected joints.

SUMMARY

Arthritis is an inflammatory condition that mainly affects the joints of the body. Two of the most common types of arthritis are *osteoarthritis* and *rheumatoid arthritis*. Osteoarthritis is caused by degeneration of cartilage in joints. Rheumatoid arthritis is a systemic, degenerative joint disease in which the body's immune system mistakenly attacks its own tissues in the joint or organs, causing an inflammatory response, leading to pain and stiffness.

Improving muscle strength and enhancing flexibility through exercise can decrease arthritis symptoms. However, health and fitness professionals must be aware of the signs and symptoms of an acute rheumatoid arthritis exacerbation. In the case of an arthritic flare-up, even flexibility exercises may not be able to be performed. In addition, exercises that cause pain to persist for more than 1 hour after exercise should be modified or eliminated from the routine. Health and fitness professionals need to be aware of the medications being taken by clients, especially oral corticosteroids and steroids.

Clients with osteoarthritis have a decrease in strength and proprioception. A loss of knee-extensor strength is a strong predictor of osteoarthritis. Symptoms of arthritis (such as joint pain and stiffness) are heightened through inactivity as a result of muscle atrophy and lack of tissue flexibility. Functional capacity and balance can be increased by progressing exercises so that they are performed in the seated position (without support) and standing.

Flexibility exercises should improve muscle strength and enhance flexibility. Static and active forms of stretching can be used and may be better tolerated from a seated or standing position. The use of self-myofascial release can be used, if tolerated. Cardiorespiratory training should begin in stage I and may progress to stage II or stage III, depending on the client's capabilities and a physician's advice. Core and balance exercises will be very important. Reactive training is not recommended. Phases 1 and 2 will be used for this population with modified repetitions (10 to 12) to avoid heavy, repetitive joint loading that increases stress to the affected joints.

Cancer

Cancer: Any of various types of malignant neoplasms, most of which invade surrounding tissues, may metastasize to several sites, and are likely to recur after attempted removal and to cause death of the patient unless adequately treated.

Cancer is the second leading cause of death in the United States with more than one-half million deaths annually, behind cardiovascular disease. It has been estimated that American men have about a 44% probability and women have a 38% probability of developing cancer during their lifetime.[79]

Because of better detection and treatment strategies, those living with cancer have increased substantially. Moreover, in recent years there have been a variety of studies that have documented the positive benefits of exercise in the treatment of cancer, including improved aerobic and muscular fitness, retention of lean body mass, less fatigue, improved quality of life, and positive effects on mood and self-concept.[80] Because cancer is not a single disease, but a collection of diseases that share the same description (with respect to cell division, accumulation, and death), its signs and symptoms vary widely. This chapter cannot do justice to the complexity of cancer. There are several excellent and descriptive resources that can be reviewed for more information.[1,3]

Medications used by clients with cancer can result in substantial adverse effects, including peripheral nerve damage, cardiac and pulmonary problems, skeletal muscle myopathy, and anemia. Clients may also experience frequent nausea. In addition, the combination of the disease and its treatments frequently result in a diminished quality of life. Health and fitness professionals must have a knowledge of and appreciation for the varied adverse effects of the treatments for cancer, as they can be substantially greater than the treatments prescribed for most other chronic diseases (Table 14-18).

Exercise is an important intervention for clients recovering from cancer. It can improve exercise tolerance, reduce the cellular risks associated with cancer, and also improve quality of life. Specifically, exercise at low to moderate intensities for moderate durations appears to have a more positive effect on the immune system (when compared with higher intensities for longer durations).[81] Research indicates that moderate to high levels of physical activity seem to be associated with decreased incidence and mortality rates for certain forms of cancer.[82]

That said, exercise programs for this population should follow the OPT™ model (Table 14-19). Assessment procedures for the individual with cancer can follow the

Table 14.18

Physiologic and Training Considerations for Individuals With Cancer

Physiologic Considerations	Considerations for Health and Fitness, Sport and Athletic Training
Fatigue and weakness is common	Aerobic exercise should be done at low-moderate intensity (40–50% of peak capacity), 3–5 days per week, using typical aerobic modes (treadmill, elliptical trainer, cycle, depending on patient preference). In particular, avoid higher-intensity training during periods of cancer treatment.
Excessive fatigue may result in overall diminished activity	Use intermittent bouts of exercise to accumulate 20–30 minutes of total aerobic exercise
Diminished immune function	Resistance training can be performed (1 set of 8–10 exercises, 10–15 repetitions to fatigue, 2–3 days per week)
Decreased lean muscle mass	Assess and provide intervention for decreased range of motion and balance

guidelines in Chapter 5 (Fitness Assessment). The specific push, pull, and overhead squat exercise should be representative of the client's ability level. A single-leg balance assessment would also be advised if a single-leg squat cannot be performed by the client. Flexibility should include static and active stretching. Self-myofascial release can be used if no complications exist that would prevent its use. Check with

Table 14.19

Basic Exercise Guidelines for Individuals With Cancer

Mode	Treadmill walking, stationary cycling, rowers, low-impact or step aerobics
Frequency	3–5 days per week
Intensity	50–70% of maximum heart rate reserve Stage I cardiorespiratory training progressing to stage II (may be reduced to 40–70% of maximum heart rate if needed)
Duration	15–30 minutes per session (may only start with 5 min)
Assessment	Push, pull, overhead squat Single-leg balance (if tolerated)
Flexibility	SMR* and static and active stretching
Resistance Training	1–3 sets of 10–15 repetitions 2–3 days per week Phases 1 and 2 of OPT™ model May use a circuit or PHA training system
Special Considerations	Avoid heavy lifting in initial stages of training Allow for adequate rest intervals and progress client slowly *Only use SMR if tolerated by the client There may be a need to start out with only 5 minutes of exercise and progressively increase, depending on the severity of conditions and fatigue

SMR, self-myofascial release; *PHA*, Peripheral Heart Action.

a physician if there is any question. Cardiorespiratory training for this population is very important, but may have to start with 5 minutes of stage I training, progressing up to 30 minutes, 3 to 5 days per week. Stage II or stage III training may be used on agreement of the client's physician.

Core and balance exercises will be essential for this population. These exercises will help in regaining stabilization necessary for activities of daily living that may have been lost (as a result of the lack of activity caused by treatments). Clients should be progressed slowly using the stabilization, strength, and power continuums. Reactive training is not recommended until the client has sufficiently progressed to performing three complete phase 1 workouts per week. Resistance training for this population will include phases 1 and 2 of the OPT™ model. Other phases may be used as the client progresses and are approved by his or her physician.

SUMMARY

Cancer is the second leading cause of death in the United States, although the number of individuals living with cancer has increased substantially. There are several positive benefits of exercise in the treatment of cancer. Exercise is an important intervention in terms of improving exercise tolerance, reducing cellular risks associated with cancer, and improving quality of life.

Medications used by clients with cancer can result in substantial adverse effects. In addition, the combination of the disease and its treatments frequently result in a diminished quality of life. The adverse effects of the treatments for cancer can be substantially greater than the treatments prescribed for most other chronic diseases.

For clients recovering from cancer, exercise that follows the OPT™ model at low to moderate intensities for moderate durations has a positive effect on the immune system. Research indicates that moderate to high levels of physical activity seem to be associated with decreased incidence and mortality rates for certain forms of cancer.

Assessment procedures for the individual with cancer can follow fitness assessment guidelines. The specific push, pull, and squat exercise should be representative of the client's ability level. A single-leg balance assessment would also be advised, if the client is capable. Flexibility should include static and active stretching. Self-myofascial release can be used if no complications exist that would prevent its use. Cardiorespiratory training for this population is very important, but may have to start with 5 minutes of stage I training, progressing up to 30 minutes, 3 to 5 days per week. Stage II or stage III training may be used on agreement of the client's physician. Core and balance exercises are essential for this population. Reactive training is not recommended until the client has progressed to three phase 1 workouts per week. Resistance training for this population will include phases 1 and 2 of the OPT™ model. Other phases may be used as the client progresses and are approved by his or her physician.

Women and Pregnancy

The physiologic differences between men and women have been well studied. The majority of observed disparities in athletic performance between men and women are explained by differences in body structure, muscle mass, and lean to fat body mass ratio and, to a lesser extent, blood chemistry. When measures are adjusted for body composition, both physiologic and performance parameters narrow considerably or completely vanish. Nonetheless, women have lower absolute measures for aerobic capacity and measures of muscular fitness (Table 14-20).

Table 14.20

Physiologic and Training Considerations for Women and Pregnancy

Physiologic Considerations	Considerations for Health and Fitness, Sport and Athletic Training
Contraindications include persistent bleeding 2nd to 3rd trimester, medical documentation of incompetent cervix or intrauterine growth retardation, pregnancy-induced hypertension, preterm rupture of membrane, or preterm labor during current or prior pregnancy	Screen carefully for potential contraindications to exercise
Decreased oxygen available for aerobic exercise	Low-moderate intensity aerobic exercise (40–50% of peak work capacity) should be performed 3–5 days per week, emphasizing non–weight-bearing exercise (e.g., swimming, cycling), although certainly treadmill or elliptical training modes may be preferred and are appropriate.
Posture can affect blood flow to uterus during vigorous exercise	Avoid supine exercise, particularly after the first trimester
Even in the absence of exercise, pregnancy may increase metabolic demand by 300 kcal per day to maintain energy balance	Advise adequate caloric intake to offset exercise effect
High-risk pregnancy considerations include individuals older than the age of 35, history of miscarriage, diabetes, thyroid disorder, anemia, obesity, and a sedentary lifestyle	There are no published guidelines for resistance, flexibility, or balance training specific to pregnancy exercise. Provided exercise intensity is below the aerobic prescription of 40–50% of peak work capacity, with careful attention to special considerations and contraindications described, adding these components may be helpful. For resistance training, if cleared by the physician, a circuit-training format is recommended, 1–3 sets of 12–15 reps per exercise, emphasizing breathing control and rest, as needed, between sets.
	Advise clothing that will dissipate heat easily during exercise
	Postpartum exercise should be similar to pregnancy guidelines, as physiologic changes that occur during pregnancy may persist for up to 6 weeks

With regard to pregnancy, there has been substantial research evaluating the effects of exercise on the physiology and health of both mother and developing fetus. Fears that the fetus may be harmed by increased blood circulation, thermoregulatory changes, or decreased oxygen supply can be minimized with appropriate precautions. The general consensus is that most recreational pursuits are appropriate for all pregnant women. Those already engaged in an exercise program before pregnancy may continue with moderate levels of exercise until the third trimester, when a logical reduction in activity is recommended.[83]

Table 14.21	
Basic Exercise Guidelines for Women and Pregnancy	
Mode	Low-impact or step aerobics that avoid jarring motions, treadmill walking, stationary cycling, and water activity
Frequency	3–5 days per week
Intensity	140 beats per minute, for beginning clients; 160 beats per minute for intermediate to advanced clients Stage I
Duration	15–30 minutes per day. There may be a need to start out with only 5 minutes of exercise and progressively increase to 30 minutes, depending on the severity of conditions
Assessment	Push, pull, overhead squat Single-leg squat or balance
Flexibility	Static, active stretching and SMR*
Resistance Training	2–3 days per week, using light loads at 12–15 repetitions Phases 1 and 2 of the OPT™ model are advised (use only phase 1 after first trimester)
Special Considerations	Avoid exercises in a prone (on stomach) or supine (on back) position after 12 weeks of pregnancy *Avoid SMR on varicose veins and areas of swelling and the inside of the lower leg, as it may be linked to premature uterine contraction.

SMR, self-myofascial release.

The gradual growth of the fetus can alter the posture of pregnant women, making flexibility and core-stabilization training important. As the mother-to-be progresses to the more advanced stages of pregnancy (second and third trimesters, or after 12 weeks), performing exercises in a prone (on stomach) or supine (on back) position is not advised. Changes also occur in the cardiovascular system, decreasing work capacity and leading to necessary alterations in the cardiorespiratory program.

In the postpartum period, there may be a tendency to rush an exercise program in an effort to return to prepregnancy physiologic and morphologic status. Fitness professionals must be careful to advise clients that the changes that occurred during pregnancy may persist for a month to a month and a half. A return to a more vigorous program should be deferred and entered into gradually.

Health and fitness professionals should follow the assessment guidelines in Chapter 5 (Fitness Assessment), using seated and standing exercises (Table 14-21). A single-leg squat assessment may be performed as well, if a woman is capable. If not, a single-leg balance assessment may be more appropriate. Flexibility exercises should be performed in a seated and standing position, especially in the second and third trimesters. Static and active stretching should be used, and self-myofascial release may also be used as tolerated. Also, self-myofascial release should not be performed on varicose veins that are sore, or on areas where there is swelling (such as the calves). Cardiorespiratory training should consist primarily of stage I and only enter stage II on a physician's advice. Reactive training is not advised for this population after the first trimester. Phases 1 and 2 of the OPT™ model may be used in the first trimester; however, in the second and third trimesters the use of only phase 1 is advised.

SUMMARY

Most disparities in athletic performance between men and women are explained by differences in body structure, muscle mass, and lean to fat body mass ratio and blood chemistry. These differences are mostly eliminated when adjustments are made for body composition.

In pregnant women, appropriate precautions can minimize the risks of increased blood circulation, thermoregulatory changes, or decreased oxygen supply. Most recreational pursuits are appropriate for all pregnant women, and moderate levels of exercise are encouraged until the third trimester. In the postpartum period, a return to a more vigorous program should be entered into gradually.

Fitness professionals should follow the assessment guidelines in Chapter 5 (Fitness Assessment), using seated or standing exercises. A single-leg squat assessment may be performed depending on the trimester. In the second and third trimester, a single-leg balance assessment may be more appropriate. Flexibility exercises should be performed in a seated and standing position, especially in the second and third trimesters. Static and active stretching should be used. Self-myofascial release can be used as long as the client avoids using the foam roll on varicose veins or anywhere there is swelling. Cardiorespiratory training should consist primarily of stage I. Reactive training is not advised for this population in the second and third trimesters. Phases 1 and 2 of the OPT™ model may be used in the first trimester. In the second and third trimesters only phase 1 is advised.

Lung Disease

Smoking has progressively declined during the last few decades. However, it is still vitally important to reinforce a continued decrease in the number of current smokers and prevent initiation of the habit. There remains an epidemiology of lung disease and its concurrent effects on so many other diagnosed chronic diseases (heart disease, cancer, and peripheral vascular disease).

Lung disease is largely broken into two major categories, obstructive and restrictive. In **restrictive lung disease** or disorders, lung tissue may be fibrotic and, thus, dysfunctional (as in the cases of pulmonary fibrosis or asbestosis). More simply, the ability to expand the lungs may be decreased as a result of any number of causes (such as fractured ribs, a neuromuscular disease, or even obesity). In **obstructive lung disease**, the lung tissue may be normal, but flows are restricted. The major obstructive lung diseases include asthma, chronic bronchitis, and emphysema. These diseases are characterized by chronic inflammation (caused primarily by smoking, although in the case of asthma may be caused by environmental irritants) and airway obstruction via mucus production. Cystic fibrosis is another disease that is characterized by excessive mucus production, but is instead a genetic disorder.

Regardless, both restrictive and obstructive lung disease result in similar impairments during exercise (Table 14-22). Problems include decreased ventilation and decreased gas exchange ability (resulting in decreased aerobic capacity and endurance, and in oxygen desaturation). Clients with lung disease experience fatigue at low levels of exercise and often have shortness of breath (or *dyspnea*). Those with emphysema are frequently underweight and may exhibit overall muscle wasting with hypertrophied neck muscles (which are excessively used to assist in labored breathing). Those with chronic bronchitis may be the opposite: overweight and barrel-chested.

In general, exercise for these clients is similar to what would be appropriate for the general population (Table 14-23). Exercise can improve functional capacity and decrease the symptoms of dyspnea in this population, among many other physiologic and psychological benefits.[84] The use of lower body cardiorespiratory and resistance training exercises seem to be best tolerated. Upper extremity exercises place an increased stress on the secondary respiratory muscles that are involved in stabilizing the upper extremities during exercise.[85] Therefore, caution

Restrictive lung disease: The condition of a fibrous lung tissue, which results in a decreased ability to expand the lungs.

Obstructive lung disease: The condition of altered airflow through the lungs, generally caused by airway obstruction as a result of mucus production.

Table 14.22

Physiologic and Training Considerations for Individuals With Lung Disease

Physiologic Considerations	Considerations for Health and Fitness, Sport and Athletic Training
Lung disease frequently is associated with other comorbidities, including cardiovascular disease	Screen for presence of other comorbidities
A decrease in the ability to exchange gas in the lungs may result in oxygen desaturation and marked dyspnea at low workloads	Whenever possible, try to ascertain the level of oxygen saturation using a pulse oximeter. Pulse oximetry values should be above 90% and certainly above 85%. Values below this level are a contraindication to continued exercise, regardless of symptoms.
Chronic deconditioning results in low aerobic fitness and decreased muscular performance	The aerobic exercise prescription should be guided by the client's shortness of breath. Workloads of 40–60% of peak work capacity, 3–5 days per week, 20–45 minutes as tolerable, may be achievable. Intermittent exercise with frequent rest breaks (at a ratio of two parts exercise to one part recovery) may be necessary to achieve sufficient overall exercise duration.
Upper extremity exercise may result in earlier onset of dyspnea and fatigue than expected, when compared with lower extremity exercise	Upper extremity exercise should be programmed carefully and modified, based on fatigue. Resistance training can be helpful; use conservative guidelines. A circuit-training in a PHA format is recommended (8–10 exercises, 1 set of 8–15 reps per exercise), emphasizing breathing control and rest as needed between sets.
Clients may have significant muscle wasting and be of low body weight (with a BMI <18)	If the client is very thin, be certain to recommend adequate caloric intake to offset exercise effects.
Clients may be using supplemental oxygen	Trainers may not adjust oxygen flow during exercise; it is considered a medication. If a client experiences unusual dyspnea or has evidence of oxygen desaturation during exercise, stop exercise and consult with the client's physician.

BMI, body mass index; *PHA*, Peripheral Heart Action.

should be used when designing programs for this population to ensure adequate rest intervals. The use of the Peripheral Heart Action (PHA) training system would be advised.

In some clients, inspiratory muscle training can specifically improve the work associated with breathing. Health and fitness professionals working with clients who have lung disease should inquire about this intervention to see whether it might augment the general exercise program. For more information, read the comprehensive guidelines regarding the exercise assessment and training of individuals with lung disease published by the American Association of Cardiovascular and Pulmonary Rehabilitation.[86]

Table 14.23

Basic Exercise Guidelines for Individuals With Lung Disease

Mode	Treadmill walking, stationary cycling, steppers, and elliptical trainers
Frequency	3–5 days per week
Intensity	40–60% of peak work capacity Stage I
Duration	Work up to 20–45 minutes
Assessment	Push, pull, overhead squat Single-leg squat or balance
Flexibility	Static and active stretching and SMR
Resistance Training	1 set of 8–15 repetitions 2–3 days per week Phase 1 of the OPT™ model are advised PHA training system is recommended
Special Considerations	Upper body exercises cause increased dyspnea and must be monitored Allow for sufficient rest between exercises

SMR, self-myofascial release; *PHA*, Peripheral Heart Action.

SUMMARY

Lung disease is largely broken into two major categories, *obstructive* and *restrictive*. In restrictive disease or disorders, lung tissue may be fibrotic and the ability to expand the lungs may be decreased owing to any number of causes. In obstructive lung disease, the lung tissue may be normal, but flows are restricted. Both types cause decreased ventilation and decreased gas exchange ability.

Clients with lung disease are often short of breath (*dyspnea*) and fatigue at low levels of exercise. Exercise can improve functional capacity and decrease the symptoms of dyspnea. In some clients, inspiratory muscle training can specifically improve the work associated with breathing.

In general, exercise for this population is similar to what would be appropriate for the general population. Lower body cardiorespiratory and resistance training exercises seem to be best tolerated. Adequate rest intervals need to be maintained. The Peripheral Heart Action training system is advised.

Intermittent Claudication/Peripheral Arterial Disease

Intermittent claudication:
The manifestation of the symptoms caused by peripheral arterial disease.

Peripheral arterial disease:
A condition characterized by narrowing of the major arteries that are responsible for supplying blood to the lower extremities.

Intermittent claudication is the name for the manifestation of the symptoms caused by peripheral arterial disease (PAD). (The term *peripheral vascular disease* is also commonly used to describe the activity-induced symptoms that characterize this disease.) Essentially, intermittent claudication is characterized by limping, lameness, or pain in the lower leg during mild exercise resulting from a decrease in blood supply (oxygen) to the lower extremities. **Peripheral arterial disease** is characterized by narrowing of the major arteries that are responsible for supplying blood to the lower extremities.

The primary limiting factor for exercise in the PAD client is, of course, leg pain. One of the problems facing the fitness professional is the ability to differentiate between those who are limited by true symptoms of true intermittent claudication

Table 14.24

Physiologic and Training Considerations for Individuals With Intermittent Claudication/PAD

Physiologic Considerations	Considerations for Health and Fitness, Sport and Athletic Training
PAD patients frequently have coexisting coronary artery disease or diabetes	For clients with coexisting coronary artery disease, do not exceed established heart rate upper limit. (Usually, this limit is established from a walking test, where leg pain is the limiting factor.) Switching modalities so that leg pain will not limit exercise may result in a higher—and possibly inappropriate—cardiac workload. If possible, a continuous format of exercise using walking is preferred. Exercise duration should be 20–30 total minutes, with continuous bouts of 10 minutes or greater, 5–7 days per week.
Smoking significantly worsens PAD and exercise tolerance	Strongly recommend smoking cessation. If a client continues to smoke, do not allow smoking for at least 1 hour before exercise.
PAD frequently results in decreased aerobic capacity and endurance	Focus on aerobic exercise activities, with an emphasis on walking.
Resistance training may improve overall physical function, but may not address limitations of PAD	Resistance exercise should be complementary, but not substituted for aerobic exercise. A circuit-training format is recommended (e.g., 8–10 exercises, 1–3 sets of 8–12 reps per exercise).
	An intermittent format of exercise may be necessary, with intensity guided by pain tolerance. Typical guidelines suggest exercise into moderate to severe discomfort, rest until subsided, and repeat until total exercise time is achieved (20–30 minutes).
	Always screen for comorbidities.

PAD, peripheral arterial disease.

versus similar leg complaints (such as tightness, cramping, and pain) that might simply be associated with deconditioning (Table 14-24). If the client has a diagnosis of PAD, the symptoms are likely to be accurate for intermittent claudication, although they still could be associated with deconditioning.[87] Consult with the client's physician concerning the condition. If pain continues during exercise, the health and fitness professional must refer the client to a licensed physician immediately.

Although experience will improve the ability of the health and fitness professional to differentiate between disease and deconditioning, in many respects it does not really matter. That is, the health and fitness professional should still develop a training regimen that attempts to improve physical function in the face of limiting factors.[88] In the case of peripheral vascular disease or deconditioning, the use of an intermittent format of exercise, with rest as necessary between exercise bouts, is similar (Table 14-25).

Table 14.25

Basic Exercise Guidelines for Individuals With Intermittent Claudication/PAD

Mode	Treadmill walking is preferred, also stationary cycling, steppers, and elliptical trainers
Frequency	3–5 days per week working up to every day
Intensity	50–85% of HR max
Duration	Work up to 20–30 minutes
Assessment	Push, pull, overhead squat Single-leg squat or balance
Flexibility	Static and active stretching
Resistance Training	1–3 sets of 8–12 repetitions 2–3 days per week Phase 1 of the OPT™ model are advised
Special Considerations	Allow for sufficient rest between exercises Workout may start with 5–10 minutes of activity Slowly progress client

Because PAD is associated with coronary heart disease and diabetes, health and fitness professionals should be aware of other existing comorbidities and be suspicious that these comorbidities may still exist, undiagnosed. Thus, physician clearance for exercise is necessary for the PAD patient.

Exercise programming should follow the OPT™ methodology, using the suggested assessment process in Chapter 5 (Fitness Assessment). The number of repetitions for the movement assessments may have to be decreased to 5 to 10, depending on the client's abilities. It will be important to make clients feel comfortable and competent with this process to ensure compliance. Static and active stretching should be used for this population. Guidelines for self-myofascial release are not known at this time, and it is suggested that it not be used in this population, unless approved by a licensed physician. Phase 1 of the OPT™ model is suggested. Repetitions may need to start at 8 to 12 (lower than indicated by these phases) and slowly progress to 12 to 20. Exercise bouts may initially start with 5 to 10 minutes of activity and progress slowly to 20 to 30 minutes.

SUMMARY

Intermittent claudication is the name for the manifestation of the symptoms caused by peripheral arterial disease (PAD). When there is increased activity of the leg muscles, PAD results in symptoms in which oxygen supply does not meet demand.

Exercise for PAD should *induce* symptoms, causing a stimulus that increases local circulation. The primary limiting factor is leg pain. The health and fitness professional must differentiate between true intermittent claudication versus similar leg complaints associated with deconditioning. If the client has a diagnosis of PAD, the symptoms are likely to be accurate for intermittent claudication, although they still could be associated with deconditioning.

Exercise in an intermittent format, with rest as necessary between exercise bouts, is recommended. Physician clearance for exercise is necessary for the PAD client.

Exercise programming should follow the OPT™ methodology, using the fitness assessment. The number of repetitions for the assessment may have to be decreased to 5 to 10, depending on the client's abilities. Static and active stretching should be used for this population. However, self-myofascial release is not recommended. Phases 1 and 2 of the OPT™ model should be used. Repetitions may need to start at 8 to 12 and slowly progress to 12 to 20. Exercise bouts may initially start with 5 to 10 minutes of activity and progress slowly to 20 to 30 minutes.

Review Questions

1 *In youth populations, the progression of aerobic training volume should not exceed what percentage per period of adaptation?*

a. 10%

b. 20%

c. 50%

2 *Select which of the following items will decrease with age in older adults.*

a. Maximum oxygen uptake

b. Percentage of body fat

c. Maximum exercise heart rate

d. Bone mass

e. Measures of pulmonary function

f. Lean body mass

3 *In overweight or obese adults, exercise capacity should be no greater than:*

a. 10 to 30% of work capacity

b. 25 to 55% of work capacity

c. 40 to 70% of work capacity

d. 60 to 80% of work capacity

4 *Clients who take β-blockers may display a skewed heart rate response to exercise.*

a. True

b. False

5 *Because of a lack of insulin in type 1 diabetes, blood sugar is not optimally delivered to the cells, which results in:*

a. Hyperglycemia

b. Hypoglycemia

6 *Symptoms should always supersede anything else as a sign to decrease or stop exercising.*

a. True

b. False

REFERENCES

1. ACSM's Exercise Management for Persons With Chronic Diseases and Disabilities, 2nd ed. Champaign, IL: Human Kinetics, 2003.
2. ACSM's Resource Manual for Guidelines for Graded Exercise and Prescription, 4th ed. Philadelphia: Lippincott Williams & Wilkins, 2001.
3. ACSM's Resources for Clinical Exercise Physiology. Philadelphia: Lippincott Williams & Wilkins, 2002.
4. Sallis JF, Patrick K, Long BJ. Overview of the International Consensus Conference on Physical Activity Guidelines for Adolescents. Pediatr Exerc Sci 1994;6:299–301.
5. US Department of Health and Human Services. Guidelines for school and community programs to promote lifelong physical activity among young people. MMWR Morb Mortal Wkly Rep 1997;46:1–36.
6. Pate RR. Physical activity for young children. President's Council on Physical Fitness and Sport Research Digest, Series 3, No. 3:1–8; 1998.
7. ACSM's Guidelines for Graded Exercise and Prescription, 6th ed. Philadelphia: Lippincott Williams & Wilkins, 2000.
8. Saltarelli W. Children. In: Ehrman JK, Gordon PM, Visich PS, Keteyian SJ (eds). Clinical Exercise Physiology. Champaign, IL: Human Kinetics, 2003:544–570.
9. Faigenbaum A, Kraemer B, Cahill B, Chandler J, Dziados J, Elfrink E, Forman M, Gaudiose M, Micheli L, Nitka M, Roberts S. Youth resistance training: position statement paper and literature review. Strength Cond J 1996;18:62–75.
10. Weltman A, Janney CA, Rians CB, Stand K, Berg B, Tippett S, Wise J, Cahill BR, Katch FI. The effects of hydraulic resistance strength training on pre-pubertal males. Med Sci Sports Exerc 1986; 18:629–638.
11. Ozmun JC, Mikesky AE, Sarburg PR. Neuromuscular adaptations following prepubescent strength training. Med Sci Sports Exerc 1994;26(4):510–514.
12. Hamill BP. Relative safety of weightlifting and weight training. J Strength Cond Res 1994;8(1):53–57.
13. Jones CS, Christensen C, Young M. Weight training injury trends. Phys Sports Med 2000;7:61–72.
14. US Consumer Product Safety Commission. National Electronic Injury Surveillance System. Washington: Director of Epidemiology, National Injury Information Clearinghouse, 1987.
15. Haff GG. Roundtable discussion: youth resistance training. Strength Cond J 2003;25(1):49–64.
16. Falk B, Tenenbaum G. The effectiveness of resistance training in children: a meta-analysis. Sports Med 1996;22:176–186.
17. Payne V, Morrow J, Johnson L. Resistance training in children and youth: a meta-analysis. Res Q Exerc Sport 1997;68:80–89.
18. Ramsay JA, Blimkie CJ, Smith K, Garner S, MacDougall JD, Sale DG. Strength training effects in prepubescent boys. Med Sci Sports Exerc 1990;22(5):605–614.
19. Milne C, Seefedlt V, Reuschlein P. Relationship between grade, sex, race, and motor development in young children. Res Q 1976;47:726.
20. Clark HH. Joint and body range of movement. Phys Fit Res Digest 1975;5:16–18.
21. Brock D, Guralnick J, Brody J. Demography and epidemiology of aging in the US. In: Schneider E, Rowe J (eds). Handbook of the Biology of Aging. San Diego: Academic Press, 1990:3–23.
22. [Anonymous] Administration on Aging 1999. http://www.aoa.dhhs.gov/aoa/stats/profile/#health
23. American Heart Association. Heart Disease and Stroke Statistics—2003 Update. Dallas: American Heart Association, 2002.
24. [Anonymous] Arthritis Foundation. Arthritis fact sheet. Atlanta, 1997.
25. Bell R, Hoshizaki T. Relationships of age and sex with joint range of motion of seventeen joint actions in humans. Can J Appl Sports Sci 1981;6:202–206.
26. Fielding JW. Presentation. Orthopedic and physical therapy seminar. September 1979. University of Cincinnati Medical Center.
27. Evans WJ. Exercise training guidelines for the elderly. Med Sci Sports Exerc 1999;31(1):12–17.
28. Larsson L, Grimby G, Karlsson J. Muscle strength and speed of movement in relation to age and muscle morphology. J Appl Physiol 1979;46;451–456.
29. Ringsberg K, Gerghem P, Johansson J, Obrant KJ. Is there a relationship between balance, gait performance and muscular strength in 75-year-old women? Age Ageing [serial online] 1999;28(3):289–293. [Abstract]
30. Luoto S, Aalto H, Taimela S, Hurri H, Pyykko I, Alaranta H. One footed and externally disturbed two footed postural control in patients with chronic low back pain and health control subjects. A controlled study with follow-up. Spine 1998;23(19):2081–2089.
31. Myers A, Young Y, Langlois J. Prevention of falls in the elderly. Bone 1996;18(Suppl):87S–101S.
32. Wescott WL, Baechle TR. Strength Training for Seniors. Champaign, IL: Human Kinetics, 1999:1–2.
33. Hides JA. Multifidus muscle recovery in acute low back patients. Ph.D. Thesis. Department of Physiotherapy, University of Queensland, 1996.
34. Hides JA, Richardson CA, Jull GA. Multifidus muscle rehabilitation decreases recurrence of symptoms following first episode low back pain. In: Proceedings of the National Congress of the Australian Physiotherapy Association, Brisbane, 1996.

35. Marks R. The effect of isometric quadriceps strength training in mid-range for osteoarthritis of the knee. Arthritis Care Res 1993;6:52–56.

36. Quirk A, Newman R, Newman K. An evaluation of interferential therapy, shortwave diathermy and exercise in the treatment of osteo-arthritis of the knee. Physiotherapy 1985;71:55–57.

37. American College of Sports Medicine. Position stand on exercise and physical activity for older adults. Med Sci Sports Exer 1998;30;992–1008.

38. Kuczmanski RJ, Flegal JM, Campbell SM, Johnson CL. Increasing prevalence of overweight among US adults. The National Health and Examination Survey, 1960 to 1991. JAMA 1994;272:205–211.

39. Schwimmer JB, Burwinkle TM, Varni JW. Health-related quality of life of severely obese children and adolescents. JAMA 2003;289(14):1813–1819.

40. Must A, Spadano J, Coakley EH, Field AE, Colditz G, Dietz WH. The disease burden associated with overweight and obesity. JAMA 1999;282(16):1523–1529.

41. Evans W, Rosenberg I. Biomarkers. New York: Simon and Schuster, 1992.

42. Meredith CN, Zackin MJ, Frontera WR, Evans WJ. Body composition and aerobic capacity in young and middle-aged endurance-trained men. Med Sci Sports Exerc 1987;19:557–563.

43. Roberts SB, Young VR, Fuss P. What are the dietary energy needs of adults? Int J Obes 1992; 16:969–976.

44. Slemenda C, Heilman DK, Brandt KD, Katz BP, Mazzuca SA, Braunstein EM, Byrd D. Reduced quadriceps strength relative to body weight. A risk factor for knee osteoarthritis in women? Arthritis Rheumatol 1998;41:1951–1959.

45. Jurimae T, Jurimae J, Pihl E. Circulatory response to single circuit weight and walking training sessions of similar energy cost in middle-aged overweight females. Clin Physiol 2000;20(2):143–149.

46. Kraemer WJ, Noble BJ, Clark MJ, et al. Physiological responses to heavy-resistance exercises with very short rest periods. Int J Sports Med 1987;8:247–251.

47. Hurley BF, Seals DR, Ehsani AA, Cartier LJ, Dalsky GP, Hagberg JM, Hollososzy JO. Effects of high-intensity strength training on cardiovascular function. Med Sci Sports Exerc 1984;16:483–488.

48. Murray D. Morbid obesity—psychosocial aspects and surgical interventions. AORN J 2003; 78(6):990–995.

49. Centers for Disease Control and Prevention. National Diabetes Fact Sheet: national estimates and general information on diabetes in the United States. Revised edition. Atlanta: U.S. Department of Health and Human Services, Centers for Disease Control and Prevention, 1998.

50. Portuese E, Orchard T. Mortality in insulin dependent diabetes. In: Harris MI, Cowie CC, Stern MP, et al. (eds). Diabetes in America. Bethesda, MD: National Institutes of Health, National Institute of Diabetes and Digestive and Kidney Diseases, 1995.

51. Pan XP, Li GW, Hu YH, Wang J, Yang W, Hu ZX, Lin J, Xiao JZ, Cao HB, Liu P, Jiang XG, Jiang YY, Wang JP, Zheng H, Zhang H, Bennet PH, Howard BV. Effects of diet and exercise in preventing NIDDM in people with impaired glucose tolerance. Diabetes Care 1997;20:537–544.

52. American College of Sports Medicine. Position stand on exercise and physical activity for older adults. Med Sci Sports Exerc. 1998;30;992–1008.

53. Hagberg JM, Ferrell RE, Dengel DR, Wilund KR. Exercise training-induced blood pressure and plasma lipid improvements in hypertensives may be genotype dependent. Hypertension 1999;34:18–23.

54. Joint National Committee of Prevention, Detection, Evaluation, and Treatment of High Blood Pressure. The sixth report of the Joint National Committee of Prevention, Detection, Evaluation, and Treatment of High Blood Pressure. Arch Int Med 1997;157:2413–2446.

55. American College of Sports Medicine Position Stand. Physical activity, physical fitness, and hypertension. Med Sci Sports Exerc 1993;25(10):i–x.

56. American Heart Association. Heart Disease and Stroke Statistics—2003 Update. Dallas: American Heart Association, 2002.

57. Centers for Disease Control and Prevention. Receipt of cardiac rehabilitation services among heart attack survivors—19 states and the District of Columbia, 2001. MMWR Morb Mortal Wkly Rep 2003;52(44):1072–1075.

58. Wenger NK, Froelicher ES, Smith LK, et al. Cardiac Rehabilitation. Clinical Practice Guideline No. 17. Rockville, MD: US Department of Health and Human Services, Public Health Service, Agency for Health Care Policy and Research, and the National Heart, Lung, and Blood Institute. AHCPR Publication No. 96–0672, October 1995.

59. Haskell WL, Alderman EL, Fair JM, Maron DJ, Mackey SF, Superko HR, Williams PT, Johnstone IM, Champagne ME, Krauss RM, et al. Effects of intensive multiple risk factor reduction on coronary atherosclerosis and clinical cardiac events in men and women with coronary artery disease: The Stanford Coronary Risk Intervention Project (SCRIP). Circulation 1994;89:975–990.

60. Ornish D, Brown SE, Scherwitz LW, Billings Armstrong WT, Ports TA, McLanahan SM, Kirkeeide RL, Braud RJ, Gould KL. Can lifestyle changes reverse coronary heart disease? The Lifestyle Heart Trial. Lancet 1990;336:129–133.

61. Hambrecht R, Niebauer J, Marburger C, Grunze M, Kalberer B, Hauer K, Schlierf G, Kubler W, Schuler G. Various intensities of leisure time physical activity in patients with coronary artery disease: effects on cardiorespiratory fitness and progression of coronary atherosclerotic lesions. J Am Coll Cardiol 1993;22:468–477.

62. Cummings S, Kelsey J, Nevitt M. Epidemiology of osteoporosis and osteoporotic fractures. Epidemiol Rev 1985;7;178–205.

63. Lindsay R. Osteoporosis. Chicago: National Osteoporosis Foundation, 1992.
64. Riggs BL, Melton LJ. Involutional osteoporosis. N Engl J Med 1986;311:1676–1686.
65. Haapasalo H, Kannus P, Sievanen H, Heinonen A, Oja P, Vuori I. Long-term unilateral loading and bone mineral density and content in female squash players. Calc Tiss Int 1994;54:249–255.
66. Kannus P, Haapasalo H, Sievanen H, Oja P, Vuori I. Site-specific effects on long-term unilateral activity on bone mineral density and content. Bone 1994;15:279–284.
67. Karlsson M, Vergnaud P, Delmas P, Obrant K. Indicators of bone formation in weight lifters. Calc Tiss Int 1995;56:177–180.
68. Courtney A, Watchel E, Myers E, Hayes W. Effects of loading rate on strength of the proximal femur. Calc Tis Int 1994;55:53–58.
69. MacRae P, Feltner M, Reinsch S. A 1-year exercise program for women: effect on falls, injury and physical performance. J Aging Phys Act 1994;2:127–142.
70. Kerr N, Morton A, Dick I, Prince R. Exercise effects on bone mass in postmenopausal women are site specific and load dependent. J Bone Mineral Res 1996;11(2):218–225.
71. Lawrence RC, Hemlick CG, Arnett FC, Deyo RA, Felson DT, Giannini EH, Heyse SP, Hirsch R, Hochberg MC, Hunder CG, Liang MH, Pillemer SR, Steen VD, Wolfe F. Estimates of the prevalence of arthritis and selected musculoskeletal disorders in the United States. Arthritis Rheum 1998;41(5):778–799.
72. Hemlick CG, Lawrence RC, Pollard RA, Lloyd E, Heyse SP. Arthritis and other rheumatic conditions: who is affected now, who will be affected later? National Arthritis Data Workgroup. Arthritis Care Res 19958(4):203–211.
73. Slemenda C, Brandt KD, Heilman DK, Mazzuca SA, Braunstein EM, Katz BP, Wolinsky FD. Quadriceps weakness and osteoarthritis of the knee. Ann Int Med 1997;17:97–104.
74. Hurley MV, Scott DL, Rees J, Newham DJ. Sensorimotor changes and functional performance in patients with knee osteoarthritis. Ann Rheum Disord 1997;56:641–648.
75. O'Reilly SC, Jones A, Muir KR, Doherty M. Quadriceps weakness in knee osteoarthritis: the effect on pain and disability. Ann Rheum Disord 1998;57:588–594.
76. Pai YC, Rogers MW, Patton J, Cain TD, Hanke TA. Static versus dynamic predictions of protective stepping following waist-pull perturbations in young and older adults. J Biomech 1998;31(12):1111–1118.
77. Hurley MV, Jones DW, Newham DJ. Arthrogenic quadriceps inhibition and rehabilitation of patients with extensive traumatic knee injuries. Clin Sci 1994;86:305–310.
78. [Anonymous] Never too late to build up your muscle. Tufts University Diet and Nutrition Letter. Tufts University 1994;12(September):6–7.
79. American Cancer Society, Cancer Facts & Figures—2003. Atlanta: American Cancer Society, 2003.
80. Courneya KS. Exercise interventions during cancer treatment: biopsychosocial outcomes. Exerc Sport Sci Rev 2001:29;60–64.
81. Woods JA, Davis JM, Smith JA, Nieman DC. Exercise and cellular innate immune function. Med Sci Sports Exerc 1999;31:57–66.
82. Segal R, Johnson D, Smith J, Colletta S, Guyton J, Woodard S, Wells G, Reid R. Structured exercise improves physical functioning in women with stages I and II breast cancer: results of a randomized controlled trial. J Clin Oncol 2001;19(3):657–665.
83. American College of Obstetricians and Gynecologists. Exercise during pregnancy and the postpartum period, ACOG Committee Opinion No. 267. Obstet Gynecol 2002;99:171–173.
84. Ries AL, Carlin BW, Carrieri-Kohlman V, et al. Pulmonary rehabilitation: joint ACCP/AACVPR evidence-based guidelines. Chest 1997;112:1363–1396.
85. Celli BR, Rassulo J, Make BJ. Dyssynchronous breathing during arm but not leg exercise in patients with chronic airflow obstruction. N Engl J Med 1986;314:1485–1490.
86. American Association of Cardiovascular and Pulmonary Rehabilitation Guidelines for Pulmonary Rehabilitation Programs, 2nd ed. Champaign, IL: Human Kinetics, 1998.
87. Greenland PG. Clinical significance, detection, and medical treatment for peripheral arterial disease. J Cardiopulm Rehabil 2002;22(2):73–79.
88. Falcone RA, Hirsch AT, Regensteiner JG, et al. Peripheral arterial disease rehabilitation. J Cardiopulm Rehabil 2003;23:170–175.

NUTRITION AND SUPPLEMENTATION

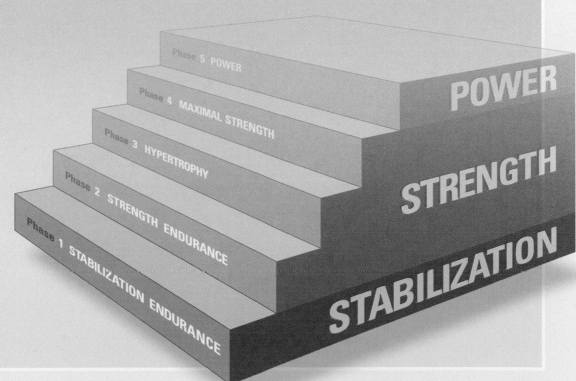

POWER

STRENGTH

STABILIZATION

Phase 5 POWER

Phase 4 MAXIMAL STRENGTH

Phase 3 HYPERTROPHY

Phase 2 STRENGTH ENDURANCE

Phase 1 STABILIZATION ENDURANCE

15

Nutrition

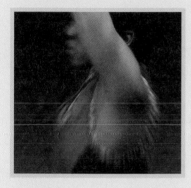

OBJECTIVES

After completing this chapter, you will be able to:

- Describe the macronutrients and their functions.
- Describe how macronutrient composition of an individual's food intake can affect satiety, compliance, daily energy expenditure, and weight control.
- Provide basic nutritional recommendations for optimizing health.
- Answer questions, handle issues, and dispel myths regarding the relationship of macronutrients to the successful alteration of body composition.

KEY TERMS

Carbohydrate	Nutrition	Protein
Lipids		

INTRODUCTION TO NUTRITION

Understanding how the kinetic chain operates and being able to design individualized integrated programs for a client is only a portion of the puzzle. NASM recognizes that a proper nutritional background is an essential component to being a well-rounded health and fitness professional. In a time when fad diets are escalating and appearance is more important than ever, it is vital that health and fitness professionals arm themselves with the hard facts about nutrition and the human body.

This text specifically explores nutritional concepts and how they relate to the kinetic chain for a variety of scenarios. This will further enable the health and fitness professional to provide a scientific rationalization for proper nutritional protocols.

Nutrition and Body Composition

DEFINITION

Nutrition: The sum of the processes by which an animal or plant takes in and uses food substances.

Nutrition is defined as the sum of the processes by which an animal or plant takes in and uses food substances.[1] This very basic definition does not begin to illuminate the role that diet plays in the health, appearance, performance, and well-being of an individual. An understanding of nutrition will be vital to the success of the health and fitness professional's clients. The proper nutrition strategy has the ability to hasten the results from the stimulus of exercise, improve health and athletic performance, reduce the risk of disease and illness, increase energy levels, and favorably alter body composition. Although the following section is designed to give the health and fitness professional an understanding of the basics of nutrition and its use in facilitating clients' goals, it is not designed to instruct on the use of diet to treat illness or high-risk individuals. It is recommended that the health and fitness professional have a network of qualified health-care professionals (doctors, dietitians, and eating-disorder specialists) in their area to whom they can refer when dealing with clients who have special needs. This can be mutually beneficial as these same health-care professionals will need qualified trainers to work with their patients when recommending exercise.

NUTRITION AND BODY COMPOSITION

There are an increasing number of overweight and obese people in the United States. A desire for a quick solution for weight loss has led to the mystification of exercise and diet and an environment ripe for promoters of quick weight-loss methods and fad diets.[2-4] Sorting through this pile of myths and inaccuracies makes the health and fitness professional's job a daunting one. Clients are coming to the health club with preconceived ideas about how they should be eating. These ideas may hinder their progress and have negative health consequences.

The facts about weight loss and gain are quite simple. Eat fewer calories than are expended and there will be a reduction in weight. Conversely, consume more calories than are expended and there will be an increase in weight.[5,6] Today's environment provides a constantly available, palatable food supply (increasing energy intake) and promotes a sedentary lifestyle (reducing energy expenditure). The facts are that we eat too much and move too little. The combination is causing America's waistline to expand.[7]

The following modules address the macronutrients (protein, carbohydrate, and fat), their uses, and recommendations, and will explore many common myths. These topics will be addressed as they relate to the common goals of altering body composition and increasing performance.

SUMMARY

Diet plays an important role in a person's health, appearance, energy, and performance as well as affecting results from exercise and overall well-being. The health and fitness professional should not instruct clients on the use of diet to treat illness or high-risk cases, but rather refer clients to qualified health-care professionals.

Clients come to health and fitness professionals with misconceptions about how they should be eating. However, the fact is that eating fewer calories than are burned will result in weight loss.

Protein

THE FUNCTION OF PROTEIN

Protein: Amino acids linked by peptide bonds.

The primary function of **protein** is to build and repair body tissues and structures. It is also involved in the synthesis of hormones, enzymes, and other regulatory peptides. Additionally, protein can be used for energy if calories or carbohydrate are insufficient in the diet.[8]

THE STRUCTURE OF PROTEIN

Proteins are made up of amino acids linked together by peptide bonds. The body uses approximately 20 amino acids to build its many different proteins.[9] These amino acids can be compared to the letters of the alphabet. Just as specific words are formed by certain sequences of letters, arranging the amino acids in different sequences yields the body's myriad of proteins (from a muscle protein like actin to proteins that make up the lens of the eye).

There are two general classes of amino acids: *essential* and *nonessential* (Table 15-1). Essential amino acids cannot be manufactured in the body (or are manufactured in insufficient amounts); therefore, they must be obtained from the food supply or some other exogenous source. There are eight essential amino acids. The second group of amino acids is termed nonessential because the body

Table 15.1

Amino Acids

Essential	Nonessential	Semiessential
Isoleucine	Alanine	Arginine
Leucine	Asparagine	Histidine
Lysine	Aspartic acid	
Methionine	Cysteine	
Phenylalanine	Glutamic acid	
Threonine	Glutamine	
Tryptophan	Glycine	
Valine	Proline	
	Serine	
	Tyrosine	

is able to manufacture them from dietary nitrogen and fragments of carbohydrate and fat.[8]

Because of their rate of synthesis within the body, arginine and histidine are considered semiessential amino acids. It appears that these amino acids cannot be manufactured by the body at a rate that will support growth (especially in children).

DIGESTION, ABSORPTION, AND UTILIZATION

Proteins must be broken down into the constituent amino acids before the body can use these building blocks for its own purposes. The fate of the amino acids after digestion and absorption by the intestines depends on the body's homeostatic needs, which can range from tissue replacement or tissue addition to a need for energy. Figure 15-1 depicts the digestion, absorption, and synthesis sequence.

As ingested proteins enter the stomach, they encounter hydrochloric acid (HCl), which uncoils (or *denatures*) the protein so that digestive enzymes can begin dismantling the peptide bonds. In addition, the enzyme pepsin begins to cleave the protein strand into smaller polypeptides (strands of several amino acids) and singular amino acids. As these protein fragments leave the stomach and enter the small intestine, pancreatic and intestinal proteases (or protein enzymes) continue to dismantle the protein fragments.

The resulting dipeptides, tripeptides, and singular amino acids are then absorbed through the intestinal wall into the enterocytes and released into the blood supply to the liver (Figure 15-2).

Once in the bloodstream, the free-form amino acids have several possible fates: they can be used for protein synthesis (building and repairing tissues or structures), immediate energy, or potential energy (fat storage).

Amino Acids for Immediate Energy

The body has a constant need for energy, and the brain and nervous system, in particular, have a constant need for glucose. If carbohydrate or total energy intake is

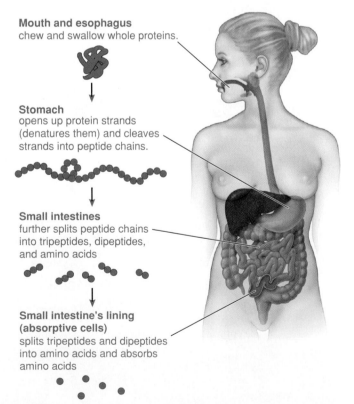

Mouth and esophagus
chew and swallow whole proteins.

Stomach
opens up protein strands (denatures them) and cleaves strands into peptide chains.

Small intestines
further splits peptide chains into tripeptides, dipeptides, and amino acids

Small intestine's lining (absorptive cells)
splits tripeptides and dipeptides into amino acids and absorbs amino acids

Figure 15.1 Protein digestion, absorption, and endogenous synthesis.

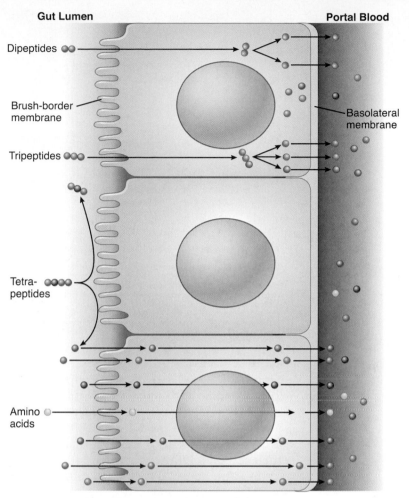

Gut Lumen

Portal Blood

Dipeptides

Brush-border
membrane

Basolateral
membrane

Tripeptides

Tetra-
peptides

Amino
acids

Figure 15.2 Amino acid absorption.

too low, the body has the ability to use amino acids (from dietary or body proteins) to provide energy.[10,11] The amino acids are first *deaminated* (or stripped of the amine group), allowing the remaining carbon skeleton to be used for the production of glucose or ketones to be used for energy. The removed amine group produces ammonia, a toxic compound, which is converted to urea in the liver and excreted as urine by the kidneys.

Amino Acids for Potential Energy (Fat)

If protein intake exceeds the need for synthesis and energy needs are met, then amino acids from dietary protein are deaminated and their carbon fragments may be stored as fat. Among Americans, protein and caloric intakes are typically well above requirements, allowing protein to contribute significantly to individuals' fat stores.[4]

PROTEIN IN FOODS

Dietary protein is the delivery vehicle for amino acids. Meats, fruits, vegetables, grains, dairy products, and even supplements supply us with the valuable building blocks of protein we need. If a food supplies all of the essential amino acids in appropriate ratios, it is called a *complete protein*. If a food source is low or lacking in one or more essential amino acid, it is called an *incomplete protein*. The essential amino acid that is missing or present in the smallest amount is called the *limiting factor* of

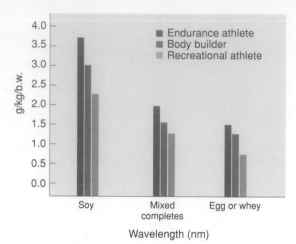

*The chart above illustrates the approximate amounts of different types of protein necessary to supply the ideal pattern of amino acids needed to satisfy the body's maintenance and growth needs. *Protein consumption beyond these amounts does not result in strength or size increases. When you exceed the amount of protein needed for growth, maintenance, or repair, your body will store it as fat or glycogen, use it for energy, or convert it to other nitrogenous compounds.

*Presuming total energy requirements are met through dietary carbohydrates and fat.

Figure 15.3   Adaptation-phase protein requirements.

that protein. Because the process of protein synthesis works on an all-or-none principle, all amino acids must be present at the site of protein manufacture, or synthesis will be reduced to the point where the cell runs out of the limiting amino acid.[12]

The ability of a protein to satisfy these essential amino acid requirements can be quantified in several ways. Terms used to rate dietary protein include protein efficiency ratio (PER), net protein utilization (NPU), and biologic value (BV).[8]

Biologic value (BV) is a measure frequently used when discussing protein sources in popular media and by supplement manufacturers. Essentially, BV is a measure of protein quality, or how well it satisfies the body's essential amino acid needs. A protein source with a higher score provides an amino acid profile that is more closely related to the needs of the human body. BV is a concept that is often misused, especially by marketers of protein supplements. One is led to believe that consuming specially prepared high-BV proteins will allow an individual who is already consuming adequate protein to build muscle to a greater degree, or more quickly. However, consuming protein above requirements will not force the body to unleash a previously untapped muscle-building capacity.[13,14] If, instead, one exclusively consumes very high BV proteins, his or her amino acid requirements would be met with less protein. Conversely, if one chooses a diet composed of mostly lower BV protein sources, the total protein requirements will increase (Figure 15-3).

FACTORS AFFECTING PROTEIN REQUIREMENTS

Exercise

Both anaerobic and aerobic exercise affect protein requirements in different ways. Exercise increases the oxidation of amino acids as well as the rate of protein turnover in lean body mass during recovery. Because different types of exercise have specific effects, an individual participating in both types of exercise may have a need for protein greater than someone involved in only one.[15,16]

Caloric Intake

Because protein can be used for tissue repair and synthesis as well as for energy, protein requirements will increase as total energy intake decreases.[17,18] As total caloric intake is reduced, energy needs may no longer be satisfied by carbohydrate and fat intake alone, necessitating that protein be used to provide energy. The goal is to satisfy the majority of energy needs with carbohydrate and fat, saving protein for tissue repair and growth. This is why carbohydrates are often referred to as protein sparing. If one does not eat adequate amounts of carbohydrate and fat (as is often seen in low-calorie or low-carbohydrate diets or during physique-competition preparation), more protein will be used for energy by default. Individuals interested in general fat loss or muscle hypertrophy have erroneously mimicked the acceptable use of a high-protein diet by a physique competitor. However, under the proper circumstances, these diets, when used temporarily, can be effective.

NEGATIVE ENERGY BALANCE

For clients pursuing body-fat reduction, body-fat loss goals require that a caloric deficit be maintained until the goal is reached. These individuals seek to modify their body composition. During a negative energy balance, amino acids are used to assist in energy production. This is called *gluconeogenesis*. Anaerobic or aerobic exercise depletes glycogen, increasing gluconeogenesis. The increase in gluconeogenesis is supported by the release of branched-chain and other amino acids from structural proteins to maintain glucose homeostasis during exercise.[19-22] The hypocaloric diet establishes less-than-optimal glycogen stores. When this is combined with increased glycogen demand during exercise, protein's energy utilization is increased.[23,24] The amount of lean body mass lost in persons in a negative energy balance can be reduced by increasing the amount of protein in the diet, leading to a more rapid return to nitrogen balance. A number of studies show that an increase in protein utilization during a hypocaloric diet will produce effects that can be exacerbated by exercise.[18,25-30]

PROTEIN AND THE BODYBUILDER

Bodybuilders during positive energy balance (off-season) should follow the same protein recommendations as strength athletes. However, during negative energy balance (used to create competition-level body-fat percentages), protein requirements may dramatically increase. To reach competitive body fat levels, calorie intake is continually lowered while exercise (such as cardiorespiratory, weight training, and posing) is increased.

Competitive levels of body fat are generally unhealthy and impossible to maintain for prolonged periods. Each component of this regimen may have additive effects on protein requirements. The body's survival mechanisms, related to increases in energy expenditure and decreases in food supply, are probably highly active during this period, forcing a continued reduction in food intake to achieve the goal.[31,32] However, because of its anabolic requirements, protein intake cannot be lowered. In fact, protein intake may have to be increased in the final weeks before competition. During this period, the body must have the option to use available food either for energy or muscle support. The body does not have a choice with dietary carbohydrate or fat, making them the only dispensable calories. Therefore, protein intake could be dramatically increased to theoretically lessen the obligatory loss of lean tissue during these drastic measures.[18-30]

It is quite common to see clients consuming the majority of their calories from protein in the final weeks before competition. However, during the off-season, athletes return to normal food intake (or protein at anabolic requirements and energy needs met primarily with carbohydrate and fats) and normal energy balance. This return to normal eating habits enables greater muscular gains than would be achieved by maintaining a high-protein intake year-round.[33-35] In fact, it appears that carbohydrate (1 g/kg), not protein, consumed within an hour after heavy resistance training inhibits muscle-protein breakdown, resulting in a positive protein balance.[36]

Protein's Effect on Satiety

In addition to the above factors, protein intake may be adjusted to aid in *satiety* (or feeling of fullness). Protein's role in satiety is an important consideration. As with all macronutrients, protein activates specific satiety mechanisms and may be more satiating than fat and carbohydrate. Protein-induced suppression of food intake in animals and humans is greater than its energy content alone. This suggests that protein has a direct effect on satiety.[37] In studies of rats and humans, a preload of protein suppressed their food intake for several hours and to a greater extent than a similar energy load of fat and carbohydrate.[38-42] Individuals seeking fat loss may benefit from the satiating properties of protein to feel full and energized throughout the day. This can assist clients in program adherence.[43,44]

PROTEIN-INTAKE RECOMMENDATIONS

The above factors can now be added to the Recommended Dietary Allowance (RDA) for protein (0.8 g/kg per day or 15 to 30% of total caloric intake), providing a range of protein recommendations for exercisers. Table 15-2 lists the appropriate recommendations for most athletes and exercisers.

The protein recommendations listed for adaptation periods are for anabolic, not necessarily total-metabolic, purposes (e.g., satiety, performance). These protein recommendations may range from 10 to 25% of total caloric intake. This not only allows for differences in goals and activity, but also for bioindividuality in terms of satiety and performance. Some people respond better to slightly higher or lower protein intakes, which may help with adherence to the amount of calories required to reach and maintain goals. Individuals eating lower amounts of protein may need supplementation. Whatever the percentage of protein ends up being, in relation to total caloric intake, the protein intake should still fall approximately within the above ranges of grams per kilogram. In other words, a small person losing fat (or hypocaloric) and exercising using strength and aerobic training may have a high percentage of protein (around 25%) but still fall in the appropriate range of absolute protein (1.2 to 2.0 g/kg per day).

Negative Side Effects Associated With Chronic Use of High-Protein Diets

For our purposes, a high-protein diet is defined as one that consists of more than 30% of total caloric intake from protein, or three times the protein RDA for athletes. Chronic consumption of a high-protein diet is generally associated with a higher intake of saturated fat and low fiber intake, both of which are risk factors for heart disease and some types of cancer.[45,46] Also, the kidneys are required to work harder to eliminate the increased urea produced.

Of genuine concern is the effect of high-protein diets on calcium status. For every gram of protein consumed above tissue maintenance, between 1 and 1.5 mg of calcium is excreted.[47-50] America's intake of calcium is notoriously poor. A high-

Table 15.2

Protein Recommendations (g/kg per day)

	Bodybuilder	Active Recreational Athlete	Endurance Athlete
Minimum acceptable intake	1.0	1.0	1.4
Adaptation period	1.6–2.0	1.2–1.8	1.6–2.0

protein diet, consumed by many sedentary Americans, certainly does not help in achieving calcium-intake goals.

In addition, the need for fluids is increased by high-protein intake. Protein requires approximately seven times the water for metabolism than carbohydrate or fat.[51] Low-carbohydrate consumption typically accompanies high-protein diets (especially for weight loss). This can lead to decreased glycogen stores, which inhibit performance and contribute to dehydration. Both of these situations will negatively affect athletic performance and overall functioning of the individual.

PROTEIN SUPPLEMENTATION

Because of protein's structure and function, protein supplementation may be the easiest to rationalize. However, in a healthy population, protein supplementation is difficult to defend, at least in its general use among athletes. The concept that "more is better" is the conventional thinking of many users of protein supplements, especially in the bodybuilding community.[52] Athletes tend to base their diet decisions on nutritional advice from their peers, nonscientific mentors, heroes, or idols, rather than the peer-reviewed, scientific literature.[53-56] No evidence has shown a constant, linear increase in muscle mass or performance related to protein intake. Thus, there is a physiologic threshold for incorporating dietary protein into fat-free mass (FFM), or for using protein as an immediate energy substrate.

Enhanced Recovery After Exercise

One defensible reason to ingest supplemental protein is to quickly get amino acids into the blood after exercise. Research has shown that the use of protein and carbohydrate supplements before and after weight training can enhance anabolic hormones compared with a nonsupplemented state.[57-59] Theoretically, this would enhance recovery, allowing the body to spend more time on building muscle rather than repair.[60-63]

Weight-Reduction Programs

Protein supplements replace whole-food proteins, eliminating unwanted calories to maintain equal or positive nitrogen balance during body-fat reduction for competitive cosmetic athletes.

Convenience

Protein supplements are used in situations when whole food is not available or is not an option (e.g., early-morning workouts).

Cost

Marketers often promote protein supplements as a lower cost-per-gram nitrogen source when compared with whole foods. In recent years, marketers have focused on building "the perfect protein." Their objective has been to enhance protein synthesis, as opposed to food protein or standard protein supplements.

Whey protein hydrolysates are the current protein-product "rage." Special processing of whey protein, which has the highest BV of any protein, yields small peptides that are absorbed faster into the enterocyte than free-form amino acids.[64] In addition, these special blends have been found to provide greater nitrogen retention and protein synthesis in starved animals, burn patients, and during enteral feeding of hospitalized patients when compared with other proteins.[65-68] The amino acid profile of whey protein (very high in branched-chain amino acids), combined with a manufacturing process that yields the ideal peptide lengths for rapid absorption, probably gives this special blend its benefits to injured, diseased, or starved recipients. The relevance of this to well-fed, healthy athletes is probably nonexistent. However, for bodybuilders, wrestlers, or other weight-conscious athletes preparing for competition (these athletes are generally underfed and overtrained at this point), these formulas offer a viable way to meet protein requirements with fewer calories.

The timing of available amino acids (before and after training), reduction of calories (while sparing nitrogen losses), convenience, and cost are all defensible benefits of protein supplements. On the other hand, if individuals meet their protein requirements (Table 15-1) and maintain desired body-fat levels, no substantial evidence exists that either using protein supplements to replace food or increasing protein intake above requirements will enhance performance or adult skeletal muscle hypertrophy.

REVIEW OF PROPERTIES OF PROTEIN

One gram of protein yields 4 calories. Protein must be broken down completely (into constituent amino acids) before it can be used.

Amino acids from protein are used by the body for the following:

- Synthesizing body-tissue protein
- Providing glucose for energy (many can be converted to glucose)
- Providing nitrogen in the form of amine groups to build nonessential amino acids
- Contributing to fat stores

Amino acids are not used to build protein under the following conditions:

- Not enough available energy from carbohydrate and fat
- Consistently low or lacking essential dietary amino acids owing to the exclusive consumption of incomplete proteins
- An excess of necessary protein

The following conditions are necessary for the body to synthesize endogenous protein:

- Availability of all essential and nonessential amino acids in proper amounts
- An adequate supply of exogenous protein (supplying amine groups, which synthesize the nonessential amino acids)
- Adequate energy-yielding carbohydrate and fat (sparing the protein)

Recommended protein intake for athletes and exercisers:

- 1 to 2.0 g/kg depending on goal, activity, protein source, and total caloric intake
- Typically falls in a range of 15 to 30% of total caloric intake

Chronic high-protein intake (greater than 2.5 times the RDA) diets can lead to:

- Calcium depletion
- Fluid imbalance
- Eventual hunger
- Slower metabolism
- Weight rebound
- Energy loss

SUMMARY

Protein primarily builds and repairs body tissues and structures. It also helps to synthesize hormones, enzymes, and other peptides, and can also be used for energy in diets lacking calories or carbohydrates.

Proteins are made up of about 20 essential and nonessential amino acids linked together by peptide bonds. Proteins must be broken down into the amino acids before the body can use them for its own purposes. The eight essential amino acids cannot be manufactured in the body. The remaining nonessentials are manufactured by the body from dietary nitrogen and fragments of carbohydrate and fat. Protein can be used by the body to create immediate energy or potential energy.

Dietary protein is the delivery vehicle for amino acids. One gram of protein yields 4 calories. Complete proteins supply all of the essential amino acids in appropriate ratios, whereas incomplete proteins are low or lacking in one or more essential amino acid. Biologic value (BV) is a measure of how well a protein satisfies the body's essential amino acid needs. One with a higher score is more closely related to the needs of the human body.

Protein requirements can be affected by anaerobic and aerobic exercise, total energy intake, caloric intake, and carbohydrate intake. During a negative energy balance (or caloric deficit), amino acids are used to assist in energy production (or gluconeogenesis), wherein protein requirements may dramatically increase. Protein intake may also be adjusted to aid in satiety in individuals seeking fat loss, who may benefit from protein by feeling full and energized throughout the day. The Recommended Dietary Allowance for protein is 0.8 g/kg per day, or 15 to 30% of total caloric intake. However, this may vary among athletes from 1.0 to 2.0 g/kg per day.

A high-protein diet consisting of more than 30% of total caloric intake from protein is associated with heart disease and some types of cancer (owing to a higher intake of saturated fat and low fiber intake), overworked kidneys (owing to elimination of the increased urea), inadequate calcium intake, and possible dehydration.

Protein supplementation is not typically recommended in general use among athletes. No substantial evidence exists that either using protein supplements to replace food or increasing protein intake above requirements will enhance performance or adult skeletal muscle hypertrophy. However, supplemental protein may be useful:

- To quickly get amino acids into the blood before and after weight training
- To replace whole-food proteins for weight loss
- In situations when whole food is not available
- For bodybuilders, wrestlers, or other weight-conscious athletes preparing for competition

Carbohydrates

THE STRUCTURE AND FUNCTION OF CARBOHYDRATES

Carbohydrates: Neutral compounds of carbon, hydrogen, and oxygen (such as sugars, starches, and celluloses), which make up a large portion of animal foods.

Carbohydrates are compounds containing carbon, hydrogen, and oxygen and are generally classified as sugars (simple), starches (complex), and fiber. The definition of sugar, as it would appear on a food label, is any monosaccharide or disaccharide.[69]

A *monosaccharide* is a single sugar unit, many of which are connected to make starches (the storage form of carbohydrates in plants) and glycogen (the storage form of carbohydrates in humans). Monosaccharides include glucose (commonly referred to as blood sugar), fructose (or fruit sugar), and galactose. *Disaccharides* (two sugar units) include sucrose (or common sugar), lactose (or milk sugar), and maltose.

Carbohydrates are a chief source of energy for all body functions and muscular exertion. This leads to a rapid depletion of available and stored carbohydrate and creates a continual craving for this macronutrient. Carbohydrates also help to regulate the digestion and utilization of protein and fat.[70,71]

DIGESTION, ABSORPTION, AND UTILIZATION

The principal carbohydrates present in food occur in the form of simple sugars, starches, and cellulose. Simple sugars, such as those in honey and fruits, are very easily digested. Double sugars, such as table sugar, require some digestive action but are not nearly as complex as starches, such as those found in whole grain. Starches require prolonged enzymatic action to be broken down into simple sugars (i.e., glucose) for utilization. Cellulose, commonly found in the skins of fruits and vegetables, is largely indigestible by humans and contributes little energy value to the diet. It does, however, provide the bulk necessary for intestinal motility and aids in elimination.[72,73]

The rate at which ingested carbohydrate raises blood sugar and its accompanying effect on insulin release is referred to as the *glycemic index* (GI). The GI for a food is determined when the particular food is consumed by itself and on an empty stomach. Mixed meals of protein, other carbohydrate, and fat can alter the glycemic effect of single foods.[74] Some fad diets place too much emphasis on the GI, stating that foods with a higher GI lead to fat storage, regardless of caloric intake. This leads to categorizing foods as "good" or "bad" based solely on their GI value. As stated earlier, weight gain or loss is related to total energy intake, not the source of the food eaten. However, as one can see in Table 15-3, foods lower on the glycemic index are good sources of complex carbohydrates, as well as being high in fiber and overall nutritional value.

Through the processes of digestion and absorption, all disaccharides and polysaccharides are ultimately converted into simple sugars such as glucose or fructose (Figure 15-4). However, fructose must be converted to glucose in the liver before it can be used for energy. Some of the glucose (or blood sugar) is used as fuel by tissues of the brain, nervous system, and muscles. Because humans are periodic eaters, a small portion of the glucose is converted to glycogen after a meal and stored within the liver and muscles. Any excess is converted to fat and stored throughout the body as a reserve source of energy. When total caloric intake exceeds output, any excess carbohydrate, dietary fat, or protein may be stored as body fat until energy expenditure once again exceeds energy input.

Table 15.3	
Glycemic Index of Select Foods	
Foods	**GI %**
Soy beans (fresh/canned), peanuts	10–19
Kidney beans, lentils, fructose	20–29
Milk (skim or whole), yogurt, tomato soup, ice cream, chickpeas, apples (Golden Delicious)	30–39
Spaghetti, sweet potato, navy beans (canned), dried peas, oranges, orange juice, porridge, oats	40–49
Sweet corn, All-Bran cereal, peas (frozen), sucrose, potato chips	50–59
Bread (white), rice (brown), muesli, bananas, raisins	60–69
Bread (whole wheat), millet, rice (white), potato	70–79
Corn Flakes, carrots, honey, potatoes (instant, mashed)	80–90
Glucose	100

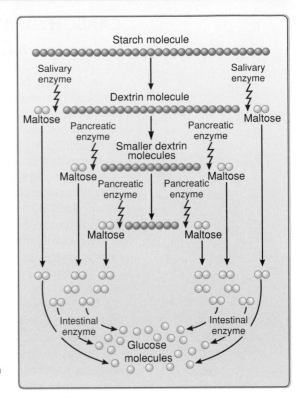

Figure 15.4 Gradual breakdown of large starch molecules by enzymes in digestion.

FIBER AND ITS ROLE IN HEALTH

One of the greatest contributions made by dietary complex carbohydrate is fiber. Higher intakes of dietary fiber are associated with lower incidence of heart disease and certain types of cancer.[75,76] Additional benefits of fiber include:[76-80]

- Provides bulk in the diet, thus increasing the satiety value of foods.
  - Some fibers also delay the emptying of the stomach, further increasing satiety.[81]
- Prevents constipation and establishes regular bowel movements.
- Maintains good intestinal motility.
  - Helps to retain the health and tone of the digestive tract muscles, therefore preventing diverticulosis, which causes the weakening of intestinal walls, then causing them to swell and distend.
- Aids in the prevention of bacterial infections of the appendix (or appendicitis).
- Helps to lower the risk of colon cancer.
- May reduce the risks of heart and artery disease by lowering blood cholesterol.
  - Certain soluble fibers bind with cholesterol compounds and are excreted from the body in the feces, lowering the body's cholesterol content.
  - Additionally, the substances produced by the bacteria's digestion of soluble fiber may help inhibit the production of cholesterol and eliminate cholesterol from the blood.
- Regulates the body's absorption of glucose (diabetics included) perhaps because fiber is believed to be capable of controlling the rate of digestion and assimilation of carbohydrates.
  - High-fiber meals have been shown to exert regulatory effects on blood glucose levels for up to 5 hours after eating.

CARBOHYDRATE AND PERFORMANCE

Carbohydrate availability is vital for maximal sports performance. When performing high-intensity, short-duration activity (anaerobic), muscular demand for energy is provided for and dependent on muscle glycogen. During endurance exercise (aerobic) performed at a moderate intensity (60% of maximal oxygen consumption [$\dot{V}O_2$ max]), muscle glycogen provides approximately 50% of energy needs. During high-intensity aerobic exercise (>79% of $\dot{V}O_2$ max), it yields nearly all of the energy needs.[82]

Duration of exercise also affects the amount of glycogen used for energy. As duration of activity increases, available glucose and glycogen diminish, increasing the reliance on fat as a fuel source. In addition, one could presume that if there is an appreciable increase in duration, there must also be a decrease in intensity, decreasing the use of glycogen.

However, this does not mean that the best way to lose body fat is to perform low-intensity activities for a long duration. If the workout contributes to a caloric deficit, the body will draw on its fat stores at some point to make up for the deficit.[83]

Ultimately, the limiting factor for exercise performance is carbohydrate availability: "Fat burns in a carbohydrate flame." That is to say, maximal fat utilization cannot occur without sufficient carbohydrate to continue Krebs cycle activity.[70,71] When an endurance athlete "hits the wall," it is the result of fatigue caused by severely lowered liver and muscle glycogen. This occurs even though there is sufficient oxygen being delivered to the muscles and an abundance of potential energy from fat stores.[84]

RECOMMENDATIONS

Endurance Exercise

The amount of carbohydrate in the diet can affect performance. High-carbohydrate diets increase the use of glycogen as fuel, whereas a high-fat diet increases the use of fat as fuel.[83] However, a high-fat diet results in lower glycogen synthesis.[85,86] This is of particular concern if the individual is consuming a reduced-energy diet.[87] For the endurance athlete, a carbohydrate-rich diet will build glycogen stores and aid in performance and recovery.[88,89] Although some studies show an increase in performance associated with the consumption of a high-fat diet, these improvements are seen in exercise performed at a relatively low intensity (less than 70% of $\dot{V}O_2$ max).[86,90] As the intensity of exercise increases, performance of high-intensity exercise will ultimately be impaired.[91-93]

A diet containing between 6 and 10 g/kg per day of carbohydrate, or approximately 60% of caloric intake, is recommended for individuals participating in endurance exercise. Complex carbohydrates (such as whole grains and fresh fruits and vegetables) should constitute the majority of calories because of their nutrient-dense (providing B vitamins, iron, and fiber) nature.

Before Exercise

It is recommended that the individual consume a high-carbohydrate meal 2 to 4 hours before exercising for more than an hour. This will allow time for appropriate gastric emptying before exercise. This is especially helpful for morning workouts when glycogen stores are lowered by as much as 80%.[83] If this is not feasible because of time constraints, a liquid meal such as a meal-replacement formula may be used. One advantage to such formulas is their quick gastric emptying time.

Some research recommends a carbohydrate intake of 1 to 4.5 g/kg, between 1 and 4 hours before exercise, respectively.[94] In this study, the group ingesting 4.5 g/kg of carbohydrate 4 hours before exercise saw performance improved by 15%.[94]

Table 15.4

Glycogen-Loading Schedule[a]

Days Before the Event	Exercise Intensity and Duration	Carbohydrate Intake
6 days out	70–75% of $\dot{V}O_2$ max, for 90 min	4 g/kg of body weight
4–5 days out	70–75% of $\dot{V}O_2$ max, for 40 min	4 g/kg of body weight
2–3 days out	70–75% of $\dot{V}O_2$ max, for 20 min	10 g/kg of body weight
1 day out	Rest	10 g/kg of body weight

[a]Athletes with diabetes or high triglycerides should consult a physician before using this plan. $\dot{V}O_2$ max, maximal oxygen consumption.

To avoid gastrointestinal distress, smaller meals should be consumed closer to the exercise session.

Carbohydrate Loading

In endurance exercise of greater than a 90-minute duration (e.g., marathon running), muscle-glycogen stores become depleted. This depletion limits the performance of endurance exercise. Carbohydrate loading, also called glycogen supercompensation, is a technique used to increase muscle glycogen before an endurance event. This practice can nearly double muscle glycogen stores, increasing endurance potential.[95]

Historically, the weeklong program includes 4 days of glycogen depletion (through a low-carbohydrate diet and exhaustive exercise), followed by 3 days of rest and a high-carbohydrate diet. This method had many drawbacks, including periods of hypoglycemia, irritability, increased susceptibility to injury, and difficulty in compliance. In 1981, one study proposed a revised method (Table 15-4) that accomplishes the same goal with greater ease of compliance and fewer side effects.[96]

During Exercise

For exercise lasting more than 1 hour, carbohydrate feedings during exercise can help supply glucose to working muscles whose glycogen stores are dwindling. This technique also maintains blood glucose levels, increasing time to exhaustion by 20 to 60 minutes.[97-100] It is recommended that endurance athletes consume between 30 and 60 g of carbohydrate every hour to accomplish this. Popular sports beverages are perfect for this goal and have the added benefit of replacing fluid losses, also benefiting performance. The replacement of carbohydrate and water has individual benefits that together are additive.

One study showed that performance during 1 hour of intense cycling was improved by 12% with the consumption of 1,330 mL (53 oz) of water containing 79 g of carbohydrate.[101] NASM concurs that consuming 600 to 1,200 mL (20 to 40 oz) per hour of fluid that contains between 4 and 8% carbohydrate will contribute to better performance for the endurance athlete.[100]

After Exercise

Repeated days of strenuous exercise take a toll on an individual's glycogen stores. A high-carbohydrate intake helps to replenish glycogen stores; however, the timing of carbohydrate ingestion can also be important to maximizing recovery. Consuming 1.5 g/kg of carbohydrate within 30 minutes of completing exercise is recommended to maximize glycogen replenishment.[102] Delaying carbohydrate intake by even 2 hours can decrease total muscle glycogen synthesis by 66%.[104] The postworkout environment may hasten glycogen repletion as a result of increased blood flow to the muscles and an increased sensitivity of the cells to the effects of insulin.[83] Additional meals of 1.5 g/kg of carbohydrate every 2 hours are recommended to completely restore muscle glycogen.[102]

For Altering Body Composition

Carbohydrate should generally make up the highest percentage of macronutrient calories when one is attempting fat loss or muscle gain. Carbohydrates provide variety, valuable nutrients, and volume to the diet. The satiating value of complex carbohydrate is especially important when one is in a caloric deficit for the goal of fat loss.[104-106] For most moderately active adults, a carbohydrate intake of between 50 and 70% is recommended. This will provide sufficient food volume and the fuel necessary for energy and productive workouts.

Despite the popularity of low-carbohydrate diets and the perpetuation of erroneous claims regarding type or time of carbohydrate intake, there is no need for one to reduce carbohydrate percentage to lose fat (see Carbohydrate and Weight Gain section). Weight loss or gain is related to total caloric intake, not the macronutrient profile of the diet. The weight lost on a low-carbohydrate diet can be attributed to two factors: low caloric intake and loss of fat-free mass (FFM).[107] When one begins dropping carbohydrate-rich foods from their diet, it is inevitable that caloric intake is reduced. Added to the caloric reduction are dwindling glycogen stores. For every gram of glucose taken out of glycogen, it brings with it 2.7 g of water.[108] This loss of muscle glycogen (including water) can be quite significant in the first week of a low-carbohydrate diet, and adds to the pounds lost on the scale. This is how low-carbohydrate fad diets can promise dramatic weight loss in such a short period. Long-term success in weight loss is associated with a realistic eating style, not one that severely limits or omits one of the macronutrients.[109]

CARBOHYDRATE AND WEIGHT GAIN: THE FACTS

A significant amount of time, energy, and resources are spent investigating the link between carbohydrate intake and the increased prevalence of obesity in Americans. The accusations are familiar: "carbohydrates make you fat;" "Americans are getting fatter, despite lower fat intakes."

Data available from the Third National Health and Nutrition Examination Survey (NHANES III), which catalogs Americans' nutrition patterns for the years 1988 through 1991, shows that percentage of calories consumed from fat has indeed dropped, from 36% (NHANES II 1976–1980) to 34% of total energy intake.[110] However, when total fat intake (grams per person per day) is measured, and not simply the percentage contributed, the data show that fat intake has remained quite constant for the past several years.[111] Additionally these data may not accurately reflect fat consumption in America, as many people underreport fat consumption owing to its negative health connotations.[69] The data from NHANES III also show an increase in total energy intake. This would support the relationship between excessive energy intake, leading to increased fat stores.

When reviewing the data on Americans' food intake, it is interesting to note that in the early 1900s, the percentage of carbohydrates consumed as energy intake was higher and consumption of fat lower than it is today, without the prevalence of obesity we now experience.[112] Only during the last two decades has there been a significant increase in obesity. The data support two primary variables responsible for this dramatic rise in obesity: an increased energy intake and a reduction in energy expenditure.[110,113] Data published in 1996 by the U.S. Department of Health and Human Services showed that 60% of American adults are not regularly active and that 25% participate in no physical activity at all.[113]

In summary, at the turn of the century, carbohydrate intake as a percentage of total energy was higher, fat as a percentage was lower, and obesity was not the problem it is today. Currently, total fat intake is higher, carbohydrate is lower, and obesity has reached epidemic proportions.[114] In addition, energy intake has increased and energy expenditure has decreased. The facts are very clear: America's increasing problem of obesity is not a direct result of carbohydrate intake, but rather of energy imbalance.

REVIEW OF THE PROPERTIES OF CARBOHYDRATES

One gram of carbohydrate yields 4 calories.

Carbohydrates provide the body with:

- Nutrition that fat and protein cannot (from complex carbohydrates)
- Satiety by keeping glycogen stores full and adding bulk to the diet
- Proper cellular fluid balance, maximizing cellular efficiency
- Proper blood sugar levels, if there is a consistent intake of low-glycemic carbohydrates
- Spare protein for building muscle

The body needs carbohydrates because:

- They are the perfect and preferred form of energy
- They constantly need to be replaced, causing a craving that must be satisfied
- Parts of the central nervous system rely exclusively on carbohydrate
- They efficiently burn and use fat and protein

Recommended carbohydrate intake:

- Daily diet should include 25 g of fiber.
- Carbohydrate intake typically should be between 50 and 70% of total caloric intake according to preference, performance, and satiety.
- Carbohydrate recommendations should be estimated after protein and fat requirements are met.
- Fruits, whole grains, and vegetables are all excellent sources of fiber.

SUMMARY

Carbohydrates are a chief source of energy for all body functions and muscular exertion. They are compounds containing carbon, hydrogen, and oxygen and are generally classified as sugars (simple), starches (complex), and fiber. A monosaccharide is a single sugar unit (such as glucose, fructose, or galactose), many of which are connected to make starches and glycogen. Disaccharides (two sugar units) include sucrose, lactose, and maltose. Carbohydrates help to regulate the digestion and utilization of protein and fat.

Glycemic index (GI) is the rate at which ingested carbohydrate raises blood sugar and affects insulin release. Foods lower on the glycemic index are good sources of complex carbohydrates, as well as being high in fiber and overall nutritional value. When total caloric intake exceeds output, any excess carbohydrate, dietary fat, or protein may be stored as body fat until needed.

Fiber is one of the greatest contributions made by dietary complex carbohydrate. Higher intakes of dietary fiber are associated with lower incidence of heart disease and certain types of cancer. In addition, fiber provides many other benefits including satiety, intestinal health, and regulation of the body's absorption of glucose.

The availability of carbohydrate is vital for maximal sports performance because the demand for energy is provided for and dependent on muscle glycogen. Duration and intensity of exercise affects the amount of glycogen used for energy. Maximal fat utilization cannot occur without sufficient carbohydrate. For the endurance athlete, a daily carbohydrate-rich diet (containing between 6 and 10 g/kg per day of carbohydrate, or approximately 60% of caloric intake) will build glycogen stores and aid in performance and recovery. It is recommended that the individual consume a high-carbohydrate meal 2 to 4 hours before exercising for more than an hour. In endurance exercise of greater than a 90-minute duration, carbohydrate loading can be used to increase muscle glycogen before an endurance event. For exercise lasting more than 1 hour, endurance athletes should consume between 30 and 60 g of carbohydrate every hour (which may consist of sports beverages). After exercise, consuming 1.5 g/kg of carbohydrate within 30 minutes is recommended. Additional meals of 1.5 g/kg of carbohydrate every 2 hours are recommended to completely restore muscle glycogen.

For fat loss or muscle gain, carbohydrates should generally make up the highest percentage of macronutrient calories. An intake between 50 and 70% is recommended. There is no need for one to reduce carbohydrate percentage to lose fat. America's increasing problem of obesity is not a direct result of carbohydrate intake, but rather one of energy imbalance.

Lipids

THE STRUCTURE OF LIPIDS

Lipids: A group of compounds that includes triglycerides (fats and oils), phospholipids, and sterols.

Lipids are a group of compounds that include *triglycerides* (fats and oils), *phospholipids,* and *sterols*. Of the lipids contained in food, 95% are fats and oils. In the body, 99% of the stored lipids are also triglycerides.[115] Structurally, triglycerides are three fatty acids attached to a glycerol backbone (Figure 15-5).

Fatty Acids

These fatty acids may be *saturated* or *unsaturated* (Figure 15-6). Unsaturated fatty acids may be further classified according to their degree of unsaturation. If the fatty acid has one double bond in its carbon chain, it is called a *monounsaturated* fatty acid. If there is more than one point of unsaturation, it is classified as a *polyunsaturated* fatty acid.

Polyunsaturated fatty acids provide important essential fatty acids (or fats that cannot be manufactured by the body but are essential for proper health and functioning).[116]

Saturated fatty acids are implicated as a risk factor for heart disease because they raise bad cholesterol levels (LDL), whereas unsaturated fats are associated with increases in good cholesterol (HDL) and decreased risk of heart disease.[117,118]

Monounsaturated fatty acids (found in olive and canola oils) and polyunsaturated fatty acids such as omega-3 fatty acids (found in cold-water fish, such as

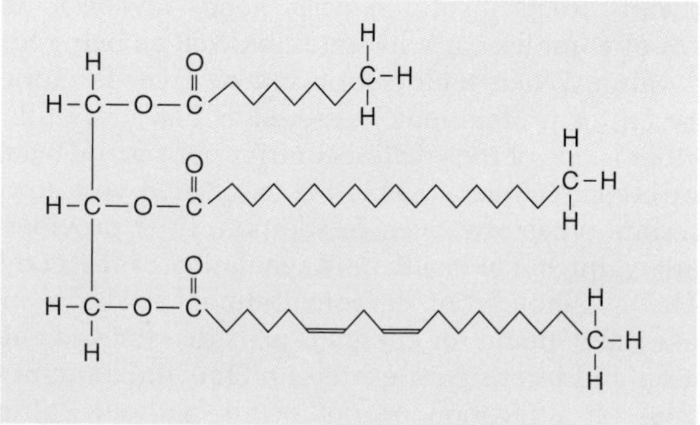

Figure 15.5 The triglyceride.

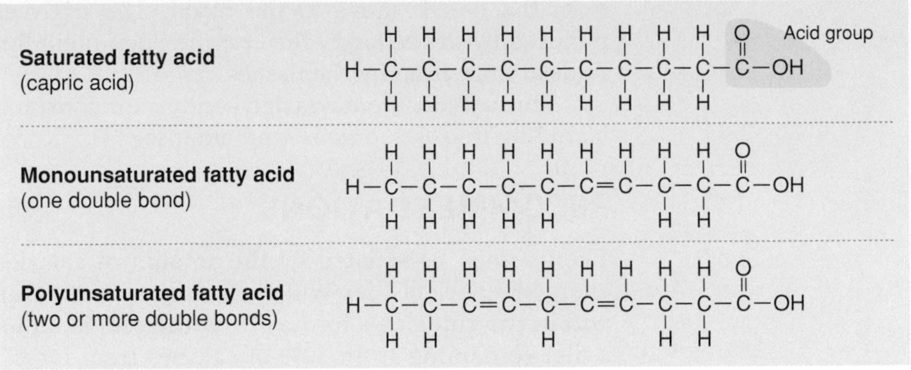

Figure 15.6 Fatty acids.

salmon) are considered to have favorable effects on blood lipid profiles and may play a role in the treatment and prevention of heart disease, hypertension, arthritis, and cancer.[117,118]

Another prevalent fatty acid in today's food supply is trans-fatty acids, the result of *hydrogenation* (or the process of adding hydrogen to unsaturated fatty acids to make them harder at room temperature and increase food shelf-life). Trans-fatty acids have been shown to increase LDL cholesterol and decrease HDL cholesterol, much like saturated fats.[119-121]

THE FUNCTION OF LIPIDS

Lipids (or fats) are the most concentrated source of energy in the diet. One gram of fat yields approximately 9 calories when oxidized, furnishing more than twice the calories per gram of carbohydrates or proteins. In addition to providing energy, fats act as carriers for the fat-soluble vitamins A, D, E, and K. Vitamin D aids in the absorption of calcium, making it available to body tissues, particularly to the bones and teeth. Fats are also important for the conversion of carotene to vitamin A.[122] Fats are involved in the following:[122]

- Cellular membrane structure and function
- Precursors to hormones
- Cellular signals
- Regulation and excretion of nutrients in the cells
- Surrounding, protecting, and holding in place organs, such as the kidneys, heart, and liver
- Insulating the body from environmental temperature changes and preserving body heat
- Prolonging the digestive process by slowing the stomach's secretions of hydrochloric acid, creating a longer-lasting sensation of fullness after a meal
- Initiating the release of the hormone cholecystokinin (CCK), which contributes to satiety

DIGESTION, ABSORPTION, AND UTILIZATION

Digestion of dietary fat starts in the mouth, moves to the stomach, and is completed in the small intestine. In the intestine, the fat interacts with bile to become emulsified so that pancreatic enzymes can break the triglycerides down into two fatty acids and a monoglyceride.

Absorption of these constituents occurs through the intestinal wall into the blood. In the intestinal wall, they are reassembled into triglycerides that are then released into the lymph in the form of a lipoprotein called *chylomicron*. Chylomicrons from the lymph move to the blood. The triglyceride content of chylomicron is removed by the action of the enzyme lipoprotein lipase (LPL), and the released fatty acids are taken up by the tissues.

Throughout the day, triglycerides are constantly cycled in and out of tissues, including muscles, organs, and adipose.

RECOMMENDATIONS

Clients must be satiated by the amount of calories necessary to allow fat loss or energy balance or they will eventually overeat. Our goal is to keep the client's diet within the guidelines for health. If the goal is fat loss or to enhance overall health, a diet containing 10 to 30% of calories from fat is recommended. Higher-fat diets are not conducive to successful weight loss or maintenance and appear to increase the ease with which the body converts ingested calories to body fat.[123-125]

Fat has a lower *thermic effect* than other macronutrients.[126] The thermic effect of a food (TEF) is the rise in metabolic rate that occurs after the food is ingested. Typically, TEF amounts to 10% of ingested calories.[116] As fat percentage in the diet increases, the amount of heat given off (TEF) decreases. Conversely, as carbohydrate percentage in the diet increases, so does the TEF. It is metabolically inexpensive to convert dietary fat to body-fat stores. Only 3% of the calories in fat are required to store it as fat. In contrast, it takes 23% of the calories in carbohydrate to convert it to body fat.[126]

Fat and Satiety

Dietary fats stimulate the release of CCK, a hormone that signals satiety. Additionally, fats slow the digestion of foods (and thus the nutrient content in the bloodstream), assisting in blood sugar stabilization. Reducing blood sugar fluctuations can contribute to satiety.

However, diets containing more than 30% of calories from fat lose the volume of food provided by higher-carbohydrate diets. In other words, both a tablespoon of oil and a large salad with nonfat dressing may contain the same amount of calories.

Because satiety is achieved by more than just total caloric intake, this low-volume, high-calorie contribution of fat may not satisfy other peripheral satiation mechanisms (chewing, swallowing, stomach distention), leading to *hyperphagia* (or overeating).[127]

FAT SUPPLEMENTATION DURING EXERCISE

In general, fat is digested and absorbed quite slowly. Long-chain triglycerides (LCT), which make up the majority of dietary fatty acids (16 to 18 carbons), must go through the process of digestion and absorption described earlier. Medium-chain triglycerides (MCT), however, are more rapidly absorbed. Additionally, they do not require incorporation into chylomicrons for transport, but can enter the systemic circulation directly through the portal vein, providing a readily available, concentrated source of energy.[128] It has been suggested that MCT could benefit endurance performance by supplying an exogenous energy source in addition to carbohydrate during exercise and increase plasma free fatty acids (FFA), sparing muscle glycogen.[129,130] Currently, there is insufficient evidence to recommend MCT supplementation for the goal of improving endurance exercise.

INSULIN RESISTANCE AND OBESITY

Proponents of high-protein, low-carbohydrate diets have profited from the erroneous assertion that carbohydrates are to blame for the increasing prevalence of metabolic syndrome (MS, or syndrome X) and therefore lead to weight gain. Metabolic syndrome is a cluster of symptoms characterized by obesity, insulin resistance, hypertension, and dyslipidemia, leading to an increased risk of cardio-vascular disease. Syndrome X is usually associated with obesity (especially abdominal), a high-fat diet, and a sedentary lifestyle.[131-134]

A common denominator associated with these factors is high levels of circulating free fatty acids (FFA). In the presence of high FFA concentrations, the body will favor their use as energy, decreasing glucose oxidation and glycogen synthesis and inhibiting glucose transport.[131] The result of this is hyperglycemia. When blood sugar levels are chronically high, insulin will also be elevated, leading to the conversion of the excess blood sugar to other products such as glyco proteins and fatty acids.

These facts alone seem to bolster the idea that carbohydrates lead to health problems. The truth is that a healthy person would need to eat an extremely high percentage of simple carbohydrates (such as sucrose) and fat, maintain a constant energy excess, or be overweight to have chronically elevated blood sugar. Although there is some evidence that there may be a genetic component that contributes to insulin resistance (IR), the condition itself will not allow for weight gain without an energy intake in excess of expenditure.[5,135,136] In fact, obesity itself is a risk factor for development of IR, not the other way around.[137]

So, what is the common cause of IR? If one constantly overeats, excess calories are stored as fat. Fat cells then increase in size. The growing fat cell itself becomes insulin resistant, and the resulting prevalence of FFA will cause the body to favor the use of fat for energy at the expense of glucose.[138] This becomes a vicious cycle.

The overweight condition leads to IR, which in turn leads to impaired glucose use. Blood sugar levels rise; insulin levels rise; and cholesterol, TG, and blood pressure rise as well. To make matters worse, the impaired ability of glucose to enter muscle cells keeps glycogen stores lower, which can increase appetite, motivating the individual to eat more, increasing fat stores, exacerbating IR, and so on.

As numerous studies point out, high-fat diets are strongly associated with obesity, thus insulin resistance and diabetes.[138-140] Of course, eating fat does not make one fat (the same applies to carbohydrate) unless it is consumed in excess of energy requirements. However, it is easier to consume excess energy (or hyperphagia) on a high-fat diet, owing to fat's high caloric density. When this high intake of dietary fat is combined with excess calories and a sedentary lifestyle, it is easy to envision an abundance of fatty acids floating around in the bloodstream.

It is much more likely that a high-fat diet leads to excess consumption of calories, obesity, IR, and eventually non–insulin-dependent diabetes mellitus than it is that carbohydrates cause IR and, as a result, obesity. The only solution is a diet containing the appropriate amount of energy, high in fibrous or starchy carbohydrates, and exercise. In fact, a study of type 2 diabetics, those with IR, and people of normal weight found that 3 weeks of a high-carbohydrate, low-fat diet and exercise program significantly lowered insulin levels.[141]

Perhaps it is convenient to place blame on carbohydrates. With obesity continuing to rise, a simple solution to the problem of America's weight gain would be welcomed. Our current environment has created a Petri dish that encourages the growth of the human organism. Highly palatable and caloric-rich food is available to most, and today's work and recreational demands do not call for much physical movement.

On the surface, the cure for obesity is simple: move more and eat less. However, the influence of societal, psychological, and physiologic factors can make putting this simple plan into action very difficult. Be that as it may, any solution will ultimately provide a way to increase energy expenditure, decrease energy consumption, or a combination of both.

REVIEW OF THE PROPERTIES OF LIPIDS

One gram of fat yields 9 calories. Fat is generally insoluble in water. Fat is present in all cells: high in adipose and nerve tissue, low in epithelial and muscle tissue. Fatty acids can be saturated, polyunsaturated, and monounsaturated.

The body needs fats for:
- Energy
- Structure and membrane function
- Precursors to hormones
- Cellular signals
- Regulation of uptake and excretion of nutrients in the cells

Recommended fat intake:
- Fat intake can range from 10 to 30%, according to performance, satiety, and palatability.
- A high polyunsaturated-to-saturated fat ratio is desirable.
- The average American's fat consumption is between 32 and 42% of total caloric intake.
- More than 30% leads to overeating (lack of food volume) and often slows metabolism.

SUMMARY

Lipids are a group of compounds that include triglycerides (fats and oils), phospholipids, and sterols. Most lipids in food and in the body are triglycerides, which are three fatty acids (saturated or unsaturated) attached to a glycerol backbone. Polyunsaturated fatty acids provide important essential fatty acids. Saturated fatty acids and trans-fatty acids are implicated as a risk factor for heart disease because they raise bad cholesterol levels (LDL), whereas unsaturated fats are associated with increases in good cholesterol (HDL) and decreased risk of heart disease.

Lipids are the most concentrated source of energy in the diet. One gram of fat yields approximately 9 calories. Lipids also regulate and excrete nutrients and act as carriers for vitamins A, D (which aids in the absorption of calcium), E, and K. Fats have many other benefits including cellular membrane structure and function, body insulation, aid in the digestive process, and satiety.

Digestion of dietary fat starts in the mouth, moves to the stomach, and is completed in the small intestine. Throughout the day, triglycerides are constantly cycled in and out of tissues.

A diet containing 10 to 30% of calories from fat is recommended for fat loss or to enhance overall health. Fat has a lower thermic effect than other macronutrients, only taking 3% of its calories to store it in the body as fat. Fat is digested and absorbed quite slowly. Thus, medium-chain triglycerides are not recommended as supplements for the goal of improving endurance exercise.

Metabolic syndrome is a cluster of symptoms characterized by obesity and insulin resistance. However, insulin resistance alone will not allow for weight gain without an energy intake in excess of expenditure. Obesity itself is a risk factor for development of insulin resistance, not the other way around.

Water

On average, an individual should consume approximately 96 ounces (3 quarts) of water per day. Those participating in a fat-loss program should drink an additional 8 ounces of water for every 25 pounds they carry above their ideal weight. Water intake should also be increased if an individual is exercising briskly or residing in a hot climate.

THE IMPORTANCE OF WATER

Water is the soup of life. It constitutes approximately 60% of the adult human body by weight. Whereas deficiencies of nutrients such as the macronutrients, vitamins, and minerals may take weeks or even years to develop, one can only survive for a few days without water. Consuming an adequate amount of water will benefit the body in the following ways:[142]

- Endocrine gland function improves.
- Fluid retention is alleviated.
- Liver functions improve, increasing the percentage of fat used for energy.
- Natural thirst returns.
- Appetite decreases significantly.
- Metabolic functions improve.
- Nutrients are distributed throughout the body.
- Body-temperature regulation improves.
- Blood volume is maintained.

WATER AND PERFORMANCE

The importance of proper hydration cannot be stressed enough. The body cannot adapt to dehydration, which impairs every physiologic function. Table 15-5 shows the effects of dehydration.

Studies have shown that a fluid loss of even 2% of body weight will adversely affect circulatory functions and decrease performance levels.[143] However, if a fairly regular daily pattern of exercise and water and food consumption is followed, average body weight will provide a very good index of the body's state of hydration. Realizing this, the organizers of certain ultradistance running events make it mandatory for competitors to weigh themselves at stations along the course and require each runner to consume enough fluid to regain a predetermined body weight before being allowed to continue.

Thirst alone is a poor indicator of how much water is needed. Athletes consistently consume inadequate fluid volume, managing to replace approximately 50% of sweat losses.[144] A good way to keep track of how much one needs to drink is to first determine his or her average daily weight (e.g., weight on waking). Use this number as the standard for the person's *euhydrated* (or normal) state. Do not begin a practice session or endurance competition until the body is at, or slightly above, its standard weight. Drink enough water, juice, or sports drinks during exercise to maintain the starting weight.

Guidelines for fluid replacement in the athlete are as follows:[145,146]

- Consume 16 oz of fluid 2 hours before exercise. An additional 8 to 16 oz may be needed if exercising in warmer weather.

Table 15.5	
Effects of Dehydration	
Decreased blood volume	Increased heart rate
Decreased performance	Sodium retention
Decreased blood pressure	Decreased cardiac output
Decreased sweat rate	Decreased blood flow to the skin
Increased core temperature	Increased perceived exertion
Water retention	Increased use of muscle glycogen

- Drink 20 to 40 oz of fluid for every hour of exercise.
- Fluids should be cold because of more rapid gastric emptying.
- If exercise exceeds 60 minutes, use of a sports drink (containing up to 8% carbohydrate) can replace both fluid and dwindling muscle glycogen stores.
- When exercising for less than 60 minutes, water is the experts' choice for fluid replacement.
- The goal is to replace sweat and urine losses.
- Ingest 20 oz of fluid for every pound of body weight lost after an exercise bout, especially if rapid rehydration is necessary, as in twice-a-day training.

SUMMARY

On average, an individual should consume approximately 96 ounces (3 quarts) of water per day. Those on fat-loss programs should drink an additional 8 ounces of water for every 25 pounds carried above ideal weight. Water intake should also be increased if an individual is exercising briskly or residing in a hot climate. The body cannot adapt to dehydration, which impairs every physiologic function. A fluid loss of even 2% of body weight will adversely affect circulatory functions and decrease performance levels.

Consuming an adequate amount of water will improve body temperature regulation, metabolic function, and endocrine gland and liver function. In addition, nutrients are distributed throughout the body, blood volume is maintained, fluid retention is alleviated, and appetite decreases significantly.

Thirst alone is a poor indicator of how much water is needed. Instead, determine average daily weight and use this number as the standard for a euhydrated state. Consume 16 oz of fluid 2 hours before exercise and drink 20 to 40 oz of fluid for every hour of exercise. Finally, ingest 20 oz of fluid for every pound of body weight lost after an exercise bout.

Altering Body Composition[147]

BASIC NUTRITION GUIDELINES FOR ALTERING BODY COMPOSITION

For Fat Loss

- Distribute protein, carbohydrate, and fat throughout the day and at each meal.
- Choose whole grains and fresh vegetables over refined grains and simple sugars (as the fiber and complexity of the starch will aid in hunger control).
- Schedule no fewer than four and as many as six meals a day. This helps to control hunger, minimize blood sugar fluctuations, and increase energy levels throughout the day.
- Avoid empty calories and highly processed foods, which contain many calories and do little to provide satiety.
- Drink a lot of water (8 to 12 cups per day).
- Have clients weigh and measure food for at least 1 week. This will make them more aware of caloric values and serving sizes, as well as decrease the likelihood of underreporting calories.

For Lean Body Mass Gain

- Eat four to six meals a day. Insulin response to a meal stimulates protein synthesis.

- Spread protein intake throughout the day to take advantage of the previous tip.
- Keep in mind the postworkout window of opportunity. Ingestion of protein and carbohydrate within 90 minutes of a workout will increase recovery and protein synthesis, maximizing gains. This may be most easily accomplished with a liquid meal-replacement formula that can be absorbed quickly owing to being predigested. Food may take several hours to digest and absorb, missing the window.
- Do not neglect the importance of carbohydrate and fat. It takes more than protein to increase lean body mass.

Review Questions

1 *Which kind(s) of fatty acids is considered to have favorable effects on blood lipid profiles and may play a role in the treatment and prevention of heart disease, hypertension, arthritis, and cancer?*

a. Monounsaturated fatty acid

b. Polyunsaturated fatty acid

c. Trans-fatty acid

2 *The _____ _____ of a food is the rise in metabolic rate that occurs after the food is ingested.*

3 *A study of type 2 diabetics (with insulin resistance) and people of normal weight found that 3 weeks of a high-carbohydrate, low-fat diet and exercise program significantly lowered insulin levels.*

a. True

b. False

4 *Water constitutes approximately what percentage of the adult human body by weight?*

5 *When exercising for less than 60 minutes, water is the experts' choice for fluid replacement.*

a. True

b. False

6 *Recommended protein intake for athletes and exercisers is:*

a. 5–20% of total caloric intake

b. 15–30% of total caloric intake

c. 30–45% of total caloric intake

7 *Recommended carbohydrate intake for adults is _____ of total caloric intake, according to preference, performance, and satlety.*

a. 10–30%

b. 30–50%

c. 50–70%

> **8** *Foods with a higher glycemic index lead to fat storage regardless of caloric intake.*
>
> *a. True*
>
> *b. False*

REFERENCES

1. Webster's Ninth New Collegiate Dictionary. Springfield, MA: Merriam-Webster Inc, 1991.
2. [Anonymous] Clinical guidelines on the identification, evaluation, and treatment of overweight and obesity in adults—the evidence report. National Institutes of Health. Obesity Res 1998;6(Suppl 2):51S–209S.
3. Walsh MF, Flynn TJ. A 54-month evaluation of a popular very low calorie diet program. J Fam Pract 1995;41(3):231–236.
4. Position of the American Dietetic Association: weight management. J Am Diet Assoc 1997; 97(1):71–74.
5. Faires VM. Thermodynamics. New York: Macmillan Company, 1967.
6. Jensen MD. Diet effects on fatty acid metabolism in lean and obese humans. Am J Clin Nutr 1998;67(3 Suppl):531S–534S.
7. Agricultural Research Service. Fat intake continues to drop; veggies, fruits still low in the US diet. Res News 1996.
8. Shils ME, Young VR. Modern Nutrition in Health and Disease, 7th ed. Philadelphia: Lea & Febiger, 1988.
9. Rose WC, Haines WJ, Warner DT. The amino acid requirements of man. V. The role of lysine, arginine, and tryptophan. J Biol Chem 1954;206:421–430.
10. Martineau A, Lecavalier L, Falardeau P, Chiasson,JL. Simultaneous determination of glucose turnover, and gluconeogenesis in humans using a double stable-isotope-labeled tracer infusion and gas chromatography-mass spectrometry analysis. Anal Biochem 1985;151(2):495–503.
11. Berdanier CD. Advanced Nutrition: Macronutrients. Boca Raton, FL: CRC Press, 1995.
12. Block RJ, Mitchell HH. Nutr Abstr Rev 1946;16:249–278.
13. Tarnopolsky MA, Atkinson SA, MacDougall JD, Chesley A, Phillip S, Schwarcz HP. Evaluation of protein requirements for trained strength athletes. J Appl Physiol 1992;73(5):1986–1995.
14. Lemon PW, Tarnolpolsky MA, MacDougall JD, Atkinson SA. Protein requirements and muscle mass/strength changes during intensive training in novice bodybuilders. J Appl Physiol 1992;73(2):767–775.
15. Keul J. The relationship between circulation and metabolism during exercise. Med Sci Sports 1973;5:209.
16. Keul J, Doll E, Keppler D. Energy Metabolism of Human Muscle. Baltimore: University Park, 1972.
17. Wahlberg JL, Leidy MK, Sturgill DJ, Hinkle DE, Ritchey SJ, Sebolt DR. Macronutrient content of a hypoenergy diet affects nitrogen retention and muscle function in weight lifters. Int J Sports Med 1988;9(4):261–266.
18. Piatti PM, Monti F, Fermo I, Baruffaldi L, Nasser R, Santambrogio G, Librenti MC, Galli-Kienle M, Pontiroli AE, Pozza G. Hypocaloric high-protein diet improves glucose oxidation and spares lean body mass: comparison to hypocaloric high-carbohydrate diet. Metabolism 1994;43(12):1481–1487.
19. Ruderman NB. Muscle amino acid metabolism and gluconeogenesis. Ann Rev Med 1975; 26:245–258.
20. Harper AE, Miller RH, Block KP. Branched-chain amino acid metabolism. Ann Rev Nutr 1984;4: 409–454.
21. Hood DA, Terjung RL. Amino acid metabolism during exercise and following endurance training. Sports Med 1990;9(1):23–35.
22. Ahlborg G, Felig P, Hagenfeldt L, Hendler R, Wahren J. Substrate turnover during prolonged exercise in man. Splanchnic and leg metabolism of glucose, free fatty acids, and amino acids. J Clin Invest 1974;53(4):1080–1090.
23. Lemon PW, Mullin JP. Effect of initial muscle glycogen levels on protein catabolism during exercise. J Appl Physiol 1980;48(4):624–629.
24. White TP, Brooks GA. [U-14C]glucose, -alanine, and -leucine oxidation in rats at rest and two intensities of running. Am J Physiol 1981;240(2):E155–E165.
25. Knapik J, Meredith C, Jones B, Fielding R, Young V, Evans W. Leucine metabolism during fasting and exercise. J Appl Physiol 1991;70(1):43–47.
26. Youn VR. Metabolic and nutritional aspects of physical exercise. Fed Proc 1985;44:341.
27. Allison JB, Bird JC. Elimination of nitrogen from the body. In: Munro HN, Allison JB (eds). Mammalian Protein Metabolism, Vol 1. New York: Academic Press, 1964.
28. Munro HN. Historical introduction: the origin and growth of our present concepts of protein metabolism. In: Munro HN, Allison JB (eds). Mammalian Protein Metabolism, Vol 1. New York: Academic Press, 1964.

29. Waterlow JC, Garlick PJ, Millward DJ. Protein Turnover in Mammalian Tissues and in the Whole Body. New York: North-Holland, 1978.

30. Kurzer MS, Calloway DH. Nitrate and nitrogen balances in men. Am J Clin Nutr 1981; 34(7):1305–1313.

31. Minghelli G, Schutz Y, Charbonnier A, Whitehead R, Jequier E. Twenty-four-hour energy expenditure and basal metabolic rate measured in a whole-body indirect calorimeter in Gambian men. Am J Clin Nutr 1990;51(4):563–570.

32. Spruce N. Plateaus and energy expenditure. Increased difficulty in attending fat or weight loss goals in healthy subjects. J Natl Intramural Recreat Sports Assoc 1997;22(1):24–28.

33. Spiller GA, Jensen CD, Pattison TS, Chuck CS, Whittam JH, Scala J. Effect of protein dose on serum glucose and insulin response to sugars. Am J Clin Nutr 1987;46(3):474–480.

34. Zawadzki KM, Yaspelkis BB 3rd, Ivy JL. Carbohydrate-protein complex increases the rate of muscle glycogen storage after exercise. J Appl Physiol 1992;72(5):1854–1859.

35. Roy BD, Tarnopolsky MA. Influence of differing macronutrient intakes on muscle glycogen resynthesis after resistance exercise. J Appl Physiol 1998;84(3):890–896.

36. Roy B, Tarnopolsky M, MacDougall J, Fowles J, Yarasheski K. Effect of glucose supplement timing on protein metabolism after resistance training. J Appl Physiol 1997;82(6):1882–1888.

37. Anderson GH, Li ET, Glanville NT. Brain mechanisms and the quantitative and qualitative aspects of food intake. Brain Res Bull 1984;12(2):167–173.

38. Gellebter AA. Effects of equicaloric loads of protein, fat and carbohydrate on food intake in the rat and man. Physiol Behav 1979;22:267–273.

39. Van Zeggeren A, Li ET. Food intake and choice in lean and obese Zucker rats after intragastric carbohydrate preloads. J Nutr 1990;120(3):309–316.

40. Li ET, Anderson GH. Meal composition influences subsequent food selection in the young rat. Physiol Behav 1982;29(5):779–783.

41. Booth DA, Chase A, Campbell AT. Relative effectiveness of protein in the late stages of appetite suppression in man. Physiol Behav 1970;5(11):1299–1302.

42. Barkeling B, Rossner S, Bjorvell H. Effects of a high-protein meal (meat) and a high-carbohydrate meal (vegetarian) on satiety measured by automated computerized monitoring of subsequent food intake, motivation to eat and food preferences. Int J Obes 1990;14(9):743–751.

43. Wurtman RJ, Wurtman JJ. Carbohydrate craving, obesity and brain serotonin. Appetite 1986;7(Suppl):99–103.

44. Drewnoski A, Oomura Y, Tarui S, Inoue S, Shmazu T (eds). Progress in Obesity Research. London: John Libbey, 1990.

45. Lichtenstein AH, Kennedy E, Barrier P, Danford D, Ernst ND, Grundy SM, Leveille GA, VanHorn L, Williams CL, Booth SL. Dietary fat consumption and health. Nutr Rev 1998;56(5 pt 2):S3–S19.

46. Hu FB, Stampfcr MJ, Manson JE, Rimm E, Colditz GA, Rosner BA, Hennekens CH, Willett WC. Dietary fat intake and the risk of coronary heart disease in women. N Engl J Med 1997;337(21):1491–1499.

47. Leiberman B. Avoiding the fracture zone: calcium. Nutr Action Heal Letter 1998;25(2):3–7.

48. Hegsted M, Linkswiler HM. Long-term effects of level of protein intake on calcium metabolism in young adult women. J Nutr 1981;111(2):244–251.

49. Kerstetter JE, Mitnick ME, Gundberg CM, Caseria DM, Ellison AF, Carpenter TO, Insogna KL. Changes in bone turnover in young women consuming different levels of dietary protein. J Clin Endocrinol Metab 1999;84(3):1025–1052.

50. Allen LH, Oddoye EA, Margen S. Protein-induced hypercalciuria: a longer term study. Am J Clin Nutr 1979;32(4):741–749.

51. Smolin LA, Grosvenor MB. Nutrition Science and Applications. Orlando: Saunders College Publishing, 1994.

52. Curtis D. Pump up your protein powder? Muscle Fitness 1991;52(10):75.

53. Parraga IM. Determinants of food consumption. J Am Diet Assoc 1990;90(5):661–663.

54. Douglas PD, Douglas JG. Nutrition knowledge and food practices of high school athletes. J Am Diet Assoc 1984;84(10):1198–1202.

55. Perron M, Endres J. Knowledge, attitudes, and dietary practices of female athletes. J Am Diet Assoc 1985;85(5):573–576.

56. Werblow JA, Fox HM, Henneman A. Nutritional knowledge, attitudes, and food patterns of women athletes. J Am Diet Assoc 1978;73(3):242–245.

57. Kraemer WJ, Volek JS, Bush JA, Putukian M, Sebastianelli WJ. Hormonal responses to consecutive days of heavy-resistance exercise with or without nutritional supplementation. J Appl Physiol 1998;85(4):1544–1555.

58. Chandler RM, Byrne HK, Patterson JG, Ivy JL. Dietary supplements affect the anabolic hormones after weight-training exercise. J Appl Physiol 1994;76(2):839–845.

59. Tarnopolsky MA, MacDougall JD, Atkinson SA. Influence of protein intake and training status on nitrogen balance and lean body mass. J Appl Physiol 1988;64(1):187–193.

60. Staron RS, Karapondo DL, Kraemer WJ, Fry AC, Gordon SE, Falkel JE, Hagerman FC, Hikida RS. Skeletal muscle adaptations during early phase of heavy-resistance training in men and women. J Appl Physiol 1994;76(3):1247–1255.

61. Tarnopolsky MA, Atkinson SA, MacDougall JD, Chesley A, Phillips S, Schwarcz HP. Evaluation of protein requirements for trained strength athletes. J Appl Physiol 1992;73(5):1986–1989.

62. Thissen JP, Ketelslegers JM, Underwood LE. Nutritional regulation of the insulin-like growth factors. Endocr Rev 1994;15(1):80–101.

63. Volek JS, Kraemer WJ, Bush JA, Incledon T, Boetes M. Testosterone and cortisol in relationship to dietary nutrients and resistance exercise. J Appl Physiol 1997;82(1):49–54.

64. Webb KE Jr. Intestinal absorption of protein hydrolysis products: a review. J Anim Sci 1990;68(9): 3011–3022.

65. Poullain MG, Cezard JP, Roger L, Mendy F. Effect of whey proteins, their oligopeptide hydrolysates and free amino acid mixtures on growth and nitrogen retention in fed and starved rats. JPEN J Parenter Enteral Nutr 1989;13(4):382–386.

66. Boza JJ, Martinez-Augustin O, Baro L, Suarez MD, Gil A. Protein v. enzymic protein hydrolysates. Nitrogen utilization in starved rats. Br J Nutr 1995;73(1):65–71.

67. Demling RH, DeSanti L. Increased protein intake during the recovery phase after severe burns increases body weight gain and muscle function. J Burn Care Rehabil 1998;19(2):161–168.

68. Stegink LD. Peptides in parenteral nutrition. In: Greene HL, Holliday MA, Munro HM (eds). Clinical Nutrition Update: Amino Acids. Chicago: American Medical Association, 1977.

69. Rolls BJ, Hill JO. Carbohydrate and Weight Management. Washington, DC: ILSI Press, 1998.

70. Turcoatte LP, Hespel PJ, Graham TE, Richter EA. Impaired plasma FFA oxidation imposed by extreme CHO deficiency in contracting rat skeletal muscle. J Appl Physiol 1994;77(2):517–525.

71. Sahlin K, Katz A, Broberg S. Tricarboxylic acid cycle intermediates in human muscle during prolonged exercise. Am J Physiol 1990;259(5 Pt 1):C834–C841.

72. Jenkins DJ, Vuksan V, Kendall CW, Wursch P, Jeffcoat R, Waring S, Mehling CC, Vidgen E, Augustin LS, Wong E. Physiological effects of resistant starches on fecal bulk, short chain fatty acids, blood lipids and glycemic index. J Am Coll Nutr 1998;17(6):609–616.

73. Lewis SJ, Heaton KW. Increasing butyrate concentration in the distal colon by accelerating intestinal transit. Gut 1997;41(2):245–251.

74. Jarvi AE, Karlstrom BE, Granfeldt YE, Bjorck IM, Vessby BO, Asp NG. The influence of food structure on postprandial metabolism in patients with non-insulin-dependent diabetes mellitus. Am J Clin Nutr 1995;61(4):837–842.

75. Anderson JW, Smith BM, Gustafson NJ. Health benefits and practical aspects of high-fiber diets. Am J Clin Nutr 1994;59(5 Suppl):1242S–1247S.

76. Wolk A, Manson JE, Stampfer MJ, Colditz GA, Hu FB, Speizer FE, Hennekens CH, Willett WC. Long-term intake of dietary fiber and decreased risk of coronary heart disease among women. JAMA 1999;281(21):1998–2004.

77. Aldoori WH, Giovanucci EL, Rockett HR, Sampson L, Rimm EB, Willett WC. A prospective study of dietary fiber types and symptomatic diverticular disease in men. J Nutr 1998;128(4):714–719.

78. Rimm EB, Ascherio A, Giovanucci E, Spiegelman D, Stampfer MJ, Willett WC. Vegetable, fruit, and cereal fiber intake and risk of coronary heart disease among men. JAMA 1996;275(6):447–451.

79. Anderson JW, Smith BM, Gustafson NJ. Health benefits and practical aspects of high-fiber diets. Am J Clin Nutr 1994;59(5 Suppl):1242S–1247S.

80. Howe GR, Benito E, Castelleto R, Cornee J, Esteve J, Gallagher RP, Iscovich JM, Deng-ao J, Kaaks R, Kune GA, et al. Dietary intake of fiber and decreased risk of cancers of the colon and rectum: evidence from the combined analysis of 13 case-controlled studies. J Natl Cancer Inst 1992;84(24):187–196.

81. Fernstrom JD, Miller GD. Appetite and Body Weight Regulation. Boca Raton, FL: CRC Press, 1994.

82. Romijn JA, Coyle EF, Sidossis LS, Gastaldelli A, Horowitz JF, Endert E, Wolfe RR. Regulation of endogenous fat and carbohydrate metabolism in relation to exercise intensity and duration. Am J Physiol 1993;265(3 Pt 1):E380–E391.

83. Berning JR, Steen SN. Nutrition for Sport and Exercise. Gaithersburg, MD: Aspen Publishers, 1998.

84. McArdle WD, Katch FI, Katch VL. Sports and Exercise Nutrition. Baltimore: Lippincott Williams & Wilkins, 1999.

85. Phinney SD, Bistrian BR, Evans WJ, Gervino E, Blackburn GL. The human metabolic response to chronic ketosis without caloric restriction: preservation of submaximal exercise capability with reduced carbohydrate oxidation. Metabolism 1983;32:769–776.

86. Lambert EV, Speechly DP, Dennis SC, Noakes, TD. Enhanced endurance in trained cyclists during moderate intensity exercise following 2 weeks adaptation to a high-fat diet. Eur J Appl Physiol 1994;69(4):287–293.

87. Pendergast DR, Horvath PJ, Leddy JJ, Venkatraman JT. The role of dietary fat on performance, metabolism, and health. Am J Sports Med 1996;24(6 Suppl):S53–S58.

88. Fallowfield JL, Williams C. Carbohydrate intake and recovery from prolonged exercise. Int J Sports Nutr 1993;3(2):150–164.

89. Simonsen JC, Sherman WM, Lamb DR, Dernbach AR, Doyle JA, Strauss R. Dietary carbohydrate, muscle glycogen, and power output during rowing training. J Appl Physiol 1991;70(4):1500–1505.

90. Lambert EV, Hawley JA, Goedecke J, Noakes TD, Dennis SC. Nutritional strategies for promoting fat utilization and delaying the onset of fatigue during prolonged exercise. J Sports Sci 1997;15(3):315–324.

91. Langfort J, Zarzeczny R, Pilis W, Nazar K, Kaciuba-Uscitko H. The effect of a low-carbohydrate diet on performance, hormonal and metabolic responses to a 30-s bout of supramaximal exercise. Eur J Appl Physiol 1997;76(2):128–133.

92. Balsom PD, Gaitanos GC, Soderlund K, Ekblom B. High intensity exercise and muscle glycogen availability in humans. Acta Physiol Scand 1999;165(4):337–345.

93. Helge JW, Richter EA, Kiens B. Interaction of training and diet on metabolism and endurance during exercise in man. J Physiol (Lond) 1996;492(Pt 1):293–306.

94. Sherman WM, Brodowicz G, Wright DA, Allen WK, Simonsen J, Dernbach A. Effects of 4 hr preexercise carbohydrate feedings on cycling performance. Med Sci Sports Exerc 1989;12:598–604.

95. Karlsson J, Saltin B. Diet, muscle glycogen, and endurance performance. J Appl Physiol 1971;31:203–206.

96. Sherman WM, Costill DL, Fink WJ, Miller JM. The effect of exercise and diet manipulation on muscle glycogen and its subsequent use during performance. Int J Sports Med 1981;2(2):114–118.

97. Coyle EF, Hagberg JM, Hurley BF, Martin WH, Ehsani AA, Holloszy JO. Carbohydrate feeding during prolonged strenuous exercise can delay fatigue. J Appl Physiol 1983;55(1 Pt 1):230–235.

98. Coyle EF, Coggan AR, Hemmert WK, Ivy JL. Muscle glycogen utilization during prolonged strenuous exercise when fed carbohydrate. J Appl Physiol 1986;61(1):165–172.

99. Wilber RL, Moffatt RJ. Influence of carbohydrate ingestion on blood glucose and performance in runners. Intl J Sports Nutr 1992;2(4):317–327.

100. American College of Sports Medicine. Position stand: exercise and fluid replacement. Med Sci Sports Exerc 1996;28:i–vii.

101. Below PR, Coyle EF. Fluid and carbohydrate ingestion independently improve performance during 1 hr of intense exercise. Med Sci Sports Exerc 1995;27(2):200–210.

102. Ivy JL, Lee MC, Broznick JT, Reed MJ. Muscle glycogen storage after different amounts of carbohydrate ingestion. J Appl Physiol 1988;65(5):2018–2023.

103. Ivy JL, Katz AL, Cutler CL, Sherman WM, Coyle EF. Muscle glycogen synthesis after exercise: effect of time of carbohydrate ingestion. J Appl Physiol 1988;64(4):1480–1485.

104. Liljeberg HG, Akergerg AK, Bjorck IM. Effect of the glycemic index and content of indigestible carbohydrates of cereal-based breakfast meals on glucose tolerance at lunch in healthy subjects. Am J Clin Nutr 1999;69(4):647–655.

105. Raben A, Tagliabue A, Christensen NJ, Madsen J, Holst JJ, Astrup A. Resistant starch: the effect on postprandial glycemia, hormonal response, and satiety. Am J Clin Nutr 1994;60(4):544–551.

106. Raben A, Christensen NJ, Madsen J, Holst JJ, Astrup A. Decreased postprandial thermogenesis and fat oxidation but increased fullness after a high-fiber meal compared with a low-fiber meal. Am J Clin Nutr 1994;59(6):1386–1394.

107. Yang MU, Van Itallie TB. Composition of weight lost during short-term weight reduction. Metabolic responses of obese subjects to starvation and low-calorie ketogenic and nonketogenic diets. J Clin Invest 1976;58(3):722–730.

108. Karlsson J, Saltin B. Lactate, ATP, and CP in working muscles during exhaustive exercise in man. J Appl Physiol 1970;29(5):596–602.

109. Shick SM, Wing RR, Klem ML, McGuire MT, Hill JO, Seagle H. Persons successful at long-term weight loss and maintenance continue to consume a low-energy, low-fat diet. J Am Diet Assoc 1998;98(4):408–413.

110. McDowell MA, Briefel RR, Alaimo K, Bischof AM, Caughman CR, Carroll MD, Loria CM, Johnson CL. Energy intakes of persons ages 2 months and over in the United States: Third National Health and Nutrition Examination Survey, Phase 1, 1988–91. Adv Data 1994;24(255):1–24.

111. Ernst ND, Obarzanek E, Clark MB, Briefel RR, Brown CD, Donato K. Cardiovascular health risks related to overweight. J Am Diet Assoc 1997;97(7 Suppl):S47–S51.

112. US Department of Agriculture, Center for Nutrition Policy and Promotion. Nutrient content of the US food supply, 1909–94. Home Economics Research Report No. 53. Washington, DC: U.S. Government Printing Office, 1997.

113. US Department of Health and Human Services. Physical activity and health: a report of the Surgeon General. Atlanta, GA: Centers for Disease Control and Prevention, 1996.

114. Flegal KM, Carroll MD, Kuczmarski RJ, Johnson CL. Overweight and obesity in the United States: prevalence and trends, 1960–1994. Int J Obes Relat Metab Disord 1998;22(1):39–47.

115. Whitney EN, Rolfes SR. Understanding Nutrition. St. Paul, MN: West Publishing, 1996.

116. Groff JL, Gropper SS, Hunt SM. Advanced Nutrition and Human Metabolism. St. Paul, MN: West Publishing, 1995.

117. Simopoulos AP. Omega-3 fatty acids in health and disease and in growth and development. Am J Clin Nutr 1991;54(3):438–463.

118. Simopoulos AP. Omega-3 fatty acids in the prevention-management of cardiovascular disease. Can J Physiol Pharmacol 1997;75(3):234–239.

119. Lichtenstein AH, Ausman LM, Jalbert SM, Schaefer EJ. Effects of different forms of dietary hydrogenated fats on serum lipoprotein cholesterol levels. N Engl J Med 1999;340(25):1933–1940.

120. Tato F. Trans-fatty acids in the diet: a coronary risk factor? Eur J Med Res 1995;1(2):118–122.

121. Ascherio A, Willett WC. Health effects of trans fatty acids. Am J Clin Nutr 1997;66(4 Suppl):1006S–1010S.

122. [NRC] National Research Council. Recommended Dietary Allowances, 10th ed. Washington, DC: National Academy Press, 1989.

123. Lissner L, Levitsky DA, Strupp BJ, Kalkwarf HJ, Roe DA. Dietary fat and the regulation of energy intake in human subjects. Am J Clin Nutr 1987;46(6):886–892.

124. Lissner L, Heitmann BL. The dietary fat: carbohydrate ratio in relation to body weight. Curr Opin Lipidol 1995;6(1):8–13.

125. Horton TJ, Drougas H, Reed GW, Peters JC, Hill JO. Fat and carbohydrate overfeeding in humans: different effects on energy storage. Am J Clin Nutr 1995;62(1):19–29.

126. Leveille GA. Isocaloric diets: effects of dietary changes. Am J Clin Nutr 1987;45(1 Suppl):158–163.

127. Stubbs RJ, Ritz P, Coward WA, Prentice AM. Covert manipulation of the ration of dietary fat to carbohydrate and energy density: effect on food intake and energy balance in free-living men eating ad libitum. Am J Clin Nutr 1995;62(2):330–337.

128. Groff JL, Gropper SS, Hunt SM. Advanced Nutrition and Human Metabolism. Minneapolis/St. Paul: West Publishing, 1995.

129. Jeukendrup AE, Saris WH, Schrauwen P, Brouns F, Wagenmakers AJ. Metabolic availability of medium-chain triglycerides coingested with carbohydrate during prolonged exercise. J Appl Physiol 1995;79(3):756–762.

130. Van Zyl CG, Lambert EV, Hawley JA, Noakes TD, Dennis SC. Effects of medium-chain triglyceride ingestion on fuel metabolism and cycling performance. J Appl Physiol 1996;80(6):2217–2225.

131. Shepherd PR, Kahn BB. Glucose transporters and insulin action—implications for insulin resistance and diabetes mellitus. N Engl J Med 1999;341(4):248–257.

132. Buemann B, Tremblay A. Effects of exercise training on abdominal obesity and related metabolic complications. Sports Med 1996;21(3):191–212.

133. Pandolfi C, Pellegrini L, Sbalzarini G, Mercantini F. Obesity and insulin resistance. Minerva Med 1994;85(4):167–171.

134. Bloomgarden ZT. Insulin resistance: current concepts. Clin Ther 1998;20(2):216–231.

135. Schraer CD, Risica PM, Ebbesson SO, Go OT, Howard BV, Mayer AM. Low fasting insulin levels in Eskimos compared to American Indians: are Eskimos less insulin resistant? Intl J Circumpolar Health 1999;58(4):272–280.

136. Beck-Nielsen H. General characteristics of the insulin resistance syndrome: prevalence and heritability. European Group for the Study of Insulin Resistance (EGIR). Drugs 1999;58(Suppl 1):7–10.

137. Pi-Sunyer FX. Medical hazards of obesity. Ann Intern Med 1993;119(7 Pt 2):655–660.

138. Grundy SM. Multifactorial causation of obesity: implications for prevention. Am J Clin Nutr 1998;67(3S):563S–569S.

139. Vaag A. On the pathophysiology of late onset non-insulin dependent diabetes mellitus. Current controversies and new insights. Dan Med Bull 1999;46(3):197–234.

140. Parekh PI, Petro AE, Tiller JM, Feinglos MN, Surwit RS. Reversal of diet-induced obesity and diabetes in C57BL/6J mice. Metabolism 1998;47(9):1089–1096.

141. Barnard RJ, Ugianskis EJ, Martin DA, Inkeles SB. Role of diet and exercise in the management of hyperinsulinemia and associated atherosclerotic risk factors. Am J Cardiol 1992;69(5):440–444.

142. Wolinsky I, Hickson JF. Nutrition in Exercise and Sport. Boca Raton, FL: CRC Press, 1994.

143. Walsh RM, Noakes TD, Hawkey JA, Dennis SC. Impaired high-intensity cycling performance time at low levels of dehydration. Int J Sports Med 1994;15(7):392–398.

144. Broad E, Burke LM, Heely P, Grundy M. Body weight changes and ad libitum fluid intakes during training and competition sessions in team sports. Int J Sport Nutr 1996;6(3):307–320.

145. Berning JR, Steen SN. Nutrition for Sport and Exercise. Gaithersburg, MD: Aspen Publishers, 1998.

146. Convertino VA, Armstrong LE, Coyle EF, Mack GW, Sawka MN, Senay LC Jr, Sherman WM. American College of Sports Medicine position stand. Exercise and fluid replacement. Med Sci Sports Exerc 1996;28(1):i–vii.

147. The Apex Fitness Group. Apex Training System: Nutritional Guidelines for Altering Body Composition.

Supplementation

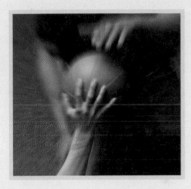

OBJECTIVES

After completing this chapter, you will be able to:

- Describe supplements and their functions.
- Understand basic supplemental recommendations for optimizing health.
- Answer questions, handle issues, and dispel myths regarding the relationship of supplements to the successful alteration of body composition.

KEY TERMS

Adequate intake (AI)

Dietary supplement

Estimated average requirement (EAR)

Recommended dietary allowance (RDA)

Tolerable upper intake level (UL)

Dietary Supplements

INTRODUCTION TO SUPPLEMENTATION

During the first half of the twentieth century, the discovery that vitamins are essential components of food (along with tremendous growth in the understanding of human nutrient needs) set the foundation for the development of dietary supplements containing vitamins and minerals.

The traditional reason for use of a dietary supplement is to provide the body with nutrients that might not be supplied adequately by a person's typical diet. Around the middle of the twentieth century, the use of dietary supplements was primarily in the form of a "one-a-day" type of vitamin-mineral supplement. Although this continues to be the most commonly used type, the rapid growth of the dietary supplement industry has led to the development of a great variety of different types of supplements. Today, dietary supplements are much more than a low-dosage vitamin-mineral pill taken by a small percentage of the population. Contemporary dietary supplements often contain numerous chemical compounds other than nutrients, and people take dietary supplements for a wide variety of reasons other than meeting nutrient needs.

The popularity of dietary supplements has grown steadily in the United States, with sales in the supplement industry booming during the 1990s. Estimates put total sales at $3.3 billion for 1990, growing to $17.7 billion in 2002.[1,2] Associated with this rapid growth, the Dietary Supplement Health and Education Act (DSHEA) was passed in 1994, providing a detailed legal definition of the term "dietary supplement." There are now new regulations for dietary supplements that are separate from the regulations for foods and drugs.[3]

WHAT IS A DIETARY SUPPLEMENT?

On the basis of the DSHEA, the U.S. Food and Drug Administration (FDA) states that a **dietary supplement** is:

- A product (other than tobacco) that is intended to supplement the diet and that bears or contains one or more of the following dietary ingredients: a vitamin, a mineral, an herb or other botanical, an amino acid
- A dietary substance for use by man to supplement the diet by increasing the total daily intake
- A concentrate, metabolite, constituent, extract, or combinations of these ingredients
- Intended for ingestion in pill, capsule, tablet, or liquid form
- Not represented for use as a conventional food or as the sole item of a meal or diet
- Labeled as a "dietary supplement"

Thus, most anything that is not already classified as a drug can be put into a pill and sold as a dietary supplement.[4]

RATIONALE FOR THE USE OF DIETARY SUPPLEMENTS

People take supplements for many reasons. Some use them to deal with or help prevent specific health problems. Others use supplements in hopes of enhancing performance in physical or mental tasks, altering body composition, stimulating metabolism, controlling appetite, or dealing with age-related changes in body structure and function.

The use of dietary supplements that contain a broad spectrum of micronutrients (in low to moderate doses) can be especially beneficial for individuals consuming

Dietary supplement: A substance that completes or makes an addition to daily dietary intake.

- Inadequate food intake (especially diets less than 1200 calories per day)
- Disordered eating patterns
  - Consuming mostly "junk" (nutrient deficient) foods
  - Avoidance of foods from specific food groups
  - Eating only one major meal each day
  - Irregular eating patterns (low-calorie diet one day, high-calorie the next)
  - Eating too much or too little protein or carbohydrate
  - Food phobias and "picky" eating
  - Financial limitations on access to a variety of wholesome foods

Figure 16.1 Common reasons why diets do not contain adequate nutrients.

diets that do not meet their needs for all nutrients.[5,6] In addition, various studies have reported that people taking a multivitamin supplement experience a reduced risk of chronic disease development.[6]

Additionally, there are specific groups who may have greater need for dietary supplements. For example, older people often do not make proper adjustments in their diets when energy needs decline with age. Although calorie needs generally drop with age, the need for protein, vitamins, and minerals does not decline.[7,8] Another group that can benefit from supplemented nutrients is women who are pregnant or breastfeeding. However, because of the potential for supplement toxicity or interactions with prescribed medications, it is extremely important for these groups to seek guidance on supplementation from qualified health professionals.[9] Whatever the goal for using a dietary supplement, the considerations for appropriate use are similar (Figure 16-1).

SUMMARY

Vitamins (and many minerals) are essential components of food and are required in very small amounts by the body. The popularity of dietary supplements has boomed in recent years. In 1994 the Dietary Supplement Health and Education Act (DSHEA) was passed, providing a detailed legal definition of the term "dietary supplement." The U.S. Food and Drug Administration (FDA) states that a dietary supplement is, basically, a labeled pill, capsule, tablet, or liquid intended to supplement the diet and contains one or more vitamin, mineral, botanical, or amino acid. Almost anything not already classified as a drug can be sold as a dietary supplement. Taking low-to-moderate dose, broad-spectrum vitamin-mineral supplements is beneficial, especially for those whose diets do not meet all micronutrient requirements. There is also a reduced risk for chronic diseases in people taking a multivitamin supplement.

Supplementation Guidelines

GENERAL GUIDELINES FOR RESPONSIBLE USE OF NUTRITIONAL DIETARY SUPPLEMENTS

Dietary supplements usually contain potent natural chemicals. Although these substances are generally safer than drugs, some precautions should be kept in mind. This section will give common guidelines for determining what quantity of a supplemental nutrient is likely to be adequate, safe, and beneficial and how much may be potentially excessive or detrimental to health.

Table 16.1

Dietary Reference Intake Publications

Nutrients Reviewed	Year of Publication
Calcium, phosphorus, magnesium, vitamin D, and fluoride[12]	1997[10]
Thiamin, riboflavin, niacin, vitamin B_6, folate, vitamin B_{12}, pantothenic acid, biotin, and choline[13]	1998[11]
Vitamin C, vitamin E, selenium, and carotenoids[14]	2000[12]
Vitamin A, vitamin K, arsenic, boron, chromium, copper, iodine, iron, manganese, molybdenum, nickel, silicon, vanadium, and zinc[15]	2002[13]
Energy, carbohydrate, fiber, fat, fatty acids, cholesterol, protein, and amino acids[16]	2005[14]
Water, potassium, sodium, chloride, and sulfate	2005

Dietary Reference Intakes

In the United States, the Food and Nutrition Board (FNB) of the Institute of Medicine, National Academy of Sciences periodically reviews the current research on nutrient needs to provide authoritative, updated recommendations for nutrient intake. In 1997, the FNB released the first in a series of publications called "Dietary Reference Intakes" with the final volumes published in 2005 (Table 16-1).

Dietary reference intake (DRI) values for nutrients provide good guidelines for what constitutes an adequate intake of a nutrient. For many nutrients, values also have been set for the amount considered to be excessive and potentially harmful. The DRIs are designed to estimate the nutrient needs of healthy people in various age and gender groups. The values also are adjusted for the special needs of women during pregnancy and lactation.

Figure 16-2 describes the DRI terminology used by the FNB. The DRIs most commonly used to evaluate or plan diets for individuals are the recommended

Estimated Average Requirement (EAR): The average daily nutrient intake level that is estimated to meet the requirement of half the healthy individuals who are in a particular life stage and gender group.

Recommended Dietary Allowance (RDA): The average daily nutrient intake level that is sufficient to meet the nutrient requirement of nearly all (97 to 98 percent) healthy individuals who are in a particular life stage and gender group.

Adequate Intake (AI): A recommended average daily nutrient intake level, based on observed (or experimentally determined) approximations or estimates of nutrient intake that are assumed to be adequate for a group (or groups) of healthy people. This measure is used when an RDA cannot be determined.

Tolerable Upper Intake Level (UL): The highest average daily nutrient intake level likely to pose no risk of adverse health effects to almost all individuals in a particular life stage and gender group. As intake increases above the UL, the potential risk of adverse health effects increases.

Figure 16.2   Dietary reference intake terminology.

dietary allowance (RDA), adequate intake (AI), and tolerable upper intake level (UL) values (described below).[15] The overall goal in designing a healthy diet is to provide nutrients at levels that represent a high probability of adequate intake (meeting RDA or AI levels) and also a low probability of excessive intake (not exceeding UL values).

Dietary Reference Intake Values and Guidelines

Table 16-2 summarizes the currently established adult DRI values for vitamins and minerals, including UL values and possible signs of excess intake of a nutrient. Except for vitamin E and magnesium, the UL values are set for total intake of each nutrient from food and supplements. The ULs for vitamin E and magnesium are set for levels of intake from supplements or pharmacologic sources only and do not include dietary intake.

Even essential nutrients are potentially toxic at some level of intake. For some nutrients, the level of intake that causes serious adverse effects is not presently known. For others, the adverse effects of excess have been documented. The effects of some nutrients can be extremely serious. Among the vitamin category of nutrients, excess vitamin A, D, and B_6 can produce serious adverse effects and are commonly available in dietary supplement form. Excess vitamin A, for example, can cause birth defects when a woman is taking too much at conception and during early pregnancy.[13] Vitamin D excess can result in the calcification of blood vessels and eventually damage the function of the kidneys, heart, and lungs.[10] Excessive intake of vitamin B_6 can cause permanent damage to sensory nerves.[11]

Excess intake of mineral elements also can cause health problems. For example, excess (and inadequate) calcium intake can increase the risk of developing kidney stones. Excess intake of iron can interfere with the absorption of other minerals (such as zinc) and can cause gastrointestinal irritation.[13]

It is important to remember that nutrient requirements and ULs are set for normal, healthy individuals. In some cases, a drug may increase or decrease the need for a nutrient. Anyone who is taking a medication may no longer fit into these DRI parameters. For example, large doses of anti-inflammatory drugs such as aspirin and ibuprofen may interfere with folic acid function and potentially increase folic acid requirements.[11,16]

With respect to ULs, the nutrient levels that are perfectly safe for normal, healthy people can be life threatening for those with specific health problems. For example, supplementation with vitamins E and K can complicate conditions for people on anticoagulant therapy (or "blood thinners").[14,15] Consequently, the use of various drugs can contraindicate the use of specific nutrient supplements, as well as the consumption of some foods high in the specific nutrient. Therefore, people with serious health problems, and especially those taking drugs for health problems, should use dietary supplements only with guidance and monitoring by a physician, pharmacist, or other health professional knowledgeable in drug-nutrient interactions.

When no UL has been established for a nutrient, it does not mean that there is no potential for adverse effects from high intake. Rather, it may just mean that too little information is currently available to establish a UL value. Complete tables of the DRI values are available at the FNB Web site (http://www.iom.edu/board). The tables include the UL values and brief descriptions of the adverse effects of excessive intake.

Another authoritative publication on ULs for nutrient intake was recently released by the Expert Group on Vitamins and Minerals of the Food Standards Agency in the United Kingdom. This publication, *Safe Upper Levels for Vitamins and Minerals*, provides "safe upper levels" (SUL) for eight nutrients and "guidance levels" for the 22 vitamins and minerals, for which data were inadequate to set an SUL.[17] These recommended ULs of intake refer specifically to intake in the form of

Table 16.2

Comparison of Dietary Reference Intake Values (for Adult Men and Women) and Daily Values for Micronutrients With the Tolerable Upper Intake Levels, Safe Upper Levels, and Guidance Levels [a]

Nutrient	RDA/AI (Men/Women) ages 31–50	Daily Value (Food Labels)	UL	SUL or Guidance Level	Selected Potential Effects of Excess Intake
Vitamin A (μg)	900/700	1,500 (5,000 IU)	3,000	1,500[c] (5,000 IU)	Liver damage, bone and joint pain, dry skin, loss of hair, headache, vomiting
β-Carotene (mg)				7 (11,655 IU)	Increased risk of lung cancer in smokers and those heavily exposed to asbestos
Vitamin D (μg)	5[b]	10 (400 IU)	50	25 (1,000 IU)	Calcification of brain and arteries, increased blood calcium, loss of appetite, nausea
Vitamin E (mg)	15	20 (30 IU)	1,000	540 (800 IU)	Deficient blood clotting
Vitamin K (μg)	120/90[b]	80	—	1,000[c]	Red blood cell damage or anemia, liver damage
Thiamin (B_1) (mg)	1.2/1.1	1.5	—	100[c]	Headache, nausea, irritability, insomnia, rapid pulse, weakness (7,000+ mg dose)
Riboflavin (B_2) (mg)	1.3/1.1	1.7	—	40[c]	Generally considered harmless; yellow discoloration of urine
Niacin (mg)	16/14	20	35	500[c]	Liver damage, flushing, nausea, gastrointestinal problems
Vitamin B_6 (mg)	1.3	2	100	10	Neurologic problems, numbness and pain in limbs
Vitamin B_{12} (μg)	2.4	6	—	2,000[c]	No reports of toxicity from oral ingestion
Folic acid (μg)	400	400	1,000	1,000[c]	Masks vitamin B_{12} deficiency (which can cause neurologic problems)
Pantothenic acid (mg)	5[b]	10	—	200[c]	Diarrhea and gastrointestinal disturbance (10,000+ mg/day)
Biotin (μg)	30[b]	300	—	900[c]	No reports of toxicity from oral ingestion
Vitamin C (mg)	90/75	60	2,000	1,000[c]	Nausea, diarrhea, kidney stones
Boron (mg)			20	9.6	Adverse effects on male and female reproductive systems
Calcium (mg)	1,000[b]	1,000	2,500	1,500[c]	Nausea, constipation, kidney stones
Chromium (μg)	35[b]	120	—	10,000[c]	Potential adverse effects on liver and kidneys; picolinate form possibly mutagenic
Cobalt (mg)				1.4[c]	Cardiotoxic effects; not appropriate in a dietary supplement except as vitamin B_{12}

Table 16.2

Comparison of Dietary Reference Intake Values (for Adult Men and Women) and Daily Values for Micronutrients With the Tolerable Upper Intake Levels, Safe Upper Levels, and Guidance Levels *a* (continued)

Nutrient	RDA/AI (Men/Women) ages 31–50	Daily Value (Food Labels)	UL	SUL or Guidance Level	Selected Potential Effects of Excess Intake
Copper (μg)	900	2,000	10,000	10,000	Gastrointestinal distress, liver damage
Fluoride (mg)	4/3*b*		10		Bone, kidney, muscle, and nerve damage; supplement only with professional guidance
Germanium				zero*c*	Kidney toxin; should not be in a dietary supplement
Iodine (μg)	150	150	1,100	500*c*	Elevated thyroid hormone concentration
Iron (mg)	8/18	18	45	17*c*	Gastrointestinal distress, increased risk of heart disease, oxidative stress
Magnesium (mg)	420/320	400	350*d*	400*c*	Diarrhea
Manganese (mg)	2.3/1.8*b*	2	11	4*c*	Neurotoxicity
Molybdenum	45	75	2,000	zero*c*	Goutlike symptoms, joint pains, increased uric acid
Nickel (μg)				260*c*	Increased sensitivity of skin reaction to nickel in jewelry
Phosphorus (mg)	700	1,000	4,000	250*c*	Alteration of parathyroid hormone levels, reduced bone mineral density
Potassium (mg)				3,700*c*	Gastrointestinal damage
Selenium (μg)	55	70	400	450	Nausea, diarrhea, fatigue, hair and nail loss
Silicon (mg)				700	Low toxicity, possibility of kidney stones
Vanadium (mg)			1.8	zero	Gastrointestinal irritation; fatigue
Zinc (mg)	11/8	15	40	25	Impaired immune function, low HDL-cholesterol

*a*Food and Nutrition Board, Institute of Medicine (U.S.). Dietary Reference Intake Tables. Available at [http://www4.nationalacademies.org/IOM/IOMHome.nsf/Pages/Food+and+Nutrition+Board].

*b*Indicates adequate intake (AI).

*c*Indicates guidance levels, set by the Expert Group on Vitamins and Minerals of the Food Standards Agency, United Kingdom. These are intended to be levels of daily intake of nutrients in dietary supplements that potentially susceptible individuals could take daily on a lifelong basis without medical supervision in reasonable safety. When the evidence base was considered inadequate to set an SUL, guidance levels were set based on limited data. SULs and guidance levels tend to be conservative, and it is possible that for some vitamins and minerals, greater amounts could be consumed for short periods without risk to health. The values presented are for a 60-kg (132-lb) adult. Consult the full publication for values expressed per kilogram of body weight. This FSA publication, *Safe Upper Levels for Vitamins and Minerals*, is available at: [http://www.foodstandards.gov.uk/multimedia/pdfs/vitmin2003.pdf].

*d*The UL for magnesium represents intake specifically from pharmacologic agents and dietary supplements in addition to dietary intake. *RDA*, recommended dietary allowance; *UL*, tolerable upper intake level; *AI*, adequate intake; *SUL*, safe upper level.

dietary supplements. The Expert Group on Vitamins and Minerals describes these terms as follows:

> The determination of SULs or Guidance Levels entails the determination of doses of vitamins and minerals that potentially susceptible individuals could take daily on a life-long basis, without medical supervision in reasonable safety. The setting of these levels provides a framework within which the consumer can make an informed decision about intake, having confidence that harm should not ensue. The levels so set will therefore tend to be conservative, and it is possible that for some vitamins and minerals larger amounts could be consumed for shorter periods without risk to health. However, there would be difficulties in deriving SULs for shorter term consumption because the available data are limited and relate to differing time periods. Although less susceptible individuals might be able to consume higher levels without risk to health, separate advice for susceptible individuals would be appropriate only if those individuals could recognize their own potential susceptibility.[17]

Values for SULs and guidance levels are included in Table 16-2, for comparison with DRI values. It is interesting to note similarities and differences in the values set by the two different approaches. Guidance levels are based on very limited data and are not meant to be confused with, or used as, SULs. However, when no UL or SUL is available, guidance levels can provide a reasonable frame of reference.

Obviously, the bottom line is that it is preferable to consume nutrients within a range that is adequate to meet the body's needs. The optimal level of intake within this adequate range is not known. Whether "optimal" is closer to the RDA and AI or to the UL for a nutrient is unknown and likely differs for the various nutrients and also may differ from one individual person to another.

SUMMARY

Most dietary supplements contain potent natural chemicals that are generally considered safer than drugs. However, some precautions for appropriate use should still be taken, and guidelines should be followed. The most recent updated recommendations for nutrient intake are presented in a series of publications called "Dietary Reference Intakes."

Dietary reference intake (DRI) values are good guidelines for adequate, excessive, and potentially harmful intakes of a nutrient for normal, healthy individuals. The overall goal in designing a healthy diet is to provide nutrients that meet recommended daily allowance or adequate intake levels and also have a low probability of exceeding tolerable upper intake levels. Optimal intake may differ for the various nutrients and also may differ from one individual person to another.

Even essential nutrients and minerals are potentially toxic at some level of intake. Nutrient levels that are perfectly safe for normal, healthy people can be altered for those taking medication and even life threatening for those with specific health problems. These clients should use dietary supplements only with guidance and monitoring by a physician, pharmacist, or other health professional knowledgeable in drug–nutrient interactions.

Labels of Dietary Supplements

UNITS OF MEASURE USED ON DIETARY SUPPLEMENT LABELS

Dietary supplement labels contain product information on "Supplement Facts" panels similar to the "Nutrition Facts" on food products (Figure 16-3). Protein, carbohydrate, and fat are generally expressed in gram quantities, whereas vitamins, minerals, amino acids, and fatty acids are generally present and expressed in milligram (mg) or microgram (mcg or µg) quantities.

Supplement Facts

Serving Size 1 Capsule

Amount per Capsule	% Daily Value
Calories 20	
Calories from fat 20	
Total Fat 2 g	3%*
Saturated Fat 0.5 g	3%*
Polyunsaturated Fat 1 g	†
Monounsaturated Fat 0.5 g	†
Vitamin A 4250 IU	85%
Vitamin D 425 IU	106%
Omega-3 fatty acids 0.5 g	†

* Percent Daily Values are based on a 2,000 calorie diet.
† Daily Value not established.

Ingredients: Cod liver oil, gelatin, water, and glycerin.

Figure 16.3 Sample supplement facts panel used on a dietary supplement label.

In addition to the nutrient amounts required on the supplement facts panel, dietary supplements must provide a "% Daily Value" for each nutrient listed. Daily values (DVs) were established specifically for food labeling and are intended to provide the consumer with a frame of reference that indicates how the amount of the nutrient present in a food or supplement compares with approximate levels of recommended intake. The DVs for vitamins and minerals are based on the 1968 RDAs for adults (using the highest of two recommended amounts, when there are differences between males and females). Thus, if a product indicates that the % DV for a nutrient is 50, it means that an adult will obtain about 50% of the amount commonly recommended on a daily basis, for that nutrient.

The amounts and DVs for nutrients listed on a supplement facts panel are the amounts present in the serving size indicated at the top of the label. In Figure 16-3, the serving size is one capsule. However, some products may indicate more than one capsule, pill, tablet, and so forth as the serving size. Many components of supplements do not have DVs. When this is the case, there is an indication "Daily Value not established" at the bottom of the panel.

Although the RDAs have been revised several times since 1968, the DVs have not changed, at the request of the food industry. When DVs are used as a general ballpark guide, they still work reasonably well. However, some issues have evolved that will likely lead to a revision in the DVs to more closely match current nutritional recommendations. For example, the DV for iron is 18 mg/day, which was based on a menstruating woman's requirement. The current RDA for a man is 8 mg/day. Consequently, when a dietary supplement provides 100% of the DV for iron, it provides more than twice the RDA for a man.

The amounts of vitamins A, D, and E are expressed on supplement labels as international units (IUs). Table 16-3 compares the RDA values for these three nutrients expressed in microgram or milligram amounts to equivalent amounts expressed in IUs. This table also illustrates that the DVs that are used as reference amounts on food and supplement nutrition labels do not equal the most current RDA values for men and women. The DV for each of these three vitamins exceeds the current RDA for adult males and females. Of particular interest, the DV for vitamin A is actually equal to the SUL value recently set by the Expert Committee on Vitamins and Minerals in the United Kingdom. Comparisons of other micronutrient DVs with current recommendations are shown in Table 16-3.

Table 16.3

Comparison of RDA Adult Values for Vitamins A, D, and E With Tolerable Upper Intake Levels, Safe Upper Levels, and Daily Values Used for Food and Supplement Labels

Vitamin	Men's RDA	Women's RDA	Adult UL/SUL	Label DV
Vitamin A (μg)	900	700	3,000/1,500	—
Vitamin A (IU)[a]	3,000	2,333	10,000/5,000	5,000
Vitamin D (μg)	5	5	50/25	—
Vitamin D (IU)	200	200	2,000/1,000	400
Vitamin E (μg)	15	15	1,000/540	—
Vitamin E (IU)[b]	22	22	1,490/800	30

[a]In the form of retinol (typically as retinyl palmitate).
[b]Based on natural vitamin E (D-α-tocopherol).

RDA, recommended dietary allowance; *UL*, tolerable upper intake level; *SUL*, safe upper level; *DV*, daily value.

SUMMARY

Dietary supplement labels contain product information on "Supplement Facts" panels, expressed in quantities of milligram (mg) or microgram (mcg or μg) or international units (IU). Also provided are "% Daily Value" (DVs) for each nutrient listed. DVs for vitamins and minerals are based on the 1968 RDAs for adults, which still work reasonably well. However, some nutrients may not match current nutritional recommendations (such as A, D, E, and iron).

Vitamin and Mineral Supplements

A great variety of dietary supplements are used to enhance overall health or reduce the risk of various diseases. The most commonly used supplement is a multiple vitamin and mineral supplement that is intended to compensate for nutrients that may be limited in a person's diet. The amounts of the various nutrients in a multiple vitamin and mineral supplement (multi-Vit/Min) that are reasonable and sensible depend on an individual's needs and their intake of nutrients from other sources. As a general rule of thumb, the safe level of most nutrients in a multi-Vit/Min should be around 100% of the DV. However, there are some notable exceptions to this general rule.

Vitamin A, if present in a supplement only as retinol (usually indicated as retinyl palmitate or vitamin A palmitate) rather than carotene, should be less than 100% of the DV. A recent study indicates that high intake of retinol, but not β-carotene, is associated with increased incidence of hip fracture in older women.[18] Also, as mentioned above, excess intake of retinol at conception and during early pregnancy increases the risk of birth defects.[19]

Concerns also exist for including large doses of β-carotene in a dietary supplement.[20] Two large intervention trials reported an increased incidence of lung cancer in smokers who were taking 20- to 30-mg/day supplements of β-carotene.[19,21] However, a large study of 22,071 physicians reported no effect on cancer incidence or mortality in those taking 50 mg/day of β-carotene and found that supplementation in those with initially low blood levels of β-carotene helped reduce the incidence of prostate cancer.[22] Still another large study conducted in China found that daily supplementation with 15 mg of β-carotene in combination with 50 μg of selenium and 30 mg of α-tocopherol was associated with a 13% reduction in cancer risk, mainly as a result of decreased incidence of gastric cancer.[23] Consequently, supplementation with β-carotene remains controversial and appears to be most clearly contraindicated in smokers.

Calcium should be at low levels or absent in a multi-Vit/Min because taking 100% of the RDA, which is 1 g (1,000 mg) of elemental calcium, would make the supplement pill too large to swallow easily. Second, for best absorption, it is preferable to consume calcium with meals, spaced throughout the day, rather than to ingest 100% of daily needs at one time.[24] Third, excess calcium consumed with other minerals can decrease the absorption of some important trace minerals.[10]

Among the B vitamins, niacin, B_6, and folic acid have UL values. For niacin and folic acid, the adult ULs are only 2.2 and 2.5 times their respective RDA values. The UL for vitamin B_6 of 100 mg is 77 times the RDA. However, the FSA Expert Group on Vitamins and Minerals SUL value for daily consumption of supplemental vitamin B_6 is only 10 mg/day.[17] At one tenth the UL value set by the U.S. Food and Nutrition Board, this value is based on the assumption that this SUL intake for supplemental B_6 is reasonably safe to consume over the lifetime of an adult.[13]

Some B vitamins (B_1, B_2, B_{12}, pantothenic acid, and biotin) do not have UL values because of a lack of data on adverse effects.[13] For these nutrients, the FSA Expert Group on Vitamins and Minerals established guidance levels that can at least provide a reasonable frame of reference (Table 16-2).[17]

Deficiencies of vitamins and minerals can impair the ability and desire to perform physical activity. In addition, many nutrient deficiencies can cause mental and emotional problems. Clearly, iron deficiency has been shown to affect both physical and mental function adversely.[25,26] Also, a deficiency of some B vitamins can affect mental functions and emotional state. Perhaps the most common example of this is caused by vitamin B_{12} deficiency, which is most commonly seen in the elderly and in those who avoid consuming animal foods.[27,28] In the elderly, mental and emotional changes caused by vitamin B_{12} deficiency are often mistaken for Alzheimer's disease and other dementias. The condition can be reversed if corrected early in the deficiency state. If not, nerve damage and dementia symptoms can be irreversible. However, correcting the deficiency will prevent further progression of the problems and potentially cause some reversal of symptoms. Because malabsorption is the usual cause of vitamin B_{12} deficiency, the usual treatment is to receive monthly injections of the vitamin. However, some research indicates that high-dose oral supplementation in the range of 200 to 2,000 μg/day may be as effective as injections.[29-31]

Selecting a multiple vitamin and mineral supplement with reasonable levels of each nutrient for an individual is not a simple task. It is not unusual to find multi-Vit/Mins with some nutrient levels that exceed the UL or SUL values. The information in Table 16-2 can provide some reasonable guidelines. Note that the upper level numbers (UL, SUL, and guidance level) for some nutrients are much closer to the RDA or AI than they are for others.

Figure 16-4 compares the DV amounts (the reference values on food and dietary supplement labels) for four nutrients to current levels of recommended intake and upper limits. Because the recommended intakes for these nutrients are relatively close to common recommendations for upper limits, people are more likely to consume excessive amounts of these nutrients from supplements and fortified foods combined.

The amount of each nutrient in a supplement that is most appropriate for an individual depends on the amount of nutrients in his or her diet. Despite claims to the contrary, today's food supply is not devoid of nutrients. Certainly it is possible to select a diet composed mostly of overly refined foods that provide limited

Vitamin A: If a dietary supplement contains 100% of the Daily Value, it contains an amount of vitamin A that is more than twice the RDA for a woman, only half of the UL, and is equal to the Guidance Level.

Vitamin D: If a dietary supplement contains 100% of the Daily Value, it contains an amount of vitamin D that is twice the AI value. The UL is only 5 times the DV, and the SUL is only 2.5 times the DV. However, recent research is likely to result in an increased DRI for vitamin D in the next revision.

Iron: If a dietary supplement contains 100% of the Daily Value, it contains an amount of iron that is equal to the RDA for women, more than twice the RDA for men. The UL is only a little over twice the DV, and the Guidance Level is 1 milligram less than the DV.

Zinc: If a dietary supplement contains 100% of the Daily Value, it contains an amount of zinc that is almost twice the RDA for women. The UL is just a little over twice the DV, and the SUL is a little less than twice the DV.

Figure 16.4 Nutrients with the greatest potential for excess dosage in dietary supplements.

amounts of vitamins and minerals and plenty of calories. However, with the plethora of fortified foods (breakfast cereals, energy bars, protein powders, and just about everything with a calcium-fortified option), it is quite possible to consume excessive amounts of some nutrients even without taking dietary supplements. Consequently, decisions to use dietary supplements should be made in the context of a typical diet, with special attention to use of foods fortified with vitamins and minerals.

CAUTION STATEMENTS ON DIETARY SUPPLEMENTS USED FOR SPECIFIC APPLICATION

1. Everyone should investigate the use of a multivitamin and mineral formula (in addition to a separate calcium supplement) to complement his or her best efforts to define and consume a proper diet.
2. Specific compounds, when ingested and manufactured properly, can allow the body to operate at full capacity, without disturbing its natural physiology.
3. Individual results during usage may be based on the physiology and psychological state of the recipient. Manufacturing methods and ingredients used may also affect results.
4. The general population should not use dietary supplements for medicinal purposes, unless recommended by a qualified health professional. Such a practitioner will have experience in treating diseases and symptoms with both prescription drugs and natural compounds and will have performed the research to choose the safest and most effective therapy.

SUMMARY

The most commonly used supplement is a multiple vitamin and mineral supplement (multi-Vit/Min) that is intended to compensate for nutrients that may be limited in a person's diet. Deficiencies of vitamins and minerals can impair ability and desire to perform physical activity and also cause mental and emotional problems.

As a general rule of thumb, the safe level of most nutrients in a multi-Vit/Min should be around 100% of the DV. However, there are some exceptions, including:

- Vitamin A (present only as retinol) should be less than 100% of the DV
- β-Carotene is contraindicated in smokers
- Calcium should be at low levels or absent in a multi-Vit/Min

People are more likely to consume excessive amounts of the following nutrients from supplements and fortified foods combined:

- Vitamin A
- Vitamin D
- Iron
- Zinc

With the plethora of fortified foods available, it is quite possible to consume excessive amounts of some nutrients even without taking dietary supplements. Consequently, decisions to use dietary supplements should be made in the context of a typical diet, with special attention to use of foods fortified with vitamins and minerals.

Review Questions

1 *Today there are separate regulations for dietary supplements from the regulations for foods and drugs.*

a. True

b. False

2 *Excess calcium consumed with other minerals inhibits the absorption of some important trace minerals.*

a. True

b. False

3 *Which of the following nutrients are not advised as a dietary supplement (choose all that apply)?*

a. Riboflavin

b. Germanium

c. Biotin

d. Cobalt

e. Calcium

f. Vitamin B$_{12}$

REFERENCES

1. Kurtzweil P. An FDA guide to dietary supplements. FDA Consum 1998;32:28–35.
2. Supplement Business Report 2002. Nutrition Business Journal, Penton Media, 2002.
3. U.S. 103rd Congress. Dietary Supplement Health and Education Act of 1994. Public Law 103–417. [http://www.fda.gov/opacom/laws/dshea.html].
4. U.S. Food and Drug Administration, Center for Food Safety and Applied Nutrition. Dietary Supplement Health and Education Act of 1994. December 1, 1995. [http://www.cfsan.fda.gov/~dms/dietsupp.html].
5. Fletcher RH, Fairfield KM. Vitamins for chronic disease prevention in adults: clinical applications. JAMA 2002;287(23):3127–3129.

6. Fairfield KM, Fletcher RH. Vitamins for chronic disease prevention in adults: scientific review. JAMA 2002;287(23):3116–3126.

7. Drewnowski A, Shultz JM. Impact of aging on eating behaviors, food choices, nutrition, and health status. J Nutr Health Aging 2001;5(2):75–79.

8. Bidlack WR, Smith CH. Nutritional requirements of the aged. Crit Rev Food Sci Nutr 1988;27(3):189–218.

9. Gunderson EP. Nutrition during pregnancy for the physically active woman. Clin Obstet Gynecol 2003;46(2):390–402.

10. Food and Nutrition Board, Institute of Medicine. Dietary Reference Intakes for Calcium, Phosphorus, Magnesium, Vitamin D, and Fluoride. Washington, DC: National Academy Press, 1997.

11. Food and Nutrition Board, Institute of Medicine. Dietary Reference Intakes for Thiamin, Riboflavin, Niacin, Vitamin B-6, Folate, Vitamin B-12, Pantothenic Acid, Biotin, and Choline. Washington, DC: National Academy Press, 1998.

12. Food and Nutrition Board, Institute of Medicine. Dietary Reference Intakes for Vitamin C, Vitamin E, Selenium, and Carotenoids. Washington, DC: National Academy Press, 2000.

13. Food and Nutrition Board, Institute of Medicine. Dietary Reference Intakes for Vitamin A, Vitamin K, Arsenic, Boron, Chromium, Copper, Iodine, Iron, Manganese, Molybdenum, Nickel, Silicon, Vanadium, and Zinc. Washington, DC: National Academy Press, 2001.

14. Food and Nutrition Board, Institute of Medicine. Dietary Reference Intakes for Energy, Carbohydrate, Fiber, Fat, Fatty Acids, Cholesterol, Protein, and Amino Acids. (prepublication copy/uncorrected proofs) Washington, DC: National Academy Press, 2002.

15. Food and Nutrition Board, Institute of Medicine. Dietary Reference Intakes: Applications in Dietary Planning. (prepublication copy/uncorrected proofs) Washington, DC: National Academy Press, 2003.

16. Baggott JE, Morgan SL, Ha T, Vaughn WH, Hine RJ. Inhibition of folate-dependent enzymes by non-steroidal anti-inflammatory drugs. Biochem J 1992;282(Pt 1):197–202.

17. Expert Group on Vitamins and Minerals. Safe Upper Levels for Vitamins and Minerals. Food Standards Agency, United Kingdom, May 2003. [http://www.foodstandards.gov.uk/multimedia/pdfs/vitmin2003.pdf].

18. Feskanich D, Singh V, Willett WC, Colditz GA. Vitamin A intake and hip fractures among post-menopausal women. JAMA 2002;287(1):47–54.

19. Albanes D, Heinonen OP, Taylor PR, et al. Alpha-tocopherol and beta-carotene supplements and lung cancer incidence in the Alpha-Tocopherol, Beta-Carotene Cancer Prevention Study: effects of baseline characteristics and study compliance. J Natl Cancer Inst 1996;88:1560–1570.

20. Pryor WA, Stahl W, Rock CL. Beta carotene: from biochemistry to clinical trials. Nutr Rev 2000;58(2 Pt 1):39–53.

21. Omen GS, Goodman G, Thornquist M, et al. The Beta-Carotene and Retinol Efficacy Trial (CARET) for chemoprevention of lung cancer in high risk populations: smokers and asbestos-exposed workers. Cancer Res 1994;54:2038–2043.

22. Cook N, Lee IM, Manson J, et al. Effects of 12 years of beta-carotene supplementation on cancer incidence in the Physician's Health Study (PHS). Am J Epidemiol 1999;149:270–279.

23. Blot WJ, Li JY, Taylor PR, et al. Nutritional intervention trials in Linxian, China: supplementation with specific vitamin/mineral combinations, cancer incidence, and disease specific mortality in the general population. J Natl Cancer Inst 1993;85:1483–1492.

24. Heaney RP, Weaver CM, Fitzsimmons ML. Influence of calcium load on absorption fraction. J Bone Miner Res 1990;5(11):1135–1138.

25. Benton D, Donohoe RT. The effects of nutrients on mood. Public Health Nutr 1999;2(3A):403–409.

26. Risser WL, Lee EJ, Poindexter HB, West MS, Pivarnik JM, Risser JM, Hickson JF. Iron deficiency in female athletes: its prevalence and impact on performance. Med Sci Sports Exerc 1988;20(2):116–121.

27. Carmel R. Current concepts in cobalamin deficiency. Annu Rev Med 2000;51:357–375.

28. Carmel R, Melnyk S, James SJ. Cobalamin deficiency with and without neurologic abnormalities: differences in homocysteine and methionine metabolism. Blood 2003;101(8):3302–3308.

29. Andres E, Kaltenbach G, Noel E, Noblet-Dick M, Perrin AE, Vogel T, Schlienger JL, Berthel M, Blickle JF. Efficacy of short-term oral cobalamin therapy for the treatment of cobalamin deficiencies related to food-cobalamin malabsorption: a study of 30 patients. Clin Lab Haematol 2003;25(3):161–166.

30. Andres E, Perrin AE, Demangeat C, Kurtz JE, Vinzio S, Grunenberger F, Goichot B, Schlienger JL. The syndrome of food-cobalamin malabsorption revisited in a department of internal medicine. A monocentric cohort study of 80 patients. Eur J Intern Med 2003;14(4):221–226.

31. Oh R, Brown DL. Vitamin B12 deficiency. Am Fam Physician 2003;67(5):979–986.

CLIENT INTERACTION AND PROFESSIONAL DEVELOPMENT

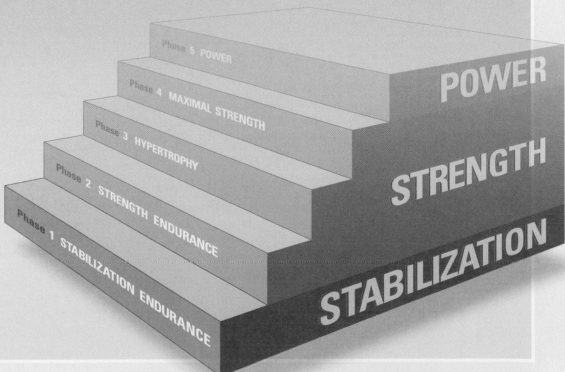

17

Behavior Modification

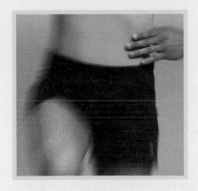

OBJECTIVES

After completing this chapter, you will be able to:

- Describe the five steps to helping clients achieve more.
- Understand positive psychology and the importance of setting goals.

KEY TERMS

Root cause analysis

INTRODUCTION TO POSITIVE PSYCHOLOGY

How To Use the New Science of Success
To Help Clients Achieve More

Successful health and fitness professionals have not only mastered exercise science, they also have a working knowledge of psychology (or the science of behavior and mind). They can keep clients motivated, they understand the psychology of peak performance, and they can help clients make lasting lifestyle changes, both inside and outside the gym. Fortunately, psychology has more tools and techniques to offer health and fitness professionals than ever before. Psychology's century-long, Freud-inspired focus on deficits and dysfunction is increasingly giving way to "positive psychology" (the scientific study of happy, successful, highly achieving people).

This chapter synthesizes the latest research on positive psychology in a very practical way. It presents a straightforward, science-based, five-step process that health and fitness professionals can use to help their clients achieve more. At each step, it offers proven tools and techniques for enhancing performance and facilitating lasting lifestyle changes.

Step One—Vision

THE SCIENCE OF CLARIFYING YOUR ULTIMATE AMBITIONS

Successful people know what they want from life. Their lives are characterized by a sense of passion, purpose, and meaning. Research confirms the physical and psychological benefits of the "vision thing." Those who are certain about what they want to accomplish are up to *six times* more likely to successfully make life changes than those who are less certain.[1] Conversely, those with conflicting goals, or those who are ambivalent about their goals, are significantly more likely to:[2,3]

- Experience depression and anxiety
- Be less happy and less satisfied with their lives
- Have more physical illnesses and doctor's visits
- Be indecisive, uncertain, and rebellious
- Be easily distracted and procrastinate
- Spend more time thinking about their goals
- Spend less time taking action toward their goals

Successful health and fitness professionals, therefore, must be adept at helping clients clarify what they really want, both in and out of the health club. When asking clients about their goals, health and fitness professionals must be able to break through top-of-mind answers, such as "get in shape," that are not helpful to health and fitness professionals or inspiring to clients. They must also be able to "reinterpret" unintentionally misleading responses. Many clients, for example, will say their goal is to "lose weight" and emphasize their need for cardiovascular workouts, when in fact they really want their bodies proportioned differently and need a regimen more focused on weight training. Clarifying a client's ultimate objectives will lead to longer, more mutually satisfying relationships for health and fitness professionals and clients alike.

Helping Clients Achieve More by Helping Them Figure Out What They Really Want

KEEP ASKING "WHY?"

Root cause analysis:
A method of asking questions on a step-by-step basis to discover the initial cause of a fault.

This process, sometimes called **root cause analysis**, helps uncover the true motivations underlying superficial answers. It's simple: just keep asking "why." Consider the health and fitness professional with two new clients, each of whom says their goal is to "lose weight." When asked, "Why?" Bob answers, "So I'll look better." The health and fitness professional may then ask Bob, "Why do you want to look better?" to which he might answer, "So I'll get more dates." When asked why she wants to lose weight, Karen answers, "So I'll have more energy." The health and fitness professional may then ask Karen, "Why do you want more energy?" to which she may answer, "So I can play sports with my kids and go hiking in Peru this summer." In this very simple example, differences in motivation and orientation become clear after asking "why" just twice. The benefits are obvious. The health and fitness professional is now better equipped to customize the fitness programs (emphasizing toning and bulk versus stamina and energy). He can better target the fitness-related articles that he regularly e-mails to his clients. When the going gets tough, he can more effectively motivate clients by reminding them of their ultimate ambitions. He can also communicate the benefits of additional sessions more persuasively. The list goes on.

VISION QUESTIONS

In addition to asking "why," try asking Vision Questions like these:

- What would you try to accomplish if you knew you couldn't fail?
- What would you do if you won the lottery?
- Who are your role models?
- What kinds of experiences do you find so engrossing that, when you engage in them, you forget about everything around you?

A few clients may find questions like these odd, so start by asking permission to pose a few "outside the box" questions, and communicate the proven benefits of the "vision thing."

SUMMARY

Successful people are certain about what they want from life and have grasped the "vision thing." Thus, health and fitness professionals must be able to help clients clarify what they truly desire, both in and out of the health club. This can be done through asking "why?" in a process called *root cause analysis*, which uncovers motivations behind superficial answers. In addition, ask "outside the box" questions about clients' vision. Clarifying a client's real objectives will lead to longer, more mutually satisfying relationships for health and fitness professionals and clients alike.

Step Two—Strategy

THE SCIENCE OF TURNING LOFTY AMBITIONS INTO CONSISTENT ACTION

Success requires a strategy for making one's vision a reality. "Flexible" thinkers who engage in higher-level visionary thinking, as well as lower-level strategic thinking, accomplish more than those who consistently think at either level alone. These "flexible" thinkers also tend to be physically healthier, with lower rates of drug and alcohol abuse.[4] In contrast, a lofty vision without a compelling strategy is associated with perfectionism, procrastination, and labels such as "a hopeless romantic." Properly set, personal goals channel effort, boost motivation, and enhance performance, but perhaps most importantly, they intensify the broader process of strategy refinement. After setting challenging goals, people think longer, harder, and more creatively about how to accomplish them.[5]

The challenge with the goal-setting literature is separating fact from fiction. Consider this goal-setting "study" described by many popular self-improvement experts. The 1953 graduating class at Yale was interviewed, and 3% had written specific goals. When reinterviewed 20 years later, the 3% who wrote goals were worth more, financially, than the other 97% combined. It's a compelling story, with one drawback: this "study" was never conducted.[6] It is a self-improvement urban legend, repeated uncritically, until accepted as truthful. In recent years, the legend has morphed; the best-selling popular fitness manual *Body for Life* recently recounted this legend as the "Harvard" study of goals.

Urban legends get repeated because they convey deeper truths, and there are, in fact, hundreds of real studies documenting the beneficial effects of goals. To maximize performance, it is best to help clients understand and use the six principles of effective goal setting summarized by the acronym *SCAMPI*.

Helping Clients Achieve More by Helping Them Set SCAMPI Goals

SPECIFIC

More than 100 published studies document that specific, challenging goals result in better performance than easy goals, no goals, or simply trying to "do your best."[7] Encourage specific goals based on the number of workouts per week, the amount of time engaging in cardiovascular exercise, and so forth.

CHALLENGING

People who set challenging goals tend to accomplish more than those setting more modest goals.[8] Setting achievable goals at the upper end of a client's ability will inspire more effort, and build more confidence when accomplished.

APPROACH

Client goals should focus on desired ends to move toward, rather than negative states to avoid. Avoidance goals conjure up memories of accidents or failures, and people with many avoidance goals are less happy, healthy, and motivated than others.[9,10]

MEASURABLE

Measuring progress toward goals allows one to ascertain whether the strategy is working.[11] Measurable goals also encourage steady progress by minimizing the tendency to conceptualize success in all-or-none terms, a tendency that leaves clients vulnerable to the "snowball effect" or letting a minor setback "snowball" into a major relapse and a total collapse.[12]

PROXIMAL

Supplementing a long-term vision with near-term, proximal goals leads to better performance, as well as a heightened sense of confidence, determination, and happiness.[13,14] A client who resolves to lose 20 pounds in the next year, for example, should set more proximal eating and exercise goals that can be reached in a week or two.

INSPIRATIONAL

Finally, goals should be inspirational in the sense that they are consistent with a client's own ideals and ambitions. People strive toward inspirational goals with greater interest and confidence, leading to enhanced performance, persistence, creativity, and self-esteem.[15]

SUMMARY

Vision is important. But more important is the strategy to make that vision a reality. Those who think on both levels tend to achieve more and be physically healthier. Strategy (and goal setting) channels effort, boosts motivation, and enhances performance.

There are six useful principles of effective goal setting, summarized by the acronym *SCAMPI*.

- S—Specific goals result in better performance.
- C—Challenging goals tend to accomplish more than modest goals.
- A—Approach to goal setting should be on desired ends to move toward.
- M—Measurable goals let a client know whether the strategy is working.
- P—Proximal, short-term goals raise sense of confidence and determination.
- I—Inspirational goals should be consistent with ideals and ambitions.

Step Three—Belief

SCIENCE OF MINIMIZING FUD (FEAR, UNCERTAINTY, AND DOUBT)

Clients must truly believe that they can implement their strategies and achieve their visions. Belief comes in many "flavors," including self-confidence, self-efficacy, locus of control, and hope. Regardless of the label, the findings are clear: belief is one of the most powerful predictors of change and success. Those who truly believe they will be successful are more likely to:[16]

- Work harder, achieve more, and perform better in many domains (from academics to sports to keeping their New Year's resolutions).
- Be happy, while more effectively tackling problems of depression, anxiety, burnout, alcoholism, smoking, and obesity.
- Set more goals and set them more effectively (in other words, based on SCAMPI principles).
- Persist vigorously in the face of obstacles and view setbacks as a source of motivation.
- Attribute failures to changeable causes (e.g., poor strategies) rather than unchangeable ones (e.g., not being smart enough).
- React better to difficult circumstances, including bad test scores, career setbacks, stressful jobs, paralyzing accidents, and chronic illnesses.
- Use more-effective coping habits, such as humor, regular exercise, and preventive care.

Helping Clients Achieve More by Helping
Them Believe in Themselves

THINK BABY STEPS

Encourage clients to start with modest goals, and increase them in small increments. Remember that goals should be challenging, but attainable.

VISUALIZATION

World-class athletes are routinely trained to visualize performing well in competitive situations, and research suggests that "mental practice" can help everyday athletes as well.[17,18] Visualization must be vivid and detailed to be effective. Envisioning broad ends like "being thinner" or "feeling stronger" may temporarily boost motivation, but greater benefits (reduced anxiety, greater confidence, and enhanced performance) result from envisioning the specific means to those ends.[19]

Of course, one must also visualize proper form and technique. Visualization enhances the performance of elite athletes, but can hamper the performance of novices because they mentally practice the wrong skills (e.g., novice basketball players mentally rehearse poor form in free-throw shooting).[20]

SCHEDULE NEGATIVITY

Many techniques can help clients battle the negative thoughts and attitudes that often undermine belief. Suggest "scheduling" negativity, perhaps setting aside time from 8:00 to 8:30 PM for self-doubt. If they find negative thoughts recurring during workouts, they should remind themselves that there will be plenty of time to plague themselves with self-doubt at 8:00 PM. Another variation involves limiting negativity to a very specific location. Although these techniques may seem "out there," research has shown that anxiety can be lessened by limiting it to 30 minutes a day and only in a "worry chair"; similarly, smoking can be reduced by limiting it to an inconvenient and uncomfortable "smoking chair."[21]

SUMMARY

Belief is extremely important for implementing strategies and achieving visions. It is one of the most powerful predictors of change and success. Those who truly believe they will be successful are more likely to be happy, work harder, perform better, set more effective goals, persist in the face of obstacles, handle failure better, and achieve more.

Belief can be fostered by having clients start with modest attainable goals, increasing them in small increments. They should also use vivid and detailed visualizations of success. Visualizing proper form and technique is important too. Finally, it may help to "schedule" negativity or confine it to a specific location.

Step Four—Persistence

THE SCIENCE OF DRIVE AND DETERMINATION

Research confirms the conventional wisdom that successful people work hard, and rebound from setbacks. In short, they persist. People who successfully maintain their New Year's resolutions for 2 years report an average of 14 slips, but they use those setbacks to strengthen their commitment.[22] Persistence is obviously crucial to weight loss, but it drives weight gain as well. The average person gains only 1 pound during holiday season, and only a pound and a half over the course of a whole year. The problem is persistence: weight goes on each year, typically staying on permanently, leading to a 10-pound weight gain in only 7 years.[23]

Helping Clients Achieve More by Helping Them Persist

REWARD SUCCESS

Rewarding oneself for success is a rarely used, but powerful technique for change. It has proven effective in aiding weight loss, smoking cessation, battling depression, boosting self-efficacy, and adhering to prescribed medical regimens.[24–26] It can start as simply as clients treating themselves to smoothies if they work out individually before their next session with you. Increase the goals and rewards gradually. For a more formal system, try the *deposit-and-refund* technique. A client who wants to lose 10 pounds could write a check to a friend for $500. The friend refunds the deposited money at the rate of $50 per pound lost. This self-reward system makes instant gratification a positive force for change ("If I lose just 1 pound, I'll get an immediate reward"), and can facilitate lasting weight loss, even after the formal reward period ends.[27]

FACILITATE NETWORKS OF EXCELLENCE

Those with supportive friends and family achieve more, live longer, and feel happier than those who are more isolated.[28,29] They also exhibit greater persistence, as supportive people close to them reward their progress, help celebrate successes, and aid in recovery from setbacks.[30,31] Encourage clients to ask for support from friends and family. They should also attempt to surround themselves with excellence, perhaps by finding equally committed workout partners (the deposit-and-refund method described above is even more effective when done as a group).[27] This will also encourage clients to publicly commit to goals, which is another potent predictor of success.

HAVE A STRATEGY FOR SETBACKS

Encourage clients to expect success, but prepare them for setbacks. A setback plan might involve identifying a friend to call in the event of a slip. Another technique involves carrying a "reminder card." Smokers who lapse while trying to quit, for example, are encouraged to look at a reassuring card that reads (in part): "Just because you slipped once does not mean that you are a failure, that you have no willpower, or that you are a hopeless addict. Look upon the slip as a single, independent event, something which can be avoided in the future with an alternative coping response."[32]

SUMMARY

Successful people succeed by working hard and rebounding from setbacks. In short, they persist. Persistence can be encouraged by rewarding success. Rewards for change may start out simply and gradually increase as goals do. A more formal system is the deposit-and-refund technique, which is best achieved with friends and groups.

Tell clients to ask for support from friends and family and find equally committed workout partners. Publicly committing to goals is another potent predictor of success. This will aid in persistence, achievement, and happiness. Their supportive network can reward their progress, help celebrate successes, and aid in recovery from setbacks. Although expecting success, clients should prepare for setbacks. To help, a setback plan is useful. The plan might be to call a friend in the event of a slip or to carry a "reminder card."

Step Five—Learning

THE SCIENCE OF MAKING COURSE CORRECTIONS

Clients must learn whether they are persisting in the right direction, and whether course corrections are necessary. The best tool for this type of learning is a process psychologists call *self-monitoring*, which simply means recording aspects of behavior and measuring progress toward goals. Keeping records of eating and exercise habits, for example, is one of the few predictors of lasting weight loss.[33] Similarly, students who keep records of their studying get better grades than those who do not. In clinical situations, self-monitoring has reduced alcohol consumption, smoking, disruptive classroom behavior, nail biting, and even hallucinations![34,35] Simply recording behavior has modest effects that diminish with time, but it can be a powerful performance-enhancing tool when combined with the first four steps of the process.[35]

Recording progress serves as a small reward when clients are doing well and as a gentle, but thought-provoking, punishment when they are doing poorly. It encourages clients to celebrate success and counteracts the natural tendency to overlook progress (as when dieters focus on times they broke their diets, overlooking all their successes). It enhances accountability and keeps clients focused on their ultimate objectives. But most of all, self-monitoring enhances learning by providing feedback on whether a client's strategy is taking her toward her vision, and it makes clear whether course corrections are necessary.

Helping Clients Achieve More by Helping Them Measure Their Progress

USE WHAT YOU ALREADY HAVE

Virtually all health and fitness professionals already record the amount of time clients spend doing cardiovascular workouts, or the amount of weight lifted in various exercises. However, most would admit they could spend more time sharing and discussing this information with clients. Jointly reviewing past data helps clients build confidence by seeing the progress they have made, and helps motivate them to achieve more. Try creating charts and graphs of a client's data that display progress visually. All the data in the world will not help clients if it only exists on a health and fitness professional's clipboard. It needs to get in clients' heads on a regular basis.

GO FURTHER

Encourage clients to take their self-monitoring to the next level by recording progress toward each of their goals on a 0-to-10 scale every day, with 0 denoting no progress and 10 representing outstanding progress. This intuitive technique works with any kind of goal and is ideal for computer graphing.

FOCUS ON "CONTROLLABLE BEHAVIORS"

Initially measure behaviors and avoid tracking physiologic "outcome measures," such as changes in weight, blood pressure, body fat, or medication needs. These measures are obviously important and should be tracked over the long term as appropriate, but they do not change immediately. Clients who measure these variables daily can quickly become discouraged and lose self-efficacy. For clients trying to lose weight, for example, encourage them not to weigh themselves for 2 or 3 weeks after beginning exercise programs.

ANALYZE THE DATA

Analyzing a client's progress data helps them to quickly ascertain which goals they are progressing toward, and which goals require new strategies or additional effort. Examining trends over time may reveal additional patterns such as "weekend snowballs" (or making solid progress toward eating and exercise goals during the week, but letting one slip snowball into periods of inactivity and overeating on weekends). This knowledge enables "course corrections"; on weekends, a client can redouble his efforts to work out, or cook healthy meals at home rather than eat out. Goal-setting software programs enable even more sophisticated analyses with point-and-click simplicity, and simplify the entry of progress data as well.

SUMMING IT UP

True success in life is not rare because of the fact that people are weak or lazy or lack willpower or fear success. Rather, true success is rare because too often people use flawed strategies for success. Across different areas of life, from weight loss to smoking cessation, from academic success to athletic excellence, those who achieve more use the best processes for change. These individuals identify more techniques for change, while using those techniques longer, more frequently, more consistently, and more thoughtfully.[36,37] The process outlined in this chapter synthesizes the most powerful tools for change known to science. Using them with clients, and with yourself, will lead to greater success for all.

SUMMARY

It is important to know whether persistence is paying off, or whether course corrections arc necessary. Self-monitoring (by recording aspects of behavior and measuring progress toward goals) is an excellent way to track this. Clients should keep records of things such as eating and exercise habits and may even want to take self-monitoring to the next level, by recording progress on a 0-to-10 scale every day. These steps encourage celebrating success and also enhance accountability. Clients stay focused on their ultimate objectives and know whether course corrections are necessary.

Health and fitness professionals should share recorded workout data with clients. It may help to create charts and graphs of data that display progress visually. Initially, measure behaviors and avoid tracking physiologic measures, because they do not change immediately. Analyzing progress data helps to quickly ascertain which goals clients are progressing toward and which goals require new strategies or additional effort.

Review Questions

1   *Those who are certain about what they want to accomplish are up to _____ times more likely to successfully make life changes than those who are less certain.*

   a. Two

   b. Six

   c. Ten

2   *Jointly reviewing past workout data helps clients build confidence by seeing the progress they have made and helps motivate them to achieve more.*

   a. True

   b. False

3 *Setting achievable goals at the <u>upper/lower</u> end of a client's ability will inspire more effort, and build more confidence when accomplished.*

4 *Success in life is rare because most people are lazy, lack willpower, or have a fear of success.*

   a. True

   b. False

REFERENCES

1. Heatherton TF, Nichols PA. Personal accounts of successful versus failed attempts at life change. Pers Soc Psychol Bull 1994;20;664–675.
2. Emmons RA, King LA. Conflict among personal strivings: immediate and long-term implications for psychological and physical well-being. J Pers Soc Psychol 1988;54;1040–1048.
3. Van Hook E, Higgins ET. Self-related problems beyond the self-concept: motivational consequences of discrepant self-guides. J Pers Soc Psychol 1988;55;625–633.
4. Pennebaker JW. Opening Up. New York: Morrow, 1994.
5. Latham GP, Locke EA. Self-regulation through goal setting. Org Behav Hum Decis Process 1991;50;212–247.
6. Tabak L. If your goal is success, don't consult these gurus. Accessed at www.fastcompany.com/online/06/cdu.html.
7. Tubbs ME. Goal setting: a meta-analytic examination of the evidence. J Appl Psychol 1986;71;474–483.
8. Latham GP, Locke EA. Self-regulation through goal setting. Org Behav Hum Decis Process 1991;50;212–247.
9. Elliot A, Sheldon K. Avoidance achievement motivation: a personal goals analysis. J Pers Soc Psychol 1997;73;171–185.
10. Singer JA, Salovey P. Motivated memory: self-defining memories, goals, and affect regulation. In: Martin LL, Tesser A (eds). Striving and Feeling: Interactions Among Goals, Affect and Self-Regulation. Mahwah, NJ: Lawrence Erlbaum Associates, 1996:229–250.
11. Becker LJ. Joint effect of feedback and goal setting on performance: a field study of residential energy conservation. J Appl Psychol 1978;63;428–433.
12. Marlatt GA. Relapse prevention: theoretical rationale and overview of the model. In: GA Marlatt, Gordon JR (eds). Relapse Prevention. New York: Guilford Press, 1985:3–70.
13. Bandura A, Simon K. The role of proximal intentions in self-regulation of refractory behavior. Cogn Ther Res 1977;1;177–193.
14. Palys TS, Little BR. Perceived life satisfaction and the organization of personal project systems. J Pers Soc Psychol 1983;44;1221–1230.
15. Ryan RM, Deci EL. Self-determination theory and the facilitation of intrinsic motivation, social development, and well-being. Am Psychol 2000;55;68–78.
16. Bandura A. Self-Efficacy: The Exercise of Control. New York: WH Freeman, 1997.
17. Suinn RM. Psychological approaches to performance enhancement. In: Asken M, May J (eds). Sports Psychology: The Psychological Health of the Athlete. New York: Spectrum, 1987:41–57.
18. Watson DL, Tharp RG. Self-Directed Behavior: Self-Modification for Personal Adjustment. Pacific Grove, CA: Brooks/Cole, 1993.
19. Pham LB, Taylor SE. From thought to action: effects of process-versus outcome-based mental simulations on performance. Pers Soc Psychol Bull 1999;25;250–260.
20. Suinn RM. Psychological approaches to performance enhancement. In: Asken M, May J (eds). Sports Psychology: The Psychological Health of the Athlete. New York: Spectrum, 1987: 41–57.
21. Watson DL, Tharp RG. Self-Directed Behavior: Self-Modification for Personal Adjustment. Pacific Grove, CA: Brooks/Cole, 1993.
22. Norcross JC, Vangarelli DJ. The resolution solution: longitudinal examination of New Year's change attempts. J Subst Abuse 1989;1;127–134.
23. You are what you eat. Psychol Today March/April 2001.
24. Stall R, Biernacki P. Spontaneous remission from the problematic use of substances: an inductive model derived from a comparative analysis of the alcohol, opiate, tobacco, and food/obesity literatures. Int J Addict 1986;21;1–23.
25. Brownell KD, Marlatt GA, Lichtenstein E, Wilson GT. Understanding and preventing relapse. Am Psychol 1986;41;765–782.
26. Epstein LH, Cluss PA. A behavioral medicine perspective on adherence to long-term medical regimens. J Consult Clin Psychol 1982;50;950–971.
27. Jeffery RW, Gerber WM, Rosenthal BS, Lindquist RA. Monetary contracts in weight control: effectiveness of group and individual contracts of varying size. J Consult Clin Psychol 1983;51;242–248.

28. House JS, Landis KR, Umberson D. Social relationships and health. Science 1988;241;540–545.
29. Kaprio J, Koskenvou M, Rita H. Mortality after bereavement: a prospective study of 95,647 widowed persons. Am J Public Health 1987;77;283–287.
30. Cohen S, Lichtenstein E. Partner behaviors that support quitting smoking. J Consult Clin Psychol 1990;58;304–309.
31. Clifford PA, Tan SY, Gorsuch RL. Efficacy of a self-directed behavioral health change program: weight, body composition, cardiovascular fitness, blood pressure, health risk, and psychosocial mediating variables. J Behav Med 1991;14;303–323.
32. Marlatt GA, Gordon JR. Relapse Prevention: Maintenance Strategies in Addictive Behavior Change. New York: Guilford, 1985.
33. National Weight Control Registry. Accessed at http://www.lifespan.org/services/bmed/wt_loss/nwcr/.
34. Kirschenbaum DS. Self-regulatory failure: a review with clinical implications. Clin Psychol Rev 1987;7;77–104.
35. Kazdin AE. Reactive self-monitoring: the effects of response desirability, goal setting, and feedback. J Consult Clin Psychol 1974;42;704–716.
36. Perri MG. Self-change strategies for the control of smoking, obesity, and problem drinking. In: Shiffman S, Wills TA (eds). Coping and Substance Use. Orlando: Academic Press, 1985: 295–317.
37. Heffernan T, Richards CS. Self-control of study behaviors: identification and evaluation of natural methods. J Counsel Psychol 1981;28;361–364.

18

Professional Development

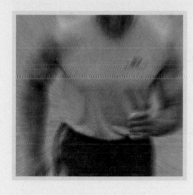

OBJECTIVES

After completing this chapter, you will be able to:

- Provide uncompromising customer service.
- Approach members and find prospective clients.
- Justify the costs of products and services.
- Know how to READ clients.
- Ask for and close a sale.

KEY TERMS

Assessment	Empathy	Rapport

Customer Service

THE PURPOSE OF A BUSINESS

It is often assumed that the primary purpose of a business is to generate a profit. Although profit is a measure for how effectively a business is run, it is not the purpose of the business itself. Rather, the purpose of a business is always to create and keep a customer.

When profit alone becomes the sole focus of the business, the source of that profit (or the customer) becomes neglected, which threatens the future of the business. Conversely, organizations (and individuals) that possess a fanatical customer focus reinvent themselves continually to provide an ever-growing level of value to their customers. Long-term profit generation is largely the result of creating and keeping customers.

The system presented in this chapter provides the health and fitness professional with a progressive, customer-focused process for creating a distinctive level of value and developing a highly successful client base. By mastering the OPT™ model, completing NASM's CPT certification, and applying the tools and solutions learned with clients, you will be able to create or greatly increase your personal level of success.

PROVIDING UNCOMPROMISING CUSTOMER SERVICE

Success depends, to a great degree, on reputation. Those known for excellence and distinction in their profession gain a competitive advantage over everyone else working in the same position.

It is essential to have a strong commitment to excellence, knowledge, and professionalism to be thought of with high regard. The best health and fitness professionals operate with the utmost level of integrity and refuse to settle for anything less than their personal best.

Establish a reputation for being adept as a health and fitness professional, then develop a reputation for uncompromising customer service. *Uncompromising customer service* means being adamant about providing an experience and level of assistance that is rarely, if ever, experienced anywhere else. Develop an obsession for becoming artistic in your approach to helping people.

All buying decisions are based on emotion. Clients have many choices regarding where to exercise. Thus, a client's choice is based on how he or she *feels* about a certain facility and its health and fitness professionals. This feeling is often based on the level of customer service received and that client's perception of the value offered. Those who adapt to uncompromising customer service as the minimum acceptable standard of professionalism will give clients positive feelings. It is clear that relationships are the most powerful competitive advantage in a service profession.

Guidelines for Uncompromising Customer Service

In everyday business, there is a tendency to get caught up in tasks and details. However, it is important to ensure that every moment is adding to clients' experience. Clients should never be thought of as an interruption of work; they are the entire purpose behind it! Keys to embodying this philosophy include:

1. Taking every opportunity to meet and greet each club member at all times, while on or off shift. Every contact is an opportunity to create a professional relationship and, eventually, make a sale.
2. Remembering to represent a positive image and high level of professionalism every minute of the day.

3. Never giving the impression that any question is inconvenient, unnecessary, or unintelligent.

4. Expressing ideas well through verbal communication, vocal tonality, and body language. All of these work together to convey a message.

5. Obsessing on opportunities to create moments that strengthen professional relationships.

6. Not merely receiving complaints, but taking ownership of them.

Successful health and fitness professionals ask themselves: "If my entire future were based on the way this one client evaluated his experience with me right now, would I change anything?" They may also ask, "Did I exceed this client's expectations?" If the answer to either of these questions is "No," committed health and fitness professionals would continue to look for ways to improve themselves. NASM's education, application, integrity, solutions, and tools are the foundation for creating "Yes" answers to these questions and providing optimum performance and results for clients.

SUMMARY

The primary purpose of a business is to create and keep customers. A customer-focused process, using the keys to uncompromising customer service, will create a distinctive level of value and develop success in finding, building, and retaining clients. Establish a reputation for excellence and distinction as a health and fitness professional, then develop a reputation for uncompromising customer service. Leave each club member with a positive impression.

A client's buying decisions are based on how he or she feels about a certain facility and its health and fitness professionals. These feelings are influenced by the level of customer service received and perception of value offered. As such, clients are never an interruption of work, but rather the entire purpose behind it. Each client's experience should be treated as if it affects the entire career of the health and fitness professional because it does.

The Customer

WHO IS THE CUSTOMER?

Clients use the services of health and fitness professionals for a variety of reasons. These range from cosmetic augmentation (appearance) and improved performance (sports-specific) to general health and increased physical capacity in activities of daily living. Whatever their reasons, the motivation is the desire to improve quality of life.

In the past decade, technology has created a lifestyle paradox. Although technology enables people to complete daily activities with greater efficiency, it has replaced everyday movement. This decline has resulted in increased dysfunction and obesity. It is obvious that the need for professional, personalized physical training is increasing. Fitness training can be a luxury, but it is moving toward becoming a necessity. In the very near future, health care will play a pivotal role in the success and growth of the health and fitness industry. NASM's certified personal trainers will be qualified to deliver the OPT™ system and tools, producing remarkable results for clients.

In today's sedentary culture, who is a potential client? Everybody! It is difficult to imagine anyone who does not have a desire to look and feel better, perform at a higher level, be healthier and more confident, enjoy a better quality of life, and reduce chronic pain.

APPROACHING POTENTIAL CLIENTS

Do not be afraid to approach clients. Remember that the health and fitness professional can change the life of a client. Openly provide that service be doing any of the following:

- Say "Hello" to every member while working each shift.
- Offer very active members a towel or water, if the club has it available.
- Roam the floor, clean up equipment, and make sure that the workout floor is impeccable and represents the highest standard of appearance.
- Do not hide behind the fitness desk, a computer, or a newspaper. Be sure to get out there and greet people at the very least.
- Simply introduce yourself by name and ask members for their names as well.
- Let members know that you are there to enrich the club experience, by attending to *any* need. Then, do it!
- By resisting the temptation to educate, your first interaction with a member is professional, pleasant, and most important, nonthreatening.
- During the next encounter, having already met, you will be in a better position to offer valuable assistance. If a member is performing an exercise incorrectly, approach the member and tell him or her about a positive benefit of that exercise. Then, offer to help that person "maximize the exercise." State that you have just attended a seminar or read a book (which should always be true) that offers an alternative to what he or she is already doing. If the member says "No, thanks," leave him or her alone. However, if he or she says "Yes," provide specific help with the exercise and articulate the benefit that the member will receive related directly to his or her goal. Continue to offer him or her assistance throughout the workout.

There are also ways that have been shown to be immediately off-putting to members. Potential clients are very unreceptive to any approach that may challenge their belief systems or judgments regarding an exercise or competencies. Avoid any of the following opening lines:

- May I make a suggestion?
- Can I recommend a better way of doing that?
- Can I show you a different technique?
- Let me show you the right way.
- Can I help you with that?
- What's your goal for that exercise?

CREATING VALUE

The increased need for personal training does not guarantee the success of all health and fitness professionals. Just because people have a need or a desire does not mean that they will take action. In the clients' minds, the value of the service must outweigh the cost. *Cost* refers to the price of the services as well as the time, effort, and commitment involved in training. In addition, individuals may have reservations created by the potential for failure. It is the health and fitness professional's personal responsibility to create and display the value of their services.

To secure a client, the health and fitness professional must use the systematic approach learned in this text to:

- Be excellent at using NASM's integrated fitness assessments (including subjective and objective information) and various movement observations to accurately assess the needs and goals of the individual.
- Have the ability to design an OPT™ training program and correctly fill out an OPT™ template.

- Explain to a client how each component of the program focuses on his or her personal goals and needs.
- Be able to safely demonstrate exercises and implement the program for a client.
- Demonstrate that the OPT™ system offers the highest benefit and explain how a client's needs will be met by it.

Clients need to believe in the health and fitness professionals they choose to work with and trust that those professionals will achieve results. The OPT™ system is a map to success and a systematic approach that ensures results.

SUMMARY

Clients use the services of health and fitness professionals for a variety of reasons, but all with the motivation to improve quality of life. In today's sedentary culture, everyone can be considered a potential client. There are countless people who desire to look and feel better, be healthier and more confident, perform better, enjoy a higher quality of life, and reduce chronic pain. Personal training is moving toward becoming a necessity and health care will soon play a pivotal role in the success and growth of the industry.

However, simply because someone has a desire to do so does not mean that person will take action. The value of personal training services must outweigh their price, time, effort, and commitment. It is the health and fitness professional's personal responsibility to create and display that value. Be proactive about approaching clients. Avoid making members feel uncomfortable by saying things such as, "Can I recommend a better way of doing that?" Instead, do things such as:

- Roaming the floor and saying "Hello" to every member, while offering towels and water and making sure that everything is tidy.
- Introducing yourself and asking members for their names, letting them know that you can help them with *any* of their needs.
- Avoiding educating an individual, at first. However, if a member is performing an exercise incorrectly, find out what it is about the exercise that is important to him or her. Then, offer to help that person "maximize the exercise." Use movement and postural observations for screening and the OPT™ model to customize the exercise and other recommendations. Continue to offer the potential client assistance throughout the workout.

To secure a client, the health and fitness professional must use OPT™ as a map to success and use its systematic approach, which ensures results by:

- Using NASM's integrated fitness assessments and movement observations to accurately assess the needs and goals of the individual.
- Designing an OPT™ training program and correctly filling out an OPT™ template.
- Explaining how the OPT™ system offers the highest benefit and how each program component focuses on personal goals and needs.
- Demonstrating exercises and implementing programs.

The READ System

The READ system was developed by NASM to guide health and fitness professionals through the process of acquiring a new client. Learning the READ system will enable you to be effective in the selling skills described in the previous module.

The acronym READ stands for:

- Rapport—Establishing positive relationships
- Empathy—Understanding what motivates each individual
- Assessment—Identifying the goals and needs of an individual
- Development—Developing the program that best meets those needs

The following text will review these components and give the health and fitness professional guidelines that make getting (and keeping) clients easier, by providing systematic steps and professional tips.

RAPPORT

Rapport: Aspect of a relationship characterized by similarity, agreement, or congruity.

Rapport is the first step in the READ system. In the beginning phases of the relationship between a health and fitness professional and client, interpersonal dynamics are more important than scientific expertise. If trust is established, communication will be open, which enables the health and fitness professional to assess the goals and needs of the client. Only then can the health and fitness professional effectively design a systematic, progressive OPT™ program and help the client reach his or her goals using proven solutions and tools.

Establishing Trust To Build Rapport

How is trust established? It is done by being honest, caring, and effective. Always keep the clients' best interest first and foremost by maintaining integrity and producing results. Once trust is established, rapport can be built.

Effective Communication To Build Rapport

Studies have shown that a mere 7% of the messages that we communicate to others are transmitted by the words we use verbally. Instead, 55% of communication is based on physiology: the way a person stands, whether or not he smiles, degree of eye contact (or lack thereof), and so forth.[1] The remaining 38% of communication is in tone of voice (Figure 18-1). What is said must be consistent with *how* it is said. Incongruent communication is not believable and therefore cannot produce a positive outcome.

People instinctively and spontaneously tend to mirror nonverbal communication patterns.[2] Body language and facial expressions affect emotions.[3] By subconsciously mirroring the physiology of others, a sensory message is sent to the brain, creating a similar emotional state. Therefore, health and fitness professionals who love their work, company, and clients and exhibit the body language that corresponds with these emotions positively affect the people around them.[4] Because all sales decisions are ultimately made on emotion, having this effect on people can open the door to initiating the relationships that a successful career is built on.

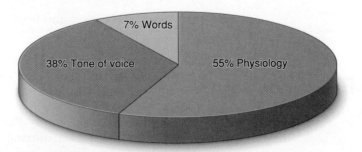

Figure 18.1   The factors affecting communication.

Creating a Presence To Build Rapport

Communication occurs constantly in a way that affects what people perceive. The most positive messages that a health and fitness professional can send (to influence the perception that people have) are represented by level of confidence, enthusiasm, and professionalism.

CONFIDENCE

Confident health and fitness professionals convey an image that it is safe to trust them because they have the experience and expertise to effectively solve problems and produce results. They keep the focus off of themselves and on the needs and goals of the client. Ethical, friendly, knowledgeable, well-spoken health and fitness professionals who have commanding presence provide reassurance to clients that they have made the right decision. This replaces anxiety with excitement.

ENTHUSIASM

In addition to confidence, enthusiasm is one of the primary components of building rapport. Enthusiasm is a positive transfer of emotion that is infectious. When every individual that a health and fitness professional comes in contact with has the impression that he is happy to see them, loves helping them, and is a friendly person, that professional becomes very approachable.

Enthusiasm means that every client should feel that the health and fitness professional is excited about the time spent with him or her and would not rather be anyplace else. The client should feel that the professional looks forward to (and is grateful for) every opportunity to assist him or her with anything.

PROFESSIONALISM

To present a manner that is congruent with the level of professionalism desired, appearance, tone of voice, and articulation are important. Driven health and fitness professionals make sure that they:

- Are dressed and groomed like highly esteemed professionals.
- Stand or sit like someone who is approachable, and do not lean on a wall or piece of equipment, sit back in a chair, or hide behind a computer.
- Smile, make eye contact, greet as many members as possible, and genuinely appear to be friendly, considerate, and happy to see clients.
- Speak clearly and deliberately, with a cheerful tone of voice.
- Feel confident in their ability to deliver OPT™ solutions.
- Truly believe that the OPT™ tools they have will accomplish any goal.

EMPATHY

Empathy: Action of awareness, understanding, and sensitivity of the thoughts, emotions, and experience of another without personally having gone through the same.

The power to positively change lives starts with the realization that it is not *what* an individual wants to achieve but *why* they want to achieve it that motivates. The second step in the READ system is empathy, which involves understanding and identifying with the thoughts or feelings of another person. This is a process of figuratively stepping in the shoes of someone else to understand their thoughts, emotions, and experiences. The process is an excellent way to shed light on a person's motivations. Thus, empathy and understanding the motivation of another person are intimately intertwined.

Motivation

Motivation is based on the forces that affect behavior. Simply stated, motivation is "a reason for doing something or behaving in some way."[5]

PRIMARY EMOTIONS GOVERNING BEHAVIOR

All decisions and actions are the result of motivation. Motivation is directed by thoughts, past experiences, interpretation of events and circumstances, what is valued, emotions, and so on.[6]

There are four essential questions to ask a client in the initial appointment:

1. What are you trying to achieve?
2. How long has this been a goal?
3. What is most important to you about achieving that?
4. What has prevented you from achieving it in the past?

The first question identifies a goal, directing the path along which each aspect of the appointment must travel. For example, a client may say that she would like to lose weight and "tone up." Her health and fitness professional would first conduct an assessment. He would inform her that the assessment will allow him to gather information necessary to individualize each component of her program to the goals of losing weight and "toning up." The health and fitness professional could explain to her how each aspect of the assessment (feet, knee, hip, shoulders, and head) helps to customize solutions that will expedite the rate and degree of changes she will experience. If, after performing the assessment, it is revealed that she has an anterior pelvic tilt and tight hip flexors, the health and fitness professional can explain to her that by individualizing the proper foam rolling and flexibility techniques for her hip flexors, there will be a profound change, increasing the "tone" in her glutes (when combined with the other components of her program).

The second question quantifies the desired result and lets the health and fitness professional know just how important the outcome may be.

The third question reveals the outcome that the client hopes to experience when that goal is achieved. The understanding of this requires empathy and understanding on the part of the health and fitness professional. It is the answer to the third question that determines why the client's goal motivates him or her. This insight is essential to having the most positive influence on a client's motivation and actions. If the client says that she has a reunion coming up and wants to look her best, integrate each component of her program with the motivation that led her to want to train in the first place. For, example: "Karen, balance training is an essential part of your program. Among other important benefits, this portion will help you to burn more calories in one workout, which will give you the potential to lose more weight in less time. So, you'll absolutely look your best in your new dress the night of your reunion."

The fourth question will help the health and fitness professional identify any foreseeable roadblocks or obstacles, and a plan can be implemented to specifically avoid them.

In addition to these questions, work on root cause analysis (explained in Chapter 17) and keep asking "Why?" The follow-up on all of these questions will help in creating a clear strategy that will achieve results.

MOTIVATIONAL STRATEGIES

It is easy to identify which emotions (positive or negative) motivate a client the most. A client may answer the first question by saying, "I want to lose weight." When prompted to answer the second question, she may respond, "Because I'm tired of feeling miserable every time I look in the mirror." She is obviously motivated to alleviate feelings of emotional suffering. However, the client may have responded to the second question by instead saying, "Because I have a family reunion coming up and I want to look great." In that case, she obviously desires to move toward the feeling of satisfaction (success, attractiveness, and admiration).

Typically, individuals who want to alleviate discontent are:

- Motivated by a fear of ridicule, rejection, failure, being unattractive, and so on.

- Motivated by the fear of the situation becoming even worse.
- Directed more by the need to avoid the feared consequences than by the attainment of the desired benefits.

Conversely, individuals who want to experience satisfaction are:

- Motivated by stated benefits.
- Driven by a desire to be better off tomorrow than they are today.
- In search of achievement, recognition, and self-satisfaction.

The bottom line is, those who use the services of a health and fitness professional do so to transform some aspect of their lives from the current state to what they desire in the future.[7,8] It is essential to get to the root cause of why they are retaining the services of a fitness professional to discover how to be of the most assistance to them.

Essentially, clients buy transformational experiences rather than a service.[9] It is the outcome they believe those services will produce for them that matters most. The health and fitness professional who does not empathize with a client will not understand his or her specific goals, nor what motivates that individual. That health and fitness professional without empathy will fail to be able to deliver the desired results or offer any value for his services.

ASSESSMENT

So far the rapport and empathy components of the READ system have been discussed. In the rapport phase of the sale, trust and a relationship were built. By empathizing, goals and the motivation behind them were understood. In the assessment phase of the sale, the objective is to uncover as many of the client's goals and needs as possible to appropriately present benefits and solutions.

The Importance of Questions

Assessment: A process of determining the importance, size, or value of something.

In the **assessment** process, direct focus onto the client and his or her specific needs and desires. The more questions are asked, the more involved a client becomes in the assessment process. In turn, the more involved he or she is in the assessment, the more ownership he or she will feel in the development of a program.[10-12]

It is important to:

1. Ask directive and nondirective questions (discussed below) that follow a systematic thought process to acquire information.
2. Listen carefully to the response. Show care and concern by being involved.
3. Repeat the client's response and paraphrase to ensure a comprehensive understanding of their needs.
4. Take detailed notes to review later.

NONDIRECTIVE QUESTIONS

Nondirective questions cannot be answered with a simple "Yes" or "No." These types of questions are also referred to as *open-ended questions*, which encourage someone to talk and give more information. Nondirective questions (such as "Why?") are perfect to use in root cause analysis. By identifying what a client wants to accomplish, the health and fitness professional can direct every component of a presentation toward the client's goal. Knowing what is most important to a client about his or her goal allows the health and fitness professional to identify the best motivational strategy.

DIRECTIVE QUESTIONS

Directive questions can only be answered with a "Yes" or a "No" response. The purpose of these questions is to establish agreement within the presentation and make sure that it stays focused on the client's goals. These questions reiterate the importance of repeating a client's responses aloud to ensure understanding.

PARAPHRASING

Paraphrasing shows a client that the health and fitness professional is listening and understands what the client is saying, which builds rapport. For example:

> Fitness Professional: Sarah, so what I hear you saying is that losing 10 pounds for your upcoming reunion is your most important goal at this time. Is that right?
> *Client: Yes.*
> Fitness Professional: Wonderful. I can create an OPT™ program that will make that goal easy to accomplish. I am so pleased that we will be working together.

DEVELOPING INDIVIDUALIZED PROGRAM RECOMMENDATIONS

The health and fitness professional's job is to demonstrate how each component of the OPT™ model is related to the client's wants, goals, and needs. Clients care about the integration of knowledge and skills that will solve their problems. Solutions, results, and retention are the products really being sold.

Each component of the OPT™ program must correlate with the solution it provides. To offer compelling solutions, health and fitness professionals must have a superior understanding of the integrated assessments, program design, solutions, and tools that make up the OPT™ model. Visit NASM's Web site at www.nasm.org to learn how to use the program design tools, which have been developed specifically to enhance health and fitness professionals' effectiveness and efficiency in delivering individualized solutions for the clients and prospects.

Features Versus Benefits

Most health and fitness professionals love the technical aspect of what they do because exercise science is the tool of the trade. However, clients are not likely to care as deeply about the technical information (or features). Their focus lies in getting results (or benefits). Health and fitness professionals must focus on benefits that specifically relate to client's goals.

The *features* of personal training programs and products are the number of sessions that they include, what materials come with the product, which assessments will be taken, and so on. The *benefits* are how the features help a client get from where they are now to where they want to be. Every time a feature is explained to the client, be sure to correlate it back to answering his or her mental question: "What's in it for me?" Clearly explain how a feature will help the client reach his or her goals.

> Fitness Professional: Sarah, I am so happy that we are training together. The OPT™ method is a revolutionary training model that will produce great results and get you in shape for your 10-year reunion. You are going to look great!

Once an individual's goals have been identified, use the following chart to correlate each component of the OPT™ program with the features it provides as well as the benefits each component will enable clients to achieve (Table 18-1).

SUMMARY

The acronym READ stands for Rapport, Empathy, Assessment, and Development.

Rapport is the aspect of a relationship characterized by similarity, agreement, or congruity. It is more important in the beginning phases of a relationship than scientific expertise. Establishing trust (by being honest, caring, and effective) opens

Table 18.1

OPT™ Program Features and Benefits

Goal	Component	Features	Benefits
Activities of daily living/quality of life	Flexibility	Improved arthrokinematics Decreased synergistic dominance Decreased relative flexibility Decreased reciprocal inhibition and arthrokinematic inhibition of stabilizers Optimal proper movement and range of motion throughout the kinetic chain	Decreased risk of injury Lowered risk of missing work, quality time with family, etc.
	Core	Inner and outer unit synergy provides proper spinal stability and movement Decreased synergistic dominance provides optimum neuromuscular efficiency, which results in acceleration, deceleration, and dynamic stabilization Attenuation of forces away from spine prevents excessive, uncontrolled intervertebral movement that can lead to injury	Greater core stability results in greater strength Lowered risk of joint injury and greater, easier movement Makes daily activities easier, less strenuous
	Balance	Improved balance and neuromuscular control during all daily activities Controlled instability transference to activities of daily living	Balance, power, and strength are all components of physical capacity, needed to meet the requirements of activities of daily living, with optimum safety and effectiveness
	Power	Develop ability to rapidly change direction and meet demands of activities of daily living	
	Strength	Optimal strength Functional strength Stabilization strength	
Tone	Flexibility	Decreased reciprocal inhibition of target areas Decreased arthrokinematic inhibition of target areas	Permits greater tone in target areas (such as the glutes)
	Core	Proper functioning of inner unit, transversus abdominis, related to "tone"	Potential for greater tone, less circumference in midsection
	Balance	Increased motor unit recruitment	Challenges and helps properly use target areas
	Power	Heightened excitability of nervous system	Potential for greater activation of desired muscles
	Strength	Endurance strength Stabilization strength Core strength	Prepares individual for progression, greater utilization of target muscles
Hypertrophy/strength	Flexibility	Improved length-tension relationships Decreased reciprocal inhibition Decreased arthrokinematic inhibition, which results in intramuscular recruitment	Greater force production and less inhibition of muscles leads to potential for greater growth
	Core	Greater neuromuscular control and stabilization strength is a biomechanically efficient position for the kinetic chain, providing optimal sensory motor integration and neuromuscular efficiency	Increased strength and ability to recruit muscles throughout the kinetic chain

(continued)

Table 18.1

(continued)

Goal	Component	Features	Benefits
	Balance Power	Increased recruitment Optimized activation of prime movers and synergists Optimum neuromuscular control, recruitment, frequency, and synchronization	A muscle can only grow if it is recruited
	Strength	Optimal strength Functional strength Stabilization strength	Greater joint stabilization permits greater activation of muscles and force production
Performance	Flexibility	Integrated flexibility continuum with program design, leading to multiplanar tissue extension, under optimum neuromuscular control, through full range of motion	All components of the program condition client for greater performance and control and reduced risk of injury (in multiple recreational and competitive sports activities)
	Core	Maintaining proper alignment of the kinetic chain during activity allows for proper deceleration of ground reaction force, gravity, and momentum Strength, neuromuscular control, endurance, and power within the lumbo-pelvic-hip complex	Increased strength and ability to recruit muscles throughout the kinetic chain
	Balance	Dynamic joint stabilization during repetitive movement Multisensory training stimulates mechanoreceptors and proprioceptors Controlled instability	
	Power	Develops ability to rapidly change direction and meet demands of sport and all functional activities Increased excitability of nervous system Optimum neuromuscular control, recruitment, frequency, and synchronization	A muscle can only grow if it is recruited
	Strength	Speed strength Relative strength Endurance strength Stabilization strength Core strength Functional strength Optimal strength	Greater joint stabilization permits greater activation of muscles and force production
Fat loss	Flexibility	Enables efficiency of inner unit and cardiorespiratory system	Potential for greater caloric expenditure
	Core	Decreased synergistic dominance enables proper activation of prime movers, increasing caloric expenditure	Increased lean tissue enables the body to burn a greater amount of calories, even when not training
	Balance Power Strength	Increased caloric expenditure Greater caloric expenditure Endurance strength Stabilization strength Core strength	

the lines of communication. This enables the health and fitness professional to assess the goals and needs of the client, leading to the design of a systematic, progressive OPT™ program. Most communication is conveyed by physiology and tone of voice. People instinctively tend to mirror these nonverbal communication patterns, which sends a sensory message to the brain, creating a similar emotional state. Therefore, health and fitness professionals who love their work, company, and clients positively affect the people around them. The most positive messages that a health and fitness professional can send are represented by a high level of confidence in themselves and the OPT™ system, approachability, genuine enthusiasm, and professionalism of appearance, tone of voice, and articulation.

Empathy involves understanding and identifying with the thoughts or feelings of another person, without personally having experienced the same things. Motivation does not come from *what* an individual wants to achieve but *why* they want to achieve it. Empathy and understanding the motivation of another person are intimately intertwined. The four essential questions to ask a client are:

1. What are you trying to achieve?
2. How long has this been a goal?
3. What is most important to you about achieving that?
4. What has prevented you from achieving it in the past?

In addition to these questions, ask "Why?" questions for root cause analysis. Individuals are either motivated by emotions of desire (the desire to experience satisfaction) or fear-driven emotions (the need to alleviate discontent). The answers to the above questions will help to create a clear strategy that will achieve results.

Clients buy transformational experiences. The outcome they believe those services will produce for them is what matters. It is essential to get to the root cause of why a client is retaining the services of a health and fitness professional to discover how to be of the most assistance to that person. This requires empathy and an understanding of motivation to deliver the desired results and offer value for services.

Assessment uncovers as many of the client's goals and needs as possible to appropriately present benefits and solutions. Questions should be asked to get the client involved in the process. It is important to ask directive (yes or no) questions to establish agreement and nondirective (open-ended) questions to get more information. Listen carefully to responses, repeat responses, paraphrase to show the client an understanding of what he or she is saying, and take notes to review later.

Developing solutions is based on demonstrating how each component of the OPT™ model is related to a client's wants, goals, and needs. Solutions, results, and retention are the products really being sold. To offer compelling solutions, health and fitness professionals must have a superior level of technical knowledge about the OPT™ system (to offer features) and understand the client (to offer benefits). Every time a benefit is explained, clearly explain how a feature will help the client reach his or her goals.

Asking for the Sale

SELLING

It is probable that a high level of customer service will, in turn, increase sales of personal training. To the health and fitness professional, that means sales to clients. However, there are many negative connotations regarding sales. Many health and fitness professionals are reluctant to ask for a sale because they associate selling with either rejection or doing something that is ethically wrong.

It is not through manipulation but concern and professionalism that sales are created. There are numerous benefits related to performance, health, self-esteem, and quality of life that can be gained though the health and fitness professional's services, using the OPT™ solutions and tools. The fact is that until a potential client makes a purchase, he or she cannot benefit from these services. The sale is the first essential step to helping a client to achieve results.

10 Steps to Success

Developing clientele depends on how well a health and fitness professional can work the floor. Do not make the mistake of relying on sales consultants to schedule all potential client orientations. That philosophy is dependent on the productivity of someone else and causes health and fitness professionals to give up control of how many presentations they are able to make each week.

Set up a plan based on a desired annual income goal. Use the following 10 steps and corresponding questions to direct the design of that plan.

STEP 1—WHAT IS THE DESIRED ANNUAL INCOME?

An annual income goal is the achievable desired sum total of monthly earnings over 12 months. After clearly identifying a desired annual income, move on to step 2.

Example: Based on her expenses and lifestyle, Christy would like to earn $40,000 annually as a health and fitness professional.

STEP 2—HOW MUCH MUST BE EARNED PER WEEK TO ACHIEVE THE ANNUAL GOAL?

Divide the desired annual income by 50 to figure out what will need to be earned on a weekly basis. (Instead of dividing by the 52 weeks in a year, use the number 50 to allow for 2 weeks of vacation, sick time, jury duty, and so on.)

Example: Christy divides $40,000 by 50, which equals $800. She knows that she will need to earn $800 each week to hit her goal.

STEP 3—TO EARN THE WEEKLY GOAL, HOW MANY SESSIONS NEED TO BE PERFORMED?

To earn the weekly amount, how many clients or sessions are needed each week? To establish this number, take the weekly goal and divide it by the amount earned per session.

Example: Christy divides $800 by $25 per hour. Now, Christy knows that she will need to perform 32 sessions per week to hit her goal.

Also, take the current average number of paid sessions performed weekly and divide it by the number of clients currently signed up.

Example: Christy currently performs 20 sessions per week and has 11 regular clients. She divides and gets a number of 1.82. So, Christy divides her goal of 32 sessions by 1.82 and can now estimate that she needs at least 18 clients to hit her income goals.

STEP 4—WHAT IS THE CLOSING PERCENTAGE?

Health and fitness professionals need to figure out their closing percentage. This number is determined by the total number of people helped on the floor compared with how many of them purchased training packages.

Example: Christy looks back at her contact log and ascertains that she has spoken to 60 members in the last 30 days. Of those 60 members, she managed to sign up 5 of them as clients. When she divides 5 by 60, she sees that her closing rate is 8%.

STEP 5—IN WHAT TIMEFRAME WILL NEW CLIENTS BE ACQUIRED?

Unrealistic timeframes will likely lead to frustration and disappointment. However, if a timeframe is set too far in the future, it will not create the sense of urgency necessary to maximize performance.

> *Example: Since she now has 11 clients and needs to have at least 18 to hit her goals, Christy decides that she wants to gain at least 7 more clients. She decides to set a time frame of 3 weeks to gain 7 new clients.*

STEP 6—HOW MANY POTENTIAL CLIENTS NEED TO BE INTERACTED WITH OVERALL TO GAIN CLIENTS WITHIN THE TIMEFRAME?

Take the desired number of new clients and divide that number by the closing percentage.

> *Example: Christy wants 7 new clients and her closing rate is 8%. She divides 7 by 8% and comes up with 87.5. Christy must have excellent contact with at least 88 members during the next 3 weeks to come close to her goal of 7 new clients.*

Break down the number of members that need to be interacted with overall into weekly increments to make the process more manageable.

> *Example: Christy needs to contact at least 88 members during the next 3 weeks. She divides 88 by 3 and realizes that she has to contact about 30 members each week.*

STEP 7—HOW MANY POTENTIAL CLIENTS NEED TO BE CONTACTED EACH DAY?

Further break down the number of members that need to be interacted with on a weekly basis into daily increments to create concrete goals for each workday.

> *Example: Christy is aiming to contact 30 members each week. She works 5 days per week. So, she divides 30 by 5 and discovers that she only needs to talk to 6 members each day. This is a much more manageable number that she originally thought.*

STEP 8—HOW MANY POTENTIAL CLIENTS NEED TO BE CONTACTED EACH HOUR OF THE DAY?

Once more, break down the number of members that need to be contacted on a daily basis into hourly increments to form easy, solid plans for each hour on the floor.

> *Example: Now that she knows she only needs to approach 6 members each day, Christy divides that number by her actual floor time. She generally conducts four 1-hour sessions each day during her 8-hour shift. She also takes a half-hour lunch and usually conducts one half-hour orientation. That leaves her with 3 hours on the floor to contact her goal of 6 members. Christy now knows that after dividing 6 by 3, she must talk to a member every 30 minutes to achieve her goals.*

For each contact in that hour, provide measurable, personalized assistance that is related to the goal of the person being approached. These contacts, even if they do not develop into sales, add to a valuable future prospect base.

STEP 9—ASK EACH MEMBER SPOKEN TO FOR HIS OR HER CONTACT INFORMATION

The NASM-certified personal trainer possesses core competencies of individualized assessment, OPT™ program design, and exercise selection. These health and fitness professionals automatically have the capacity to provide a personalized, results-oriented experience for any member they make a connection with.

If a good level of rapport has been built with a member, do not be afraid to ask him or her for their contact information. Offer to develop a few exercises to help him or her achieve the goals discussed. Contact the member and arrange a time to assist him or her in implementing the new exercises during his or her next visit to the club.

STEP 10—FOLLOW UP

It should be clear by now that every exercise is an assessment. Regardless of the exercise that a member was doing on the floor, write down what you saw according to the five kinetic chain checkpoints in general movement and postural observations. Write and keep detailed notes on each member.

Within 24 hours, mail the member a hand-written thank-you card for the time they spent with you in the club. This is classy and considerate, causing members to remember a specific health and fitness professional.

Give the card 2 to 3 days to arrive, and then call the member 1 week from initial contact. During the call, work toward the following goals:

- Make sure the member got the card.
- Thank him or her personally for his or her time.
- Let the member know that you have thought about his or her goals and would like to go over some exercises that will be helpful.
- Be clear that it will only take about 10 minutes the next time he or she is in the club.
- Determine the next time he or she is coming to the club.
- Schedule an informal appointment during his or her next visit.

When you see the member again, be sure to:

- Implement a couple of the exercises on the floor and explain how they relate to the member's goal.
- Offer the member a more-thorough assessment, an individualized program design, and a single training session to maximize the results he or she is currently seeing.
- Directly ask the member to sign up for a package of sessions.

Asking for the Sale

Most sales are lost because they are not asked for. Failure to close a sale comes down to one or more of the following four reasons:

1. There was not enough value built into the sale.
2. An insufficient level of rapport makes the potential client hesitant to go ahead.
3. The health and fitness professional did not affirmatively ask for the sale.
4. The potential client legitimately does not have the ability to pay.

The first three can be directly controlled. Many health and fitness professionals are able to offer high value and have outstanding personalities, but do not ask for the sale because they fear rejection.

After following the above 10 steps and then directly asking for the sale, 9 of 10 members will say, "No." That may seem incredibly discouraging. However, even with a 10% closing ratio, thousands of health and fitness professionals in the industry have been able to develop a steady clientele. If the health and fitness professional has established rapport, had empathy for why the client's goals are important to him or her, conducted a thorough assessment, and made the right program recommendations, then rejection is considerably less likely. For example:

Fitness Professional: Sarah, we have outlined what is most important to you and developed the OPT™ program to get you there. Let's go through the OPT™ template and I'll explain all the parts to you. Ask me any questions that come up. Once you feel like you understand it, let's get started today.

When a potential client says "Yes" to a product, program, or personal training package, go through the following steps:

1. Finish the sales transaction.
2. Schedule the client's first appointment within 48 hours.
3. Send the client a thank-you card within 24 hours.
4. Call to confirm before the first appointment.
5. Go over the client's goals again and briefly reiterate how he or she will achieve those goals.
6. Congratulate the client and acknowledge him or her for taking the first step in achieving his or her goals.

If a potential client declines to take the appointment or purchase services:

- Remain professional and helpful.
- Thank the potential client for participating in the session.
- Make sure to have the potential client's contact information.
- Ask to call him or her in a couple of weeks to check on program status.
- Send a thank-you card immediately.
- Schedule a follow-up call in 14 days in a daily planner.
- Every 30 days, send information that pertains to the potential client's goals (such as pertinent points from article clippings, trade journals, fitness Web sites, and so forth).
- Make sure to follow through on all of the above tasks.
- Keep a record of all points of contact.

Successful health and fitness professionals keep in consistent contact. They understand that a "No" today is not a "No" indefinitely. They realize that contacts equal opportunity and that the more contacts they make, the more opportunity they will have to change lives. Finally, these individuals know that the greater the number of people who consider them "expert" resources, the larger their referral base will be.

SUMMARY

Health and fitness professionals must work the floor and greet members to develop rapport, build relationships, and eventually close sales. Use the 10-step plan to work toward an overall goal:

1. Choose a desired annual income.
2. Determine how much must be earned per week to achieve the annual goal.
3. Figure out how many sessions need to be performed to earn the weekly goal (and how many clients are needed for those sessions).
4. Calculate closing percentage.
5. Decide in what timeframe new clients will be acquired.
6. Determine the number of potential clients that need to be interacted with overall to gain clients within the timeframe. Figure out a weekly contact rate based on that number.
7. Break down the weekly contact rate into daily increments.
8. Further break down the daily contact rate into the number of hourly contacts.
9. Ask each contact for his or her contact information.

10. Follow up with a thank-you card and a call, and schedule an informal appointment during the member's next visit.

Most sales are lost, because they are not asked for. The sale is the first essential step to helping a client benefit from the health and fitness professional's services. Rejection is much less likely when the health and fitness professional has established rapport, built a relationship, had empathy for why the client's goals are important to him or her, conducted a thorough assessment, and made the right OPT™ program recommendations. Whether a potential client says "Yes" or "No" to a product, it is important to remain professional and helpful, get the potential client's contact information, send out a thank-you card immediately, call to check in, stay in contact, make sure to follow through, and finally, keep a record of all points of contact. A "No" today is not a "No" indefinitely. Having a large base of people who consider a health and fitness professional an "expert" resource will surely increase his or her referral base. More contacts create more opportunities.

Review Questions

1 *What are most buying decisions based on?*

a. Price

b. Emotion

c. Recommendation

2 *In the client's mind, the value of a health and fitness professional's services must outweigh their cost.*

a. True

b. False

3 *What percentage of communication is based on physiology?*

a. 7

b. 38

c. 55

REFERENCES

1. Richardson J. The Magic of Rapport: How You Can Gain Personal Power in Any Situation. Miami Beach, FL: Meta Publishing, 1987.
2. Gray P. Psychology, 2nd ed. New York: Worth Publishers, 1994:234–236.
3. Ekman P. Facial expressions of emotion: new findings, new questions. Psychol Sci 102–105.
4. Goleman D, Boyatzis R, McKee A. Primal Leadership: Realizing the Power of Emotional Intelligence. Boston: Harvard Business School Press, 2002.
5. Encarta World English Dictionary; 2000.
6. Kassin S. Psychology, 3rd ed. New York: Prentice-Hall, 2001:299–325.
7. O'Connor J. Leading With NLP: Essential Leadership Skills for Influencing and Managing People. Thorstons Publishers, 1999.
8. Aristotle. Nicomachean Ethics: Book One; the Highest Good: Happiness. Classics of Western Philosophy, 4th ed. Indianapolis: Hackett Publishing. 1977:277–281.
9. Pine J, Gilmore JH. The Experience Economy; Work Is Theatre and Every Business Is a Stage. Boston: Harvard Business School Press, 1999.
10. Tracy B. The Psychology of Selling (audiocassette). Illinois: Nightingale Content, 1985:Cassette 4, tracks 7, 8.
11. Rackham N. Spin Selling. New York: McGraw-Hill, 1988:14–17.
12. Jolles RL. Customer Centered Selling; Eight Steps to Success From the World's Best Sales Force. New York: Fireside Publishers, 2000:91–101.

Glossary

A

A-Band: The region of the sarcomere where myosin filaments are predominantly seen with minor overlap of the actin filaments.

Abduction: A movement in the frontal plane away from the midline of the body.

Acceleration: When a muscle exerts more force than is being placed on it, the muscle will shorten. Also known as a concentric contraction or force production.

Acidosis: The accumulation of excessive hydrogen that causes increased acidity of the blood and muscle.

Actin: One of the two major myofilaments, actin is the "thin" filament that acts along with myosin to produce muscular contraction.

Action Potential: Nerve impulse that allows neurons to transmit information.

Active Flexibility: The ability of agonists and synergists to move a limb through the full range of motion while their functional antagonist is being stretched.

Active Stretching: The process of using agonists and synergists to dynamically move the joint into a range of motion.

Acute Variables: Important components that specify how each exercise is to be performed.

Adaptive: Capable of changing for a specific use.

Adduction: Movement in the frontal plane back toward the midline of the body.

Adenosine Triphosphate (ATP): Energy storage and transfer unit within the cells of the body.

Adequate Intake (AI): A recommended average daily nutrient intake level, based on observed (or experimentally determined) approximations or estimates of nutrient intake that are assumed to be adequate for a group (or groups) of healthy people. This measure is used when an RDA cannot be determined.

Advanced Stage: The second stage of the dynamic pattern perspective theory when learners gain the ability to alter and manipulate the movements more efficiently to adapt to environmental changes.

Aerobic: Activities requiring oxygen.

Afferent Neurons: (Also known as sensory neurons.) They gather incoming sensory information from the environment and deliver it to the central nervous system.

Agility: The ability to accelerate, decelerate, stabilize, and change direction quickly, while maintaining proper posture.

Agonist: Muscles that are the primary movers in a joint motion. Also known as prime movers.

Alarm Reaction Stage: The first stage of the GAS, the initial reaction to a stressor.

Altered Reciprocal Inhibition: The concept of muscle inhibition, caused by a tight agonist, which inhibits its functional antagonist.

Amortization Phase: The electromechanical delay a muscle experiences in the transition from eccentric (reducing force and storing energy) to concentric (producing force) muscle action.

Anaerobic: Activities that do not require oxygen.

Anaerobic Threshold: The point during high-intensity activity when the body can no longer meet its demand for oxygen and anaerobic metabolism predominates; also called lactate threshold.

Anatomic Locations: Refers to terms that describe locations on the body.

Annual Plan: Generalized training plan that spans 1 year to show when the client will progress between phases.

Antagonist: Muscles that act in direct opposition to agonists (prime movers).

Anterior: Refers to a position on the front or toward the front of the body.

Aortic Semilunar Valve: Controls blood flow from the left ventricle to the aorta going to the entire body.

Appendicular Skeleton: The portion of the skeletal system that includes the upper and lower extremities.

Arteries: Vessels that transport blood away from the heart.

Arterioles: Medium-sized arteries that further divide into smaller arteries.

Arthritis: Chronic inflammation of the joints.

Arthrokinematics: The motions of joints in the body.

Arthrokinetic Dysfunction: A biomechanical and neuromuscular dysfunction in which forces at the joint are altered, resulting in abnormal joint movement and proprioception.

Arthrokinetic Inhibition: The neuromuscular phenomenon that occurs when a joint dysfunction inhibits the muscles that surround the joint.

Articulation: Junctions of bones, muscles, and connective tissue at which movement occurs. Also known as a joint.

Assessment: A process of determining the importance, size, or value of something.

Association Stage: Fitt's second stage in which learners become more consistent with their movement with practice.

Atherosclerosis: Clogging, narrowing, and hardening of the body's large arteries and medium-sized blood vessels. Atherosclerosis can lead to stroke, heart attack, eye problems, and kidney problems.

Atmospheric Pressure: Everyday pressure in the air.

Atrioventricular Valves: Allow for proper blood flow from the atria to the ventricles.

Atrium: A smaller chamber located superiorly on either side of the heart.

Augmented Feedback: Information provided by some external source such as a fitness professional, videotape, or a heart rate monitor.

Autogenic Inhibition: The process when neural impulses sensing tension are greater than the impulses causing muscle contraction. Stimulation of the Golgi tendon organ overrides the muscle spindle.

Autonomous Stage: Fitt's third stage of motor learning in which the learner has refined the skill to a level of automation.

Axial Skeleton: The portion of the skeletal system that consists of the skull, rib cage, and vertebral column.

Axon: A cylindric projection from the cell body that transmits nervous impulses to other neurons or effector sites.

B

Balance: The ability to sustain or return the body's center of mass or line of gravity over its base of support.

Ball-and-Socket Joint: Most-mobile joints that allow motion in all three planes. Examples would include the shoulder and hip.

Basal Ganglia: A portion of the lower brain that is instrumental in the initiation and control of repetitive voluntary movements such as walking and running.

Bicuspid (Mitral) Valve: Two cusps control the blood flow from the left atrium to the left ventricle.

Bioenergetic Continuum: Three main pathways used by the kinetic chain to produce ATP.

Bioenergetics: The study of energy in the human body.

Biomechanics: The study of mechanics in the human body.

Bipenniform Muscle Fibers: Muscle fibers that are arranged with short, oblique fibers that extend from both sides of a long tendon. An example would be the rectus femoris.

Blood Vessels: Form a closed circuit of hollow tubes that allow blood to be transported to and from the heart.

Brainstem: The link between the sensory and motor nerves coming from the brain to the body and vice versa.

C

Calories: The energy contained in food, measured in kilocalories, often described simply as calories. A unit of measurement of heat. The amount of heat required to raise the temperature of 1 gram of water by 1°C.

Cancer: Any of various types of malignant neoplasms, most of which invade surrounding tissues, may metastasize to several sites, and are likely to recur after attempted removal and to cause death of the patient unless adequately treated.

Capillaries: Arterioles that branch out into a multitude of microscopic vessels.

Carbohydrate: Organic compounds of carbon, hydrogen, and oxygen, which include starches, cellulose, and sugars, and are an important source of energy. All carbohydrates are eventually broken down in the body to glucose, a simple sugar.

Cardiac Muscle: Heart muscle.

Cardiac Output ($\dot{Q}$): Heart rate × stroke volume, the overall performance of the heart.

Cardiorespiratory (CR) System: The combination of the cardiovascular and respiratory systems that provides the tissues of the kinetic chain with oxygen, nutrients, protective agents, and a means to remove waste byproducts.

Cardiorespiratory Training: Any physical activity that involves and places stress on the cardiorespiratory system.

Cardiovascular Control Center (CVC): Directs impulses that will either increase or decrease cardiac output and peripheral resistance based on feedback from all structures involved.

Cardiovascular System: The system composed of the heart, blood vessels, and blood.

Cell Body: The portion of the neuron that contains the nucleus, lysosomes, mitochondria, and a Golgi complex.

Central Controller: Controls heart rate, left ventricular contractility, and arterial blood pressure by manipulating the sympathetic and parasympathetic nervous systems.

Central Nervous System: The portion of the nervous system that consists of the brain and spinal cord.

Cerebellum: A portion of the lower brain that compares sensory information from the body and the external environment with motor information from the cerebral cortex to ensure smooth coordinated movement.

Cerebral Cortex: A portion of the central nervous system that consists of the frontal lobe, parietal lobe, occipital lobe, and temporal lobe.

Cervical Spine: The area of the spine containing the seven vertebrae that compose the neck.

Chain: A system that is linked together or connected.

Chemoreceptors: Sensory receptors that respond to chemical interaction (smell and taste).

Circuit Training System: This consists of a series of exercises that an individual performs one after another with minimal rest.

Co-contraction: Muscles contract together in a force-couple.

Cognitive Stage: Fitt's first stage of motor learning that describes how the learner spends much of the time thinking about what they are about to perform.

Collagen: A protein that is found in connective tissue that provides tensile strength. Collagen, unlike elastin, is not very elastic.

Compound-Sets: Involve the performance of two exercises for antagonistic muscles. For example a set of bench presses followed by cable rows (chest/back).

Concentric: When a muscle exerts more force than is being placed on it, the muscle will shorten. Also known as acceleration or force production.

Conduction Passageway: Consists of all the structures that air travels through before entering the respiratory passageway.

Condyles: Projections protruding from the bone to which muscles, tendons, and ligaments can attach. Also known as a process, epicondyle, tubercle, and trochanter.

Condyloid Joint: A joint where the condyle of one bone fits into the elliptical cavity of another bone to form the joint. An example would include the knee joint.

Contralateral: Refers to a position on the opposite side of the body.

Controlled Instability: Training environment that is as unstable as can safely be controlled by an individual.

Core: The center of the body and the beginning point for movement. Refers to the lumbo-pelvic-hip complex, thoracic spine, and cervical spine.

Core Strength: The ability of the lumbo-pelvic-hip complex musculature to control an individual's constantly changing center of gravity.

Coronal Plane: An imaginary plane that bisects the body to create front and back halves. Also known as the frontal plane.

Corrective Exercise Training (CET): The first phase of the OPT model is designed to correct muscle imbalances, joint dysfunctions, neuromuscular deficits, and postural distortion patterns. It is also designed to recondition each individual and improve total kinetic chain structural integrity.

Corrective Flexibility: Designed to improve muscle imbalances and altered arthrokinematics.

Creatine Phosphate: A high-energy phosphate molecule that is stored in cells and can be used to resynthesize ATP immediately.

Cumulative Injury Cycle: A cycle whereby an injury will induce inflammation, muscle spasm, adhesions, altered neuromuscular control, and muscle imbalances.

D

Davis's Law: States that soft tissue models along the line of stress.

Decelerate: When the muscle is exerting less force than is being placed on it, the muscle lengthens. Also known as an eccentric muscle action or force reduction.

Deconditioned: Refers to a state in which a person has muscle imbalances, decreased flexibility, or a lack of core and joint stability.

Dendrites: A portion of the neuron that is responsible for gathering information from other structures.

Depression: A flattened or indented portion of bone, which could be a muscle attachment site. Also known as a fossa.

Diabetes: Chronic metabolic disorder, caused by insulin deficiency, which impairs carbohydrate usage and enhances usage of fats and proteins.

Dietary Supplement: A substance that completes or makes an addition to daily dietary intake.

Diffusion: The process of getting oxygen from the environment to the tissues of the body.

Distal: Refers to a position farthest from the center of the body or point of reference.

Dorsal: Refers to a position on the back or toward the back of the body.

Dorsiflexion: When applied to the ankle, the ability to bend at the ankle, moving the front of the foot upward.

Drawing-In Maneuver: Activation of the transverse abdominis, multifidus, pelvic floor muscles, and diaphragm to provide core stabilization.

Dynamic Functional Flexibility: Multiplanar soft tissue extensibility with optimal neuromuscular efficiency throughout the full range of motion.

Dynamic Joint Stabilization: The ability of the stabilizing muscles of a joint to produce optimum stabilization during functional, multiplanar movements.

Dynamic Pattern Perspective (DPP): The theory that suggests that movement patterns are produced as a result of the combined interactions among many systems (nervous, muscular, skeletal, mechanical, environmental, past experiences, and so forth).

Dynamic Range of Motion: The combination of flexibility and neuromuscular efficiency.

Dynamic Stabilization: When a muscle is exerting force equal to the force being placed on it. Also known as an isometric contraction.

Dynamic Stretching: Uses the force production of a muscle and the body's momentum to take a joint through the full available range of motion.

E

Eccentric: When the muscle is exerting less force than is being placed on it, the muscle lengthens. Also known as deceleration, or force reduction.

Effectors: Any structure innervated by the nervous system, including organs, glands, muscle tissue, connective tissue, blood vessels, bone marrow, and so forth.

Efferent Neurons: Neurons that transmit nerve impulses from the brain or spinal cord to the effector sites such as muscles or glands. Also known as motor neurons.

Elastin: A protein that is found in connective tissue that has elastic properties.

Empathy: Action of awareness, understanding, and sensitivity of the thoughts, emotions, and experience of another without personally having gone through the same.

Endocrine System: The system of glands in the human body that is responsible for producing hormones.

Endomysium: The deepest layer of connective tissue that surrounds individual muscle fibers.

Endurance Strength: The ability to produce and maintain force for prolonged periods.

Energy: The capacity to do work.

Energy-Utilizing: When energy is gathered from an energy-yielding source by some storage unit (ATP) and then transferred to a site that can use this energy.

Enjoyment: The amount of pleasure derived from performing a physical activity.

Epicondyle: Projections protruding from the bone to which muscles, tendons, and ligaments can attach. Also known as a condyle, process, tubercle, and trochanter.

Epimysium: A layer of connective tissue that is underneath the fascia and surrounds the muscle.

Equilibrium: A condition of balance between opposed forces, influences, or actions.

Erythrocytes: Red blood cells.

Estimated Average Requirement (EAR): The average daily nutrient intake level that is estimated to meet the requirement of half the healthy individuals who are in a particular life stage and gender group.

Eversion: A movement in which the inferior calcaneus moves laterally.

Excess Postexercise Oxygen Consumption (EPOC): The state in which the body's metabolism is elevated after exercise.

Excitation-Contraction Coupling: The process of neural stimulation creating a muscle contraction.

Exercise Order: Refers to the order in which the exercises are performed during a workout.

Exercise Selection: The process of choosing exercises for program design.

Exhaustion: The result of prolonged stress or stress that is intolerable to a client.

Exhaustion Stage: The third stage of the GAS, when prolonged stress or stress that is intolerable to a client will cause distress.

Expert Stage: The third stage of the dynamic pattern perspective model in which the learner now focuses on recognizing and coordinating their joint motions in the most efficient manner.

Expiratory: Exhalation.

Explosive Strength: The ability to develop a sharp rise in force production once a movement pattern has been initiated.

Extensibility: Capability of being elongated or stretched.

Extension: A straightening movement in which the relative angle between two adjacent segments increases.

External Feedback: Information provided by some external source such as a fitness professional, videotape, or a heart rate monitor.

F

Fan-Shaped Muscle: A muscular fiber arrangement that has muscle fibers span out from a narrow attachment at one end to a broad attachment at the other end. An example would be the pectoralis major.

Fascia: The outermost layer of connective tissue that surrounds the muscle.

Fascicle: A grouping of muscle fibers that house myofibrils.

Fast Twitch Fibers: Muscle fibers that can also be characterized by the term type IIA and IIB. These fibers contain fewer capillaries, mitochondria, and myoglobin. These fibers fatigue faster than type I fibers.

Fats: One of the three main classes of foods and a source of energy in the body. Fats help the body use some vitamins and keep the skin healthy. They also serve as energy stores for the body. In food, there are two types of fats, saturated and unsaturated.

Feedback: The utilization of sensory information and sensorimotor integration to aid the kinetic chain in the development of permanent neural representations of motor patterns.

Flat Bones: A classification of bone that is involved in protection and provides attachment sites for muscles. Examples include the sternum and scapulae.

Flexibility: The normal extensibility of all soft tissues that allow the full range of motion of a joint.

Flexibility Training: Physical training of the body that integrates various stretches in all three planes of motion to produce the maximum extensibility of tissues.

Flexion: A bending movement in which the relative angle between two adjacent segments decreases.

Force: The interaction between two entities or bodies that results in either the acceleration or deceleration of an object.

Force-Couples: The synergistic action of muscles to produce movement around a joint.

Force-Velocity Curve: The ability of muscles to produce force with increasing velocity.

Formed Elements: Refers to the cellular component of blood that includes erythrocytes, leukocytes, and thrombocytes.

Fossa: A depression or indented portion of bone, which could be a muscle attachment site. Also known as a depression.

Frequency: The number of training sessions in a given time frame.

Frontal Lobe: A portion of the cerebral cortex that contains structures necessary for the planning and control of voluntary movement.

Frontal Plane: An imaginary plane that bisects the body to create front and back halves.

Fructose: Known as fruit sugar; a member of the simple sugars carbohydrate group found in fruits, honey and syrups, and certain vegetables.

Functional Efficiency: The ability of the nervous and muscular systems to move in the most efficient manner while placing the least amount of stress on the kinetic chain.

Functional Flexibility: Integrated, multiplanar, soft tissue extensibility with optimum neuromuscular control through the full range of motion.

Functional Strength: The ability of the neuromuscular system to perform dynamic eccentric, isometric, and concentric contractions efficiently in a multiplanar environment.

Fusiform: A muscular fiber arrangement that has a full muscle belly that tapers off at both ends. An example would include the biceps brachii.

G

General Adaptation Syndrome (GAS): A syndrome in which the kinetic chain responds and adapts to imposed demands.

Generalized Motor Program (GMP): A motor program for a distinct category of movements or actions, such as overhand throwing, kicking, or running.

General Warm-Up: Consists of movements that do not necessarily have any movement specificity to the actual activity to be performed.

Gliding Joint: A nonaxial joint that moves back and forth or side to side. Examples would include the carpals of the hand and the facet joints.

Glycemic Index: A ranking of carbohydrate-containing foods based on the food's effect on blood sugar compared with a standard reference food's effect.

Glycogen: The complex carbohydrate molecule used to store carbohydrates in the liver and muscle cells. When carbohydrate energy is needed, glycogen is converted into glucose for use by the muscle cells.

Golgi Tendon Organs: Located within the musculotendinous junction and sensitive to changes in muscular tension and rate of tension change.

Goniometric Assessment: Technique measuring angular measurement and joint range of motion.

Gravity: The attraction between earth and the objects on earth.

Ground Reaction Force (GRF): The equal and opposite force that is exerted back onto the body with every step that is taken.

H

Heart Rate (HR): The rate at which the heart pumps.

Hemoglobin: Oxygen-carrying component of red blood cells and also gives blood its red color.

Hierarchical Theories: Theories that propose all planning and implementation of movement result from one or more higher brain centers.

Hinge Joint: A uniaxial joint that allows movement in one plane of motion. Examples would include the elbow and ankle.

Hobbies: Activities that a client may partake in regularly, but which may not necessarily be athletic in nature.

Homeostasis: The ability or tendency of an organism or a cell to maintain internal equilibrium by adjusting its physiologic processes.

Human Movement Science: The study of functional anatomy, functional biomechanics, motion learning, and motor control.

Hypercholesterolemia: Chronic high levels of cholesterol in the bloodstream.

Hyperglycemia: Abnormally high blood sugar.

Hyperlipidemia: Elevated levels of blood fats (e.g., triglycerides, cholesterol).

Hypertension: Raised systemic arterial blood pressure, which, if sustained at a high enough level, is likely to induce cardiovascular or end-organ damage.

Hypertrophy: Enlargement of skeletal muscle fibers in response to overcoming force from high volumes of tension.

H-Zone: The area of the sarcomere where only myosin filaments are present.

I

I-Band: The area of the sarcomere where only actin filaments are present.

Inferior: Refers to a position below a reference point.

Insertion: The part of a muscle by which it is attached to the part to be moved—compare with origin.

Inspiratory: Inhalation.

Insulin: A protein hormone released by the pancreas that helps glucose move out of the blood and into the cells in the body, where the glucose can be used as energy and nourishment.

Integrated Cardiorespiratory Training: Training that involves and places a stress on the cardiorespiratory system.

Integrated Fitness Profile: A systematic problem-solving method that provides the fitness professional with a basis for making educated decisions about exercise and acute variable selection.

Integrated Flexibility Training: A multifaceted approach integrating various flexibility techniques to achieve optimum soft tissue extensibility in all planes of motion.

Integrated Performance Paradigm: This paradigm states that to move with precision, forces must be reduced (eccentrically), stabilized (isometrically), and then produced (concentrically).

Integrated Stabilization Training (IST): A phase of the OPT model designed to create optimum levels of stabilization strength and postural control.

Integrated Training: A concept that applies all forms of training such as integrated flexibility training, integrated cardiorespiratory training, neuromuscular stabilization (balance), core stabilization, and reactive neuromuscular training (power) and integrated strength training.

Integrative (Function of Nervous System): The ability of the nervous system to analyze and interpret the sensory information to allow for proper decision-making to produce the appropriate response.

Intensity: The level of demand that a given activity places on the body.

Intermittent Claudication: The manifestation of the symptoms caused by peripheral arterial disease.

Internal Feedback: The process whereby sensory information is used to reactively monitor movement and the environment.

Internal Rotation: Rotation of a joint toward the middle of the body.

Interneurons: Transmit nerve impulses from one neuron to another.

Intermuscular Coordination: The ability of the neuromuscular system to allow all muscles to work together with proper activation and timing between them.

Intramuscular Coordination: The ability of the neuromuscular system to allow optimal levels of motor unit recruitment and synchronization within a muscle.

Intrapulmonary Pressure: Pressure within the thoracic cavity.

Inversion: A movement in which the inferior calcaneus moves medially.

Ipsilateral: Refers to a position on the same side of the body.

Irregular Bones: A classification of bone that has its own unique shape and function, which does not fit the characteristics of the other categories. Examples include the vertebrae and pelvic bones.

Isometric: When a muscle is exerting force equal to the force being placed on it. Also known as dynamic stabilization.

J

Joint: Junctions of bones, muscles, and connective tissue at which movement occurs. Also known as an articulation.

Joint Motion: Movement in a plane occurs about an axis running perpendicular to the plane.

Joint Receptors: Receptors surrounding a joint that respond to pressure, acceleration, and deceleration of the joint.

Joint Stiffness: Resistance to unwanted movement.

K

Kinetic: Force.

Kinetic Chain: The combination and interrelation of the nervous, muscular, and skeletal systems.

Knowledge of Performance (KP): A method of feedback that provides information about the quality of the movement pattern performed.

Knowledge of Results (KR): A method of feedback after the completion of a movement to inform the client about the outcome of their performance.

Kyphosis: Exaggerated outward curvature of the thoracic region of the spinal column resulting in a rounded upper back.

L

Lactic Acid: An acid produced by glucose-burning cells when these cells have an insufficient supply of oxygen.

Lateral: Refers to a position relatively farther away from the midline of the body or toward the outside of the body.

Lateral Flexion: The bending of the spine (cervical, thoracic, or lumbar) from side to side.

Law of Acceleration: Acceleration of an object is directly proportional to the size of the force causing it, in the same direction as the force, and inversely proportional to the size of the object.

Law of Action-Reaction: Every force produced by one object onto another produces an opposite force of equal magnitude.

Law of Gravitation: Two bodies have an attraction to each other that is directly proportional to their masses and inversely proportional to the square of their distance from each other.

Law of Thermodynamics: Weight reduction can only take place when there is more energy burned than consumed.

Length-Tension Relationship: Refers to the length at which a muscle can produce the greatest force.

Leukocytes: White blood cells.

Ligament: Primary connective tissue that connects bone-to-bone to provide stability, proprioception, guidance, and limitation of joint motion.

Limit Strength: The maximum force a muscle can produce in a single contraction.

Long Bones: A characteristic of bone that has a long cylindric body with irregular or widened bony ends. Examples include the clavicle and humerus.

Longitudinal Muscle Fiber: A muscle fiber arrangement in which its fibers run parallel to the line of pull. An example would include the sartorius.

Lower-Brain: The portion of the brain that includes the brainstem, the basal ganglia, and the cerebellum.

Lower-Extremity Postural Distortion: An individual who has increased lumbar lordosis and an anterior pelvic tilt.

Lumbar Spine: The portion of the spine, commonly referred to as the small of the back. The lumbar portion of the spine is located between the thorax (chest) and the pelvis.

Lumbo-Pelvic-Hip Complex: Involves the anatomic structures of the lumbar, thoracic, and cervical spines, the pelvic girdle, and the hip joint.

Lumbo-Pelvic-Hip Postural Distortion: Altered joint mechanics in an individual that lead to increased lumbar extension and decreased hip extension.

M

Maximal Oxygen Consumption ($\dot{V}O_2$ max): The highest rate of oxygen transport and utilization achieved at maximal physical exertion.

Maximal Strength: The maximum force an individual's muscle can produce in a single voluntary effort, regardless of the rate of force production.

Mechanical Specificity: The specific muscular exercises using different weights and movements that are performed to increase strength or endurance in certain body parts.

Mechanoreceptors: Sensory receptors that respond to mechanical forces.

Medial: Refers to a position relatively closer to the midline of the body.

Mediastinum: The area where the heart is positioned obliquely in the center of the chest or thoracic cavity lying between the spine posteriorly and the sternum anteriorly and flanked by the lungs.

Metabolic Specificity: The specific muscular exercises using different levels of energy that are performed to increase endurance, strength, or power.

Metabolism: The amount of energy (calories) the body burns to maintain itself. Metabolism is the process in which nutrients are acquired, transported, used, and disposed of by the body.

Mitochondria: The mitochondria are the principal energy source of the cell. Mitochondria convert nutrients into energy as well as doing many other specialized tasks.

M-Line: The portion of the sarcomere where the myosin filaments connect with very thin filaments called titin and create an anchor for the structures of the sarcomere.

Mode: Type of exercise performed.

Momentum: The product of the size of the object (mass) and its velocity (speed with which it is moving).

Monthly Plan: Generalized training plan that spans 1 month and shows which phases will be required each day of each week.

Motor Behavior: The manner in which the nervous, skeletal, and muscular systems interact to produce an observable mechanical response to the incoming sensory information from the internal and external environments.

Motor Control: The involved structures and mechanisms that the nervous system uses to gather sensory information and integrate it with previous experiences to produce a motor response.

Motor (Function of Nervous System): The neuromuscular response to sensory information.

Motor Learning: The integration of motor control processes with practice and experience that lead to relatively permanent changes in the capacity to produced skilled movements.

Motor Neurons: Neurons that transmit nerve impulses from the brain or spinal cord to the effector sites such as muscles or glands. Also known as efferent neurons.

Motor Unit: A motor neuron and the muscle fibers that it innervates.

Multipenniform: Muscles that have multiple tendons with obliquely running muscle fibers.

Multiple-Set System: The system consists of performing multiple sets of the same exercise.

Multisensory Condition: Training environment that provides heightened stimulation to proprioceptors and mechanoreceptors.

Muscle Action Spectrum: The range of muscle actions that include concentric, eccentric, and isometric actions.

Muscle Fiber Arrangement: Refers to the manner in which the fibers are situated in relation to the tendon.

Muscle Fiber Recruitment: Refers to the recruitment pattern of muscle fiber or motor units in response to creating force for a specific movement.

Muscle Imbalance: Alteration of muscle length surrounding a joint.

Muscle Spindles: Microscopic intrafusal fibers that are sensitive to change in length and rate of length change.

Muscular Development Training (MDT): A phase of the OPT model that is designed to improve the cross-sectional area and alter body composition.

Muscular Endurance: The ability of the body to produce low levels of force and maintain them for extended periods of time.

Muscle Hypertrophy: Characterized by the increase in the cross-sectional area of individual muscle fibers and believed to result from an increase in the myofibril proteins.

Myofibrils: A portion of muscle that contains myofilaments.

Myofilaments: The contractile components of muscle, actin and myosin.

Myosin: One of the two major myofilaments known as the thick filament that works with actin to produce muscular contraction.

N

Nervous System: A conglomeration of billions of cells specifically designed to provide a communication network within the human body.

Neural Adaptation: An adaptation to strength training in which muscles are under the direct command of the nervous system.

Neuromuscular Efficiency: The ability of the neuromuscular system to allow agonists, antagonists, stabilizers, and neutralizers to work synergistically to produce, reduce, and dynamically stabilize the entire kinetic chain in all three planes.

Neuromuscular Junction: The point at which the neuron meets the muscle to allow the action potential to continue its impulse.

Neuromuscular Specificity: The specific muscular exercises using different speeds and styles that are performed to increase neuromuscular efficiency.

Neuron: The functional unit of the nervous system.

Neurotransmitters: Chemical messengers that cross the neuromuscular junction to trigger the appropriate receptor sites.

Neutralizer: Muscles that counteract the unwanted action of other muscles.

Nociceptors: Sensory receptors that respond to pain.

Novice Stage: The first stage of the dynamic pattern perspective model in which the learner simplifies movements by minimizing the specific timing of joint motions, which tends to result in movement that is rigid and jerky.

O

Obesity: The condition of subcutaneous fat exceeding the amount of lean body mass.

Obstructive Lung Disease: The condition of altered air flow through the lungs, generally caused by airway obstruction, as a result of mucus production.

Occipital Lobe: A portion of the cerebral cortex that deals with vision.

Optimal Strength: The ideal level of strength that an individual needs to perform functional activities.

Optimum Performance Training: A systematic, integrated, and functional training program that simultaneously improves an individual's biomotor abilities and builds high levels of functional strength, neuromuscular efficiency, and dynamic flexibility.

Origin: The more fixed, central, or larger attachment of a muscle—compare with insertion.

Osteoarthritis: Arthritis in which cartilage becomes soft, frayed, or thins out as a result of trauma or other conditions.

Osteopenia: A decrease in the calcification or density of bone as well as reduced bone mass.

Osteoporosis: Condition in which there is a decrease in bone mass and density as well as an increase in the space between bones, resulting in porosity and fragility.

Overtraining: Excessive frequency, volume, or intensity of training, resulting in fatigue (which is also caused by a lack of proper rest and recovery).

Oxygen Uptake: The usage of oxygen by the body.

P

Parietal Lobe: A portion of the cerebral cortex that is involved with sensory information.

Pattern Overload: Repetitive physical activity that moves through the same patterns of motion, placing the same stresses on the body over time.

Perception: The integrating of sensory information with past experiences or memories.

Periodization: Division of a training program into smaller, progressive stages.

Perimysium: The connective tissue that surrounds fascicles.

Peripheral Arterial Disease: A condition characterized by narrowing of the major arteries that are responsible for supplying blood to the lower extremities.

Peripheral Heart Action System (PHA): A variation of circuit training in which the client performs an upper body exercise followed by a lower body exercise and repeats.

Peripheral Nervous System: Twelve cranial and 31 pairs of spinal nerves that provide a connection for the nervous system to activate different bodily organs and relay information from the bodily organs back to the brain, providing a constant update of the relation between the body and the environment.

Photoreceptors: Sensory receptors that respond to light (vision).

Physical Activity Readiness Questionnaire (PAR-Q): A questionnaire that has been designed to help qualify a person for low-to-moderate-to-high activity levels.

Pivot Joint: Allows movement in predominately the transverse plane; examples would include the atlantoaxial joint at the base of the skull and between the radioulnar joint.

Plane of Motion: Refers to the plane (sagittal, frontal, or transverse) in which the exercise is performed.

Plantarflexion: Ankle motion such that the toes are pointed toward the ground.

Plasma: Aqueous liquidlike component of blood.

Plyometrics: Exercise that enhances muscular power through quick, repetitive eccentric and concentric contractions of muscles.

Posterior: Refers to a position on the back or toward the back of the body.

Posterior Pelvic Tilt: A movement in which the pelvis rotates backward.

Postural Distortion Patterns: Predictable patterns of muscle imbalances.

Postural Equilibrium: The ability to efficiently maintain balance throughout the body segments.

Posture: Position and bearing of the body for alignment and function of the kinetic chain.

Power: The ability to exert maximal force in the shortest amount of time.

Pregnancy: The condition of a female who contains an unborn child within the body.

Preprogrammed: Activation of muscles in healthy people that occurs automatically and independently of other muscles before movement.

Principle of Individualism: Refers to the uniqueness of a program to the client for whom it is designed.

Principle of Overload: Implies that there must be a training stimulus provided that exceeds the current capabilities of the kinetic chain to elicit the optimal physical, physiologic, and performance adaptations.

Principle of Progression: Refers to the intentional manner in which a program is designed to progress according to the physiologic capabilities of the kinetic chain and the goals of the client.

Principle of Specificity: The kinetic chain will specifically adapt to the type of demand placed on it. Also known as the SAID principle.

Processes: Projections protruding from the bone to which muscles, tendons, and ligaments can attach. Also known as condyle, epicondyle, tubercle, and trochanter.

Program Design: A purposeful system or plan put together to help an individual achieve a specific goal.

Pronation: A triplanar movement that is associated with force reduction.

Proprioception: The cumulative neural input from the sensory afferents to the central nervous system.

Proprioceptively Enriched Environment: An environment that challenges the internal balance and stabilization mechanisms of the body.

Protein: Amino acids linked by peptide bonds, which consist of carbon, hydrogen, nitrogen, oxygen, and usually sulfur, and that have several essential biologic compounds.

Proximal: Refers to a position nearest the center of the body or point of reference.

Pulmonary Arteries: Deoxygenated blood is pumped from the right ventricle to the lungs through these arteries.

Pulmonary Capillaries: Surround the alveolar sacs. As oxygen fills the sacs it diffuses across the capillary membranes and into the bloodstream.

Pulmonary Semilunar Valve: Controls blood flow from the right ventricle to the pulmonary arteries going to the lungs.

Pyramid System: Involves a triangle or step approach that either progress up in weight with each set or decreases weight with each set.

Pyruvate: A byproduct of anaerobic glycolysis.

Q

Quadrilateral Muscle Fiber: An arrangement of muscle fibers that is usually flat and four-sided. An example would include the rhomboid.

Quickness: The ability to react and change body position with maximum rate of force production, in all planes of motion, from all body positions, during functional activities.

R

Range of Motion: Refers to the range that the body or bodily segments move during an exercise.

Rapport: Aspect of a relationship characterized by similarity, agreement, or congruity.

Rate Coding: Muscular force can be amplified by increasing the rate of incoming impulses from the motor neuron after all prospective motor units have been activated.

Rate of Force Production: Ability of muscles to exert maximal force output in a minimal amount of time.

Reactive Strength: The ability of the neuromuscular system to switch from an eccentric contraction to a concentric contraction quickly and efficiently.

Reactive Training: Exercises that use quick, powerful movements involving an eccentric contraction immediately followed by an explosive concentric contraction.

Recommended Dietary Allowance (RDA): The average daily nutrient intake level that is sufficient to meet the nutrient requirement of nearly all (97 to 98%) healthy individuals who are in a particular life stage and gender group.

Recreation: A client's physical activities outside of their work environment.

Relative Flexibility: When the body seeks the path of least resistance during functional movement patterns.

Relative Strength: The maximum force that an individual can generate per unit of body weight, regardless of the time of force development.

Repetition: One complete movement of a particular exercise.

Repetition Tempo: The speed with which each repetition is performed.

Resistance Development Stage: The second stage of the GAS, when the body increases its functional capacity to adapt to the stressor.

Respiratory Passageway: Collects the channeled air coming from the conducting passageway.

Respiratory Pump: Moves air in and out of the body.

Respiratory System: The system of the body responsible for taking in oxygen, excreting carbon dioxide, and regulating the relative composition of the blood.

Rest Interval: The time taken to recuperate between sets or exercises.

Restrictive Lung Disease: The condition of a fibrous lung tissue, which results in a decreased ability to expand the lungs.

Rheumatoid Arthritis: Arthritis primarily affecting connective tissues, in which there is a thickening of articular soft tissue and extension of synovial tissue over articular cartilages that have become eroded.

Roll: The joint motion that depicts the rolling of one joint surface on another. Examples would include that of the femoral condyles over the tibial condyles during a squat.

Root Cause Analysis: A method of asking questions on a step-by-step basis to discover the initial cause of a fault.

Rotary Motion: Movement of an object or segment around a fixed axis in a curved path.

S

Saddle Joint: One bone is shaped as a saddle, the other bone is shaped as the rider; the only example is in the carpometacarpal joint in the thumb.

Sagittal Plane: An imaginary plane that bisects the body into right and left halves.

Sarcolemma: A plasma membrane that surrounds muscle fibers.

Sarcomere: The functional unit of muscle, repeating sections of actin and myosin.

Sarcoplasm: Cell components that contain glycogen, fats, minerals, and oxygen that are contained within the sarcolemma.

Self-Myofascial Release: Another form of flexibility that focuses on the fascial system in the body.

Self-Organization: This theory, which is based on the dynamic pattern perspective, provides the body with the ability to overcome changes that are placed on it.

Semilunar Valves: Allow for proper blood flow from the ventricles to the aorta and pulmonary arteries.

Sensation: The process whereby sensory information is received by the receptor and transferred either to the spinal cord for reflexive motor behavior or to higher cortical areas for processing.

Sensorimotor Integration: The ability of the nervous system to gather and interpret sensory information to anticipate, select, and execute the proper motor response.

Sensors: Provide feedback from the effectors to the central controller and cardiovascular control system. They include baroreceptors, chemoreceptors, and muscle afferents.

Sensory Feedback: The process whereby sensory information is used to reactively monitor movement and the environment.

Sensory (Function of Nervous System): The ability of the nervous system to sense changes in either the internal or external environment.

Sensory Neurons: Neurons that gather incoming sensory information from the environment delivered to the central nervous system. Also known as afferent neurons.

Set: A group of consecutive repetitions.

Short Bones: A classification of bone that appears cubical in shape. Examples include the carpals and tarsals.

Single-Set System: The individual performs one set of each exercise, usually 8 to 12 repetitions at a slow, controlled tempo.

Skeletal System: The portion of the kinetic chain that comprises the bones of the body.

Skin-Fold Caliper: An instrument with two adjustable legs to measure thickness of a skin fold.

Slide: The joint motion that depicts the sliding of a joint surface across another. Examples would include the tibial condyles moving across the femoral condyles during a knee extension.

Sliding Filament Theory: The proposed process by which the contraction of the filaments within the sarcomere takes place.

Slow Twitch Fibers: Another term for type I muscle fibers, fibers that are characterized by a greater amount of capillaries, mitochondria, and myoglobin. These fibers are usually found to have a higher endurance capacity than fast twitch fibers.

Specific Warm-Up: Consists of movements that more closely mimic those of the actual activity.

Speed: The ability to move the body in one intended direction as fast as possible.

Speed Strength: The ability of the neuromuscular system to produce the greatest possible force in the shortest possible time.

Spin: Joint motion that depicts the rotation of one joint surface on another. Examples would include the head of the radius rotating on the end of the humerus during pronation and supination of the forearm.

Split-Routine System: A system that incorporates training an individual's body parts with a high volume on separate days.

Stability: The ability of the body to maintain postural equilibrium and support joints during movement.

Stabilization Endurance: The ability of the stabilization mechanisms of the kinetic chain to sustain proper levels of stabilization to allow for prolonged neuromuscular efficiency.

Stabilization Strength: Ability of the stabilizing muscles to provide dynamic joint stabilization and postural equilibrium during functional activities.

Stabilizer: Muscles that support or stabilize the body while the prime movers and the synergists perform the movement patterns.

Starting Strength: The ability to produce high levels of force at the beginning of a movement.

Static Stretching: Passively taking a muscle to the point of tension and holding the stretch for 20 seconds.

Strength: The ability of the neuromuscular system to provide internal tension and exert force against external resistance.

Strength Endurance: The ability of the body to repeatedly produce high levels of force for prolonged periods.

Stroke Volume (SV): The amount of blood that is pumped out with each contraction of a ventricle.

Structural Efficiency: The structural alignment of the muscular and skeletal systems that allows the body to be balanced in relation to its center of gravity.

Subjective: Information that is provided by a client.

Sucrose: Often referred to as table sugar, it is a molecule made up of glucose and fructose.

Sulcus: A groove in a bone that allows a soft structure to pass through.

Superior: Refers to a position above a reference point.

Superset System: Uses a couple of exercises performed in rapid succession of one another.

Supination: A triplanar motion that is associated with force production.

Supine: Lying on one's back.

Synarthrosis Joint: A joint without any joint cavity and fibrous connective tissue. Examples would include the sutures of the skull and the symphysis pubis.

Synergist: Muscles that assist prime movers during functional movement patterns.

Synergistic Dominance: When synergists take over function for a weak or inhibited prime mover.

Synovial Joints: This type of joint is characterized by the absence of fibrous or cartilaginous tissue connecting the bones. Examples include the ball-and-socket joint, the hinge joint, and the saddle joint.

T

Temporal Lobe: A portion of the cerebral cortex that deals with hearing.

Tendon: Connective tissue that attaches muscle to bone and provides an anchor for muscles to exert force.

Tendonitis: An inflammation in a tendon or the tendon covering.

Thoracic Spine: The 12 vertebrae in mid torso that are attached to the rib cage.

Time: The length of time an individual is engaged in a given activity.

Tolerable Upper Intake Level (UL): The highest average daily nutrient intake level likely to pose no risk of adverse health effects to almost all individuals in a particular life stage and gender group. As intake increases above the UL, the potential risk of adverse health effects increases.

Torque: The ability of any force to cause rotation around an axis.

Training Duration: The time frame from the start of the workout to the finish.

Training Frequency: The number of training sessions that are conducted during a given period.

Training Intensity: An individual's level of effort compared with their maximum effort.

Training Plan: The specific outline, created by a health and fitness professional to meet a client's goals, that details the form of training, length of time, future changes, and specific exercises to be performed.

Training Volume: The total amount of work performed within a specified time period.

Transfer-of-Training Effect: The more similar the exercise is to the actual activity, the greater the carryover into real-life settings.

Transverse Plane: An imaginary plane that bisects the body to create upper and lower halves.

Tricuspid Valve: Controls the blood flow from the right atrium to the right ventricle.

Tri-Sets System: A system very similar to supersets, the difference being three exercises back to back to back with little to no rest in between.

Trochanter: Projections protruding from the bone to which muscles, tendons, and ligaments can attach. Also known as a condyle, process, tubercle, and epicondyle.

Tubercle: Projections protruding from the bone to which muscles, tendons, and ligaments can attach. Also known as a condyle, process, epicondyle, and trochanter.

Type: The type or mode of physical activity that an individual is engaged in.

U

Unipenniform Muscle Fiber: Muscle fibers that are arranged with short, oblique fibers that extend from one side of a long tendon. An example would include the tibialis posterior.

Upper-Extremity Postural Distortion: An individual who exhibits a forward head, rounded shoulder posture.

V

Veins: Vessels that transport blood back to the heart.

Ventilation: The actual process of moving air in and out of the body.

Ventral: Refers to a position on the front or toward the front of the body.

Ventricles: Larger chambers located inferiorly on either side of the heart.

Venules: Vessels that collect blood from the capillaries.

Vertical Loading: A circuit style of training that involves a series of exercises being performed in succession.

$\dot{V}O_2$ Max: The highest volume of oxygen a person can consume during exercise. Often used as a predictor of potential in endurance sports.

W

Weekly Plan: Training plan of specific workouts that spans 1 week to show which exercises are required each day of the week.

Appendix

Cardiopulmonary Resuscitation (CPR)

WHEN TO PERFORM CPR

CPR is indicated in a person who is not breathing (or, is "apneic") and has no pulse. Adult CPR is administered to any person 8 years of age or older. Children are classified as 1 to 8 years of age and infants are 0 to 1 years of age. There are differences in the application and procedures of adult, child, and infant CPR. This is why instruction on the techniques of CPR is vital to its efficient and effective execution. If the rescuer has difficulty in remembering the steps in CPR, frequently dispatchers can provide this information, as well as what to do in special circumstances.

CPR starts with recognition of the emergency and then ensuring your own personal safety. Always survey the surroundings for existing hazards *before* helping someone. Any time blood or body fluids could be present, use appropriate infection-control techniques (gloves, masks, eyewear, gowns, and so forth). Don't become part of the problem by becoming injured. Avoid being exposed to communicable diseases.

After taking safety precautions, the victim is checked for responsiveness. Determining that the adult victim is indeed unresponsive, 911 should be called. Then, the ABCs should be performed. The ABCs of CPR stand for airway, breathing, and circulation (and are discussed in greater detail below).

THE ABCs OF CPR

The A step in CPR checks for a victim's open airway. This is accomplished by opening the airway with either a head tilt–chin lift (for nontraumatic conditions) or the jaw-thrust when trauma is suspected. The head tilt–chin lift is performed by placing one hand on the victim's forehead with the fingers of the other hand under the mandible (chin). Make sure to stay off the soft tissues of the chin, and apply gentle pressure to the forehead to tilt the victim's head back, thus opening the airway. The jaw-thrust maneuver is performed when trauma is suspected. It is accomplished by placing the fingers from both hands under the angles of the jaw and the thumbs on both cheekbones or mask. Gentle pressure is then applied to push the jaw upward without hyperextending the cervical spine. This process allows the tongue to be lifted off the back of the throat (as it is attached to the jaw) without moving the head or neck. This technique takes practice. The rescuer then looks for chest rise, listens for air movement, and feels for air exchange.

The B signifies breathing. After the rescuer has determined no air exchange has occurred, then artificial respirations are administered. Mouth-to-mouth or mouth-to-mask respirations involve giving two slow breaths, watching for chest rise, and feeling for the ease of airflow. When performing mouth-to-mouth, the rescuer gently pinches the nose of the adult or child victim closed and makes a seal with their mouth over the mouth of the victim. (Infants require mouth-to–mouth-and-nose.) Many different types of barrier devices are available to perform mouth-to-mask. Whatever barrier device is chosen, the rescuer must be familiar with its use before real-world application. Artificial respirations for adults are 1.5 to 2 seconds each, for children and infants, 1 to 1.5 seconds. If only performing rescue breaths, the ratio in adults is 1 breath given every 5 seconds and in children and infants, 1 breath given every 3 seconds. If the breaths do not go in (signified by lack of chest rise and resistance), then the head is repositioned and administration of breaths is attempted again. If still unsuccessful, then a foreign body is most likely blocking the airway. The scenario will then involve the procedures needed for foreign body in airway removal.

If the breath is successfully administered, then the next step consists of the C: checking for signs of circulation (such as coughing, moving, breathing, or the presence of a carotid pulse). If no signs of circulation are present, then the rescuer provides chest compressions. Adult compressions are given over the lower half of the sternum and artificially cause the flow of blood throughout the body with each compression. The compression site, depth, rate, and ratio to breaths for one-rescuer CPR for adults is as follows: on the lower half of the sternum (avoiding the xiphoid process), use two hands to compress the chest 1.5 to 2 inches at a rate of about 100 compressions/min and with a ratio of 15 compressions and 2 ventilations. For children apply compressions in the same CPR site as adults with one hand at a depth of 1 to 1.5 inches at a rate of about 100 compressions/min and a ratio of 5 compressions and 1 ventilation. For infants the compression site is between the nipples, midsternum, using the middle and ring finger to compress the chest 0.5 to 1 inch in depth at a rate of at least 100 compressions/min with a ratio of 5 compressions and 1 ventilation. Becoming comfortable with application and management of age-dependent differences in CPR and foreign body airway obstruction (FBAO) requires supervised practice with a qualified instructor. Chest compressions can provide up to 30% of normal cardiac output.

ADULT CPR PERFORMANCE CHECKLIST

1. Check the scene for hazards.
2. Take personal safety and infection-control precautions.
3. Check for responsiveness.
   a. Touch the person and ask, "Are you okay?"
   b. If there is no response, continue on.
4. Activate the EMS system.
   a. You (or another person) should call 911 or another emergency response number.
   b. If available, get an AED. (When the AED arrives, use it in conjunction with CPR, as listed in the AED performance checklist below.)
5. Open the airway.
   a. If *no trauma* is suspected, use the *head tilt–chin lift* method.
   b. If *trauma* is suspected, use the jaw-thrust maneuver.

6. Check for breathing.

   a. Look, listen, and feel for chest rise.

   b. If the person is breathing adequately, place them in the recovery position.

   c. If breathing is not present, give two slow breaths.

   d. Watch for chest rise and fall. If there is no chest movement, reposition the head and try again. If still unsuccessful, perform foreign body airway maneuvers.

7. Check for circulation.

   a. Assess carotid pulse or check for other signs of circulation: moving, coughing, or talking.

   b. If signs of circulation are present but the person is not breathing, give one breath every 5 seconds.

   c. Reassess signs of circulation in about 1 minute. If no signs are present, continue on.

8. Begin compressions.

   a. Place the heel of one hand in the center of the person's chest, over the *lower half of the sternum*. Place the other hand on top of the first and deliver compressions, at a depth of *1.5 to 2 inches*.

   b. Perform 15 compressions at a rate of approximately *100 times per minute*.

   c. Perform *four cycles of 15 compressions and 2 ventilations* (1 minute).

9. Reassess circulation.

   a. If no breathing or pulse is present, continue CPR.

   b. If pulse is present but there is no breathing, provide rescue breaths.

REFERENCES

1. Bergeron J, Bizjak G. Brady's First Responder, 6th ed. Prentice Hall, 2001. (The ABC's of CPR.)
2. National Safety Council. CPR and AED, 4th ed. Jones and Bartlett Publishers, 2002.
3. American Heart Association. BLS Instructor's Manual. 2000.

APPENDIX B

Administering First Aid

If possible, obtain vital signs (respiratory rate, pulse, and blood pressure) while waiting for responders. Also, attempt to obtain pertinent information (such as patient's full name, date of birth, home address, the events leading up to the injury or illness, what occurred during the event, chief complaint, medicines, allergies, past medical history, and so on). Ask permission to share this information with responders, before doing so.

Do not perform any interventions that require special knowledge for which you are not trained (i.e., splinting, and so forth). Persons suspected of injuries or illness (such as the ones listed below) should always seek the advice of a physician.

SUSPECTED INJURIES OR ILLNESSES

Fractures, Sprains, Strains, and Dislocations

Often, it is difficult to determine the extent of an injury in the field. Signs and symptoms can be seen in various combinations: pain, swelling, deformity, tenderness, crepitus (or, bone ends grinding together), redness, bruising or discoloration, and loss of movement. If any indications of **impaired circulation or nerve damage** exist (such as numbness, tingling, weak or absent pulses, cool, pale skin, or inability to sense touch distal to the injury site), this is a **true emergency**! This information should immediately be relayed to the dispatcher.

1. Expose the area for visualization, unless doing so could cause further injury.
2. Control major bleeding. If possible, cover any open wounds with sterile dressings.
3. Prevent further movement of the injury. If trained to do so, immobilize the joints above and below the injury site using splints, cravats, pillows, and so forth. Remember to check for signs of adequate distal sensation and circulation before and after applying splints!
4. To reduce pain and swelling, apply ice or cold packs, but do not place them directly on the skin.
5. Cover the patient to preserve body heat, as needed.

If someone is suspected of having a spinal fracture, do not move the person or allow him or her to move, unless he or she needs to be protected from immediate danger. Monitor the ABCs and control life-threatening bleeding (if present). If you must open the person's airway, remember to use the jaw-thrust maneuver rather than the head tilt–chin lift method.

External Bleeding

Most external bleeding will be effectively controlled with direct pressure. However, if the bleeding persists despite the use of direct pressure, the following methods can be used. Remember not to remove dressings once they are in place. Removing them will disrupt the clotting process.

1. Apply direct pressure, using a gloved hand and, if possible, a sterile dressing.
2. If the bleeding continues, apply a pressure dressing.
3. If the bleeding continues, continue with pressure and elevate the area.
4. If still unsuccessful, find and use appropriate pressure points.
5. As a last resort, apply a tourniquet.

Shock

Patients can experience shock for many different reasons including problems with the heart, vessels, and blood volume. If a person experiences weakness; dizziness; thirst; cool, pale, clammy skin; decreased levels of consciousness; and nausea and vomiting, follow the steps below.

1. Assist the person into the shock position:
   a. Lying down, with feet above the level of the heart.
   b. Cover with blankets to preserve adequate body temperature.
2. Do not give the person anything by mouth.
3. If he or she becomes unconscious, perform ABCs. Administer rescue breathing or CPR, as needed. If CPR is not needed but the person remains unconscious, place him or her on one side and be alert for vomiting.

Fainting or Syncope

There are many causes of fainting, some serious and some not so serious. It is never normal to faint. Frequently, an underlying problem can be complicated with trauma associated from a resulting fall. If you suspect someone is about to faint, instruct them to sit down on the floor, and place them in the shock position. Monitor their ABCs and preserve body temperature with blankets.

Seizures

Most people who suffer from seizures will have a history of epilepsy or previous head trauma. They will be aware when the seizure is about to begin. First aid for a seizure involves the following:

1. Protect the person from further harm by helping him or her to the floor and working to prevent injuries while the seizure is occurring.
2. Do not allow anyone to try to place anything in the mouth, such as a bite block.
3. Monitor the ABCs and note the length of the seizure. Also note if the seizure stops and then begins again without the person regaining consciousness. *This constitutes a true emergency*!
4. Preserve modesty by covering the person with sheets or blankets, as often-times seizures will cause a voiding of the bladder or bowels.

Insulin Shock

Persons who experience insulin shock will have a history of diabetes. The onset of insulin shock is quick and causes a variety of signs and symptoms, including irritability, weakness, shakiness, decreased levels of consciousness, and cool, pale, moist skin. If left untreated, it will lead to unconsciousness and death. If the person is awake and alert, you can assist him or her by providing nondiet colas, fruit juices, hard candies, or tubes of oral glucose. If the person is not conscious or alert, do not give anything by mouth. The best way to avoid a severe reaction is prevention.

Asthma Attacks

Suspect an asthma attack in someone experiencing labored breathing, shortness of breath, wheezes, tightness in the chest, increased respirations, changes in skin color, restlessness, or anxiousness. If someone is suffering an asthma attack and can only speak in one- or two-word sentences, this indicates a very serious attack, which should be immediately relayed to the dispatcher. It is helpful to pass along what medicine is in a person's inhaler and how many times the person has used it.

1. Confirm that no foreign bodies are causing the breathing difficulty.
2. Confirm the cause is not an existing exposure to an allergen. If this is the case, safely remove the substance or move the patient.
3. Most patients will naturally sit or stand in a tripod position (arms outstretched and leaning forward). Allow them to sit or stand however they feel most comfortable.
4. Be supportive.
5. Monitor ABCs.

Heart Attacks

Suspect someone could be having a heart attack if he or she experiences chest pain; pressure, heaviness, or squeezing that radiates to the arms (typically the left), neck, jaw, or back; shortness of breath; cool, pale, sweaty skin; and nausea or vomiting.

1. Prevent further exertion.
2. Provide a position of comfort.

3. Give emotional support.

4. Ask the person if he or she took any nitroglycerin. If so, ask how many.

5. Monitor ABCs.

Stroke

Strokes are caused by broken or blocked blood vessels in the brain, causing brain damage. The best way to help someone suffering from a stroke is recognition. If someone has a severe headache, numbness or paralysis on one side of the body, slurred speech, visual disturbances, or decreased level of consciousness, call 911 immediately.

1. Place the person in a position of comfort, or the recovery position if he or she is having trouble swallowing.

2. Protect paralyzed limbs from injury.

3. Remain calm and be reassuring.

4. Do not give the person anything by mouth.

5. Monitor ABCs.

Choking

Signs and symptoms of choking include inability to breathe, talk, or cough. People who are choking will typically hold their hands to their throats. For adults and children:

1. Stand behind the person.

2. Wrap your arms under his or her armpits and around the waist.

3. Make a fist and place it just above his or her umbilicus (just above the belly button). Put your other hand on top of your fist.

4. Deliver deliberate, rapid, upward thrusts.

5. Continue until the object is dislodged or the person becomes unconscious.

6. If they become unconscious, assist them to the floor and place them supine.

7. Use the tongue-jaw lift to open the mouth and look for an object. Perform a finger sweep if you see something.

8. Open the airway. Attempt two ventilations.

9. If unsuccessful, reposition the head and try again.

10. Straddle the person. Place your hands one on top of the other in the same location (as in the standing position) and deliver five abdominal thrusts.

11. If still unsuccessful, repeat steps 7, 8, 9, and 10.

Heat Exhaustion and Heat Stroke

The differences in heat exhaustion and heat stroke are outlined below:

Heat Exhaustion	Heat Stroke
Moist, pale, normal, or cool skin	Hot, dry skin (sometimes moist)
Muscle cramps	Altered level of consciousness
Heavy perspiration	Little or no perspiration
Exhaustion, dizziness	Weakness
Weak pulse	Full, rapid pulse

Someone suffering from heat exhaustion should be removed from the hot environment to a cool area. Place in the shock position or the recovery position (if not alert or nauseated). Loosen or remove clothing. Cool with fanning, but do not induce shivering. Alert persons may sip water. Ease muscle cramps with moist towels or gentle massage if the person has no history of circulatory problems.

Someone suffering heat stroke needs to be cooled, but not so rapidly as to induce shivering. Remove him or her from the hot environment and place in a cool environment in the shock position. Loosen or remove clothing. Pour cool water over wet wrappings. Fan the patient and use wrapped cold packs in the armpits and groin.

REFERENCES

1. Bergeron J, Bizjak G. Brady's First Responder, 6th ed. Prentice Hall, 2001. (The ABC's of CPR.)
2. National Safety Council. CPR and AED, 4th ed. Jones and Bartlett Publishers, 2002.
3. American Heart Association. BLS Instructor's Manual. 2000.

APPENDIX C

AED (Automated External Defibrillators)

MANUAL VERSUS AUTOMATED DEFIBRILLATORS

When the word *defibrillator* is used, most minds conjure images of manual defibrillators like the ones frequently seen on prime-time television. *Manual defibrillators* are used by EMS providers who have received in-depth instruction on cardiac arrhythmia recognition and management. In the prehospital field, these individuals are typically paramedics.

First responders, EMTs, and the general public are trained to use *automated external defibrillators*. AEDs can be fully automated or semiautomated. Semiautomated machines require the rescuer to press buttons to assist the machine in analyzing rhythms or delivering shocks, whereas fully automated machines only require the rescuer to turn the device on and correctly place the pads. Whether fully automated or semiautomated, these machines are programmed to recognize heart arrhythmias and deliver therapeutic shocks when appropriate.

AEDs AND CARDIAC ARRHYTHMIAS

When operating normally, the heart has its own electrical system that works to induce the pumping function of the heart. Cardiac arrhythmias are abnormalities in this electrical system, which inhibit normal pumping function. Normal electrical rhythms most often produce a heartbeat, but the presence of a normal rhythm does not always equate to mechanical activity.

In cases of cardiac arrest, the most common arrhythmias or electrical disturbances consist of asystole, pulseless electrical activity, ventricular fibrillation, and pulseless ventricular tachycardia. All of these rhythms prevent the heart from pumping. Unfortunately, neither pulseless electrical activity nor asystole are shockable rhythms. However, ventricular fibrillation and pulseless ventricular tachycardia are shockable and can be treated with the use of an AED.

WHEN NOT TO USE AN AED

Patients younger than 8 years of age or less than 55 pounds should not be defibrillated with an adult defibrillator. It is important to note that AED manufacturers are starting to provide special pediatric pads for use in children, but do not assume all AEDs are equipped with children's pads.

AEDs should be applied to those persons who are in cardiac arrest (i.e., unresponsive, no respirations, and no pulse). If you suspect that a person might go into cardiac arrest, keep the AED nearby and apply when cardiac arrest is confirmed.

Special circumstances can affect the use of AEDs. This is why it is very important that fitness professionals receive training in the use of AEDs by a qualified instructor before real-world application. Contact your local fire department, community college, area hospital, the American Heart Association, or the AED Instructor Foundation. All of these agencies either directly offer CPR and AED training or can recommend qualified area instructors.

ADULT AED PERFORMANCE CHECKLIST

1. Check the scene for hazards.
2. Take personal safety and infection-control precautions.
3. Confirm unresponsiveness.
4. Activate the EMS system and retrieve the AED.
   a. If possible, send someone else to accomplish these tasks.
5. Perform ABCs.
   a. Confirm that no breathing or circulation is present.
6. Start CPR.
7. When unit arrives, turn on the AED.
8. Follow the verbal prompts given by the machine.
9. Attach pads to the patient's bare chest.
   a. Correct placement is often illustrated on the pads.
10. When instructed, stop CPR and allow the machine to analyze.
    a. Some machines require the rescuer press an "analyze" button, and other machines are fully automated.
    b. *Ensure that no one is touching the patient when analyzing or shocking!*
11. If instructed, press the "shock" button.
    a. Some machines are fully automated and do not require the rescuer to press a button.
12. Repeat this step, as instructed.
    a. The machine may indicate to shock up to 3 times.
13. Reassess ABCs.
14. If no pulse, perform CPR for 1 minute.
15. Repeat the analyzing and shock steps, as instructed, while ensuring that no one touches the patient. Follow the voice prompts. Reassess ABCs and provide CPR as needed.
16. If the machine states "no shock advised," reassess ABCs.
    a. If there is no pulse, continue CPR.
    b. If pulse is regained, ensure adequate breathing.
    c. If inadequate or no breathing is present, perform rescue breaths.
    d. If breathing is adequate and pulse is present, place the patient in the recovery position.
17. Continue to monitor the patient for changes.

REFERENCES

1. Bergeron J, Bizjak G. Brady's First Responder, 6th ed. Prentice Hall, 2001. (The ABC's of CPR.)
2. National Safety Council. CPR and AED, 4th ed. Jones and Bartlett Publishers, 2002.
3. American Heart Association. BLS Instructor's Manual. 2000.

APPENDIX D

Body-Composition Formulas

Table A4.1					
Young Women 17–26					
Abdomen					
Inches	**Constant A**	**Inches**	**Constant A**	**Inches**	**Constant A**
20.00	26.74	26.00	34.76	32.00	42.78
20.25	27.07	26.25	35.09	32.25	43.11
20.50	27.41	26.50	35.43	32.50	43.45
20.75	27.74	26.75	35.76	32.75	43.78
21.00	28.07	27.00	36.10	33.00	44.12
21.25	28.41	27.25	36.43	33.25	44.45
21.50	28.74	27.50	36.76	33.50	44.78
21.75	29.08	27.75	37.10	33.75	45.12
22.00	29.41	28.00	37.43	34.00	45.45
22.25	29.74	28.25	37.77	34.25	45.79
22.50	30.08	28.50	38.10	34.50	46.12
22.75	30.41	28.75	38.43	34.75	46.46
23.00	30.75	29.00	38.77	35.00	46.79
23.25	31.08	29.25	39.10	35.25	47.12
23.50	31.42	29.50	39.44	35.50	47.46
23.75	31.75	29.75	39.77	35.75	47.79
24.00	32.08	30.00	40.11	36.00	48.13
24.25	32.42	30.25	40.44	36.25	48.46
24.50	32.75	30.50	40.77	36.50	48.80
24.75	33.09	30.75	41.11	36.75	49.13
25.00	33.42	31.00	41.44	37.00	49.46
25.25	33.76	31.25	41.78	37.25	49.80
25.50	34.09	31.50	42.11	37.50	50.13
25.75	34.42	31.75	42.45	37.75	50.47

(continued)

Young Women 17–26 (continued)

Abdomen

Inches	Constant A	Inches	Constant A	Inches	Constant A
38.00	50.80	45.50	60.82	53.00	70.84
38.25	51.13	45.75	61.15	53.25	71.17
38.50	51.47	46.00	61.48	53.50	71.51
38.75	51.80	46.25	61.82	53.75	71.84
39.00	52.14	46.50	62.15	54.00	72.17
39.25	52.47	46.75	62.49	54.25	72.51
39.50	52.81	47.00	62.82	54.50	72.84
39.75	53.14	47.25	63.15	54.75	73.18
40.00	53.47	47.50	63.49	55.00	73.51
40.25	53.80	47.75	63.82	55.25	73.85
40.50	54.13	48.00	64.16	55.50	74.18
40.75	54.47	48.25	64.49	55.75	74.51
41.00	54.80	48.50	64.82	56.00	74.85
41.25	55.14	48.75	65.16	56.25	75.18
41.50	55.47	49.00	65.49	56.50	75.52
41.75	55.80	49.25	65.83	56.75	75.85
42.00	56.14	49.50	66.16	57.00	76.18
42.25	56.47	49.75	66.49	57.25	76.52
42.50	56.81	50.00	66.83	57.50	76.85
42.75	57.14	50.25	67.16	57.75	77.19
43.00	57.47	50.50	67.50	58.00	77.52
43.25	57.81	50.75	67.83	58.25	77.85
43.50	58.14	51.00	68.17	58.50	78.19
43.75	58.48	51.25	68.50	58.75	78.52
44.00	58.81	51.50	68.83	59.00	78.86
44.25	59.14	51.75	69.17	59.25	79.19
44.50	59.48	52.00	69.50	59.50	79.52
44.75	59.81	52.25	69.84	59.75	79.86
45.00	60.15	52.50	70.17	60.00	80.19
45.25	60.48	52.75	70.50		

Table A4.2

Young Women 17–26

Thigh

Inches	Constant B	Inches	Constant B	Inches	Constant B	Inches	Constant B
14.00	29.13	20.75	43.17	27.50	57.21	34.25	71.26
14.25	29.65	21.00	43.69	27.75	57.73	34.50	71.78
14.50	30.17	21.25	44.21	28.00	58.26	34.75	72.30
14.75	30.69	21.50	44.73	28.25	58.78	35.00	72.82
15.00	31.21	21.75	45.25	28.50	59.30	35.25	73.34
15.25	31.73	22.00	45.77	28.75	59.82	35.50	73.86
15.50	32.25	22.25	46.29	29.00	60.34	35.75	74.38
15.75	32.77	22.50	46.81	29.25	60.86	36.00	74.90
16.00	33.29	22.75	47.33	29.50	61.38	36.25	75.42
16.25	33.81	23.00	47.85	29.75	61.90	36.50	75.94
16.50	34.33	23.25	48.37	30.00	62.42	36.75	76.46
16.75	34.85	23.50	48.89	30.25	62.94	37.00	76.98
17.00	35.37	23.75	49.41	30.50	63.46	37.25	77.50
17.25	35.89	24.00	49.93	30.75	63.98	37.50	78.02
17.50	36.41	24.25	50.45	31.00	64.50	37.75	78.54
17.75	36.93	24.50	50.97	31.25	65.02	38.00	79.06
18.00	37.45	24.75	51.49	31.50	65.54	38.25	79.58
18.25	37.97	25.00	52.01	31.75	66.06	38.50	80.10
18.50	38.49	25.25	52.53	32.00	66.58	38.75	80.62
18.75	39.01	25.50	53.05	32.25	67.10	39.00	81.14
19.00	39.53	25.75	53.57	32.50	67.62	39.25	81.66
19.25	40.05	26.00	54.09	32.75	68.14	39.50	82.18
19.50	40.57	26.25	54.61	33.00	68.66	39.75	82.70
19.75	41.09	26.50	55.13	33.25	69.18	40.00	83.22
20.00	41.61	26.75	55.65	33.50	69.70		
20.25	42.13	27.00	56.17	33.75	70.22		
20.50	42.65	27.25	56.69	34.00	70.74		

Table A4.3

Young Women 17–26

Forearm

Inches	Constant C	Inches	Constant C	Inches	Constant C
6.00	25.86	12.50	53.88	19.00	81.90
6.25	26.94	12.75	54.96	19.25	82.98
6.50	28.02	13.00	56.04	19.50	84.05
6.75	29.10	13.25	57.11	19.75	85.13
7.00	30.17	13.50	58.19	20.00	86.21
7.25	31.25	13.75	59.27	20.25	87.29
7.50	32.33	14.00	60.35	20.50	88.37
7.75	33.41	14.25	61.42	20.75	89.45
8.00	34.48	14.50	62.50	21.00	90.53
8.25	35.56	14.75	63.58	21.25	91.61
8.50	36.64	15.00	64.66	21.50	92.69
8.75	37.72	15.25	65.73	21.75	93.77
9.00	38.79	15.50	66.81	22.00	94.85
9.25	39.87	15.75	67.89	22.25	95.93
9.50	40.95	16.00	68.97	22.50	97.01
9.75	42.03	16.25	70.04	22.75	98.09
10.00	43.10	16.50	71.12	23.00	99.17
10.25	44.18	16.75	72.20	23.25	100.25
10.50	45.26	17.00	73.28	23.50	101.33
10.75	46.34	17.25	74.36	23.75	102.41
11.00	47.41	17.50	75.43	24.00	103.49
11.25	48.49	17.75	76.51	24.25	104.57
11.50	49.57	18.00	77.59	24.50	105.65
11.75	50.65	18.25	78.67	24.75	106.73
12.00	51.73	18.50	79.74	25.00	107.81
12.25	52.80	18.75	80.82		

Note: Percent fat = Constant A + Constant B − Constant C − 19.6.
For athletic people, the age correction is 22.6.

Table A4.4

Older Women (27–50)

Abdomen

Inches	Constant A	Inches	Constant A	Inches	Constant A	Inches	Constant A	Inches	Constant A
25.00	29.69	32.25	38.30	39.50	46.90	46.75	55.51	54.00	64.12
25.25	29.98	32.50	38.59	39.75	47.20	47.00	55.81	54.25	64.42
25.50	30.28	32.75	38.89	40.00	47.50	47.25	56.11	54.50	64.71
25.75	30.58	33.00	39.19	40.25	47.79	47.50	56.40	54.75	65.01
26.00	30.87	33.25	39.48	40.50	48.09	47.75	56.70	55.00	65.31
26.25	31.17	33.50	39.78	40.75	48.39	48.00	57.00	55.25	65.60
26.50	31.47	33.75	40.08	41.00	48.69	48.25	57.29	55.50	65.90
26.75	31.76	34.00	40.37	41.25	48.98	48.50	57.59	55.75	66.20
27.00	32.06	34.25	40.67	41.50	49.28	48.75	57.89	56.00	66.49
27.25	32.36	34.50	40.97	41.75	49.58	49.00	58.18	56.25	66.79
27.50	32.65	34.75	41.26	42.00	49.87	49.25	58.48	56.50	67.09
27.75	32.95	35.00	41.56	42.25	50.17	49.50	58.78	56.75	67.38
28.00	33.25	35.25	41.86	42.50	50.47	49.75	59.07	57.00	67.68
28.25	33.55	35.50	42.15	42.75	50.76	50.00	59.37	57.25	67.98
28.50	33.84	35.75	42.45	43.00	51.06	50.25	59.67	57.50	68.28
28.75	34.14	36.00	42.75	43.25	51.36	50.50	59.96	57.75	68.57
29.00	34.44	36.25	43.05	43.50	51.65	50.75	60.26	58.00	68.87
29.25	34.73	36.50	43.34	43.75	51.95	51.00	60.56	58.25	69.17
29.50	35.03	36.75	43.64	44.00	52.25	51.25	60.86	58.50	69.46
29.75	35.33	37.00	43.94	44.25	52.54	51.50	61.15	58.75	69.76
30.00	35.62	37.25	44.23	44.50	52.84	51.75	61.45	59.00	70.06
30.25	35.92	37.50	44.53	44.75	53.14	52.00	61.75	59.25	70.35
30.50	36.22	37.75	44.83	45.00	53.44	52.25	62.04	59.50	70.65
30.75	36.51	38.00	45.12	45.25	53.73	52.50	62.34	59.75	70.95
31.00	36.81	38.25	45.42	45.50	54.03	52.75	62.64	60.00	71.24
31.25	37.11	38.50	45.72	45.75	54.33	53.00	62.93		
31.50	37.40	38.75	46.01	46.00	54.62	53.25	63.23		
31.75	37.70	39.00	46.31	46.25	54.92	53.50	63.53		
32.00	38.00	39.25	46.61	46.50	55.22	53.75	63.82		

Table A4.5

Older Women (27–50)

Thigh

Inches	Constant B	Inches	Constant B	Inches	Constant B	Inches	Constant B
14.00	17.31	20.75	25.66	27.50	34.00	34.25	42.35
14.25	17.62	21.00	25.97	27.75	34.31	34.50	42.66
14.50	17.93	21.25	26.28	28.00	34.62	34.75	42.97
14.75	18.24	21.50	26.58	28.25	34.93	35.00	43.28
15.00	18.55	21.75	26.89	28.50	35.24	35.25	43.58
15.25	18.86	22.00	27.20	28.75	35.55	35.50	43.89
15.50	19.17	22.25	27.51	29.00	35.86	35.75	44.20
15.75	19.47	22.50	27.82	29.25	36.17	36.00	44.51
16.00	19.78	22.75	28.13	29.50	36.48	36.25	44.82
16.25	20.09	23.00	28.44	29.75	36.79	36.50	45.13
16.50	20.40	23.25	28.75	30.00	37.09	36.75	45.44
16.75	20.71	23.50	29.06	30.25	37.40	37.00	45.75
17.00	21.02	23.75	29.37	30.50	37.71	37.25	46.06
17.25	21.33	24.00	29.68	30.75	38.02	37.50	46.37
17.50	21.64	24.25	29.98	31.00	38.33	37.75	46.68
17.75	21.95	24.50	30.29	31.25	38.64	38.00	46.98
18.00	22.26	24.75	30.60	31.50	38.95	38.25	47.29
18.25	22.57	25.00	30.91	31.75	39.26	38.50	47.60
18.50	22.87	25.25	31.22	32.00	39.57	38.75	47.91
18.75	23.18	25.50	31.53	32.25	39.88	39.00	48.22
19.00	23.49	25.75	31.84	32.50	40.19	39.25	48.53
19.25	23.80	26.00	32.15	32.75	40.49	39.50	48.84
19.50	24.11	26.25	32.46	33.00	40.80	39.75	49.15
19.75	24.42	26.50	32.77	33.25	41.11	40.00	49.46
20.00	24.73	26.75	33.08	33.50	41.42		
20.25	25.04	27.00	33.38	33.75	41.73		
20.50	25.35	27.25	33.69	34.00	42.04		

Table A4.6

Older Women (27–50)

Calf

Inches	Constant C	Inches	Constant C	Inches	Constant C
10.00	14.46	16.75	24.22	23.50	33.98
10.25	14.82	17.00	24.58	23.75	34.34
10.50	15.18	17.25	24.94	24.00	34.70
10.75	15.54	17.50	25.31	24.25	35.07
11.00	15.91	17.75	25.67	24.50	35.43
11.25	16.27	18.00	26.03	24.75	35.79
11.50	16.63	18.25	26.39	25.00	36.15
11.75	16.99	18.50	26.75	25.25	36.51
12.00	17.35	18.75	27.11	25.50	36.87
12.25	17.71	19.00	27.47	25.75	37.23
12.50	18.08	19.25	27.84	26.00	37.59
12.75	18.44	19.50	28.20	26.25	37.95
13.00	18.80	19.75	28.56	26.50	38.31
13.25	19.16	20.00	28.92	26.75	38.67
13.50	19.52	20.25	29.28	27.00	39.03
13.75	19.88	20.50	29.64	27.25	39.39
14.00	20.24	20.75	30.00	27.50	39.75
14.25	20.61	21.00	30.37	27.75	40.11
14.50	20.97	21.25	30.73	28.00	40.47
14.75	21.33	21.50	31.09	28.25	40.83
15.00	21.69	21.75	31.45	28.50	41.19
15.25	22.05	22.00	31.81	28.75	41.55
15.50	22.41	22.25	32.17	29.00	41.91
15.75	22.77	22.50	32.54	29.25	42.27
16.00	23.14	22.75	32.90	29.50	42.63
16.25	23.50	23.00	33.26	29.75	42.99
16.50	23.86	23.25	33.62	30.00	43.35

Note: Percent fat = Constant A + Constant B − Constant C − 18.4.
    For athletic people, the age correction is 21.4.

Table A4.7

Young Men (17–26)

Upper Arm

Inches	Constant A	Inches	Constant A	Inches	Constant A
10.00	37.01	16.75	61.99	23.50	86.95
10.25	37.94	17.00	62.97	23.75	87.88
10.50	38.86	17.25	63.84	24.00	88.81
10.75	39.79	17.50	64.77	24.25	89.73
11.00	40.71	17.75	65.69	24.50	90.66
11.25	41.64	18.00	66.62	24.75	91.58
11.50	42.56	18.25	67.54	25.00	92.51
11.75	43.49	18.50	68.47	25.25	93.43
12.00	44.41	18.75	69.40	25.50	94.36
12.25	45.34	19.00	70.32	25.75	95.28
12.50	46.26	19.25	71.25	26.00	96.21
12.75	47.19	19.50	72.17	26.25	97.13
13.00	48.11	19.75	73.10	26.50	98.06
13.25	49.04	20.00	74.02	26.75	98.98
13.50	49.96	20.25	74.95	27.00	99.91
13.75	50.89	20.50	75.87	27.25	100.83
14.00	51.82	20.75	76.80	27.50	101.76
14.25	52.74	21.00	77.72	27.75	102.68
14.50	53.67	21.25	78.65	28.00	103.61
14.75	54.59	21.50	79.57	28.25	104.54
15.00	55.52	21.75	80.50	28.50	105.46
15.25	56.44	22.00	81.42	28.75	106.39
15.50	57.37	22.25	82.34	29.00	107.31
15.75	58.29	22.50	83.26	29.25	108.24
16.00	59.22	22.75	84.18	29.50	109.16
16.25	60.14	23.00	85.10	29.75	110.09
16.50	61.07	23.25	86.03	30.00	111.01

Table A4.8

Young Men (17–26)

Abdomen

Inches	Constant B	Inches	Constant B	Inches	Constant B	Inches	Constant B
28.00	36.74	36.25	47.57	44.50	58.38	52.75	69.20
28.25	37.07	36.50	47.89	44.75	58.71	53.00	69.53
28.50	37.40	36.75	48.22	45.00	59.04	53.25	69.86
28.75	37.73	37.00	48.55	45.25	59.37	53.50	70.19
29.00	38.05	37.25	48.88	45.50	59.70	53.75	70.52
29.25	38.38	37.50	49.21	45.75	60.02	54.00	70.84
29.50	38.71	37.75	49.54	46.00	60.35	54.25	71.17
29.75	39.04	38.00	49.86	46.25	60.68	54.50	71.50
30.00	39.37	38.25	50.19	46.50	61.01	54.75	71.83
30.25	39.69	38.50	50.52	46.75	61.34	55.00	72.16
30.50	40.02	38.75	50.85	47.00	61.66	55.25	72.48
30.75	40.35	39.00	51.18	47.25	61.99	55.50	72.81
31.00	40.68	39.25	51.50	47.50	62.32	55.75	73.14
31.25	41.01	39.50	51.83	47.75	62.65	56.00	73.47
31.50	41.33	39.75	52.16	48.00	62.97	56.25	73.80
31.75	41.66	40.00	52.49	48.25	63.30	56.50	74.12
32.00	41.99	40.25	52.82	48.50	63.63	56.75	74.45
32.25	42.32	40.50	53.14	48.75	63.96	57.00	74.78
32.50	42.65	40.75	53.47	49.00	64.29	57.25	75.11
32.75	42.97	41.00	53.80	49.25	64.61	57.50	75.43
33.00	43.30	41.25	54.13	49.50	64.94	57.75	75.76
33.25	43.63	41.50	54.46	49.75	65.27	58.00	76.09
33.50	43.96	41.75	54.78	50.00	65.60	58.25	76.42
33.75	44.29	42.00	55.11	50.25	65.93	58.50	76.75
34.00	44.61	42.25	55.43	50.50	66.25	58.75	77.07
34.25	44.94	42.50	55.76	50.75	66.58	59.00	77.40
34.50	45.27	42.75	56.09	51.00	66.91	59.25	77.73
34.75	45.60	43.00	56.42	51.25	67.24	59.50	78.06
35.00	45.93	43.25	56.74	51.50	67.57	59.75	78.39
35.25	46.25	43.50	57.07	51.75	67.89	60.00	78.71
35.50	46.58	43.75	57.40	52.00	68.22		
35.75	46.91	44.00	57.73	52.25	68.55		
36.00	47.24	44.25	58.06	52.50	68.88		

Table A4.9

Young Men (17–26)

Forearm

Inches	Constant C	Inches	Constant C	Inches	Constant C
10.00	54.30	15.25	82.80	20.50	111.31
10.25	55.65	15.50	84.16	20.75	112.67
10.50	57.01	15.75	85.52	21.00	114.02
10.75	58.37	16.00	86.88	21.25	115.38
11.00	59.73	16.25	88.23	21.50	116.74
11.25	61.08	16.50	89.59	21.75	118.10
11.50	62.44	16.75	90.95	22.00	119.45
11.75	63.80	17.00	92.31	22.25	120.80
12.00	65.16	17.25	93.66	22.50	122.15
12.25	66.51	17.50	95.02	22.75	123.50
12.50	67.87	17.75	96.38	23.00	124.85
12.75	69.23	18.00	97.74	23.25	126.21
13.00	70.59	18.25	99.09	23.50	127.57
13.25	71.94	18.50	100.45	23.75	128.92
13.50	73.30	18.75	101.81	24.00	130.28
13.75	74.66	19.00	103.17	24.25	131.64
14.00	76.02	19.25	104.52	24.50	133.00
14.25	77.37	19.50	105.88	24.75	134.35
14.50	78.73	19.75	107.24	25.00	135.71
14.75	80.09	20.00	108.60		
15.00	81.45	20.25	109.95		

Note: Percent fat = Constant A + Constant B − Constant C − 10.2.
For athletic people, the age correction is 14.2.

Table A4.10

Older Men (27–50)

Buttocks

Inches	Constant A	Inches	Constant A	Inches	Constant A	Inches	Constant A
35.00	36.68	41.50	43.49	48.00	50.30	54.50	57.11
35.25	36.94	41.75	43.75	48.25	50.56	54.75	57.37
35.50	37.20	42.00	44.02	48.50	50.83	55.00	57.63
35.75	37.46	42.25	44.28	48.75	51.09	55.25	57.90
36.00	37.73	42.50	44.54	49.00	51.35	55.50	58.16
36.25	37.99	42.75	44.80	49.25	51.61	55.75	58.42
36.50	38.25	43.00	45.06	49.50	51.87	56.00	58.68
36.75	38.51	43.25	45.32	49.75	52.13	56.25	58.94
37.00	38.78	43.50	45.59	50.00	52.39	56.50	59.21
37.25	39.04	43.75	45.85	50.25	52.66	56.75	59.47
37.50	39.30	44.00	46.12	50.50	52.92	57.00	59.73
37.75	39.56	44.25	46.37	50.75	53.18	57.25	59.99
38.00	39.82	44.50	46.64	51.00	53.44	57.50	60.25
38.25	40.08	44.75	46.89	51.25	53.70	57.75	60.52
38.50	40.35	45.00	47.16	51.50	53.97	58.00	60.78
38.75	40.61	45.25	47.42	51.75	54.23	58.25	61.04
39.00	40.87	45.50	47.68	52.00	54.49	58.50	61.30
39.25	41.13	45.75	47.94	52.25	54.75	58.75	61.56
39.50	41.39	46.00	48.21	52.50	55.01	59.00	61.83
39.75	41.66	46.25	48.47	52.75	55.28	59.25	62.09
40.00	41.92	46.50	48.73	53.00	55.54	59.50	62.35
40.25	42.18	46.75	48.99	53.25	55.80	59.75	62.61
40.50	42.44	47.00	49.26	53.50	56.06	60.00	62.87
40.75	42.70	47.25	49.52	53.75	56.32		
41.00	42.97	47.50	49.78	54.00	56.59		
41.25	43.23	47.75	50.04	54.25	56.85		

Older Men (27–50)

Abdomen

Inches	Constant B	Inches	Constant B	Inches	Constant B	Inches	Constant B
32.00	28.66	39.25	35.15	46.50	41.64	53.75	48.13
32.25	28.88	39.50	35.38	46.75	41.86	54.00	48.35
32.50	29.11	39.75	35.59	47.00	42.09	54.25	48.58
32.75	29.33	40.00	35.82	47.25	42.31	54.50	48.80
33.00	29.55	40.25	36.05	47.50	42.54	54.75	49.03
33.25	29.78	40.50	36.27	47.75	42.76	55.00	49.25
33.50	30.00	40.75	36.49	48.00	42.98	55.25	49.47
33.75	30.22	41.00	36.72	48.25	43.21	55.50	49.70
34.00	30.45	41.25	36.94	48.50	43.43	55.75	49.92
34.25	30.67	41.50	37.17	48.75	43.66	56.00	50.15
34.50	30.89	41.75	37.39	49.00	43.88	56.25	50.37
34.75	31.12	42.00	37.62	49.25	44.10	56.50	50.59
35.00	31.35	42.25	37.87	49.50	44.33	56.75	50.82
35.25	31.57	42.50	38.06	49.75	44.55	57.00	51.04
35.50	31.79	42.75	38.28	50.00	44.77	57.25	51.26
35.75	32.02	43.00	38.51	50.25	45.00	57.50	51.49
36.00	32.24	43.25	38.73	50.50	45.22	57.75	51.71
36.25	32.46	43.50	38.96	50.75	45.45	58.00	51.94
36.50	32.69	43.75	39.18	51.00	45.67	58.25	52.16
36.75	32.91	44.00	39.41	51.25	45.89	58.50	52.38
37.00	33.14	44.25	39.63	51.50	46.12	58.75	52.60
37.25	33.36	44.50	39.85	51.75	46.34	59.00	52.83
37.50	33.58	44.75	40.08	52.00	46.56	59.25	53.05
37.75	33.81	45.00	40.30	52.25	46.79	59.50	53.28
38.00	34.03	45.25	40.52	52.50	47.01	59.75	53.50
38.25	34.26	45.50	40.74	52.75	47.24	60.00	53.72
38.50	34.48	45.75	40.97	53.00	47.46		
38.75	34.70	46.00	41.19	53.25	47.68		
39.00	34.93	46.25	41.41	53.50	47.91		

Table A4.12					
Older Men (27–50)					
Forearm					
Inches	**Constant C**	**Inches**	**Constant C**	**Inches**	**Constant C**
8.00	24.02	13.75	41.27	19.50	58.53
8.25	24.76	14.00	42.03	19.75	59.28
8.50	25.52	14.25	42.77	20.00	60.03
8.75	26.26	14.50	43.53	20.25	60.78
9.00	27.02	14.75	44.27	20.50	61.53
9.25	27.76	15.00	45.03	20.75	62.28
9.50	28.52	15.25	45.77	21.00	63.03
9.75	29.26	15.50	46.53	21.25	63.78
10.00	30.02	15.75	47.28	21.50	64.53
10.25	30.76	16.00	48.03	21.75	65.28
10.50	31.52	16.25	48.78	22.00	66.03
10.75	32.27	16.50	49.53	22.25	66.78
11.00	33.02	16.75	50.28	22.50	67.53
11.25	33.77	17.00	51.03	22.75	68.28
11.50	34.52	17.25	51.78	23.00	69.03
11.75	35.27	17.50	52.54	23.25	69.78
12.00	36.02	17.75	53.28	23.50	70.52
12.25	36.77	18.00	54.04	23.75	71.27
12.50	37.53	18.25	54.78	24.00	72.02
12.75	38.27	18.50	55.53	24.25	72.77
13.00	39.03	18.75	56.28	24.50	73.52
13.25	39.77	19.00	57.03	24.75	74.27
13.50	40.53	19.25	57.78	25.00	75.02

Note: Percent fat = Constant A + Constant B − Constant C − 15.0.
For athletic people, the age correction is 19.0.

APPENDIX E

Percent of One Rep Maximum (IRM) Conversion

Weight	30%	40%	50%	55%	60%	65%	70%	75%	80%	85%	90%
5	2	2	3	3	3	3	4	4	4	4	5
10	3	4	5	6	6	7	7	8	8	9	9
15	5	6	8	8	9	10	11	11	12	13	14
20	6	8	10	11	12	13	14	15	16	17	18
25	8	10	13	14	15	16	18	19	20	21	23
30	9	12	15	17	18	20	21	23	24	26	27
35	11	14	18	19	21	23	25	26	28	30	32
40	12	16	20	22	24	26	28	30	32	34	36
45	14	18	23	25	27	29	32	34	36	38	41
50	15	20	25	28	30	33	35	38	40	43	45
55	17	22	28	30	33	36	39	41	44	47	50
60	18	24	30	33	36	39	42	45	48	51	54
65	20	26	33	36	39	42	46	49	52	55	59
70	21	28	35	39	42	46	49	53	56	60	63
75	23	30	38	41	45	49	53	56	60	64	68
80	24	32	40	44	48	52	56	60	64	68	72
85	26	34	43	47	51	55	60	64	68	72	77
90	27	36	45	50	54	59	63	68	72	77	81
95	29	38	48	52	57	62	67	71	76	81	86
100	30	40	50	55	60	65	70	75	80	85	90
105	32	42	53	58	63	68	74	79	84	89	95
110	33	44	55	61	66	72	77	83	88	94	99
115	35	46	58	63	69	75	81	86	92	98	104
120	36	48	60	66	72	78	84	90	96	102	108
125	38	50	63	69	75	81	88	94	100	106	113
130	39	52	65	72	78	85	91	98	104	111	117
135	41	54	68	74	81	88	95	101	108	115	122
140	42	56	70	77	84	91	98	105	112	119	126
145	44	58	73	80	87	94	102	109	116	123	131
150	45	60	75	83	90	98	105	113	120	128	135
155	47	62	78	85	93	101	109	116	124	132	140
160	48	64	80	88	96	104	112	120	128	136	144
165	50	66	83	91	99	107	116	124	132	140	149
170	51	68	85	94	102	111	119	128	136	145	153

(continued)

Weight	30%	40%	50%	55%	60%	65%	70%	75%	80%	85%	90%
175	53	70	88	96	105	114	123	131	140	149	158
180	54	72	90	99	108	117	126	135	144	153	162
185	56	74	93	102	111	120	130	139	148	157	167
190	57	76	95	105	114	124	133	143	152	162	171
195	59	78	98	107	117	127	137	146	156	166	176
200	60	80	100	110	120	130	140	150	160	170	180
205	62	82	103	113	123	133	144	154	164	174	185
210	63	84	105	116	126	137	147	158	168	179	189
215	65	86	108	118	129	140	151	161	172	183	194
220	66	88	110	121	132	143	154	165	176	187	198
225	68	90	113	124	135	146	158	169	180	191	203
230	69	92	115	127	138	150	161	173	184	196	207
235	71	94	118	129	141	153	165	176	188	200	212
240	72	96	120	132	144	156	168	180	192	204	216
245	74	98	123	135	147	159	172	184	196	208	221
250	75	100	125	138	150	163	175	188	200	213	225
255	77	102	128	140	153	166	179	191	204	217	230
260	78	104	130	143	156	169	182	195	208	221	234
265	80	106	133	146	159	172	186	199	212	225	239
270	81	108	135	149	162	176	189	203	216	230	243
275	83	110	138	151	165	179	193	206	220	234	248
280	84	112	140	154	168	182	196	210	224	238	252
285	86	114	143	157	171	185	200	214	228	242	257
290	87	116	145	160	174	189	203	218	232	247	261
295	89	118	148	162	177	192	207	221	236	251	266
300	90	120	150	165	180	195	210	225	240	255	270
305	92	122	153	168	183	198	214	229	244	259	275
310	93	124	155	171	186	202	217	233	248	264	279
315	95	126	158	173	189	205	221	236	252	268	284
320	96	128	160	176	192	208	224	240	256	272	288
325	98	130	163	179	195	211	228	244	260	276	293
330	99	132	165	182	198	215	231	248	264	281	297
335	101	134	168	184	201	218	235	251	268	285	302
340	102	136	170	187	204	221	238	255	272	289	306

(continued)

(continued)

Weight	30%	40%	50%	55%	60%	65%	70%	75%	80%	85%	90%
345	104	138	173	190	207	224	242	259	276	293	311
350	105	140	175	193	210	228	245	263	280	298	315
355	107	142	178	195	213	231	249	266	284	302	320
360	108	144	180	198	216	234	252	270	288	306	324
365	110	146	183	201	219	237	256	274	292	310	329
370	111	148	185	204	222	241	259	278	296	315	333
375	113	150	188	206	225	244	263	281	300	319	338
380	114	152	190	209	228	247	266	285	304	323	342
385	116	154	193	212	231	250	270	289	308	327	347
390	117	156	195	215	234	254	273	293	312	332	351
395	119	158	198	217	237	257	277	296	316	336	356
400	120	160	200	220	240	260	280	300	320	340	360
405	122	162	203	223	243	263	284	304	324	344	365
410	123	164	205	226	246	267	287	308	328	349	369
415	125	166	208	228	249	270	291	311	332	353	374
420	126	168	210	231	252	273	294	315	336	357	378
425	128	170	213	234	255	276	298	319	340	361	383
430	129	172	215	237	258	280	301	323	344	366	387
435	131	174	218	239	261	283	305	326	348	370	392
440	132	176	220	242	264	286	308	330	352	374	396
445	134	178	223	245	267	289	312	334	356	378	401
450	135	180	225	248	270	293	315	338	360	383	405
455	137	182	228	250	273	296	319	341	364	387	410
460	138	184	230	253	276	299	322	345	368	391	414
465	140	186	233	256	279	302	326	349	372	395	419
470	141	188	235	259	282	306	329	353	376	400	423
475	143	190	238	261	285	309	333	356	380	404	428
480	144	192	240	264	288	312	336	360	384	408	432
485	146	194	243	267	291	315	340	364	388	412	437
490	147	196	245	270	294	319	343	368	392	417	441
495	149	198	248	272	297	322	347	371	396	421	446
500	150	200	250	275	300	325	350	375	400	425	450
505	152	202	253	278	303	328	354	379	404	429	455
510	153	204	255	281	306	332	357	383	408	434	459
515	155	206	258	283	309	335	361	386	412	438	464

(continued)

Weight	30%	40%	50%	55%	60%	65%	70%	75%	80%	85%	90%
520	156	208	260	286	312	338	364	390	416	442	468
525	158	210	263	289	315	341	368	394	420	446	473
530	159	212	265	292	318	345	371	398	424	451	477
535	161	214	268	294	321	348	375	401	428	455	482
540	162	216	270	297	324	351	378	405	432	459	486
545	164	218	273	300	327	354	382	409	436	463	491
550	165	220	275	303	330	358	385	413	440	468	495
555	167	222	278	305	333	361	389	416	444	472	500
560	168	224	280	308	336	364	392	420	448	476	504
565	170	226	283	311	339	367	396	424	452	480	509
570	171	228	285	314	342	371	399	428	456	485	513
575	173	230	288	316	345	374	403	431	460	489	518
580	174	232	290	319	348	377	406	435	464	493	522
585	176	234	293	322	351	380	410	439	468	497	527
590	177	236	295	325	354	384	413	443	472	502	531
595	179	238	298	327	357	387	417	446	476	506	536
600	180	240	300	330	360	390	420	450	480	510	540
605	182	242	303	333	363	393	424	454	484	514	545
610	183	244	305	336	366	397	427	458	488	519	549
615	185	246	308	338	369	400	431	461	492	523	554
620	186	248	310	341	372	403	434	465	496	527	558
625	188	250	313	344	375	406	438	469	500	531	563
630	189	252	315	347	378	410	441	473	504	536	567
635	191	254	318	349	381	413	445	476	508	540	572
640	192	256	320	352	384	416	448	480	512	544	576
645	194	258	323	355	387	419	452	484	516	548	581
650	195	260	325	358	390	423	455	488	520	553	585
655	197	262	328	360	393	426	459	491	524	557	590
660	198	264	330	363	396	429	462	495	528	561	594
665	200	266	333	366	399	432	466	499	532	565	599
670	201	268	335	369	402	436	469	503	536	570	603
675	203	270	338	371	405	439	473	506	540	574	608
680	204	272	340	374	408	442	476	510	544	578	612
685	206	274	343	377	411	445	480	514	548	582	617

(continued)

(continued)

Weight	30%	40%	50%	55%	60%	65%	70%	75%	80%	85%	90%
690	207	276	345	380	414	449	483	518	552	587	621
700	210	280	350	385	420	455	490	525	560	595	630
705	212	282	353	388	423	458	494	529	564	599	635
710	213	284	355	391	426	462	497	533	568	604	639
715	215	286	358	393	429	465	501	536	572	608	644
720	216	288	360	396	432	468	504	540	576	612	648
725	218	290	363	399	435	471	508	544	580	616	653
730	219	292	365	402	438	475	511	548	584	621	657
735	221	294	368	404	441	478	515	551	588	625	662
740	222	296	370	407	444	481	518	555	592	629	666
745	224	298	373	410	447	484	522	559	596	633	671
750	225	300	375	413	450	488	525	563	600	638	675
755	227	302	378	415	453	491	529	566	604	642	680
760	228	304	380	418	456	494	532	570	608	646	684
765	230	306	383	421	459	497	536	574	612	650	689
770	231	308	385	424	462	501	539	578	616	655	693
775	233	310	388	426	465	504	543	581	620	659	698
780	234	312	390	429	468	507	546	585	624	663	702
785	236	314	393	432	471	510	550	589	628	667	707
790	237	316	395	435	474	514	553	593	632	672	711
795	239	318	398	437	477	517	557	596	636	676	716
800	240	320	400	440	480	520	560	600	640	680	720
805	242	322	403	443	483	523	564	604	644	684	725
810	243	324	405	446	486	527	567	608	648	689	729
815	245	326	408	448	489	530	571	611	652	693	734
820	246	328	410	451	492	533	574	615	656	697	738
825	248	330	413	454	495	536	578	619	660	701	743
830	249	332	415	457	498	540	581	623	664	706	747
835	251	334	418	459	501	543	585	626	668	710	752
840	252	336	420	462	504	546	588	630	672	714	756
845	254	338	423	465	507	549	592	634	676	718	761
850	255	340	425	468	510	553	595	638	680	723	765
855	257	342	428	470	513	556	599	641	684	727	770
860	258	344	430	473	516	559	602	645	688	731	774
865	260	346	433	476	519	562	606	649	692	735	779

(*continued*)

Weight	30%	40%	50%	55%	60%	65%	70%	75%	80%	85%	90%
870	261	348	435	479	522	566	609	653	696	740	783
875	263	350	438	481	525	569	613	656	700	744	788
880	264	352	440	484	528	572	616	660	704	748	792
885	266	354	443	487	531	575	620	664	708	752	797
890	267	356	445	490	534	579	623	668	712	757	801
895	269	358	448	492	537	582	627	671	716	761	806
900	270	360	450	495	540	585	630	675	720	765	810
905	272	362	453	498	543	588	634	679	724	769	815
910	273	364	455	501	546	592	637	683	728	774	819
915	275	366	458	503	549	595	641	686	732	778	824
920	276	368	460	506	552	598	644	690	736	782	828
925	278	370	463	509	555	601	648	694	740	786	833
930	279	372	465	512	558	605	651	698	744	791	837
935	281	374	468	514	561	608	655	701	748	795	842
940	282	376	470	517	564	611	658	705	752	799	846
945	284	378	473	520	567	614	662	709	756	803	851
950	285	380	475	523	570	618	665	713	760	808	855
955	287	382	478	525	573	621	669	716	764	812	860
960	288	384	480	528	576	624	672	720	768	816	864
965	290	386	483	531	579	627	676	724	772	820	869
970	291	388	485	534	582	631	679	728	776	825	873
975	293	390	488	536	585	634	683	731	780	829	878
980	294	392	490	539	588	637	686	735	784	833	882
985	296	394	493	542	591	640	690	739	788	837	887
990	297	396	495	545	594	644	693	743	792	842	891
995	299	398	498	547	597	647	697	746	796	846	896
1000	300	400	500	550	600	650	700	750	800	850	900

APPENDIX F

One Rep Maximum (IRM) Conversion

Pounds	10	9	8	7	6	5	4	3	2
5	7	6	6	6	6	6	6	5	5
10	13	13	13	12	12	11	11	11	11
15	20	19	19	18	18	17	17	16	16
20	27	26	25	24	24	23	22	22	21
25	33	32	31	30	29	29	28	27	26
30	40	39	38	36	35	34	33	32	32
35	47	45	44	42	41	40	39	38	37
40	53	52	50	48	47	46	44	43	42
45	60	58	56	55	53	51	50	49	47
50	67	65	63	61	59	57	56	54	53
55	73	71	69	67	65	63	61	59	58
60	80	77	75	73	71	69	67	65	63
65	87	84	81	79	76	74	72	70	68
70	93	90	88	85	82	80	78	76	74
75	100	97	94	91	88	86	83	81	79
80	107	103	100	97	94	91	89	86	84
85	113	110	106	103	100	97	94	92	89
90	120	116	113	109	106	103	100	97	95
95	127	123	119	115	112	109	106	103	100
100	133	129	125	121	118	114	111	108	105
105	140	135	131	127	124	120	117	114	111
110	147	142	138	133	129	126	122	119	116
115	153	148	144	139	135	131	128	124	121
120	160	155	150	145	141	137	133	130	126
125	167	161	156	152	147	143	139	135	132
130	173	168	163	158	153	149	144	141	137
135	180	174	169	164	159	154	150	146	142
140	187	181	175	170	165	160	156	151	147
145	193	187	181	176	171	166	161	157	153
150	200	194	188	182	176	171	167	162	158
155	207	200	194	188	182	177	172	168	163
160	213	206	200	194	188	183	178	173	168
165	220	213	206	200	194	189	183	178	174

(continued)

Pounds	10	9	8	7	6	5	4	3	2
170	227	219	213	206	200	194	189	184	179
175	233	226	219	212	206	200	194	189	184
180	240	232	225	218	212	206	200	195	189
185	247	239	231	224	218	211	206	200	195
190	253	245	238	230	224	217	211	205	200
195	260	252	244	236	229	223	217	211	205
200	267	258	250	242	235	229	222	216	211
205	273	265	256	248	241	234	228	222	216
210	280	271	263	255	247	240	233	227	221
215	287	277	269	261	253	246	239	232	226
220	293	284	275	267	259	251	244	238	232
225	300	290	281	273	265	257	250	243	237
230	307	297	288	279	271	263	256	249	242
235	313	303	294	285	276	269	261	254	247
240	320	310	300	291	282	274	267	259	253
245	327	316	306	297	288	280	272	265	258
250	333	323	313	303	294	286	278	270	263
255	340	329	319	309	300	291	283	276	268
260	347	335	325	315	306	297	289	281	274
265	353	342	331	321	312	303	294	286	279
270	360	348	338	327	318	309	300	292	284
275	367	355	344	333	324	314	306	297	289
280	373	361	350	339	329	320	311	303	295
285	380	368	356	345	335	326	317	308	300
290	387	374	363	352	341	331	322	314	305
295	393	381	369	358	347	337	328	319	311
300	400	387	375	364	353	343	333	324	316
305	407	394	381	370	359	349	339	330	321
310	413	400	388	376	365	354	344	335	326
315	420	406	394	382	371	360	350	341	332
320	427	413	400	388	376	366	356	346	337
325	433	419	406	394	382	371	361	351	342
330	440	426	413	400	388	377	367	357	347
335	447	432	419	406	394	383	372	362	353
340	453	439	425	412	400	389	378	368	358

(*continued*)

Pounds	10	9	8	7	6	5	4	3	2
345	460	445	431	418	406	394	383	373	363
350	467	452	438	424	412	400	389	378	368
355	473	458	444	430	418	406	394	384	374
360	480	465	450	436	424	411	400	389	379
365	487	471	456	442	429	417	406	395	384
370	493	477	463	448	435	423	411	400	389
375	500	484	469	455	441	429	417	405	395
380	507	490	475	461	447	434	422	411	400
385	513	497	481	467	453	440	428	416	405
390	520	503	488	473	459	446	433	422	411
395	527	510	494	479	465	451	439	427	416
400	533	516	500	485	471	457	444	432	421
405	540	523	506	491	476	463	450	438	426
410	547	529	513	497	482	469	456	443	432
415	553	535	519	503	488	474	461	449	437
420	560	542	525	509	494	480	467	454	442
425	567	548	531	515	500	486	472	459	447
430	573	555	538	521	506	491	478	465	453
435	580	561	544	527	512	497	483	470	458
440	587	568	550	533	518	503	489	476	463
445	593	574	556	539	524	509	494	481	468
450	600	581	563	545	529	514	500	486	474
455	607	587	569	552	535	520	506	492	479
460	613	594	575	558	541	526	511	497	484
465	620	600	581	564	547	531	517	503	489
470	627	606	588	570	553	537	522	508	495
475	633	613	594	576	559	543	528	514	500
480	640	619	600	582	565	549	533	519	505
485	647	626	606	588	571	554	539	524	511
490	653	632	613	594	576	560	544	530	516
495	660	639	619	600	582	566	550	535	521
500	667	645	625	606	588	571	556	541	526
505	673	652	631	612	594	577	561	546	532
510	680	658	638	618	600	583	567	551	537
515	687	665	644	624	606	589	572	557	542

(continued)

Pounds	10	9	8	7	6	5	4	3	2
520	693	671	650	630	612	594	578	562	547
525	700	677	656	636	618	600	583	568	553
530	707	684	663	642	624	606	589	573	558
535	713	690	669	648	629	611	594	578	563
540	720	697	675	655	635	617	600	584	568
545	727	703	681	661	641	623	606	589	574
550	733	710	688	667	647	629	611	595	579
555	740	716	694	673	653	634	617	600	584
560	747	723	700	679	659	640	622	605	589
565	753	729	706	685	665	646	628	611	595
570	760	735	713	691	671	651	633	616	600
575	767	742	719	697	676	657	639	622	605
580	773	748	725	703	682	663	644	627	611
585	780	755	731	709	688	669	650	632	616
590	787	761	738	715	694	674	656	638	621
595	793	768	744	721	700	680	661	643	626
600	800	774	750	727	706	686	667	649	632
605	807	781	756	733	712	691	672	654	637
610	813	787	763	739	718	697	678	659	642
615	820	794	769	745	724	703	683	665	647
620	827	800	775	752	729	709	689	670	653
625	833	806	781	758	735	714	694	676	658
630	840	813	788	764	741	720	700	681	663
635	847	819	794	770	747	726	706	686	668
640	853	826	800	776	753	731	711	692	674
645	860	832	806	782	759	737	717	697	679
650	867	839	813	788	765	743	722	703	684
655	873	845	819	794	771	749	728	708	689
660	880	852	825	800	776	754	733	714	695
665	887	858	831	806	782	760	739	719	700
670	893	865	838	812	788	766	744	724	705
675	900	871	844	818	794	771	750	730	711
680	907	877	850	824	800	777	756	735	716
685	913	884	856	830	806	783	761	741	721
690	920	890	863	836	812	789	767	746	726

(*continued*)

Pounds	10	9	8	7	6	5	4	3	2
695	927	897	869	842	818	794	772	751	732
700	933	903	875	848	824	800	778	757	737
705	940	910	881	855	829	806	783	762	742
710	947	916	888	861	835	811	789	768	747
715	953	923	894	867	841	817	794	773	753
720	960	929	900	873	847	823	800	778	758
725	967	935	906	879	853	829	806	784	763
730	973	942	913	885	859	834	811	789	768
735	980	948	919	891	865	840	817	795	774
740	987	955	925	897	871	846	822	800	779
745	993	961	931	903	876	851	828	805	784
750	1000	968	938	909	882	857	833	811	789
755	1007	974	944	915	888	863	839	816	795
760	1013	981	950	921	894	869	844	822	800
765	1020	987	956	927	900	874	850	827	805
770	1027	994	963	933	906	880	856	832	811
775	1033	1000	969	939	912	886	861	838	816
780	1040	1006	975	945	918	891	867	843	821
785	1047	1013	981	952	924	897	872	849	826
790	1053	1019	988	958	929	903	878	854	832
795	1060	1026	994	964	935	909	883	859	837
800	1067	1032	1000	970	941	914	889	865	842
805	1073	1039	1006	976	947	920	894	870	847
810	1080	1045	1013	982	953	926	900	876	853
815	1087	1052	1019	988	959	931	906	881	858
820	1093	1058	1025	994	965	937	911	886	863
825	1100	1065	1031	1000	971	943	917	892	868
830	1107	1071	1038	1006	976	949	922	897	874
835	1113	1077	1044	1012	982	954	928	903	879
840	1120	1084	1050	1018	988	960	933	908	884
845	1127	1090	1056	1024	994	966	939	914	889
850	1133	1097	1063	1030	1000	971	944	919	895
855	1140	1103	1069	1036	1006	977	950	924	900
900	1200	1161	1125	1091	1059	1029	1000	973	947
905	1207	1168	1131	1097	1065	1034	1006	978	953

(*continued*)

Pounds	10	9	8	7	6	5	4	3	2
910	1213	1174	1138	1103	1071	1040	1011	984	958
915	1220	1181	1144	1109	1076	1046	1017	989	963
920	1227	1187	1150	1115	1082	1051	1022	995	968
925	1233	1194	1156	1121	1088	1057	1028	1000	974
930	1240	1200	1163	1127	1094	1063	1033	1005	979
935	1247	1206	1169	1133	1100	1069	1039	1011	984
940	1253	1213	1175	1139	1106	1074	1044	1016	989
945	1260	1219	1181	1145	1112	1080	1050	1022	995
950	1267	1226	1188	1152	1118	1086	1056	1027	1000
955	1273	1232	1194	1158	1124	1091	1061	1032	1005
960	1280	1239	1200	1164	1129	1097	1067	1038	1011
965	1287	1245	1206	1170	1135	1103	1072	1043	1016
970	1293	1252	1213	1176	1141	1109	1078	1049	1021
975	1300	1258	1219	1182	1147	1114	1083	1054	1026
980	1307	1265	1225	1188	1153	1120	1089	1059	1032
985	1313	1271	1231	1194	1159	1126	1094	1065	1037
990	1320	1277	1238	1200	1165	1131	1100	1070	1042
995	1327	1284	1244	1206	1171	1137	1106	1076	1047
1000	1333	1290	1250	1212	1176	1143	1111	1081	1053

Answer Key

CHAPTER 1
1. c
2. True
3. Stabilization, strength, and power
4. Strength
5. Phase 5: Power Training

CHAPTER 2
1. a, iii; b, i; c, ii
2. a, i; b, iii; c, iv; d, ii
3. a, iv; b, i; c, ii; d, iii
4. b
5. a

CHAPTER 3
1. Heart, blood, and blood vessels
2. c
3. ATP-CP system
4. Right, left

CHAPTER 4
1. Frontal plane
2. a
3. d
4. a
5. b

CHAPTER 5
1. c
2. c, d, e, g
3. Dynamic
4. Zone 1
5. b

CHAPTER 6
1. d
2. Cumulative injury cycle
3. a
4. Static stretching, self-myofascial release
5. a

CHAPTER 7
1. Decreases
2. True
3. Calories
4. b, c
5. False

CHAPTER 8
1. b
2. a
3. a, ii; b, iii; c, i; d, ii
4. b
5. b

CHAPTER 9
1. a
2. d
3. b
4. a
5. c
6. b
7. b

CHAPTER 10
1. b
2. Maximal; minimal
3. c
4. a
5. c
6. b
7. a, d

CHAPTER 11
1. b
2. a
3. Backside mechanics

CHAPTER 12

1. c
2. b
3. b
4. b
5. b

CHAPTER 13

1. a
2. Phases 1, 2, and 5
3. b
4. d
5. a
6. b and e

CHAPTER 14

1. a
2. a, c, d, e, f
3. d
4. a
5. a
6. a

CHAPTER 15

1. a, b
2. Thermic effect
3. True
4. 60%
5. True
6. b
7. c
8. b

CHAPTER 16

1. a
2. a
3. b, d

CHAPTER 17

1. b
2. a
3. Upper
4. b

CHAPTER 18

1. b
2. a
3. c

Index

Page numbers in *italics* denote figures; those followed by "t" denote tables

stabilization, 291–292
strength, 293–294
Chest pass, rotation, 211
Chest press
ball dumbbell, 291
barbell, 294
flat dumbbell, 293
Children
adults vs., physiologic differences
between, 376–378
automated external defibrillator
contraindications, 513–514
cardiopulmonary resuscitation of, 508
exercise guidelines for, 376, 377t, 379t
maximum oxygen uptake in, 377, 377t
movement assessments in, 378
obesity in, 376, 382
resistance training in, 378
summary of, 381
Choking, 512
Cholecystokinin, 438
Chordae tendineae, 42
Chromium, 454t
Chronic diseases (see also specific disease)
in adult population, 5
description of, 106
Chylomicrons, 437–438
Circuit training, 189–190, 282–283, 285
Circulation assessments, 508
Circumduction, 26
Circumference measurements, 114,
114–115
Client
ambitions of, 466–467
approaching of, 480
belief in success, 469–470
communication with, 482
goal setting by, 467–469
initial appointment with, 484
motivation of, 483–485
negativity by, 470
questions to ask, 484
rapport with, 482–483, 486, 489
SCAMPI goals for, 468–469
selling of services to, 489–494
Cobalt, 454t
Collagen, 28, 148
Communication, 482
Complete protein, 423
Complex carbohydrates, 432
Compound-sets, 282
Concentric contraction, 68
Conduction passageway, 48
Condyle, 23, 23
Condyloid joint, 25, 25, 28t
Confidence, 483
Contralateral, 60
Controllable behaviors, 472
Cool-down
application of, 177–178
benefits of, 177
duration of, 176–177, 179
flexibility during, 177
purpose of, 176
summary of, 179
Copper, 455t
Core (see also Lumbo-pelvic-hip complex)
definition of, 198

divisions of, 198
inefficient
description of, 199
illustration of, 200
low back pain and, 200
muscles of, 198, 199t
summary of, 199–200
weakness in, 199, 200
Core movement system
description of, 198
muscles of, 199t, 203
Core stabilization system
description of, 198
muscles of, 199t, 202
training of, 200–203, 205–207
Core training
cervical spine position during, 201
drawing-in maneuver, 201, 202
evidence to support, 202
of hypertensive client, 389
levels of, 203–205
obesity reductions through, 383
of osteoporosis clients, 398
power-based, 210–213
program for
design of, 203–213, 214t
implementation of, 214
requirements for, 202–203
strength-based, 207–210
Coronary heart disease, 391–395
Corrective flexibility, 149, 151t, 167
CPR (see Cardiopulmonary resuscitation)
Creatine phosphate, 332
Cumulative injuries, 147, 147–148
Customer service, 478–479
Customers, 479–481
Cystic fibrosis, 407

D
Daily values, 457
Davies test, 129, 129
Davis's law, 148
Deconditioned, 6
Defibrillator (see Automated external
defibrillator)
Dehydration, 441t
Deltoids, 83
Dendrites, 17, 17
Deposit-and-refund technique, 471
Depressions, 22, 22
Descending aorta, 42
Diabetes, 385–388, 439
Diaphragm, 78
Diastolic pressure, 110
Diet
high-carbohydrate, 432
high-protein, 426–427
hypocaloric, 425
low-carbohydrate, 434
Dietary reference intakes, 452–456,
454t–455t
Dietary supplements
annual expenditures on, 450
cautions for, 460
definition of, 450
guidelines for, 451–456
labels on, 456–458

rationale for using, 450–451
for seniors, 451
vitamins, 458–461
Directive questions, 485–486
Disaccharides, 429
Diseases, 5
Dislocations, 509–510
Distal, 59
Diuretics, 107t–108t
Dorsiflexion, 60, 62
Drawing-in maneuver, 201, 202
DRI (see Dietary reference intakes)
Dumbbell exercises
ball dumbbell chest press, 291
ball dumbbell row, 297
flat dumbbell chest press, 293
lunge to two-arm dumbbell press, 288
prone ball dumbbell triceps extensions,
310
seated shoulder press, 303
seated two-arm dumbbell biceps curl,
308
single-leg dumbbell curl, 306
supine ball dumbbell triceps extensions,
309
Durnin-Womersley formula, 112, 113t
DV (see Daily values)
Dynamic functional flexibility, 141
Dynamic joint stabilization, 221
Dynamic postural assessments (see
Postural assessments)
Dynamic range of motion, 141
Dynamic resistance training, 332
Dynamic stretching
definition of, 164
description of, 150
medicine ball chop and lift, 167
multiplanar lunge, 165
prisoner squat, 164–165
single-leg squat touchdown, 166
summary of, 168
tube walking, 166–167
Dysfunctional breathing, 53
Dyspnea, 409

E
Eccentric contraction, 63–65, 68t
Efferent neurons, 17
Elastin, 28–29
Empathy, 483–485, 489
Endomysium, 30, 30
Endurance training
carbohydrates for, 432
intensity of, 331
repetitions for, 329
sets for, 330
stabilization, 9, 342–343
strength, 10, 345t–346t, 345–346
Energy
amino acids for, 422–423
carbohydrates for, 429, 434
negative energy balance, 425
oxygen and, 51–52
Energy-utilizing reaction, 51
Energy-yielding process, 51
Enjoyment, 180–181
Enthusiasm, 483